Managing the Veterinary Cancer Patient:

A PRACTICE MANUAL

Gregory K. Ogilvie, DVM
Diplomate ACVIM
(Specialties of Internal Medicine and Oncology)
Associate Professor and Medical Oncologist/Internist
Comparative Oncology Unit
Department of Clinical Sciences
College of Veterinary Medicine and Biomedical Sciences
Colorado State University
Fort Collins, Colorado

Antony S. Moore, MVSc
Diplomate ACVIM
(Specialty of Oncology)
Associate Professor and Medical Oncologist
Tufts University School of Veterinary Medicine
North Grafton, Massachusetts

Designed and Published by Veterinary Learning Systems

Credits:

Bioillustrator: *Jackie Dial, MS, Fort Collins, Colorado*

Library of Congress Card Number: 94-061975

ISBN 1-884254-20-9

Copyright © 1995
Veterinary Learning Systems Co., Inc.
Trenton, New Jersey

First published 1995
Second printing 1996

Group Publisher: *Antoinette B. Passaretti*
Copy Editor: *Kevin L. Stone*
Designer: *Jeanne M. Mistretta*
Typesetter: *Karen J. Oswald*
Production Supervisor: *Elizabeth A. Lang*

To Karla and Torrie:
The roses of my life

Gregory K. Ogilvie

❧

To Catriona Moore:
For her courage and grace

Antony S. Moore

ACKNOWLEDGMENTS

This book would not have been possible without the direct and indirect input of a number of very important people. The list must start with a very special friend, an accomplished clinician–scientist, a veterinary oncologist, a true renaissance man, and the co-author of this book: Dr. Antony S. Moore. Without Tony's authorship, this work would not have met its goal of being a practical and up-to-date resource for the progressive practicing veterinarian. These pages reflect Tony's critical eye, humor, and intelligence. For those who do not know this remarkable man, he is, among many other things, an accomplished academician, athlete, gardener, apiarist, connoisseur of fine foods and wine, lover and collector of old books, and above all, a kind and sensitive human being.

A second person who must not go unnoticed is the book's magnificent bioillustrator, Jackie Dial, who breathed life into many sections of the book with her artistry and editorial skill. She allowed us to fulfill our dream of adding motion to the written page to assist the reader in understanding complex procedures and ideas. Jackie has been through each and every page of the text with her critical eye and sharp pencil. More than that, she has been an unrestrained source of kind criticism, boundless enthusiasm, and special friendship.

Each page of this book has been critically reviewed by a small army of people too numerous to mention at Colorado State University and Veterinary Learning Systems. My thanks to all of them, with special thoughts of appreciation for the extraordinary efforts of Dr. Kim Selting and Ms. Kelly Erickson at Colorado State University. A special thanks must go to three people at Veterinary Learning Systems. The first is Toni Passaretti, group publisher, who believed in our dream and made sure that the dream stayed alive. Next is Ruth Savitz, who infused humor, excitement, and enthusiasm into the editing process. Finally, thank you to Kevin Stone, whose attention to detail made the final product so magnificent.

The pages of this book directly or indirectly reflect the knowledge, experience, and wisdom of a number of people who have impacted my life tremendously: Drs. H. L. Hopkinson and Wendel Hutchinson, who kindled my dreams of becoming a veterinarian; Dr. Susan Cotter, my residency tutor, who guided my development and taught me to doubt the obvious; Dr. Ralph Richardson, whose special friendship and guidance as a mentor and colleague is irreplaceable; Dr. S. J. Withrow, the best oncologic surgeon our profession will ever know and a man who gave me the freedom, friendship, and wealth of information to complete this book; Dr. Edward L. Gillette, a patient scientist and radiation therapist and that special teacher who began the program at Colorado State University that has nurtured and fostered my professional growth; and Drs. Rod Straw, Dennis Macy, Sue LaRue, and Barbara Powers who have contributed significantly to this book with their support, knowledge, and friendship. The pages of this book also reflect the enthusiasm and knowledge of medical residents and veterinary students who kept me running to keep up with them while I attempted to provide them with some mentorship. Special recognition goes to former and current medical oncology residents and friends: Drs. Donna Vicini, M. K. Klein, David Vail, Robyn Elmslie, Steve Atwater, Joyce Obradovich, Phyllis Ciekot, Phillip Bergman, Elizabeth McNiel, Karina Valerius, and Susan Lana.

Last, but not least, a special acknowledgment must go to my parents, Bev and Stan, who continue to foster my growth and independence to this day; my grandfather, Jeff Snider, a third parent and ageless friend who nurtured my demand for excellence; and finally, my wife Karla and daughter Torrie, who have enslaved my heart and granted me the time and opportunity to complete this book.

Gregory K. Ogilvie

ACKNOWLEDGMENTS

My interest in treating cancer in cats and dogs has developed slowly over the years. It began with a realization that telling an owner that there was nothing we could do for their aged pet with cancer was, at best, frustrating and, at worst, an easy way out from what could be a highly emotional ordeal for myself, the animal, and the client. I could not have been further from the truth on the latter point. Treating a pet with cancer is an emotional ordeal—but not in a negative way. Some of the dogs and cats I have treated have become my friends, as have their owners. Even though most of my patients die, I have the comfort of knowing that when I perform euthanasia, they usually know and trust me. That trust extends to their owners, who are the most dedicated and compassionate people as a group I have had the pleasure to meet. The veterinarian who decides to treat cancer in animals should find it challenging, at times frustrating, but ultimately rewarding to provide an extension of the quality of life for the patient and the owner. I hope this book goes at least part of the way to providing the practical basis for veterinarians to manage their cancer patients.

I would like to acknowledge my colleague and friend, Greg Ogilvie, for the support he has given me throughout the writing of this book. It is rare that one finds an individual who can work 12 hours a day, bike 150 miles in a weekend, and yet have time for a family as well as writing a book. I cannot begin to express my admiration for this man, and I am honored to be his co-author in this endeavor.

The production of this book would not have been possible without the support, care, and attention of numerous people. Specifically, Kevin Stone, Ruth Savitz, and Toni Passaretti from Veterinary Learning Systems who provided encouragement, expertise, and deadlines. Robert Brown, medical bioillustrator at Tufts University School of Veterinary Medicine, spent hours helping to devise, arrange, and produce graphics and photographs for the book. Colleagues who lent transparencies of animals, their tumors, and various imaging modalities include John Berg, Amy Tidwell, Dominique Penninck, Susan Cotter, Anne Evans, Bruce Madewell, and Gordon Theilen. These transparencies add significantly to the section on specific types of tumors and represent the finest of years of collecting such photographs by these individuals. I am grateful to be able to use them here. I am also grateful to the library staff at Tufts for all their help.

This seems like the ideal forum to thank a group of people who influenced the way I think about, diagnose, and treat animals with cancer. Either as mentors or as contemporaries in the field of veterinary science, they have all encouraged my interest and supported my endeavors. Thanks go to David Watson and Brian Farrow, who guided me through an internship in clinical studies at the University of Sydney and sowed the first seeds of clinical competence in what must have seemed pretty fallow ground; Max Zuber, who remains, in my opinion, one of the best all-around veterinarians with whom I have worked; Bruce Madewell and Susan Cotter, whose collective experience and knowledge of veterinary oncology I have been lucky enough to share a small portion of; and Alain Theon and John Berg, who have kept me honest in my investigations into, and sweeping generalizations about, cancer in companion animals. I also want to thank the residents in veterinary oncology at Tufts University: David Ruslander, Angela Frimberger, and Carrie Wood, whose enthusiasm, new ideas, and constant challenges have kept my interest in oncology growing over the past six years. Particular thanks go to Angela Frimberger for her scrupulous editing.

In the writing of a book, it is easy to lose objectivity. For me, the encouragement and help given by Tara Temple was invaluable. Deb L'Heureux, the best oncology technician money can buy, co-wrote the section on administration of chemotherapy. Deb is the consummate oncology technician who loves the work and the animals and never misses an opportunity to sing a song.

Special thanks go to Trena Haroutunian, who painstakingly typed and retyped the manuscript, compiled a list of more than 1000 references, made deadlines, and yet never once complained.

Antony S. Moore

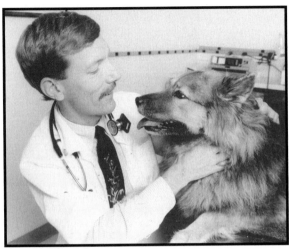

Photograph by William A. Cotton

Dr. Gregory K. Ogilvie is Associate Professor and Medical Oncologist/Internist at the Comparative Oncology Unit, Colorado State University. He is board certified in the specialties of Internal Medicine and Oncology, American College of Veterinary Internal Medicine. Dr. Ogilvie is author of more than 140 publications and is the recipient of many awards, including the Arnold O. Beckman Research Award, 1985; List of Outstanding Teachers, University of Illinois, 1985, 1986, and 1987; Norden Distinguished Teacher Award, 1987 and 1988; Beecham Award for Research Excellence, 1989; Purina Small Animal Research Award, 1992; MSD AgVet Award for Creativity in Teaching, 1992; SCAVMA Award for "Dedication to Students and the Profession," 1993 and 1994; and AVMA/AKC Award for Research Excellence, 1994. Research interests in the areas of nutrition and cancer, development of new chemotherapeutics, hematopoietic growth factors, and biological response modifiers have resulted in many major grants, including support from the National Cancer Institute and National Institutes of Health. Dr. Ogilvie is a certified ski instructor and enjoys camping and long-distance bicycle riding. Since 1987, he has been a counselor at the Sky High Hope Camp for children with cancer.

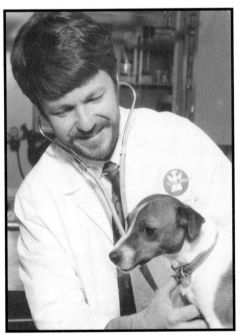

Photograph by Robert Brown

Dr. Antony S. Moore is an Associate Professor and Medical Oncologist at Tufts University School of Veterinary Medicine, North Grafton, Massachusetts. He is board certified in the specialty of Oncology, American College of Veterinary Internal Medicine. Dr. Moore received his veterinary degree from the University of Sydney, Australia and a Master's degree in feline hematology from the same institution. In 1988, he received the Robert S. Brodey Clinical Research Award for veterinary clinical oncology. Dr. Moore was recently the Course Director for the Sydney University Postgraduate Committee in Veterinary Science course entitled, Treatment of Cancer in Companion Animals. Research interests include multiple drug resistance in neoplastic disease and utilization of chemotherapy for treatment of cancer in animals. Outside interests include open-water scuba diving, underwater photography, hiking, contemporary fiction, book collecting, and running. (Pictured with Dr. Moore is his Jack Russell terrier, Arthur.)

This handbook is designed to provide veterinary practitioners with clinically relevant details about the diagnosis and management of the veterinary cancer patient in an easy-to-read format. The table of contents is divided into the five major sections and includes all chapters. Each chapter is organized and subdivided by major headings, which facilitate easy access to practical information and the most common problems encountered in clinical veterinary oncology. A clinical briefing is included at the beginning of each chapter to give the reader information about the most commonly asked clinical questions. Key points are also included throughout the text to reinforce facts that, in many cases, are critical to the successful management of the veterinary cancer patient.

The first section on **Biopsy** is devoted to important diagnostic procedures that can be performed in private practice. This step-by-step, highly illustrated section provides the busy practitioner with an easy reference guide for executing diagnostic methods that are essential for the management of the cancer patient. Also included in the chapter on Clinical Cytology and Neoplasia is a section of 24 color slides that will assist the practitioner in general cytologic interpretation.

The second section on **Common Therapeutic and Supportive Procedures** details practical and important information that is needed to treat and support an animal with cancer. These include such therapeutic modalities as safe handling and administration of chemotherapeutic agents as well as the use of biological response modifiers, cryotherapy, and hyperthermia. Management of complications of cancer in small animals, such as pain, vomiting, and side effects of treatment, are discussed. Information about the nutritional needs of animals with cancer is provided. Also helpful is an appendix at the end of the chapter that lists the toxicities of some commercially available anticancer drugs and hormones.

The third section on **Oncologic Emergencies** is essential for veterinarians who deal with cancer. This "bottom line" section focuses on the diagnosis and treatment of life-threatening problems that can arise during the course of cancer and its treatment. Tables provide easy access to drugs and dosages that may be needed in an emergency situation.

The fourth section focuses on the diagnosis and management of **Paraneoplastic Syndromes**. These problems may complicate the management of animals with cancer. In many cases, the successful diagnosis and management of paraneoplastic conditions can impact the patient's quality of life and survival as much as the management of the malignant condition itself.

The final section is directed at the **Management of Specific Diseases**. Extraordinary efforts have been made to provide only the most important, up-to-date, and clinically relevant data to assist the practitioner in understanding how to determine the extent of a cancer and how best to treat the affected animal. To facilitate quick and easy access, each disease is listed at the top of every page of its corresponding chapter.

This manual is a comprehensive reference guide to the management of the most common natural cause of death in dogs and cats: cancer. Our hope is that it will provide an easy-to-use, practical resource for the progressive practitioner who seeks the very best for his or her patient.

The authors, editors, and publisher of this manual have made every effort to ensure that all therapeutic modalities are recommended in accordance with accepted standards at the time of publication and that all drug dosages and regimens are correct. Nevertheless, anyone not familiar with cancer treatment should consult a veterinary oncologist before administering or prescribing any form of cancer treatment.

G. K. Ogilvie
A. S. Moore

CONTENTS

CONTENTS

CONTENTS

CONTENTS

CONTENTS

CONTENTS

CONTENTS

CLINICAL BRIEFING: THEORY AND PRACTICE	
Indications	A biopsy should be performed prior to definitive therapy if: 1) the results will alter the type of therapy to be employed or 2) the results will influence the owner's willingness to treat their pet
Guidelines	• A biopsy should be performed after consultation with the surgeon who will perform the definitive surgery • Obtain as large a sample as possible • Do not use electrocautery or surgical instruments that crush or otherwise damage tissues • Ensure the tissue is adequately fixed in 10% buffered neutral formalin • Place each biopsy in a separate, properly labeled container • Submit the entire lesion that has been resected and prepared properly for fixation whenever possible • Consider submitting portions of the lesion for culture and sensitivity or alternate analysis • Submit the biopsy to a highly qualified veterinary pathologist

The biopsy is one of the most important procedures performed when evaluating a pet with cancer. Biopsy results must be interpreted carefully in conjunction with results of other diagnostic procedures such as blood work, radiographs, and other imaging modalities. An accurately obtained biopsy specimen is only of value if it is taken and prepared properly and then interpreted by a highly trained pathologist who is willing to use all of the clinical information available to arrive at an accurate diagnosis.

Several types of biopsies exist. A small core of tissue is obtained with a *needle core biopsy*. A portion of the tumor is removed (generally at the junction of normal and abnormal tissue) for an *incisional* or *"wedge" biopsy*. Incisional biopsies are preferred in cases in which punch or needle biopsies cannot provide adequate tissue. Regardless, the biopsy must be performed so that it will not compromise subsequent curative resection. The entire tumor is removed in an *excisional biopsy*, which is preferred in cases in which knowledge of the tissue type would not change the definitive procedure (e.g., a solitary lung mass or a splenic mass).

A biopsy should be performed prior to definitive therapy if (1) the results will alter the type of therapy to be employed or (2) the results will influence the owner's willingness to treat the pet.[1] For example, with a biopsy result of a benign sebaceous adenoma, a clinician can confidently proceed to perform a small resection, but if the biopsy result reveals that the mass is a moderately anaplastic grade II mast cell tumor, a more aggressive, wide surgical resection with 2- to 3-cm margins around the periphery of the tumor is required, and adjunctive therapy may be recommended. For financial or emotional reasons, some owners may be willing to treat a dog with a benign sebaceous adenoma but not a more malignant mast cell tumor.

GUIDELINES[1,2]

1. *Biopsies do not negatively influence survival.* The myth that biopsy causes cancer cells to spread throughout the body, resulting in an early demise of the patient, is not supported in the scientific literature.

2. *A biopsy should be performed after consultation with the surgeon who will perform the definitive surgery.* This ensures that the lesion and the entire biopsy tract are removed to allow adequate resection of the mass without "spilling" or "seeding" tumor cells into the surgical field. That is to say, if a carcinoma or a sarcoma is suspected, a biopsy should not be performed unless an overall plan for definitive therapy is made, because the biopsy procedure can "seed" the operative field with tumor cells if the principle of *en bloc* dissection is violated. In addition, the biopsy incision should be oriented to cause the least amount of tension on the skin, which will make a subsequent definitive surgical procedure easier. With some exceptions, the direction of the incision should be made just like the stripes on a tiger to minimize skin tension and maximize the amount of tissue that can be removed around the tumor (Figure 1-1).

3. *Obtain as large a sample as possible to enhance correct diagnosis by the pathologist.* As just noted, the juncture of normal and abnormal tissue is an ideal site for tissue procurement. Osteosarcoma is an exception; biopsy specimens should be taken from the center of these tumors because the periphery of the lesion is composed primarily of reactive bone. Ulcerated, necrotic tissue should never be biopsied.

4. *The original architecture of the removed tissue should be maintained; therefore, electrocautery or surgical instruments that crush or otherwise damage tissues should not be used.*

5. *Ensure that the tissue is fixed adequately in 10% buffered neutral formalin (1 part tissue to 10 parts fixative).* Fresh tissue should be placed in fixative for 24 to 48 hours. Ten percent buffered formalin is preferred by most pathologists; however, fixatives such as Zenker's or Bouin's can be used for special purposes,

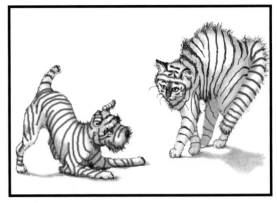

Figure 1-1: *When a biopsy or definitive procedure is performed, an incision should be made to minimize tension on the skin. Generally, incisions are made "like the stripes on a tiger" to minimize skin tension and maximize the amount of tissue that can be removed around the tumor.*

such as for the eye. For best results, tissue should not be wider than 1 cm to ensure proper exposure to the fixative. The tissue can be cut like a loaf of bread to allow proper exposure of the tissue to the fixative (Figure 1-2). The exception to this rule is brain tissue, which can be fixed intact. Very thin samples should be avoided because the fixation process can distort the tissue architecture. Mailing costs can be reduced by sending adequately fixed tissues in just enough formalin to keep the tissues moist. Tissues that are adequately fixed in formalin can be placed in sealable sandwich bags with a formalin-saturated paper towel or sponge. The tissue should not be exposed to heat, cold, or water at any time.

6. *Each biopsy specimen should be placed into a separate, properly labeled container.* The container should be labeled on the sides instead of the lid to prevent mislabeling if container tops are switched. If multiple biopsies are performed, all containers should be labeled before the procedure is

> **KEY POINT:**
>
> *Whenever possible, the person doing the definitive surgery is the person who should do the initial biopsy. If this is not possible, the surgeon who will do the definitive surgery should be consulted prior to biopsy.*

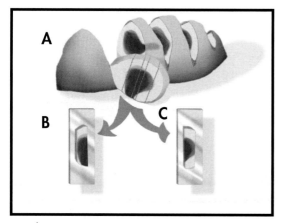

*Figure 1-2: Tissues greater than 1 cm in diameter should be incompletely sliced like a loaf of bread, leaving one side uncut to retain the tumor's spatial relationship (**A**). The slices should be 1 cm apart to allow adequate fixation. Note that the ability of the pathologist to determine whether the margins are free of tumor (tumor noted as darkest area) may depend on where the representative sample was taken from the biopsy specimen (**B**) and how it was placed on a microscope slide (**C**). Therefore, submit the entire, properly fixed and prepared biopsy specimen with a detailed history and description for the most accurate results.*

begun to reduce the chance of confusing samples.

7. *When possible, all resected tissue should be prepared properly and submitted for proper fixation.* This will enable the pathologist to examine the tissue for completeness of removal ("clean" or "dirty" margins). Trimming the biopsy specimen or submitting only a small section means that this valuable information may be lost. Alternatively, the margins of interest may be inked or marked with suture and submitted separately from the primary tumor, which is also submitted for analysis.

8. *After a tissue is biopsied, consideration should be given to submitting portions for culture and sensitivity or alternate analysis (e.g., electron microscopy).* For best results, it is essential to plan what types of samples are to be submitted and analyzed before beginning the biopsy. Once the tissue is in the formalin, other tests or analyses may not be possible.

9. *Biopsy specimens should be submitted to a highly qualified veterinary pathologist who is willing to work with the clinician.* The pathologist should be given a detailed history and a complete account of all relevant clinical material. Margins should be identified with ink or suture. The pathologist will then have all the information necessary to make an accurate diagnosis. If the pathologist's diagnosis does not fit the clinical picture, the clinician and pathologist together should reevaluate the case, including the histopathology. This cooperative interaction is essential for the patient's benefit.

CONTRAINDICATIONS

In each case, the risks and benefits of the biopsy should be evaluated and clearly described to the owner. In most cases, the risks are minimal. Uncontrollable hemorrhage is the most common complication with all biopsy procedures except, perhaps, bone marrow aspiration and biopsy. Therefore, before each biopsy, hemostatic abnormalities should be identified and corrected. Infection at the local biopsy site or sepsis is an uncommon but serious problem that must be avoided by strict aseptic technique. Lastly, a biopsy should not be performed if it would put the success of a definitive procedure at risk. For example, an incisional biopsy of a primary lung tumor may contaminate the entire chest cavity with tumor cells; therefore, primary lung tumors are usually removed and biopsied with one definitive surgery.

BIOPSY AS A PRELUDE TO DEFINITIVE THERAPY

A palpable persistent mass or dominant nodule is the most common indication for biopsy as a prelude to definitive therapy.[1-3] Because the accuracy and sensitivity of diagnostic tests are improving, biopsies are being performed with increasing frequency to clarify the etiology of nonpalpable masses.

When developing a diagnostic strategy for a pet with cancer, the clinician must consider the subsequent management of the disease.[3] The first step in management of most palpable lesions is *fine-needle aspiration cytology.* If the cytologic diagnosis strongly suggests a malignant condition, a definitive procedure such as surgery can be planned. Fine-needle aspiration cytology also can confirm the presence of

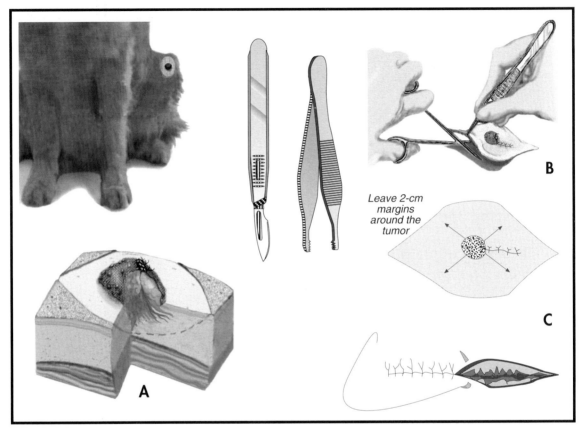

Leave 2-cm margins around the tumor

Figure 1-3: *This figure demonstrates removal of the site of a previous biopsy. The entire previous surgical field, including all tissues or tissue planes that may have been disturbed (**A**), is removed by the definitive surgery. Note that this involves making an elliptical "bird's-eye" incision (**B**) and going at least one fascial layer below the tumor and obtaining wide surgical margins laterally (**C**). The surgeon should not leave any portion of the tumor or any tissue that was disrupted by the previous biopsy.*

a benign process, eliminating the need for further diagnostic steps. If fine-needle aspiration cytology is not definitive, then an open biopsy should be performed, guided by the surgeon who will perform the indicated surgery. Prior to a biopsy procedure, standard staging procedures can be performed to identify any concurrent disease and any clinically evident metastatic disease. Staging is accomplished by certain diagnostic tests that determine the extent of the neoplastic disorder. The staging scheme differs for each neoplastic disease, but tests used often include a complete blood count, biochemical profile, urinalysis, chest radiographs, and cytologic evaluation of region-

al lymph nodes. Discussions about appropriate staging schemes are included in the chapters reviewing specific diseases.

Each biopsy should be performed with the assumption that the lesion is malignant. Therefore, the biopsy should be done so that the entire surgical field, including all tissues or tissue planes that may have been disturbed, can be removed by a subsequent surgery. Second surgeries performed to remove the tumor and surrounding tissues frequently involve going at least one fascial layer below the tumor and all tissues disturbed by the previous surgery (Figure 1-3).

REFERENCES

1. Withrow SJ: Biopsy principles, in Withrow SJ, MacEwen EG (eds): *Clinical Veterinary Oncology.* Philadelphia, JB Lippincott, 1989, pp 53–57.
2. Morrison WB, Hamilton TA, Hahn KA, et al: Diagnosis of neoplasia, in Slatter D (ed): *Textbook of Small Animal Surgery,* ed 2. Philadelphia, WB Saunders, 1993, pp 2036–2048.
3. Wolmark N: Biopsy as a prelude to a definitive operative therapy for breast cancer, in Wittes RE (ed): *Manual of Oncologic Therapeutics 1991/1992.* Philadelphia, JB Lippincott, 1991, pp 5–8.

CLINICAL BRIEFING: SKIN BIOPSY	
Methods	**Benefits**
Punch Biopsy	Outpatient diagnostic procedure; quick and simple
Incisional Biopsy	Diagnostic and allows surgeon to plan definitive procedure properly
Excisional Biopsy	Potentially therapeutic and diagnostic
Needle Core Biopsy	Outpatient diagnostic procedure; quick and simple

A skin biopsy is essential to diagnose and evaluate potentially malignant skin conditions. *Punch, incisional, excisional,* and *needle core biopsies* are employed.[1-3]

PUNCH BIOPSY[1-3]

Biopsy punches are disposable. They are available in diameters ranging from 2 mm to 6 mm. Generally, larger biopsy specimens are preferred so that the pathologist has adequate tissue to make a histologic diagnosis. When possible, the junction between normal and abnormal tissue should be biopsied. Punch biopsies are usually inadequate to obtain tissue below the dermis; subcutaneous fat is rarely obtained in the average punch biopsy of the skin.

Indication: Any dermal or epidermal lesion of unknown etiology.
Contraindications: Coagulopathies.
Benefits: General anesthesia is not required; outpatient procedure.
Limitation: The small tissue samples obtained may not be diagnostic.
Equipment: 2% lidocaine; Baker's biopsy instrument; suture; standard surgical instruments.
Technique (Figure 1-4):
1. The hair is clipped, and the surgery site is prepared with a surgical scrub.
2. Using a 25-ga needle, approximately 2 to 3 ml of

the local anesthetic agent, lidocaine, is injected around the lesion. It is important to make sure that injection of the lidocaine does not distort or disturb the normal architecture of the tissue to be biopsied.
3. The biopsy area is scrubbed a final time after the lidocaine is injected.
4. The skin is stretched between the thumb and index finger.
5. The biopsy punch is placed at a right angle to the skin surface.
6. The punch is rotated in one direction; at the same time, firm downward pressure is applied until the subcutis is reached.
7. The punch is angled almost parallel with the skin while still applying pressure along the long axis of the biopsy punch.
8. The punch is rotated to sever at least part of the base of the biopsied material.
9. The punch is removed.
10. The core of tissue is gently elevated with the point of a needle, and the base is severed with a scalpel or iris scissors.
11. One to two sutures are placed to close the defect.

INCISIONAL BIOPSY[1-3]

In some cases, an incisional biopsy is preferred to a punch biopsy because larger sections of tissue can be

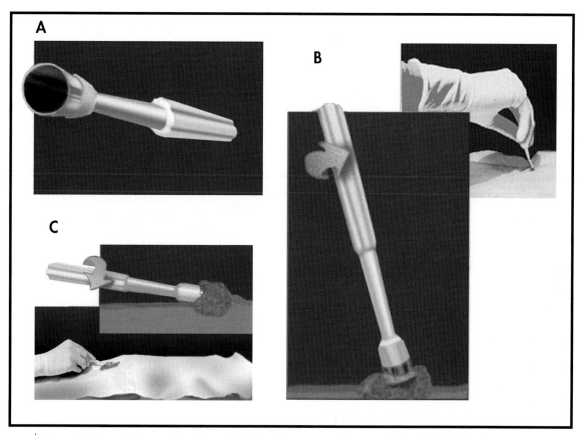

Figure 1-4: *A punch biopsy procedure is begun by injecting lidocaine around the area to be biopsied. The skin is then stretched between the thumb and index finger. The biopsy punch (e.g., Baker's biopsy punch [**A**]) is placed at a right angle to the skin surface (**B**). The punch is rotated in one direction; at the same time, firm downward pressure is applied until the subcutis is reached. The punch is then angled almost parallel with the skin while still applying pressure along the long axis of the biopsy punch (**C**). The punch is rotated to sever at least part of the base of the biopsied material. The punch is removed, and the core of tissue is gently elevated with the point of a needle and severed at the base with a scalpel.*

obtained for histologic diagnosis. In addition, if the lesion is biopsied at the junction of the normal and abnormal tissue, a "wedge" of tissue is obtained that retains a larger section of the tissue's architecture. This makes it easier for the histopathologist to see characteristics of malignancy, such as invasion of normal tissue.

Indication: Any dermal, epidermal, or subcutaneous lesion of unknown etiology.

Contraindications: Coagulopathies. Patients at high risk for general anesthesia.

Benefit: The large tissue sample that can be obtained often results in an accurate diagnosis.

Limitations: General anesthesia is often needed. Not a definitive procedure.

Equipment: Standard surgical instruments; suture material.

Technique (Figure 1-5):

1. Routine screening tests are performed to identify problems such as coagulopathies and metabolic disease. Then, the animal is placed under general anesthesia.

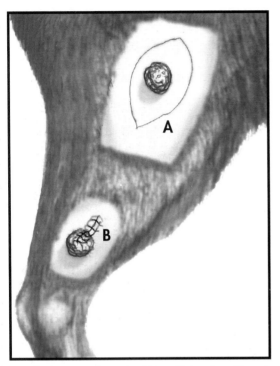

Figure 1-5: An excisional biopsy (**A**) is performed by making an elliptical incision around the tumor for subsequent removal. An incisional biopsy (**B**) is made by removing a portion of normal and neoplastic tissue. Keep in mind that the entire tumor and the biopsy tract will have to be removed by a definitive surgical procedure. The bottom lesion has been sutured and shows that a piece of normal and neoplastic tissue was excised for histopathologic analysis.

2. The hair is clipped, and the surgery site is prepared with a surgical scrub.
3. After the region is draped, an elliptical or wedge incision is made at the margin of the normal and abnormal tissue. Care is taken to obtain adequate tissue and to ensure that a subsequent definitive surgery can remove the tumor and the incisional biopsy area successfully.
4. Vessels going to and from the tissue to be biopsied are carefully identified and ligated.
5. The specimen is lifted and severed at the base with either scissors or a scalpel blade.
6. The incision is sutured for closure.

EXCISIONAL BIOPSY[1-3]

An excisional biopsy should be performed when tissue is required for a histologic diagnosis on a lesion that is small enough and in an anatomic location to permit wide surgical removal without compromising the normal tissue around it (e.g., cutaneous papilloma on the lateral abdominal wall <0.5 cm in diameter) . In general, an excisional biopsy is preceded by at least fine-needle aspiration cytology to give the surgeon as much information as possible about the characteristics of the tumor prior to removal. For example, a mast cell tumor or a soft tissue sarcoma requires wide surgical margins (2 to 3 cm), whereas a sebaceous cyst or sebaceous adenoma can be excised with smaller margins.

Indication: Any dermal, epidermal, or subcutaneous lesion of unknown etiology.
Contraindications: Coagulopathies. Patients at high risk for general anesthesia.
Benefit: The large tissue sample that can be obtained often results in an accurate diagnosis.
Limitation: Requires general anesthesia.
Equipment: Standard surgical instruments; suture material.
Technique (Figure 1-5):
1. This biopsy is performed in the same manner as an incisional biopsy except the lesion is excised completely, with adequate margins.

NEEDLE CORE BIOPSY

Needle core biopsy generally is safe and quick and can be performed on an awake, cooperative patient on an outpatient basis.[1] The histopathologic results generally are more accurate than those of fine-needle aspiration cytology but are not as accurate as the results of an excisional biopsy.

Indication: Skin or subcutaneous lesion of unexplained etiology.
Contraindications: Coagulopathies.
Benefit: General anesthesia is not required, so the procedure can be performed on an outpatient basis.
Limitation: The small tissue samples that are obtained may not be diagnostic.

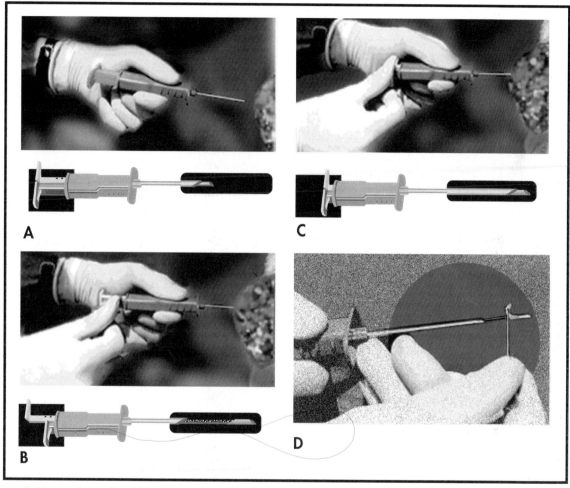

Figure 1-6: *A needle core biopsy is accomplished by making a stab incision through the skin with a no. 11 surgical blade after the skin and underlying structures are anesthetized locally with 2 to 3 ml of lidocaine. A needle biopsy instrument is then advanced through the skin to the periphery of the lesion (**A**). The stylet is advanced into the tissue to be biopsied (**B**), and the outer cannula is advanced over the stylet to "cut" off the tissue left in the notch of the stylet (**C**). The entire instrument is removed from the incision, and the tissue is teased out of the stylet using a 22-ga needle (**D**).*

Equipment: No. 11 surgical blade; 2% lidocaine; needle biopsy instrument.

Technique (Figure 1-6):

1. The cutaneous or subcutaneous lesion is grasped by an assistant and immobilized, and the biopsy site is prepared with surgical scrub for an aseptic procedure.

2. Approximately 2 to 3 ml of 2% lidocaine is injected around the lesion to be biopsied while trying not to disturb the architecture of the tissue to be evaluated with the lidocaine.

3. Using a no. 11 surgical blade, a stab incision is made in the skin to allow easy entry of the needle core biopsy instrument.

4. The needle core biopsy instrument is advanced through the incision to the outer portion of the lesion to be biopsied. In the case of the skin, the instrument is just entered into the tissue to be biopsied.

5. At least three to five biopsy specimens are taken of the suspect tissue through the same stab incision.

6. The needle biopsy specimens are fixed in 10% buffered formalin, as described previously. A separate container should be used for each lesion that is biopsied.

7. The stab incision is sutured only if indicated.

REFERENCES

1. Withrow SJ: Biopsy principles, in Withrow SJ, MacEwen EG (eds): *Clinical Veterinary Oncology.* Philadelphia, JB Lippincott, 1989, pp 53–57.
2. Morrison WB, Hamilton TA, Hahn KA, et al: Diagnosis of neoplasia, in Slatter D (ed): *Textbook of Small Animal Surgery,* ed 2. Philadelphia, WB Saunders, 1993, pp 2036–2048.
3. Sober AJ: Skin biopsy in the diagnosis and management of malignancy, in Wittes RE (ed): *Manual of Oncologic Therapeutics 1991/1992.* Philadelphia, JB Lippincott, 1991, pp 1–5.

CLINICAL BRIEFING: LYMPH NODE BIOPSY

Methods	Benefits
Lymph Node Excision	Pathologist can evaluate complete nodal architecture
Needle Core Biopsy	Outpatient diagnostic procedure; quick and simple

Lymph node biopsy is often important in the diagnosis, staging, and proper therapeutic management of the pet with cancer.[1-3] A biopsy often is performed after fine-needle aspiration cytology suggests the presence of disease. Despite the accuracy of fine-needle aspiration cytology in determining certain diseases such as lymphoma, mast cell tumors, and the presence of metastatic solid tumors, a histopathologic diagnosis is always recommended prior to initiation of therapy. In each case, adequate tissue must be obtained for histopathologic diagnosis and for special stains, if indicated. When possible, the submandibular lymph nodes should be avoided; they often are reactive in the normal animal because they drain the oral cavity, where the bacterial count usually is quite high. These reactive cells are sometimes misdiagnosed as neoplastic cells. If a carcinoma or a sarcoma is suspected, a biopsy should not be performed unless an overall plan for definitive therapy is made because the biopsy procedure can "seed" the operative field with tumor cells if the principle of *en bloc* dissection is violated. As with all biopsies, the surgeon who will perform the definitive surgery should be consulted prior to the biopsy to ensure that incisions are properly placed for a subsequent definitive procedure.

LYMPH NODE EXCISION

The type of biopsy selected will depend on each case; however, an excisional biopsy should be performed when possible[1-3] because this biopsy allows the pathologist to determine the architecture of the entire lymph node and to determine whether capsular invasion exists. This is especially valuable when lymphoma must be differentiated from lymph node hyperplasia.

Lymph node excisions are performed commonly in dogs that have lymphadenopathy, especially when lymphoma or other malignant conditions are suspected. A lymph node that is not easily seen or palpated by the casual observer should be considered for removal. Hair should be clipped prior to surgery; however, the amount of hair clipped should not be excessive, because animals on chemotherapy often have slow hair regrowth. In addition, antineoplastic agents can cause alopecia, which makes the surgical site observable for weeks to months after the procedure.

Indication: Lymphadenopathy of unexplained etiology.

Contraindications: Coagulopathies; patients who are at high risk for complications due to anesthesia.

Benefit: An accurate histopathologic diagnosis can be obtained because the entire lymph node architecture is present for evaluation.

Limitation: Requires general anesthesia.

Equipment: Standard surgical instruments.

Technique (Figure 1-7):

1. The animal is placed under general anesthesia after routine screening tests are performed to identify problems such as coagulopathies and metabolic disease.
2. The hair is clipped, and the surgical site is prepared with a surgical scrub.
3. After the region is draped, an incision is made over the enlarged lymph node.

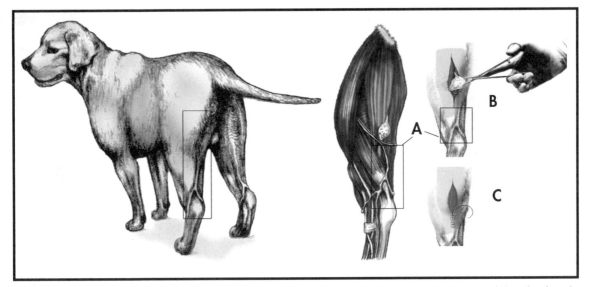

Figure 1-7: *Removal of the popliteal lymph node is accomplished by making an incision over the lymph node and then identifying the popliteal artery for ligation. Care is taken to avoid the saphenous vein (**A**). The lymph node in the capsule is bluntly dissected and removed (**B**). The subcutaneous tissue and skin are closed routinely (**C**).*

4. Care is taken to identify and ligate vessels going to and from the lymph node to be excised.
5. After the lymph node is removed, subcutaneous tissue is closed with absorbable suture, and the skin is closed with either absorbable or nonabsorbable suture.
6. The removed lymph nodes should then be "bread-sliced" to allow adequate exposure to 10% formalin. Care is taken to ensure that there is at least 1 part tissue for 10 parts formalin.

NEEDLE CORE BIOPSY

Needle core biopsy generally is safe and quick. It can be performed on an awake, cooperative patient.[1] The histopathologic results generally are more accurate than those of fine-needle aspiration cytology but are not as accurate as the results of an excisional biopsy.

Indication: Lymphadenopathy of unexplained etiology.
Contraindications: Coagulopathies.
Benefit: General anesthesia is not required, so the procedure can be performed on an outpatient basis.

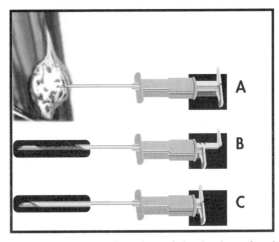

Figure 1-8: *Needle core biopsy of a lymph node is performed after the skin and nearby structures are anesthetized with approximately 2 to 3 ml of lidocaine. Using a no. 11 surgical blade, a stab incision is made in the skin to allow easy entry of the needle core biopsy instrument. The needle core biopsy instrument is then advanced through the incision and into the capsule of the enlarged lymph node for subsequent biopsy (**A**). The inner cannula is advanced first (**B**), followed by the outer portion, which cuts the tissue and leaves a biopsy sample in the needle (**C**). At least three to five biopsy specimens are taken through the same stab incision.*

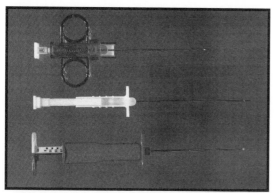

Figure 1-9A

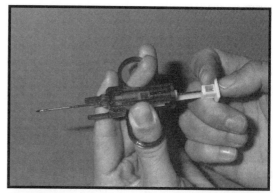

Figure 1-9B

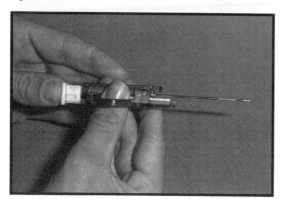

Figure 1-9C

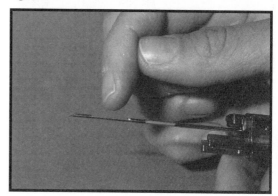

Figure 1-9D

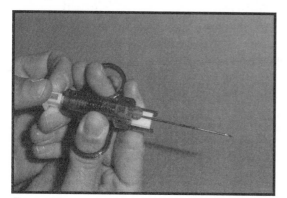

Figure 1-9E

Figure 1-9: *Examples of different types of needle core biopsy instruments (A). A spring-loaded biopsy instrument can be used with one or two hands. The instrument is first "cocked" by pulling back the handle (B); the inner cannula is advanced into the tumor (C) so that the notched portion of the stylet will fill with tissue (D). The spring-loaded outer portion of the biopsy instrument is then "fired" (E), resulting in quick advancement of the outer portion of the instrument over the piece of tumor that is within the recessed area of the inner stylet.*

Limitation: The small tissue samples obtained may not be diagnostic.

Equipment: No. 11 surgical blade; 2% lidocaine; needle biopsy instrument.

Technique (Figures 1-8 and 1-9):
1. The lymph node is grasped by an assistant and held firmly against the overlying skin; the biopsy site is prepared as noted in steps 1 and 2 for lymph

node excision.

2. Approximately 2 to 3 ml of 2% lidocaine is injected under the skin overlying the enlarged lymph node.

3. Using a no. 11 surgical blade, a stab incision is made in the skin to allow easy entry of the needle core biopsy instrument.

4. The needle core biopsy instrument is advanced through the incision and into the capsule of the enlarged lymph node.

5. At least three to five biopsy specimens of the lymph node are taken through the same stab incision.

6. The needle biopsy specimens are fixed in 10%

buffered formalin. A separate container should be used for each lesion that is biopsied.

7. The stab incision is sutured only if indicated.

REFERENCES

1. Withrow SJ: Biopsy principles, in Withrow SJ, MacEwen EG (eds): *Clinical Veterinary Oncology.* Philadelphia, JB Lippincott, 1989, pp 53–57.

2. Morrison WB, Hamilton TA, Hahn KA, et al: Diagnosis of neoplasia, in Slatter D (ed): *Textbook of Small Animal Surgery,* ed 2. Philadelphia, WB Saunders, 1993, pp 2036–2048.

3. Avis F: Lymph node biopsy, in Wittes RE (ed): *Manual of Oncologic Therapeutics 1991/1992.* Philadelphia, JB Lippincott, 1991, pp 8–9.

CLINICAL BRIEFING: RESPIRATORY TRACT BIOPSY

Thoracic Cavity

Methods	Benefits
Bronchoscopy	Visualization of lesions and a directed biopsy allows more accurate diagnosis
Transthoracic Aspirate	Quick, simple, and inexpensive method of diagnosing pleural or pulmonary lesions
Transtracheal Wash	Relatively quick and simple method of diagnosing some lesions confined to the airways

Nasal Cavity

Methods	Benefits
Bronchoscopy	Visualization of lesion and a biopsy especially valuable to differentiate tumor from fungal rhinitis
Cannula Biopsy	Large core biopsy samples acquired, maximizing accurate diagnosis
Curette Biopsy	Biopsy method especially valuable for cats and small dogs

THORACIC CAVITY DIAGNOSTICS

Bronchoscopy is used commonly to diagnose primary lung tumors in humans; however, in veterinary practice, lung tumors are not often diagnosed successfully with this approach.[1-5] This may be because primary lung tumors of the dog and cat rarely arise from the major airways. Transtracheal washes, therefore, are not often successful in obtaining primary or metastatic tumors of the pulmonary parenchyma. Primary lung tumors of dogs and cats are often limited to the pulmonary parenchyma; therefore, they must be accessed via techniques that can sample pulmonary tissue from outside the airways. Bronchoscopy is helpful in the diagnosis of metastatic neoplastic conditions that shed tumor cells into the major airways and is of great value in nonneoplastic conditions of the lungs and major airways.[1-4] When bronchoscopy does not successfully obtain diagnostic cells or tissue from lesions of the peripheral pulmonary parenchyma, samples often can be obtained successfully from transthoracic needle aspiration, with or without imaging guidance. When this method fails, an open biopsy via thoracotomy may be successful. Biopsy of nasal tumors frequently involves the use of different instruments, including a straw attached to a syringe or a bone curette. Although biopsy through a bronchoscope or a cystoscope is relatively easy to accomplish, the size of the tissue sample obtained through these instruments often is inadequate for an accurate diagnosis. In part, this is because the tissue removed by these methods is superficial and the underlying true histopathology frequently is obscured by septic inflammation.

Bronchoscopy[1,2,4]

The flexible fiberoptic bronchoscope has super-

SELECTION OF AN ENDOSCOPE

The endoscope should
(1) have an instrument port and channel

(2) be at least bidirectional

(3) bend more than 100 degrees in at least one direction

(4) have an external light source

Cytology brushes, biopsy forceps, and graspers that can pass through the instrument port with the endoscope in a flexed position should be available.

Adult or pediatric endoscopes ≤ 5 mm in diameter can be inserted into the trachea of most dogs and cats.

---

seded the rigid bronchoscope. The latter instrument limits lung visualization and is not as effective in obtaining significant amounts of diagnostic tissue as fiberoptic bronchoscopy. The fiberoptic bronchoscope permits wide visualization of the respiratory tract. In addition, a wide variety of brushes, biopsy instruments, and grasping forceps can be introduced through the bronchoscope to obtain tissue or cytologic samples. It is estimated that more than 90% of all tumors located in the airways and 50% of the peripheral lung tumors can be diagnosed with this modality.[1-5] The benefits of bronchoscopic imaging and biopsies include the ability to explore a large portion of the lungs and to obtain tissue or cells from extremely localized areas. Disadvantages include the need for general anesthesia, inability to obtain tissue samples larger than those that can be brought through a 1- to 2-mm channel, and the complication of secretions from the respiratory tract that obscure visualization. When possible, multiple biopsy specimens should be obtained to increase the probability of an accurate diagnosis. If large pieces of tissue are obtained, the tissue should not be brought through the biopsy channel of the endoscope. Instead, with the biopsy instrument still extended through the biopsy port, the endoscope is removed from the trachea and endotracheal tube.

Indications: Any disease that appears to involve the airways or alveoli. This includes, but is not limited to, primary or metastatic lung tumors.

Contraindications: Coagulopathies. Patients at high risk for general anesthesia, including patients with limited pulmonary function.

Benefits: Relatively minimal risk. Noninvasive.

Limitations: Requires general anesthesia. The small tissue samples that are obtained may not be diagnostic.

Equipment: There are many fiberoptic endoscopes on the market for performance of bronchoscopy. Adapters can be used to pass the bronchoscope down into the respiratory tract with oxygen and inhalant anesthetic gases.

Technique:

1. After tests have been carried out to ensure the absence of life-threatening diseases, general anesthesia with endotracheal intubation is performed.

2. After the patient is well oxygenated, a y-piece adapter specifically designed for bronchoscopy is attached between the endotracheal tube and the anesthesia machine. One end of the y-piece adapter is attached to the endotracheal tube while the other end is fixed to the anesthesia machine. The open end is available to pass the bronchoscope down through the y-piece into the endotracheal tube and down the trachea.

3. The bronchoscope is inserted through the y-piece and down the trachea. If the bronchoscope com-

promises adequate endotracheal space for normal respiration, oxygen, with or without anesthetic gases, can be advanced down the bronchoscope. A systematic exploration of the respiratory tree is initiated.

4. Suspect lesions are first sampled with the cytology brush for evaluation and then biopsied for histopathology. If a diffuse lesion is suspected, then bronchoalveolar lavage is performed by introducing a catheter down the bronchoscope into the area to be sampled. Sterile saline (12–20 ml 0.9% NaCl) is then injected into the area and immediately withdrawn for culture and cytologic evaluation. This procedure can be repeated several times.

Complications: Rare. Can include bleeding, which usually stops spontaneously. If brisk bleeding persists, introducing a Fogarty balloon catheter to occlude the opening is recommended. In humans, the risk of pneumothorax is reported to be less than 1%; when it occurs, it is usually preceded by a transbronchial biopsy of peripheral lymph nodes.

Transthoracic Aspirate[2–4]

Transthoracic aspiration cytology and thoracentesis are procedures to remove or sample pleural fluid or tissue within the lung for diagnostic or therapeutic reasons. Fluoroscopy generally is used to guide the biopsy of pulmonary, parenchymal, pleural, and mediastinal lesions. Whenever tissue or fluid is present in the thorax, ultrasonography can be used instead of fluoroscopy. In those cases that cannot be defined clearly by fluoroscopy or ultrasonography, computerized tomography (CT) can be used to guide tissue sampling. In one study that included over 400 percutaneously biopsied pulmonary lesions, the accuracy of the procedure was determined to be 96.5%.[4]

Indications: Any masses, lesions, or fluid accumulations within or around the pulmonary parenchyma that are not near or associated with the heart or blood vessels.

Contraindications: Coagulopathies, poor pulmonary reserve, and pulmonary arterial hypertension. Complications are rare (<10%) but include hemothorax and pneumothorax. Placement of a chest tube generally resolves these problems.

Benefit: Cells or fluid can be acquired with limited risk and without a thoracotomy.

Limitations: Requires general anesthesia or tranquilization. May cause pneumothorax or hemothorax.

Equipment: 2% lidocaine; 12-ml syringe; 22-ga 1.5-inch needle.

Technique (Figure 1-10):

1. After routine screening tests have been performed to identify problems such as coagulopathies, metabolic disease, or organ failure, the animal is placed under general anesthesia or tranquilized.

2. The lesions are identified with fluoroscopy, ultrasonography, or CT. The hair is clipped, and the surgical site is prepared with a surgical scrub. A surgical drape is placed to enhance sterility.

3. If tranquilization is used, the skin and underlying tissue up to the pleura are anesthetized with 2% lidocaine (3 to 5 ml).

4. A 22-ga needle attached to a 12-ml syringe is advanced through the skin and intercostal muscles using fluoroscopic, ultrasonographic, or CT-guided imaging. Care is taken to avoid the heart and great vessels. If fluid is to be sampled, a three-way stopcock is attached between the syringe and needle to facilitate removal of large amounts of fluid.

5. Tissue is aspirated while the needle is advanced through the lesion. The pressure is eliminated prior to removing the needle from the

> ## KEY POINTS:
>
> *Extreme care should be used to prevent overinflation of the lungs or overdosing the patient on inhalant anesthetic gases.*
>
> ---
>
> *Patients at high risk for general anesthesia, including patients with limited pulmonary function, should be excluded from this procedure.*

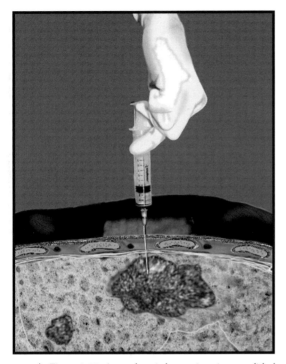

Figure 1-10: A transthoracic lung aspirate is accomplished with a 22-ga needle attached to a 12-ml syringe, which is advanced through the skin and intercostal muscles using fluoroscopic, ultrasonographic, or CT guidance. If fluid is to be sampled, a three-way stopcock is attached between the syringe and needle to facilitate removal of large amounts of fluid. Tissue is quickly aspirated while the needle is advanced through the lesion. The pressure is eliminated prior to removing the needle from the mass and chest cavity.

quent submission to a clinical pathologist for analysis.

6. The patient is watched carefully for respiratory difficulty for several hours. Ideally, a chest radiograph is taken to insure that hemothorax or pneumothorax has not developed after the procedure. The patient is then rested for 24 to 48 hours.

NASAL BIOPSY[1,4]

A nasal biopsy should be considered for every dog and cat with facial deformity, unilateral or bilateral epistaxis, or epiphora of unknown etiology. A nasal tumor or fungal rhinitis must be suspected in many of these cases. A biopsy is required in each case before appropriate therapy can be recommended. Dogs and cats can be biopsied using equipment that is relatively inexpensive and quite effective. Although fiberoptic examinations and nasal flushes are valuable in some cases, they are not as rewarding as nasal cannula or curette biopsy techniques. Regardless of the procedure, general anesthesia is required for both dogs and cats. Medium and large dogs are biopsied effectively using a cannula biopsy method. Small dogs and cats are biopsied effectively using a bone curette. Both species are biopsied through the external nares to reduce the need for surgical exposure through the skin, which could contaminate these structures with tumor cells from the nasal cavity.

Indication: Any undiagnosed nasal problem, especially when the animal has epiphora and unilateral to bilateral epistaxis.

Contraindications: Coagulopathies. Patients at high risk for general anesthesia.

Benefit: The large tissue sample that can be obtained often results in an accurate diagnosis.

Limitation: Requires general anesthesia.

Equipment: 12-ml syringe; straw that will fit securely over a sovereign catheter; needle hub. Sovereign catheters have a straw that is used to cover the catheter and needle. This can be assembled to make a biopsy instrument. A small- to medium-sized bone curette is used for small dogs and cats.

mass and chest cavity. To prevent injury of normal lung tissue, the needle is inserted and the mass aspirated over a relatively short period. The syringe is then removed from the needle and filled with air. After the needle is re-attached to the syringe, the material in the needle is forcefully expelled onto a clean microscope slide. If indicated, the material is gently spread over the slide to obtain a single layer of cells for subsequent analysis. If fluid is removed, slides are made, and fluid is saved for culture and sensitivity. The remaining fluid is saved in an EDTA tube and a red top tube without anticoagulant for subse-

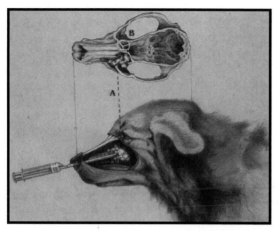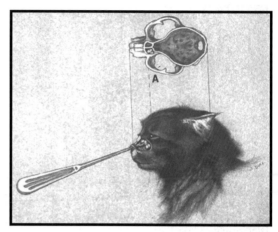

Figure 1-11: *A nasal biopsy can be accomplished in medium to large dogs with a large-bore (3–5 mm) plastic cannula. This cannula is fixed to the hub of a needle that has had the metal portion removed with a knife or old scissors. The cannula/needle hub is then fixed to a 12-ml syringe. The entire apparatus is passed up the nostril and directed into the tumor. The biopsy instrument should never pass further caudal than the medial canthus of either eye (**A**) to prevent it from entering the cribriform plate and the brain (**B**). The tumor is entered forcefully, and suction is applied to core and aspirate the tumor effectively. The apparatus is removed from the nasal cavity, and the tumor is then ejected out of the cannula by forcefully expelling a syringe full of air through the needle hub and cannula. Cats and small dogs can be biopsied using the same landmarks and procedures. Instead of using the cannula method, a small- to medium-sized bone curette is used to "scoop up" the tumor. (Left: From Ogilvie GK, LaRue SM: Canine and feline nasal and paranasal sinus tumors. Vet Clin North Am Small Anim Pract 22:1133–1145, 1992; with permission. Right: From Elmslie RE, Ogilvie GK: Solitary extranodal lymphomas: Presentation and management, in August JR (ed):* Consultations in Feline Internal Medicine, *ed 2. Philadelphia, WB Saunders, 1994, pp 547–552; with permission.)*

Technique (Figure 1-11):

1. The animal is placed under general anesthesia after routine screening tests have been performed to identify problems, such as coagulopathies, metabolic disease, or organ failure.
2. The nasal lesion is identified with skull radiographs or CT. The most valuable skull radiograph is an intraoral exposure, which is best made with non-screen film placed inside the mouth to allow imaging of the caudal aspect of the nasal cavity. General anesthesia is required for this procedure.
3. Three to 5 ml of 2% lidocaine can be flushed up into the biopsy site by placing a tomcat catheter or soft catheter without the needle in place through the nasal passage to the level of the lesion. This may

reduce local discomfort and allow a lighter plane of anesthesia.

4. Medium to large dogs can be biopsied with a large-bore (3–5 mm) plastic cannula. The cannula is fixed to the hub of a needle that has the metal portion removed. The cannula/needle hub is then fixed to a 12-ml syringe. The entire apparatus is then passed up the nostril and directed into the tumor. It is essential to "pre-measure" from the nares to the medial canthus of the eye and either cut the straw off at the proper length or mark it with tape. The tumor is then entered forcefully, and suction is applied to core and aspirate the tumor effectively. The apparatus is removed from the nasal cavity, and the tumor is ejected out of the cannula by forcefully expelling a syringe full of air through the needle

> **KEY POINT:**
>
> *The biopsy instrument should never pass further caudal than the medial canthus of either eye to prevent entering the cribriform plate and the brain.*

hub and cannula. A similar technique using cup-type mare uterine biopsy forceps can be used with similar results. The tumor, which usually is white to yellow, should be placed into formalin for subsequent analysis.

5. Cats and small dogs can be biopsied using the same landmarks and procedures. Instead of using the cannula method, a small- to medium-sized bone curette is used to "scoop up" the tumor.

6. Mild to moderate hemorrhage is expected and will subside within a relatively short period. If hemorrhage is excessive, ipsilateral carotid artery ligation should assist in reducing the bleeding. Hematocrit levels should be monitored hourly until all bleeding has stopped.

REFERENCES

1. Withrow SJ: Biopsy principles, in Withrow SJ, MacEwen EG (eds): *Clinical Veterinary Oncology.* Philadelphia, JB Lippincott, 1989, pp 53–57.
2. Morrison WB, Hamilton TA, Hahn KA, et al: Diagnosis of neoplasia, in Slatter D (ed): *Textbook of Small Animal Surgery*, ed 2. Philadelphia, WB Saunders, 1993, pp 2036–2048.
3. Martini N: Diagnostic procedures relating to the thorax, in Wittes RE (ed): *Manual of Oncologic Therapeutics 1991/1992.* Philadelphia, JB Lippincott, 1991, pp 9–10.
4. Westcott JL: Direct percutaneous needle aspiration of localized pulmonary lesions: Results in 422 patients. *Radiology* 137:31–35, 1985.
5. Withrow SJ: Diseases of the respiratory system, in Withrow SJ, MacEwen EG (eds): *Clinical Veterinary Oncology.* Philadelphia, JB Lippincott, 1989, pp 215–233.

CLINICAL BRIEFING: BONE MARROW ASPIRATION AND BIOPSY

Methods	Benefits
Illinois or Rosenthal Needle Aspirate	Relatively quick and simple outpatient procedure for obtaining marrow for cytology
Jamshidi Needle Biopsy	Simple method of obtaining marrow core aspirates and biopsies in anesthetized patient

Bone marrow aspiration and biopsy are essential procedures for determining cytologic and histologic abnormalities of the bone marrow caused by a wide variety of neoplastic, infectious, and myelodysplastic conditions.[1-3] A bone marrow aspirate and biopsy are indicated when an abnormality in blood cell production is suspected or when attempting to stage an animal with a hematopoietic malignancy.

Bone marrow aspiration is performed to acquire a monolayer of cells for individual evaluation.[1-3] To identify a wide variety of malignant and nonmalignant disorders, Romanovsky (including Wright's and Giemsa) stains are preferred. When the cytologic diagnosis of a cell type is not certain, additional special stains, including myeloperoxidase, Sudan black, and periodic acid-Schiff, can be used. Bone marrow biopsies are beneficial for determining bone marrow cellularity, the presence and extent of fibrosis or granulomatous conditions, and the presence of non-hematopoietic malignancies.

Indications: Blood cell production abnormality. Staging procedure for a hematopoietic or non-hematopoietic malignancy.

Contraindications: Coagulopathies.

Benefits: Aspiration can provide a sample for individual cell analysis, whereas a biopsy can provide tissue to analyze cellularity, architecture, and content. Often, this can be done with local anesthesia, with or without systemic analgesia and/or tranquilization.

Limitation: Single sample may not be representative of the entire bone marrow.

Equipment: No. 11 surgical blade; 2% lidocaine; 12-ml syringe; 16- or 18-ga Illinois or Rosenthal bone marrow needle; microscope slides; EDTA container.

Technique[1-3] (Figure 1-12):

1. The hair is clipped, and the bone marrow aspiration site is prepared with a surgical scrub. Preferred sites and patient positioning include:
   - dorsocranial or lateral aspects of iliac crest (patient is in sternal recumbency)
   - greater trochanter of the femur (patient is in lateral recumbency)
   - greater tubercle of the proximal aspect of the head of the humerus (patient is in lateral recumbency)
2. Using a 25-ga needle, approximately 2 to 3 ml of the local anesthetic agent, lidocaine, is injected in and around the site where the bone marrow needle is to be introduced. Care is taken to deposit lidocaine in and around all of the tissues that extend from the skin to the bone.
3. The biopsy area is scrubbed a final time after the lidocaine is injected. A surgical drape should be applied for sterility.
4. The bone marrow site is identified, the skin is stretched between the thumb and index finger, and a small stab incision is made with a no. 11 surgical blade in the area blocked with lidocaine.
5. The bone marrow needle with the stylet in place is advanced through the stab incision and

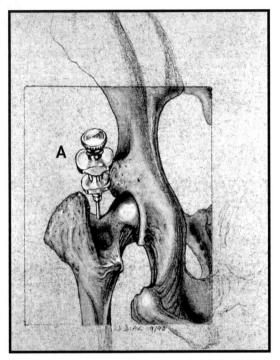

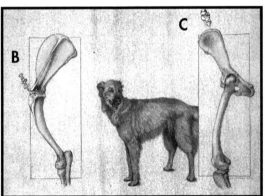

Figure 1-12: Three ideal locations for bone marrow aspiration are the greater trochanter of the femur (**A**), the greater tubercle of the proximal aspect of the head of the humerus (**B**), and the dorsocranial aspect of the iliac crest (**C**). A bone marrow sample is acquired by advancing a bone marrow needle with the stylet in place through one stab incision in the skin. With the stylet in place, the 1-inch, 16- to 18-ga bone marrow needle is advanced into the bone using a corkscrew motion. When the needle is fixed in the bone, the stylet is removed and the syringe is affixed. The bone marrow sample (1 ml) is then aspirated briskly into the 12-ml syringe and placed on slides or in a 1.5-ml EDTA tube.

through the skin, subcutaneous tissue, and muscle down to the bone. It is crucial to keep the stylet in place because it has a tendency to back out during the procedure. A 1- to 1.5-inch-long, 16-ga Illinois or Rosenthal bone marrow needle is preferred for dogs, and a 1-inch-long, 18-ga Illinois or Rosenthal needle is preferred for cats. After a sample is obtained for cytologic evaluation, a Jamshidi needle is used to collect a biopsy specimen, if required.

6. With the stylet in place, the bone marrow needle is advanced into the bone, using a corkscrew motion. The instrument should not be allowed to wobble and should be fixed firmly into the bone like a nail that has been securely hammered into wood. When the needle is firmly fixed in the bone, the stylet is removed and the syringe is affixed. Many clinical pathologists suggest rinsing the syringe and bone marrow needle with EDTA before the procedure to reduce clotting of the bone marrow sample.

7. The bone marrow sample is aspirated briskly into the 12-ml syringe; usually, 1 ml of marrow is adequate. The aspiration may be accompanied by a few seconds of pain, but this cannot be prevented.

8. If a sample is not obtained, the stylet is replaced in the bone marrow needle, and the instrument is then advanced further into the bone for a second attempt at aspirating marrow contents.

9. Once marrow has been obtained, smears are prepared. This can be done in a number of ways:
   - The marrow and blood are expelled into a small Petri dish. The marrow-rich spicules are placed on a slide or coverslip and then spread between slides or coverslips to make a monolayer of cells.
   - A portion of the marrow sample is placed on the proximal portion of the slide; the slide is tipped downward to allow the blood to run down and off the slide. The spicules and heavier nucleated cells do not run off and are used for subsequent slide preparation.
   - Marrow can be spread into a monolayer like an ordinary blood smear.

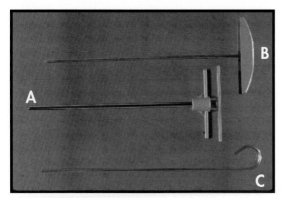

Figure 1-13: *A Jamshidi biopsy needle (**A**) with the stylet (**B**) removed from the biopsy instrument is shown. The Jamshidi is used to acquire a bone marrow core sample for histopathology. The stylet is kept in place until the needle is seated in bone. After the stylet is removed, the needle is advanced 1 to 2 inches. The instrument is then rocked back and forth in two directions at 90° to each other to "break" the piece of bone off at the base while it is within the needle. The needle is removed, and the biopsy specimen is pushed from the front of the needle out the back with a smaller wire stylet (**C**).*

The first two methods may enhance the ability to evaluate the nucleated cell population of the bone marrow specimen.

10. A biopsy can be obtained with the Jamshidi needle after aspiration is performed (Figure 1-13).

For biopsy, the stylet is kept out of the needle. After the aspiration, the instrument is advanced in the method described earlier. The needle is then rocked back and forth in two directions at 90° to each other. In humans, premedication usually is not necessary, because pain usually is minimal if local anesthesia is adequate. The purpose of the rocking movement is to sever the bone in the needle from its base. The biopsy instrument is then removed, and a smaller wire obturator is used to retrograde the biopsy piece out of the top end of the biopsy instrument. Cytology and histopathology can be performed on this tissue.

11. Direct pressure should be applied to the site for several minutes to prevent hematoma formation.

REFERENCES

1. Withrow SJ: Biopsy principles, in Withrow SJ, MacEwen EG (eds): *Clinical Veterinary Oncology.* Philadelphia, JB Lippincott, 1989, pp 53–57.
2. Morrison WB, Hamilton TA, Hahn KA, et al: Diagnosis of neoplasia, in Slatter D (ed): *Textbook of Small Animal Surgery,* ed 2. Philadelphia, WB Saunders, 1993, pp 2036–2048.
3. Lee EJ, Schiffer CA: Bone marrow aspiration and biopsy, in Wittes RE (ed): *Manual of Oncologic Therapeutics 1991/1992.* Philadelphia, JB Lippincott, 1991, pp 24–26.

CLINICAL BRIEFING: LOWER UROGENITAL TRACT BIOPSY

Bladder

Methods	Benefits
Cystotomy Bladder Biopsy	Surgical procedure allows for visual staging of tumor with biopsy
Suction Capsule Biopsy Method	Large biopsy samples can be obtained with this self-contained instrument
Open-End Catheter Bladder Biopsy	Relatively inexpensive procedure for obtaining biopsy
Flexible or Rigid Fiberoptic Bladder Biopsy	Visualization of lesion and direction of biopsy enhances diagnosis

Prostate

Methods	Benefits
Transabdominal Needle Core Biopsy	Relatively simple to perform; outpatient procedure
Transrectal Needle Core Biopsy	May allow more direct access to prostate with more accurate biopsy

Biopsies of the lower urogenital tract are common procedures for the practitioner. Bladder tumors can be biopsied by laparotomy or with less invasive procedures such as using cystoscopy and a Quinton biopsy capsule.[1,2] The prostate can be biopsied percutaneously, especially when guided with concurrent ultrasonographic or CT images, or per rectum.[1,2] Testicular biopsies can be performed by castration, transscrotal biopsy, or fine-needle aspiration cytology.[1]

BIOPSY OF THE BLADDER

Patients with micro- or gross hematuria, with or without stranguria and dysuria, that is not resolved with antibiotic therapy must be evaluated for a bladder tumor.[1,2] Transitional cell carcinoma is the most common bladder tumor in dogs; it is uncommon in cats. Other differentials, including uroliths, must be ruled out. In each case, a biopsy is required to make an appropriate diagnosis. Prior to the biopsy, a double-contrast cystogram and/or bladder ultrasonogra-phy is essential to localize and characterize the lesion. The most common methods for nonsurgical biopsy of the bladder are cystoscopy with a rigid or flexible fiberoptic endoscope or with a suction capsule biopsy instrument that allows the tissue to be aspirated into a biopsy chamber at the end of the flexible instrument. The tissue is subsequently cut off with a small wire that acts as a blade, which is located within the biopsy instrument. A cheaper method is to use an open-ended urinary catheter that is advanced against the tumor; the tumor is vigorously aspirated into the catheter and the entire instrument is then retracted, hopefully with a piece of tumor within the catheter lumen.

Suction Capsule or Catheter Biopsy Technique[1,2]

Indication: Any undiagnosed persistent bladder problem, especially when the animal has cystitis or hematuria, that is unresponsive to standard therapy.

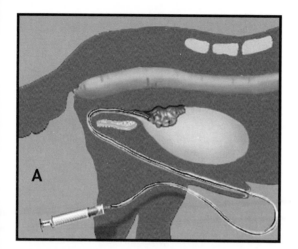

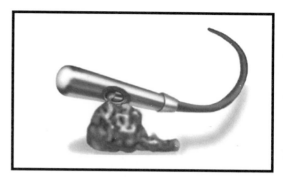

Figure 1-15: A capsule biopsy instrument can be used to suction a piece of tumor into a side chamber. The piece of tissue suctioned into the chamber is then severed by a wire that is contained within the instrument. The tissue is retrieved by withdrawing the instrument.

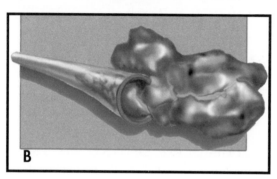

Figure 1-14: Biopsy of a bladder tumor can be accomplished by advancing a catheter with an open end into the tumor (A). Suction is applied to aspirate a plug of tumor into the catheter (B). The catheter is removed while suction is maintained to ensure that the tissue stays in the catheter.

Contraindications: Coagulopathies. Patients at high risk for general anesthesia. This technique is difficult to perform in male dogs and cats.

Benefit: Fairly large tissue samples can be obtained that often result in an accurate diagnosis.

Limitations: Requires general anesthesia and is easier to perform in medium to large dogs. In smaller male dogs, the relatively small size of the urethral diameter through the os penis may limit these techniques.

Equipment: 12-ml syringe and urinary catheter or a suction capsule biopsy instrument.

Technique (Figures 1-14 and 1-15):

1. After routine screening tests have been performed to identify problems such as coagulopathies, metabolic disease, or organ failure, the animal is placed under general anesthesia.
2. The bladder or urethral lesion is identified with ultrasonography or a double-contrast cystogram.
3a. **Catheter technique** (Figure 1-14): Medium to large dogs can be biopsied with a large-bore (12- to 13-ga) open-ended urinary catheter. The catheter should be "pre-measured" so the length to be advanced does not exceed the measurement from the area of the distal urethra to the level of the tumor, which generally is not further forward than the caudal two mammary glands. This reduces the risk of bladder perforation. The open-ended catheter is then advanced through the urethra and then forcefully into the tumor. This is best accomplished with ultrasonographic or fluoroscopic guidance or by palpating the mass per abdomen or per rectum. Once the tumor has been entered, suction is applied while the instrument is withdrawn. Tissue that has been suctioned up into the catheter and torn off during removal of the catheter is expelled and placed in 10% formalin for subsequent fixation and analysis.
3b. **Suction capsule biopsy instrument technique:** Suction capsule (e.g., Quinton) biopsy instru-

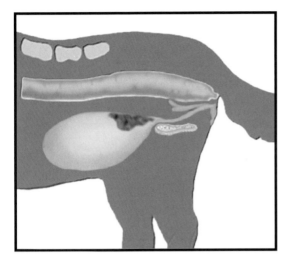

against the tumor, suction is applied to aspirate the tissue into the capsule. The self-contained wire that acts as a knife is then activated to sever the biopsied tissue from the main tumor for subsequent retrieval.

Fiberoptic or Rigid Cystoscopic Biopsy[1,2]

Indications: Any diseases that appear to involve the urethra or bladder.

Contraindications: Coagulopathies. Patients at high risk for general anesthesia, including patients with limited pulmonary function.

Benefits: Relatively minimal risk. Noninvasive.

Limitation: Requires general anesthesia.

Equipment: There are many fiberoptic endoscopes on the market for performance of cystoscopy. Pediatric bronchoscopes are often good choices. The endoscope should have an instrument port and channel, be at least bidirectional, bend more than 100 degrees in at least one direction, and have an external light source. Cytology brushes and biopsy forceps of a size and type that will pass through the instrument port with the bronchoscope in a flexed position should be available. Pediatric bronchoscopes ≤ 5 mm in diameter can be inserted into the urethra of most female dogs and large male cats that have had a perineal urethrostomy.

Technique (Figure 1-16):

1. After tests are done to ensure the absence of life-threatening diseases, general anesthesia or other chemical restraint is performed. General anesthesia is used in any animal suspected of being uncooperative.

2. The distance from the distal aspect of the urethra to the area of the tumor is pre-measured to ensure that the rigid or fiberoptic instrument is not advanced too far, which would result in a perforated bladder.

3. Using aseptic technique, the rigid or flexible fiberoptic endoscope is inserted through the urethra by identifying the urethral papilla visually or by inserting the tip of the instrument blindly with digital guidance. Urine is suctioned off, and a judicious amount of air is insufflated into the

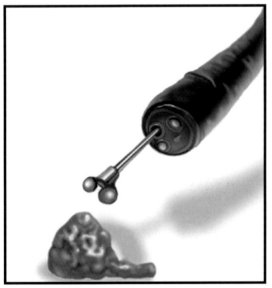

Figure 1-16: A bladder tumor biopsy via flexible endoscopy is performed by first locating the tumor and then taking several "pinch" biopsies through the endoscope.

ments are used in exactly the same way as described with the catheter biopsy method except that the biopsy port is on the side (Figure 1-15). Therefore, the operator must direct the instrument so that the biopsy port is directed toward the tumor. Once the biopsy port is bladder to enhance visualization of any pathology.

4. Suspect lesions are first sampled with the cytology brush for cytology and then biopsied for histopathology. If a diffuse lesion is suspected, random samples are acquired. After biopsies are performed, the air is suctioned off, and the instrument is removed.

Complications: Very rare. Can include bleeding, which usually stops spontaneously, and bladder rupture.

BIOPSY OF THE PROSTATE[1]

The suspicion of a prostatic mass is almost always secondary to a mass identified on abdominal or rectal examination and after prostatic ultrasonography or abdominal radiography. A tumor of the prostate should always be suspected in a male dog, especially if the prostate is firm, asymmetrical, fixed to nearby tissues, and calcified on radiographs. Diagnosis can be made by fine-needle aspiration cytology; exploratory surgery and biopsy; transabdominal biopsy with a needle biopsy instrument, with or without ultrasonographic guidance; and transrectal needle biopsy methods. The latter two methods are outlined because they are easy to perform and highly accurate.

Needle Core Biopsy[1,2]

This type of biopsy is usually safe and quick. With proper analgesia and tranquilization, it can be performed on an awake, cooperative patient. The histopathologic results generally are more accurate than fine-needle aspirate cytology but less accurate than an open biopsy.

Indication: Prostatomegaly of unexplained etiology.
Contraindications: Coagulopathies, prostatic abscess.
Benefit: General anesthesia is not routinely required; however, it should be considered for uncooperative patients.

Limitations: The small tissue samples that are obtained may not be diagnostic. Perforation of the urethra or rupture of a prostatic abscess can lead to life-threatening complications.

Equipment: No. 11 surgical blade; 2% lidocaine; needle biopsy instrument.

Technique:

1. The prostate is brought close to the nearby abdominal wall via abdominal palpation by an assistant. The organ is held firmly against the abdominal wall, and the biopsy site is prepared for surgery.

2. Approximately 2 to 3 ml of the local anesthetic agent, lidocaine, is injected under the skin overlying the prostate.

3. A stab incision is made in the skin using a no. 11 surgical blade to allow easy entry of the needle core biopsy instrument.

4. The needle core biopsy instrument is then advanced through the incision and into the capsule of the prostate. The accuracy of the biopsy is enhanced by using an ultrasound probe covered with a sterile glove, lubricating the biopsy site with sterile ultrasound gel, and imaging the prostate to direct the biopsy.

5. Several biopsy specimens of the prostate are removed through the same stab incision.

6. The needle biopsy specimens are fixed in 10% buffered formalin in the manner described previously. Separate containers should be used for specimens of each different lesion that is biopsied.

7. The stab incision is sutured if indicated.

Transrectal Needle Core Biopsy of the Prostate

Like the transabdominal biopsy technique, the transrectal prostatic biopsy method generally is safe and quick. With proper analgesia and tranquilization, it can be performed

> **KEY POINT:**
>
> *Care should be taken to prevent overinflation and rupture of the bladder. In addition, biopsies should be taken with the understanding that the bladder wall is likely to be friable due to the presence of the underlying disease.*

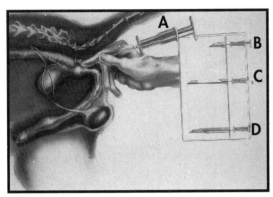

Figure 1-17: *A transrectal needle core biopsy is performed by placing a gloved index finger over the end of the biopsy needle; a finger cut from another glove is then placed over the needle tip and the overlying index finger. The outer portion of this finger cover is lubricated and inserted rectally (**A**). The prostate is pushed up and back by the operator or an assistant and held into position for biopsy. The needle core biopsy instrument is advanced through the glove cover, rectum, and outer capsule of the prostate (**B**). The inner stylet is then advanced into the tissue (**C**), and the outer cannula is advanced over the stylet to cut off the tissue (**D**). Several biopsy specimens of the prostate are taken through the same stab incision. The needle biopsy specimens are fixed in 10% buffered formalin, as described previously.*

on an awake, cooperative patient. The histopathologic results generally are more accurate than fine-needle aspiration cytology but less accurate than an open biopsy. The rectum must be evacuated prior to the procedure. Surprisingly, abscess formation is not a common complication of this method.

Indication: Prostatomegaly of unexplained etiology.
Contraindications: Coagulopathies, prostatic abscess.
Benefit: General anesthesia is not routinely required, but it should be considered for uncooperative patients.
Limitation: The small tissue samples that are obtained may not be diagnostic.

Equipment: Surgical glove; a finger of a surgical glove; 2% lidocaine; needle biopsy instrument.
Technique (Figure 1-17):

1. Approximately 2 to 3 ml of the local anesthetic agent, lidocaine, is injected into the distal rectum and colon using a lubricated syringe without a needle attached. The patient should receive appropriate tranquilizers, analgesics, or general anesthesia.

2. The gloved index finger is placed over the end of the biopsy needle; the finger of another glove is then placed over the needle tip and the overlying index finger. The outer portion of this finger cover is lubricated. The index finger, overlying the needle tip, is covered with the glove finger; the tip is then inserted into the rectum. The prostate is pushed up and back by the operator or an assistant and held in position for biopsy.

3. The needle core biopsy instrument is advanced through the glove cover, rectum, and outer capsule of the prostate. The accuracy of the biopsy is enhanced by covering an ultrasound probe with a sterile glove, lubricating the biopsy site with sterile ultrasound gel, and imaging the prostate to direct the biopsy.

4. Several biopsy specimens of the prostate are taken through the same stab incision.

5. The needle biopsy specimens are fixed in 10% buffered formalin, as described previously. Separate containers should be used for each different lesion that is biopsied.

KEY POINT:

Perforation of the urethra or rupture of a prostatic abscess, although very rare, can lead to life-threatening complications during or after a transrectal needle core biopsy of the prostate. Localized abscess formation must be considered as an unlikely complication.

REFERENCES

1. Withrow SJ: Biopsy principles, in Withrow SJ, MacEwen EG (eds): *Clinical Veterinary Oncology.* Philadelphia, JB Lippincott, 1989, pp 53–57.
2. Morrison WB, Hamilton TA, Hahn KA, et al: Diagnosis of neoplasia, in Slatter D (ed): *Textbook of Small Animal Surgery,* ed 2. Philadelphia, WB Saunders, 1993, pp 2036–2048.

CLINICAL BRIEFING: DIGESTIVE SYSTEM BIOPSY

Oral Biopsy

Methods	Benefits
Excisional Biopsy	Diagnostic and therapeutic; requires knowledge of extent of disease prior to surgery
Incisional Biopsy	Diagnosis allows logical planning of definitive therapeutic procedure

Upper and Lower Gastrointestinal Biopsy

Methods	Benefits
Surgical Exploration and Biopsy	Allows visual determination of extent of disease and directed biopsy
Fiberoptic Endoscopic Biopsy	Allows visualization of tract noninvasively; useful for specifically directing biopsy

Liver Biopsy

Methods	Benefits
Surgical Exploration	Allows visual determination of extent of disease and directed biopsy
Transabdominal Percutaneous Liver Biopsy	Relatively easy and inexpensive method for blindly obtaining liver tissue
Keyhole Liver Biopsy	Allows liver to be isolated and stabilized for blind biopsy
Laparoscopy	Allows direct visualization of abdominal contents and visually directed biopsy

Surgical exploration and biopsy remains the most complete method of exploring the digestive system. The oral cavity is readily accessible; however, biopsy is crucial not only to obtain a definitive diagnosis but also to ensure that definitive surgery can be performed subsequently with minimal cosmetic and functional alterations to the patient.[1] Surgical exploration of the abdomen and chest is more invasive than fiberoptic endoscopy and may be associated with greater risks. Although exploratory surgery has many benefits, endoscopic examination of the gastrointestinal (GI) tract is a common, effective, low-risk means of diagnosing malignant conditions of this organ system.[1–5] In addition, with endoscopy, benign conditions that mimic malignancy can be identified for subsequent treatment.[1,5] Flexible fiberoptic endoscopes can be used to examine all areas of the esophagus, stomach, proximal duodenum, rectum, and colon. Rigid endoscopes or proctoscopes can be used to examine portions of the esophagus, rectum, and most of the descending colon. Laparoscopy has the advantage of evaluating many organs of the abdomen with very little trauma to the patient. The techniques of oral biopsy, upper and lower GI endoscopy, and abdominal laparoscopy will be discussed separately.

BIOPSY OF THE ORAL CAVITY[3]

Biopsy of the oral cavity lesion is essential because almost all of the tumors of this structure have differing prognoses and treatments despite similar gross appearances. Before any oral lesion is biopsied, radiographs should be taken to determine the presence of bone invasion. This is essential information for the pathologist and the surgeon. For example, a pathologist would consider a diagnosis of a low-grade fibrosarcoma rather than a fibroma if radiographs suggested the presence of bone involvement, despite the fact that the biopsy finding was consistent with a diagnosis of fibroma. Similarly, a mandibulectomy or a maxillectomy would be mandatory as a surgical approach if bone was involved. Whenever a tooth is removed in an older dog, a biopsy should be considered to rule out the presence of cancer as an underlying cause. Before a biopsy is planned, the surgeon who will perform the definitive procedure should be consulted to ensure that the biopsy does not compromise the success of the procedure or the health of the patient. If the biopsy involves tissues that are essential for closure or if the tumor is potentially seeded into an area that is too large to resect, a successful outcome of the definitive procedure is prevented. Although an excisional biopsy is an option, an incisional biopsy is more frequently performed to guide the extent of a definitive procedure.

Indication: Oral mass of unexplained etiology.
Contraindications: Coagulopathies. Patients at high risk for general anesthesia.
Benefit: An accurate histopatholog-

ic evaluation can be obtained because part or all of the oral mass can be sampled.
Equipment: Standard surgical instruments.
Technique:

1. After routine screening tests have been performed to identify problems such as coagulopathies and metabolic disease, the animal is placed under general anesthesia. An endotracheal tube with a properly fitting cuff is secured to prevent aspiration of blood or other oral contents.
2. The oral mass is radiographed. When possible, intraoral radiographs should be acquired in addition to other views. More specific details are outlined in the chapter on Tumors of the Oral Cavity.
3. An incision is made over the oral mass, and a section of the lesion is taken at the junction of normal and abnormal tissue. Care is taken not to biopsy through normal lip or skin, as this may be needed for reconstructive techniques. Options include excisional or incisional biopsy procedures.
4. Any bleeding that occurs is stopped with ligation, cautery, or, in the case of an open bone biopsy, bone wax. Bleeding usually subsides within 5 to 10 minutes.
5. After the oral mass is removed, surrounding tissue is sutured if possible. Keep in mind that the oral cavity is a contaminated area.
6. The oral tumor should then be "bread-sliced" to allow adequate exposure to 10% formalin. There should be at least 1 part tissue for 10 parts formalin.

KEY POINT:

Despite the fact that the oral cavity is a contaminated area, infection is rarely a significant problem after oral surgery.

UPPER GASTROINTESTINAL ENDOSCOPY[5]

Indications for upper gastrointestinal endoscopy include, but are not limited to, regurgitation, dysphagia, retching, nausea, vomiting, hematemesis, diarrhea, melena, and any mass-like lesions identified in the esophagus, stomach, or upper duodenum. In humans, the diagnostic accuracy of flexible endoscopic biopsies is approximately 95%. Accuracy is highest with intraluminal diseases regardless of whether they are focal or diffuse, benign or malignant. Less diagnostic accuracy is seen with infiltrating cancers such as lymphoma, in which a full-thickness biopsy often is required to make a diagnosis. In addition, endoscopy is ideal for rechecks of an intraluminal lesion. A veterinary pathologist who is interested and experienced in examining endoscopic biopsies is essential to the success of this type of diagnostic procedure.

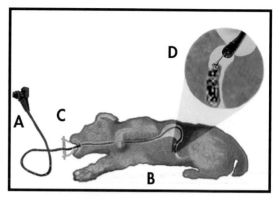

Figure 1-18: A flexible endoscope (*A*) can be used to localize, characterize, and biopsy esophageal, gastric, or upper duodenal (*B*) tumors or lesions. The animal is given general anesthesia and is placed on its right side. A mouth gag (*C*) is used. In each case, multiple biopsy specimens (*D*) should be acquired to ensure that an accurate diagnosis is made.

Indications: Any diseases that appear to involve the esophagus, stomach, or upper duodenum.

Contraindications: Coagulopathies. Patients at high risk for general anesthesia.

Benefits: Minimal risk. Noninvasive.

Limitations: Requires general anesthesia. Biopsy samples are superficial and therefore pathologists may miss deeper pathology.

Equipment: There are many fiberoptic endoscopes on the market for performance of upper GI endoscopy. The flexible fiberoptic endoscope should have an instrument port and channel, be at least bidirectional, bend more than 100 degrees in at least one direction, and have an external light source, suction, and water insufflation capability. Cytology brushes, biopsy forceps, and graspers that will pass through the instrument port with the endoscope in a flexed position should be available. Adult or pediatric fiberoptic endoscopes 5 to 8 mm in diameter and longer than 150 cm can be inserted into the duodenum of most dogs and cats.

Technique (Figure 1-18):

1. Animals should be fasted for 6 to 8 hours before upper GI endoscopy. After tests are performed to ensure the absence of life-threatening diseases, general anesthesia with endotracheal intubation is performed. A mouth gag is used to prevent the patient from biting on the endoscope.

2. The endoscope is inserted through the mouth and down into the esophagus. Carbon dioxide or air is insufflated into the structure to be examined. If excessive fluid is encountered, it is aspirated. A systematic examination of the esophagus, lower esophageal sphincter, stomach, and proximal duodenum is performed.

4. Suspect lesions are first sampled with the cytology brush for cytology and then biopsied for histopathology. A minimum of five biopsy samples are acquired for histopathologic analysis.

Complications: Very rare. Can include bleeding, which usually stops spontaneously. If brisk bleeding persists, introducing a Fogarty balloon catheter to occlude the bleeding vessel is recommended. In humans, the risk of perforation of the bowel is reported to be less than 0.1%. If perforation occurs, emergency surgery should be performed.

LOWER INTESTINAL ENDOSCOPY[1,4]

In selected patients, indications for endoscopic evaluation of the rec-

KEY POINT:

Care must be taken to avoid overdistention when performing upper GI endoscopy, as this can result in compromised blood return to the heart and rupture of the stomach or intestines.

tum, colon, and, possibly, the ileum include diarrhea, dyschezia, constipation, and a mass of the lower intestinal tract. Because it allows greater visualization of the colon and rectum, lower intestinal flexible fiberoptic endoscopy is surpassing rigid sigmoidoscopy in popularity. The rigid scope is more effective in evaluating the large bowel. Both instruments provide a means of examining the mucosal surface of the entire large bowel in great detail. Pinch biopsies can be taken for subsequent evaluation by a veterinary histopathologist. A trained endoscopist with proper equipment can perform polypectomies by removing premalignant adenomas or carcinomas in situ. Although the procedure is best accomplished with the patient under general anesthesia, chemical tranquilization with analgesia may be adequate for selected patients.

Indications: Any diseases that appear to involve the colon or rectum, especially those of the mucosal surface.

Contraindications: Coagulopathies. Patients at high risk for general anesthesia or tranquilization. Animals with fulminant, severe colitis may be at increased risk for perforation.

Benefits: Minimal risk. Noninvasive.

Limitations: Requires general anesthesia or tranquilization with analgesia. This procedure generally is only effective for diagnosing diseases that affect the lumen of the colon or rectum.

Equipment: There are many fiberoptic endoscopes on the market for performance of lower GI endoscopy. The flexible fiberoptic endoscope should have an instrument port and channel, be at least bidirectional, bend more than 100 degrees in at least one direction, and have an external light source, suction, and water insufflator. Adult or pediatric fiberoptic endoscopes 5 to 8 mm in diameter and longer than 1 meter can be inserted into the colon and advanced to the level of the cecum of most dogs and cats. A skilled operator can occasionally pass the scope into the ileum. The rigid scope should be 25 cm in length and have a light source. Cytology brushes, biopsy forceps, and graspers that can pass through the instrument port with the flexible fiberoptic endoscope in a flexed position should be available. These same biopsy instruments can be used with a rigid scope; mare uterine biopsy instruments should be used with extreme care because of the high risk of perforating the colon or rectum.

Technique (Figure 1-19):

1. Patient preparation requires a 24- to 36-hour fast and administration of warm water enemas or a gastrointestinal lavage solution that contains polyethylene glycol as the main nonabsorbed solute (e.g., Golytely®, Braintree Laboratories, Inc., Braintree, MA; Colyte®, Endlaw Preparations, Inc., Farmington, NY) at a dosage of 12 ml/lb via orogastric tube twice, 1 hour apart, 12 to 18 hours before endoscopy. If the latter is used, administering metoclopramide 30 minutes before the solution is administered may decrease distention and nausea. Care should be taken not to administer phosphate-containing enemas (e.g., "Fleet®" enemas) to cats due to the potential for inducing serious, adverse effects, including acute collapse and death. The patient is given the opportunity to eliminate all fecal material before the procedure is performed. After tests are performed to ensure the absence of life-threatening diseases, general anesthesia or tranquilization is performed.

2. The endoscope is inserted through the anus and into the colon. Insufflation of CO_2 or air allows adequate visualization of the colon and proximal rectum. If liquid material is present, it is suctioned out. The lower GI tract is systematically examined.

3. Suspect lesions are first sampled with the cytology brush for cytology and then biopsied for histopathology. A minimum of five biopsy samples are acquired for histopathologic analysis.

Complications: Very rare. Can include bleeding, which usually stops spontaneously. If brisk bleeding persists, the introduction of a Fogarty balloon catheter to occlude the bleeding vessels is recommended. In humans, the risk of perforating the bowel is reported to be less than 0.5%. If bowel perforation occurs, emergency surgery should be performed.

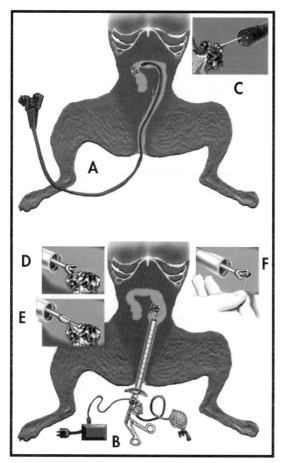

Figure 1-19: *Colonoscopy can be performed with either a flexible endoscope (**A**) or a rigid proctoscope (**B**). The flexible fiberoptic endoscope is more effective for exploring the area of the ileococcolic junction and the transverse colon. The biopsy instrument is extended through the biopsy port to take small pinch biopsies (**C**) in the transverse colon. The rigid endoscope may be more effective for draining the colon of blood and for introducing larger biopsy instruments. Larger biopsy specimens can be taken from the descending colon by extending rigid biopsy instruments (**D**) to the lesion to be biopsied. The tissue is grasped (**E**), and a piece is obtained (**F**).*

LIVER BIOPSY[1-3]

A liver biopsy is a common procedure to determine the histologic characteristics of a tumor or a nonmalignant condition after laboratory work and routine imaging methods have determined that the liver is

abnormal.[1-4] The accuracy of a liver biopsy is enhanced with ultrasonographic or fluoroscopic guidance.[2,4] More accurate biopsies are being performed as CT becomes more commonly used in veterinary practice. Other methods of obtaining a liver biopsy include direct visualization by laparoscopy, open surgical biopsy, and an unguided "blind" percutaneous biopsy that is most accurate when diffuse liver disease is suspected. In all types of liver biopsies, the most common complication is bleeding from the biopsy site. Therefore, before a liver biopsy is performed, a platelet count and an activated clotting time (ACT) or a one-step partial thromboplastin time (OSPTT) and an activated partial thromboplastin time (APTT) should be performed to identify patients that may be at high risk for bleeding after the procedure.

Transabdominal Percutaneous Liver Biopsy[1-3]

Indication: Malignant and nonmalignant liver disease.

Contraindications: Coagulopathies.

Benefits: Aspiration can provide a sample for individual cell analysis, whereas a biopsy can provide tissue to analyze cellularity, architecture, and content. Often can be done with local anesthesia, systemic analgesia, and tranquilization. If there are any concerns about the patient's ability to lie quietly on its back, general anesthesia should be performed.

Limitation: Single sample may not be representative of the entire liver.

Equipment: Standard surgical instruments; needle biopsy instrument.

Technique (Figure 1-20):

1. An area of hair 4 to 6 cm in diameter, encompassing the xyphoid process and the ventral left costal arch, is clipped, and the liver biopsy site is prepared with a surgical scrub. The patient should be positioned in dorsal recumbency, and its right side should be tilted slightly down toward the table surface. Ideally, the caudal aspect of the animal should be lowered to allow the liver to "fall" caudally for easier access by the biopsy procedure.

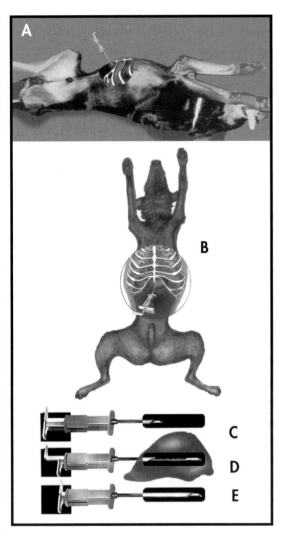

2. Using a 25-ga needle, approximately 2 to 3 ml of the local anesthetic agent, lidocaine, is injected in and around the site where the biopsy needle is to be introduced.
3. The area to be biopsied is scrubbed a final time after the lidocaine is injected. A surgical drape can be applied for sterility.
4. The operator puts on sterile gloves and then makes a small stab incision with a no. 11 surgical blade at a point adjacent and to the left of the tip of the xyphoid process and the left costal arch.
5. A needle core biopsy instrument is advanced in the subcutaneous tissue and then just through the abdominal wall.
6. At least one biopsy specimen is obtained; one piece of tissue is submitted for bacterial culture and sensitivity and the others are submitted for histopathology and for special analyses such as for copper.
7. The patient is placed sternally and is observed for 24 to 48 hours for signs of bleeding or other complications. This technique has a 94% chance of obtaining diagnostic quality tissue and has a mortality rate of approximately 1%.

Keyhole Liver Biopsy[1-4]

In the keyhole method, after the patient is prepared using the same methods as noted previously, a sterile gloved index finger is inserted through the abdominal musculature at the same site that is used for the percutaneous biopsy technique, and the abdominal wall is bluntly dissected. After the finger is introduced into the abdomen through this blunt dissection, the liver is palpated and stabilized against the abdominal wall for subsequent biopsy, as noted previously.

Laparoscopic Liver Biopsy[1-3]

Laparoscopic liver biopsy takes approximately 5 to 10 minutes from the time the abdomen is insufflated to the time of closure. With this method, the liver can be directly visualized for specific localization of lesions in the liver. The method is well described[1-3] and varies slightly depending on the equipment used.

Figure 1-20: A liver biopsy can be acquired with a needle core biopsy instrument, which is advanced through a skin incision, through the subcutaneous tissue, and then just through the abdominal wall. The biopsy needle is directed slightly craniad and to the animal's left (*A* and *B*). At this point, to prevent lacerating the liver and underlying structures, the biopsy instrument should be advanced no more than 1 to 3 cm into the abdomen to the liver (*C*). The inner stylet is then advanced into the liver (*D*), and the outer cannula is advanced over the stylet to cut off the tissue (*E*). If ultrasonography is available, it is used to direct the biopsy equipment. At least one biopsy specimen is obtained, and one piece of tissue is submitted for bacterial culture and sensitivity and the others for histopathology and for special analyses such as for copper.

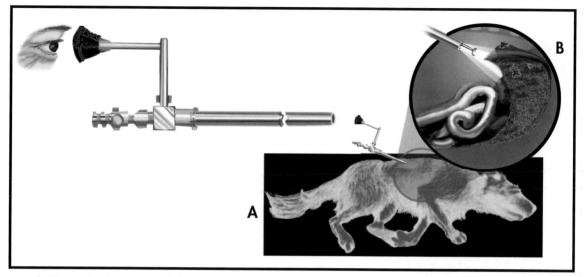

Figure 1-21: *Laparoscopy is ideal for visually characterizing the health and structure of many abdominal organs, including the liver. In addition, it is effective for directing a biopsy instrument to localized lesions. The laparoscope is advanced through an area bordered on the right side below the lateral spinous processes of the lumbar vertebrae and caudal to the last rib (**A**). The liver is identified, and a biopsy instrument is advanced to acquire at least one sample (**B**).*

Using either general or local anesthesia with tranquilizers and analgesics, the site for insertion of the laparoscope can be on the midline, or, more commonly, the right lateral abdominal wall just caudal to the ribs and ventral to the lateral spinous processes, depending on the area of the abdomen that is to be explored and biopsied.

Indications: Malignant and nonmalignant liver disease. Determining the extent of neoplastic processes.

Contraindications: Coagulopathies. Animals with significantly compromised cardiovascular or respiratory systems. Because insufflation of the abdomen can reduce venous return to the heart and compress the diaphragm, the ability to inspire with ease is compromised.

Benefits: Biopsy can be selectively performed to acquire tissue to analyze cellularity, architecture, and content. In selected cases, the procedure can be done with local anesthesia, systemic analgesia, and tranquilization. If there are any concerns about the patient's ability to lie quietly, general anesthesia should be performed.

Limitations: Small biopsy samples may not be representative of the entire liver. This procedure allows visualization of lesions on the surface of all visible organs; therefore, lesions below the surfaced of the organ may be overlooked.

Equipment: Standard surgical instruments; laparoscope and laparoscopic biopsy instruments.

Technique (Figure 1-21):
1. General anesthesia or tranquilizers with analgesic properties (e.g., atropine and oxymorphone) are administered.

KEY POINT:

To prevent lacerating the liver and underlying structures, the biopsy needle is directed slightly craniad and to the animal's left; the biopsy instrument should be advanced no more than 1 to 3 cm. Ultrasonography, if available, is used to direct the biopsy equipment.

2. If a lateral approach is used, the patient is placed with the left side down. If the patient is tranquilized, gentle but firm restraint of the limbs is applied so that the patient cannot change position during the procedure, ideally with an assistant nearby to calm the animal. The hair is clipped and prepared with a surgical scrub from the ninth rib to the caudal flank and from the dorsal to the ventral midline on the right side. The animal is draped.

3. If tranquilization is used, approximately 2 to 3 ml of the local anesthetic agent, lidocaine, is injected in and around the site where the laparoscope and any biopsy needles are to be introduced.

4. A Verres needle is inserted into the right side, below the lateral spinous processes of the lumbar vertebrae and caudal to the last rib, into the peritoneal cavity. After it is determined that the needle is not in a hollow viscus or blood vessel, CO_2 or nitrous oxide is used to insufflate the abdomen to 10 to 15 mmHg. The placement of the Verres needle can be checked by injecting saline and aspirating material through the needle to check for blood, bowel contents, or urine.

5. A small incision (0.5–1 cm) is made ventral to the lumbar muscles and caudal to the costal arch on the right side. The trocar and cannula assembly is then pushed into the gas-filled abdomen through the incision. The Verres needle is removed. The trocar is removed, and the laparoscope that is attached to the CO_2 or nitrous oxide insufflator and light source is advanced through the cannula to visualize the liver and other abdominal organs.

If visualization is obscured by blood or other material, the laparoscope (but not the outer cannula) is removed and cleaned in a bowl of saline.

6. A biopsy needle is advanced through the laparoscope or through a separate puncture site nearby. The alligator or needle biopsy instrument is directed to the sites of interest by direct visualization. Five to six biopsy specimens are taken; at least one is submitted for bacterial culture and sensitivity and another is submitted for copper stains, if indicated.

7. After the biopsy sites are observed for several minutes for excessive bleeding, the CO_2 is evacuated, the instrument is removed from the abdominal cavity, and the small incision is sutured with simple interrupted absorbable sutures.

REFERENCES

1. Morrison WB, Hamilton TA, Hahn KA, et al: Diagnosis of neoplasia, in Slatter D (ed): *Textbook of Small Animal Surgery*, ed 2. Philadelphia, WB Saunders, 1993, pp 2036–2048.

2. Lightdale CJ: Liver biopsy, in Wittes RE (ed) *Manual of Oncologic Therapeutics 1991/1992*. Philadelphia, JB Lippincott, 1991, pp 20–22.

3. Jones BD, Hitt M, Hurst T: Hepatic biopsy. *Vet Clin North Am Small Anim Pract* 15:39–64, 1985.

4. Withrow SJ: Biopsy principles, in Withrow SJ, MacEwen EG (eds): *Clinical Veterinary Oncology*. Philadelphia, JB Lippincott, 1989, pp 53–57.

5. Lightdale CJ: Upper gastrointestinal endoscopy, in Wittes RE (ed): *Manual of Oncologic Therapeutics 1991/1992*. Philadelphia, JB Lippincott, 1991, pp 14–15.

CLINICAL BRIEFING: CLINICAL CYTOLOGY AND NEOPLASIA

Methods of Biopsy	Benefits
Fine-Needle Aspiration Cytology: "Needle-On" Technique	Negative pressure ideal when cells difficult to exfoliate
Fine-Needle Aspiration Cytology: "Needle-Off" Technique	Lack of negative pressure reduces chance for dilution of cells of interest with blood or fluid
Impression Smears	Increase chances for obtaining many representative cells and may indirectly reveal architecture and associated cells of mass
Tissue Scrapings	Ideal for sarcomas and other tissues that exfoliate poorly

Cytology is a valuable diagnostic tool for making a diagnosis, directing the management of the cancer patient, and providing a prognosis. A histopathologic diagnosis also is important for the evaluation of a cancer patient, but histopathology is often interpreted with increased accuracy if the results are combined with the results of cytology. First, a representative sample must be obtained. Virtually every part of the body can be sampled. Second, the sample must be adequately prepared. Finally, the sample must be accurately interpreted. The attending clinician must at least ensure that the sample is representative of the tissue of interest.

SAMPLE COLLECTION
Fine-Needle Aspiration
This method is used to acquire tissue or fluid from almost any part of the body with minimal risk.

Solid Tissues[1–3]
Indication: Any condition suspected as being benign or malignant.
Contraindications: Coagulopathies. Any abscessed or neoplastic tissue that may rupture, spill into, and contaminate a body cavity.

Benefits: Aspiration can be selectively performed to acquire cells to analyze cellularity and cell morphology, with or without the direction of imaging modalities such as ultrasonography or fluoroscopy. In most cases, the procedure can be done on an outpatient basis without any anesthesia. If there are any concerns about the patient's ability to lie quietly when a deep abdominal organ is to be sampled, general anesthesia should be performed.
Limitation: Small samples may not be representative of the entire tissue of interest.
Equipment: The materials needed are a 3-, 6-, or 12-ml syringe, a 22-ga needle with sufficient length to sample the tissue of interest, microscope slides, proper staining materials, and a microscope.
Technique:
1. The mass to be sampled is identified and immobilized.
2. The skin is then cleaned with surgical soap and alcohol if an abdominal cavity is to be entered. Superficial skin lesions can be cleaned with alcohol.
3. The needle is advanced into the tissue and partially withdrawn several times, with or without the syringe attached (Figure 1-22), in several different

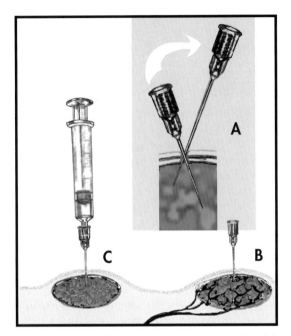

Figure 1-22: *Fine-needle aspiration is performed by advancing the needle into the tissue and partially withdrawing it several times (**A**), with or without the syringe attached, in several different directions through the same entry point in the skin. The "needle-off" method (**B**) is ideal for vascular tissues, whereas the "needle-on" technique (**C**) is ideal for tissues that do not exfoliate well, such as soft tissue sarcomas. When using the needle attached to the syringe, suction is applied as the needle is advanced through the tissue in several different directions.*

All negative pressure is then released before the needle is withdrawn from the tissue. The objective is to fill the needle with cells. The sampling is discontinued if blood or other tissue is noted in the hub of the needle or in the syringe. With both methods, the syringe is filled with air before the needle filled with cells is attached, and the cellular contents of the needle are forcefully expelled onto clean glass slides.

4. If the "needle-on" method is used, all negative pressure is released before the needle is withdrawn from the tissue. The objective is to fill the needle with cells. The sampling is discontinued if blood or other tissue is noted in the hub of the needle or in the syringe.

5. The needle is then removed from the syringe. The syringe is filled with air before it is re-attached, and the cellular contents of the needle are forcefully expelled onto clean glass slides.

6. A "squash-prep" is then made by placing two slides on top of each other in a perpendicular orientation so that only the weight of the upper slide "squashes" the cells as they are pulled apart. The result is a smear of fluid or tissue on both slides.

7. Slides also can be made by spreading a drop of fluid like a blood smear. That is, the drop of fluid is spread across the primary slide by placing a second slide at a 45° angle to it. The slide that is at an angle is then backed into the sample so that the acute angle is facing it. The angled slide is then firmly and smoothly pushed along the slide until the entire sample is distributed. The best smears can be obtained when the sample is relatively small; this precludes making a thick smear.

Abdominal Paracentesis[1]

Indication: Any fluid within the abdominal cavity.

Contraindications: Coagulopathies.

Benefits: Aspiration of the abdominal cavity can be selectively performed to acquire fluid, with or without the direction of imaging modalities such as ultrasonography or fluoroscopy. In most cases, the procedure can be done on an outpatient basis, with or without local anesthesia.

Limitations: Fluid analysis may not be diagnostic for an underlying malignancy. Fluid may leak into subcutaneous sites or completely through the skin. Injury to the bowel or other organs is rare but possible.

Equipment: The materials needed are a 12-ml syringe, a 22-ga needle, microscope slides, proper staining materials, and a microscope.

directions through the same entry point in the skin. The "needle-off" method is ideal for vascular tissues such as thyroid tumors, because blood may be aspirated when suction is applied, diluting the tumor cells. The "needle-on" technique is ideal for tissues that do not exfoliate well, such as soft tissue sarcomas. If a syringe with the needle is used, suction is applied as the needle is advanced through the tissue in several different directions.

Technique:

1. To reduce the probability of accidentally aspirating the spleen, abdominal paracentesis should be performed at a site 3 to 5 cm caudal to the umbilicus and to the right of midline. The area is clipped and prepared with surgical scrub and alcohol.
2. Local anesthesia is optional.
3. The syringe is filled with 1.5 ml of air. The needle on the syringe is then advanced slowly into the abdominal cavity. Negative pressure is gently applied after the abdominal wall is penetrated. If no fluid is acquired, 0.5 ml of air is injected into the abdomen to clear the needle of any blockage. Negative pressure is applied once more. The procedure is repeated with the needle in different positions or depths within the abdominal cavity.

Thoracentesis[13]

Indication: Any fluid within the thoracic cavity.
Contraindications: Coagulopathies.
Benefits: An aspiration of the abdominal cavity can be selectively performed to acquire fluid with or without the direction of imaging modalities such as ultrasonography or fluoroscopy. In most cases, the procedure can be done on an outpatient basis, with or without local anesthesia.
Limitations: Fluid analysis may not be diagnostic for an underlying malignancy. Fluid may leak into subcutaneous sites or completely through the skin. Alternatively, a pneumothorax may develop. Injury to the lung or heart is rare but possible.
Equipment: The materials needed are a 12-ml syringe, a three-way stopcock, a 22-ga needle, microscope slides, proper staining materials, and a microscope.
Technique:

1. Ideally, the animal should be standing and quiet. The site for thoracentesis varies depending on the site of the fluid but is commonly around the seventh or eighth intercostal spaces. The area is clipped and prepared with surgical scrub and alcohol.
2. Local anesthesia is optional.
3. The needle on the syringe is advanced slowly into the thoracic cavity just anterior to the nearby rib to prevent hitting the intercostal arteries, which are located just caudal to the ribs. The bevel should face the pleural lining. Negative pressure is gently applied after the pleural space is entered. The three-way stopcock can be used to prevent air from leaking into the chest while syringes are changed to drain the chest.
4. Once a sample is acquired, it is put into EDTA and into a culturette for bacterial culture and sensitivity if indicated. Slides also can be made directly, or the fluid can be centrifuged to concentrate the cells for subsequent analysis.

Impressions and Scraping Techniques[1–3]

Cells can be acquired from masses once they are removed from the patient by doing impressions of the tissue or by actually scraping cells from that tissue. Impression smears are ideal for lymph nodes, whereas scrapings are optimum for tissues that do not exfoliate easily, such as soft tissue sarcomas.

Indications: Almost any tissue that may be abnormal that has been removed from the patient. Occasionally, an ulcerated mass on the patient can be sampled by making an impression or by scraping cells from its surface.
Contraindications: None known.
Benefits: An impression is ideal for indirectly acquiring information about the cell types involved as well as providing some idea of cellular architecture within the mass itself. If done correctly, the cells may be less traumatized than when "squash preps" are made.
Limitation: Small samples may not be representative of the entire tissue of interest.
Equipment: The materials needed are a surgical blade, Brown-Adson forceps, microscope slides, proper staining materials, and a microscope.
Technique:
Impressions

1. A freshly removed piece of tissue is blot-dried before it is transected in half to obtain a flat surface for performing the impressions. The surface should be smaller than the slide to allow multiple impressions.

TABLE 1-1
Inflammatory processes

Type of Inflammation	Characterization
Acute	Greater than 70% of the inflammatory cells are neutrophils; the neutrophils can be well preserved, hypersegmented, toxic, or lysed
Chronic active	Approximately 30% to 50% of the inflammatory cell population are plasma cells and monocytes; neutrophils are also present in significant numbers in a chronic active inflammatory condition
Chronic or granulomatous	Mononuclear inflammatory cells and macrophages predominate

2. The cut surface is then blotted on an absorbent surface such as a paper towel.
3. Several impressions are made on each slide.

Scrapings

1. The tissue is dried and blotted to allow any blood or fluid to be removed. The surface of the tissue is then gently scraped with a new surgical blade, and the cells on the blade are gently smeared across the slide.

Slide Preparation

At least one slide from every site should be saved for possible submission to a clinical pathologist. In each case, slides should be prepared with utmost care. Tumor cells often are very fragile and easily disrupted. After the slides are made, one representative slide should be stained and examined to insure that it is likely to be diagnostic. The most frequently used stains in the clinic or laboratory are Wright's–Giemsa, new methylene blue, and Papanicolaou stains. An adaptation of the Wright's stain (Diff-Quik®) is commonly used in veterinary practice; it can be performed in a 15-second, three-step procedure. In addition, the stain is very effective in providing good cytoplasmic detail. The new methylene blue stain also is easy to perform and provides good nuclear detail. The Papanicolaou stain is more labor-intensive and generally is used only in a clinical pathology laboratory. This staining technique provides excellent cellular morphology.

GENERAL CYTOLOGIC INTERPRETATION[1-3]

Detailed interpretation of cytology requires considerable experience and knowledge of normal cellular morphology. The practitioner will often need to call upon the expertise of a clinical pathologist to make subtle diagnoses. With practice, the practitioner can determine whether a sample is likely to have adequate cellularity for subsequent diagnosis by an expert in the field. In addition, with experience, inflammation can be differentiated from neoplasia, which can be of great value for directing other diagnostic tests. In any case, the cytology should be interpreted in combination with other clinical information such as the physical examination and results of radiographs and blood work. The limitations of all diagnostic tests, including cytology, should be realized.

Each sample should be evaluated in a routine fashion. First, the slide is reviewed with the 10× objective to ensure adequate cellularity and staining. Once all the slides are reviewed, representative clusters of cells are evaluated at 100× (oil immersion). The cells are then assessed to determine whether they represent normal tissue (Color Figure 1), an inflammatory process (Color Figure 2), hyperplasia, or neoplasia (Color Figures 3 to 24).

An inflammatory process (Table 1-1) can be divided somewhat arbitrarily into acute, chronic active, or chronic or granulomatous inflammation based on the presence or absence of neutrophils, monocytes, plasma cells, eosinophils, and differentiated macrophages.

(continues on page 47)

COLOR FIGURE LEGENDS

Color Figure 1: Cytology from a normal lymph node. Note that small lymphocytes predominate.

Color Figure 2: Nondegenerate neutrophils, macrophages, and erythrocytes predominate in this lymph node aspirate diagnostic for an inflammatory condition. It is important to differentiate hyperplasia or inflammation from neoplasia. Hyperplasia principally differs from normal tissue in that hyperplastic cells exhibit the features of cytoplasmic activity and are cytologically immature. Therefore, reactive or hyperplastic cells may have more basophilic cytoplasm, and the nuclei may be larger than in normal cells. One key differentiating feature is that hyperplastic cells have a fairly constant nuclear/cytoplasmic ratio, whereas neoplastic tissue does not.

Color Figures 3–13: Round cell or discrete cell tumors have round to oval cells with well-defined cytoplasmic borders. They include lymphoma, histiocytoma, transmissible venereal tumor, mast cell tumors, and plasma cell tumors.

    Color Figures 3–5: These three photomicrographs are representative of lymphoma. Color Figure 3 is from a cutaneous lymphoma from a dog, whereas Color Figure 4 is from an anterior mediastinum of a cat. Note the mitotic figures and the prominent nucleoli that are characteristic features of malignancy. The cells are characterized as being made up of a monotonous population of large, poorly differentiated lymphoid cells with scanty blue cytoplasm, dense nuclear margins, and round to slightly irregularly shaped nuclei, generally with at least one nucleolus. Some cells may have azurophilic granules. Lymphoma cells usually resemble lymphoblasts, although in a few rare cases they can be very well differentiated and resemble normal lymphocytes. A biopsy is required to confirm the diagnosis of each case of lymphoma, especially small cell or well-differentiated lymphoma.

    Color Figures 6 and 7: Cytology from hairless, red, raised lesions from two young dogs, later diagnosed histopathologically as histiocytomas. Cytologically, these tumors are composed of a uniform population of round cells that resemble monocytes and epithelioid cells that are 10 to 25 μm in diameter. Nuclei appear benign cytologically, although they may vary in size and shape. The pale cytoplasm of these cells varies in amount from cell to cell and is surrounded by a distinct cytoplasm. Histiocytomas can resemble transmissible venereal tumors, but the former show more variation in nuclear and cytoplasmic shape.

Color Figure 8: Transmissible venereal tumor (TVT) cells are round, approximately 15 to 30 μm in diameter, and have round to oval nuclei that may be placed eccentrically within the cytoplasm. The nuclear chromatin generally is coarsely granular. A single prominent nucleolus often is present. The cytoplasm is distinguished as being relatively abundant, moderately basophilic, and, often, vacuolated. Plasma cells, lymphocytes, and macrophages often are seen within a TVT cell. TVT cells can be distinguished from lymphoma cells because they have more abundant cytoplasm. Compared to histiocytomas, TVTs have a more uniformly round nucleus and cytoplasm.

Color Figure 9: This is the cytology from the bone marrow of a dog with a monoclonal gammopathy in the serum, Bence Jones proteins in the urine, and multiple "punched out" lytic bone lesions consistent with a diagnosis of a plasma cell tumor, also known as multiple myeloma. Note the round cell tumor cells with eccentric nuclei. The cytoplasm of plasma cells often contains a perinuclear halo that is actually immunoglobulin prior to release from the cell.

Color Figures 10, 11, and 12: Mast cell tumors from dogs. Mast cells are round and vary in size from 10 to 40 μm in diameter. They have eccentric round to oval nuclei that may be hidden by variable numbers of fine to coarse blue-black to reddish-purple granules. Histopathology is necessary to grade the tumor, which is essential to give a prognosis.

Color Figure 13: Melanomas are considered by some to be a discrete cell tumor. Others believe the tumor has characteristics of both epithelial and mesenchymal cells. Because melanomas often have intracytoplasmic granules, they must be differentiated from mast cell tumors. With most stains, the granules are black or brown and irregular in shape and size. They are often small and are described as dust-like. The granules are often noted extracellularly because they are released from some cells.

Color Figure 14: Cytology from a lipoma. Adipocytes range from very large cells that are fully distended with fat to collapsed cells with lacy cytoplasm. This photomicrograph shows fully distended adipocytes with small, eccentric nuclei.

Color Figures 15–19: Epithelial cell tumors easily exfoliate in clusters, clumps, or sheets of oval to round cells. The cells may arrange into a ductular or acinar pattern around a central lumen, and the cytoplasm may contain a secretory product.

Color Figure 15: Cells from a perianal adenoma of an intact male dog. These cells exfoliate readily into clusters, are often described as hepatoid in appearance, and are characterized as having an abundant, foamy pale cytoplasm and eccentric or centrally located round to oval nuclei that may vary in size.

Color Figure 16: Carcinoma cells from a transtracheal wash of a dog later determined to have a bronchogenic carcinoma. Note the large, round cells with prominent nucleoli that exhibit criteria of malignancy.

Color Figure 17: Carcinoma from a cat with an intestinal tumor. Note the round cells, some with multiple nuclei, multinucleated cells, and variable nuclear to cytoplasmic ratios and other indications of malignancy.

Color Figure 18: Cytology from a mammary mass confirmed histologically as a mammary adenocarcinoma. Note the secretory product within some cells and the attempt of some cells at maintaining a duct-like arrangement. The secretory contents often make the cells resemble signet rings, which is characteristic of many carcinomas.

Color Figure 19: Cytology from a Poodle with small, raised, pedunculated fleshy masses determined histologically to be sebaceous adenomas. Note the sheets or clusters of round cells with abundant cytoplasm that are relatively uniform in size and shape with few mitotic figures.

Color Figure 20: This cytology is obtained from a mass located within the skin and determined to be a sebaceous cyst. Note the amorphous debris and the unstained area in the center, characteristic of a cholesterol cleft commonly seen in these masses.

Color Figures 21–24: Sarcomas or mesenchymal tumors exfoliate with difficulty. They have individual cells or disorganized clusters. The cells are recognized as being spindle-shaped and have cytoplasmic extensions with ill-defined cytoplasmic borders.

Color Figures 21 and 22: Fine-needle aspiration of an oral mass (Color Figure 21) and a submandibular lymph node (Color Figure 22) from a dog with an oral fibrosarcoma. The cells are usually seen alone or in disorganized clusters. The cytoplasm is often indistinct and spindle-shaped.

Color Figure 23: Cells from a dog with a hemangiopericytoma. Note the poorly defined cytoplasmic borders, the nucleoli, and wispy, streaming cytoplasm. In some cases, some cells appear to form a whirling pattern that may distinguish them from other mesenchymal tumors.

Color Figure 24: Cells from a dog with osteosarcoma. The cells from an osteosarcoma are often spindle-shaped and have abundant foamy basophilic cytoplasm that forms a spindle shape surrounding a variably sized nucleus, with coarse chromatin and variable numbers of nuclei. Sometimes, these cells have an eosinophilic substance within the cytoplasm that occasionally may be noted extracellularly as an osteoid matrix. Normal osteoblasts may be seen in conjunction with the malignant cells.

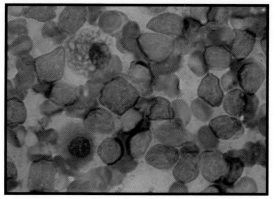

Color Figure 1.

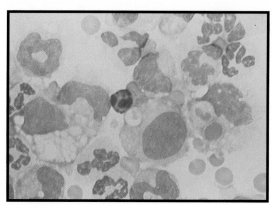

Color Figure 2.

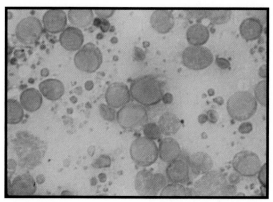

Color Figure 3.

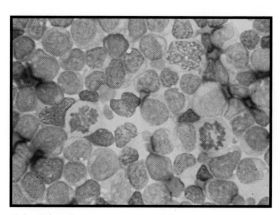

Color Figure 4.

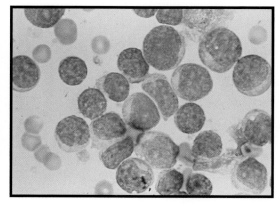

Color Figure 5.

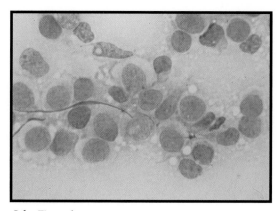

Color Figure 6.

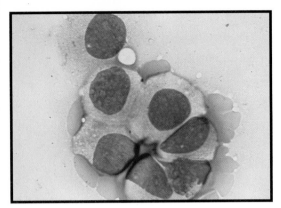

Color Figure 7.

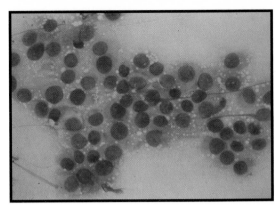

Color Figure 8.

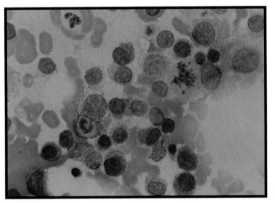

Color Figure 9.

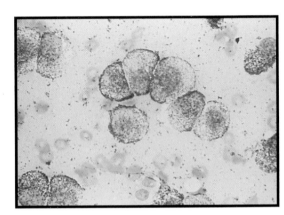

Color Figure 10.

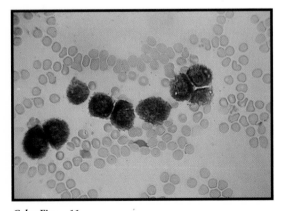

Color Figure 11.

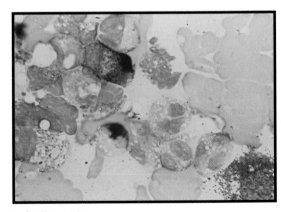

Color Figure 12.

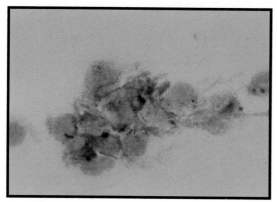

Color Figure 13.

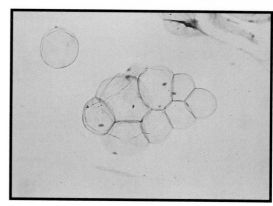

Color Figure 14.

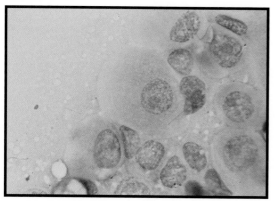

Color Figure 15.

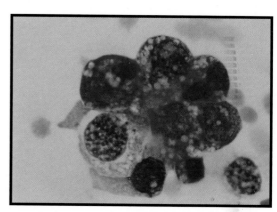

Color Figure 16.

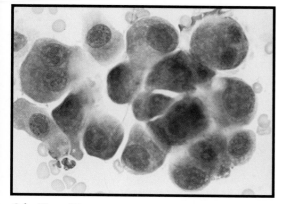

Color Figure 17.

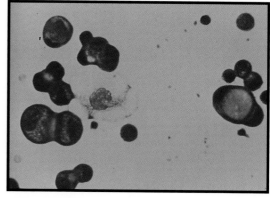

Color Figure 18.

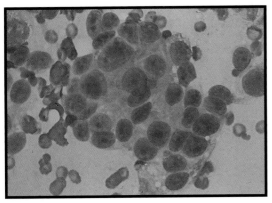

Color Figure 19.

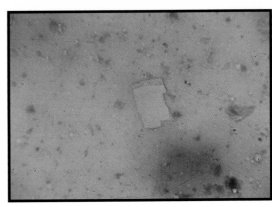

Color Figure 20.

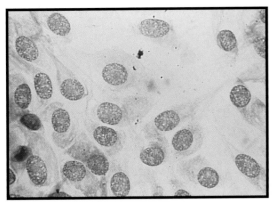

Color Figure 21.

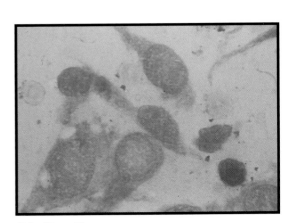

Color Figure 22.

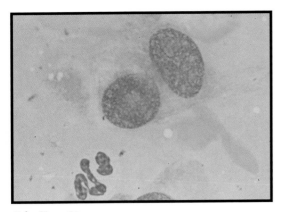

Color Figure 23.

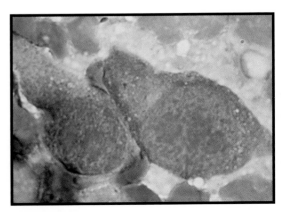

Color Figure 24.

(continued from page 40)

Acute inflammation can be diagnosed when greater than 70% of the inflammatory cells are neutrophils. The neutrophils can be well preserved, hypersegmented, toxic, or lysed. Chronic active inflammation can be diagnosed when 30% to 50% of the inflammatory cell population are plasma cells and monocytes. Chronic inflammatory responses are those in which mononuclear inflammatory cells and macrophages predominate. If epithelioid or inflammatory giant cells are present, the condition is considered to be granulomatous.

It is important to differentiate hyperplasia from neoplasia. Hyperplasia principally differs from normal tissue in that hyperplastic cells exhibit the features of cytoplasmic activity and are cytologically immature. Therefore, reactive or hyperplastic cells may have more basophilic cytoplasm, and the nuclei may be larger than in normal cells. One key differentiating feature is that hyperplastic cells have a fairly constant nuclear/cytoplasmic ratio, whereas neoplastic tissue does not.

The diagnosis of neoplasia is made on the cytologic characteristics of nuclear, cytoplasmic, and structural features. In brief, the criteria for malignancy are:[1-3]

Nuclear:
- Marked variation in nuclear size
- Marked variation in nuclear/cytoplasmic ratio
- Irregular nuclear membrane
- Variable sized, irregular nucleoli
- Irregular chromatin that clumps
- Abnormal mitotic figures

Cytoplasmic:
- Vacuolization
- Basophilia with Wright's stain
- Irregular and indistinct cytoplasmic boundaries
- Variable cytoplasmic amount from cell to cell

Structural:
Discrete Cell Neoplasms: Round Cell Tumors
(Color Figure 12)

- Round to oval cells
- Easy to exfoliate individual cells
- Well-defined cytoplasmic margins

Carcinomas: Epithelial Cell Tumors
(Color Figures 15–19)
- Cells easily exfoliate in clusters, clumps, or sheets
- Oval to round cells
- May arrange in ductular or acinar pattern around a central lumen
- Cytoplasm may contain a secretory product

Sarcomas: Connective Tissue Tumors
(Color Figures 21–24)
- Difficult to exfoliate
- Individual cells or disorganized clusters
- Spindle-shaped cells
- Cytoplasmic extensions with ill-defined cytoplasmic borders

CYTOLOGY OF SPECIFIC NEOPLASMS
Once a neoplastic process is suspected using the criteria just noted, the cells are examined and categorized into:
- Benign or malignant
- Carcinomas, sarcomas, or discrete cell tumors
- Specific cell type
- Degree of differentiation

The references noted at the end of this section are excellent resources to further understand clinical veterinary cytology.[1-3] A brief description of some of the more common tumors diagnosed cytologically in veterinary medicine follows. In each case, a biopsy should be done to confirm the cytologic diagnosis.

Discrete Cell Neoplasms: Round Cell Tumors
(Color Figures 3–12)

Round cell tumors are commonly seen in veterinary medicine; they have unique distinguishing features that make them identifiable cytologically. Round cell tumors include lymphoma, mast cell tumors, plasma cell

> ### KEY POINT:
>
> *Hyperplasia is difficult to differentiate from neoplasia in many cases. Whenever there is a question, a biopsy should be performed.*

tumors, transmissible venereal tumors, and histiocytomas. They are all round, have well-defined cytoplasmic borders, and are easily exfoliated into single cells because of their lack of cell-to-cell attachments. The following is a brief description of some distinguishing features of specific types of round cell tumors:

Mast Cell Tumors *(Color Figures 10–12)*

Mast cell tumors are commonly found in the skin, spleen, liver, lymph node, and bone marrow of affected dogs and cats. Mast cell tumors commonly contain eosinophils and fibroblasts. They are round and vary in size from 10 to 40 μm in diameter. Staining reveals eccentric round to oval nuclei that may be hidden by variable numbers of fine to coarse blue-black to reddish-purple granules. Diff-Quik® staining may not stain the granules effectively. Normal mast cells can be seen in a variety of inflammatory conditions; however, they are usually accompanied by neutrophils and macrophages.

Lymphoma *(Color Figures 3–5)*

Lymphoma is usually found in lymph nodes, liver, spleen, bone marrow, and, occasionally, extranodal sites such as the skin. The cells are characterized as being made up of a monotonous population of large, poorly differentiated lymphoid cells with scanty blue cytoplasm, dense nuclear margins, and round to slightly irregularly shaped nuclei, generally with at least one nucleolus. Some lymphoma cells may have azurophilic granules upon staining. Lymphoma cells usually resemble lymphoblasts, although in a few rare cases they can be very well differentiated and resemble normal lymphocytes; a biopsy is required to confirm the diagnosis of small cell or well-differentiated lymphoma. Indeed, a histologic diagnosis is always recommended when lymphoma is tentatively diagnosed cytologically. In each case, lymphoma must be differentiated from lymphoid hyperplasia that is characterized by the presence of lymphocytes in all stages of differentiation; however, the immature cells such as lymphoblasts and prolymphocytes are increased in numbers when compared to a normal lymph node. Mitotic figures may be increased in number in hyperplastic lymph nodes, but the appearance of mitotic figures is normal.

Plasma Cell Tumor

Cutaneous plasma cell tumors are benign solitary tumors of the skin that are most commonly localized to the skin, digits, lips, and ears. The cells from these tumors are oval to round with round nuclei and coarse, clumped chromatin. A single, relatively small nucleolus may be identified within each nucleus. The mitotic activity generally is low due to the benign nature of this condition. The amount of basophilic cytoplasm in these cells varies.

Plasma cell tumors from dogs with multiple myeloma appear cytologically like immature plasma cells (Color Figure 9). These tumors must not be confused with plasma cell tumors of the skin because they have different biological behavior, prognosis, and treatment. Cells from these tumors vary in size and cytoplasmic basophilia; binucleated and trinucleated cells are common. The more mature cells may have an eccentric nucleus and a round to oval cytoplasm, which may have a perinuclear halo consistent with an active cell producing immunoglobulin.

Histiocytoma *(Color Figures 6 and 7)*

The histiocytoma is a benign tumor that is commonly seen in young dogs. It is apparent clinically as a hairless, raised lesion that may be ulcerated and inflamed. Cytologically, the tumor is composed of a uniform population of round cells, which resemble monocytes, and epithelioid cells that are 10 to 25 μm in diameter. Nuclei appear benign cytologically, although they may vary in size and shape. The pale cytoplasm of these cells varies in amount from cell to cell and is surrounded by a distinct cytoplasm. Histiocytomas can resemble transmissible venereal tumors, but the former show more variation in nuclear and cytoplasmic shape. Histiocytomas can be difficult to differentiate from the cells identified in chronic inflammatory lesions.

Transmissible Venereal Tumor *(Color Figure 8)*

Transmissible venereal tumors (TVTs) usually are

found around the genitalia and, occasionally, in the mouths or around the heads of younger, sexually active dogs. The lesions often are cherry red in color and very friable to the touch. Cytologically, the tumor cells are round, approximately 15 to 30 μm in diameter, and have round to oval nuclei that may be eccentrically placed within the cytoplasm. The nuclear chromatin generally is coarsely granular. A single prominent nucleolus often is present. The cytoplasm is distinguished as being relatively abundant in quantity and moderately basophilic; it often is vacuolated. Plasma cells, lymphocytes, and macrophages are often seen when these tumor cells are present. TVTs can be distinguished from lymphoma cells because they have more abundant cytoplasm. TVTs have a more uniformly round nucleus and cytoplasm than histiocytomas.

Melanoma (Color Figure 13)

Melanomas are considered by some to be a discrete cell tumor. Others believe the tumor has characteristics of both epithelial and mesenchymal cells. This neoplastic process is common in dogs but uncommon in cats. The lesion may be pigmented or amelanotic. As expected, pigmented lesions are almost black in color, whereas amelanotic lesions may be pink or white. Because melanomas often have intracytoplasmic granules, they must be differentiated from mast cell tumors. With most stains, the granules are black or brown and irregular in shape and size. The granules are often noted extracellularly because they are released from some cells. The melanoma can be composed of round cells, epithelioid cells, or cells can be spindle-shaped; sometimes, there are cells of different shapes within the same tumor. Malignant melanomas must be differentiated from mast cell tumors and macrophages that contain hemosiderin.

Epithelial Cell Tumors: Carcinomas
(Color Figures 13–15)

Epithelial cell tumors are found throughout the body. Regardless of whether they originate from the lung (Color Figure 16), the intestine (Color Figure 17), or the mammary gland (Color Figure 18) they all have similar characteristics, including easy exfoliation of cells in clusters, clumps, or sheets; oval to round cells; ductular or acinar arrangement around a central lumen; and cytoplasm that may contain a secretory product. This secretory product may induce a "signet ring" appearance because the nucleus is eccentrically located within the cytoplasm. An experienced pathologist might be able to classify the tumor as a carcinoma; a clinical pathologist may be able to differentiate the cells further. The following are some characteristics of epithelial cell tumors commonly seen in veterinary practice.

Mammary Adenocarcinoma (Color Figure 18)

Cytologic interpretation of the cells from a mammary adenocarcinoma are classic for any adenocarcinoma. The cells often are arranged in clusters and exhibit cytoplasmic basophilia and variable nuclear/cytoplasmic ratios. Mitotic figures are common; some cells may be distended with a cytoplasmic product forming a "signet ring" appearance.

Sebaceous Gland Tumor (Color Figure 19)

These small, fleshy tumors of the skin of older dogs often are pedunculated, and they are almost always benign. The cells have a high nuclei/cytoplasm ratio with a scant basophilic cytoplasm. The cells do not have criteria for malignancy. The nucleus usually is centrally located. The cytoplasm is abundant and foamy.

Squamous Cell Carcinoma

Squamous cell carcinomas occur throughout the body in dogs and cats and often have a different biologic behavior depending on the location of the tumor. They may be ulcerated and therefore may have an inflammatory component mixed with a bacterial infection. Squamous cell carcinomas often exfoliate into clusters; however, they are just as likely to be individual cells. The cells of this tumor may vary morphologically depending on the degree of differentiation. The more anaplastic cells are small and round with a basophilic cytoplasm, which often contains hyperchromatic nuclei. Cells in an intermediate stage of differentiation are larger, with more abundant, paler cytoplasm. The nuclei generally are large and have marked clumps of chromatin. More mature cells actually show signs of forming keratin, which may be seen in the extracellular space. The more mature cells may have cytoplasmic borders that appear quite angular due to keratinization. An inflammatory response is often seen in conjunction with the tumor cells. As with all aspirates, a histologic sample is essential to confirm the diagnosis.

Perianal Adenoma (Color Figure 15)

Perianal gland adenomas are common tumors seen primarily in intact male dogs; they occasionally occur in female dogs with hyperadrenocorticism. These raised, hairless tumors of the perianal glands are often small and multiple, but they may become very large. Cytologically, perianal gland adenomas may resemble perianal gland adenocarcinomas; therefore, a biopsy using parameters such as invasion of the basement membrane is essential to differentiate between the two types. Cytologically, these cells exfoliate readily into clusters, are often described as hepatoid in appearance, and are characterized as having an abundant, foamy pale cytoplasm and eccentric or centrally located round to oval nuclei that may vary in size.

Intracutaneous Cornifying Epithelioma or Inclusion Cysts (Color Figure 12)

These two benign conditions of the skin often are cytologically indistinguishable. The intracutaneous cornifying epithelioma often occurs in Norwegian Elkhounds. Inclusion cysts can be seen in any breed. The tumors are actually cavities within the skin that contain keratinized cellular debris. They may open and drain to the outside. Cytologically, they are composed of epithelial cells, keratin debris, and cholesterol crystals.

Sarcomas: Connective Tissue Tumors
(Color Figures 21–24)

Connective tissue tumors exfoliate poorly and therefore may be difficult to diagnose cytologically. Cytologic diagnosis of a sarcoma is reasonably straightforward; however, specifically distinguishing connective tissue tumors may not be possible.

Soft Tissue Sarcomas (Color Figures 21–23)

Soft tissue sarcomas occur anywhere on the dog's body. Hemangiopericytomas (Color Figure 23) often are found on the extremities of dogs and occasionally are found in cats. All soft tissue sarcomas have a relatively low probability for metastasis and are locally invasive. The cells exfoliate poorly and usually are seen alone or in disorganized clusters. The cytoplasm often is indistinct and spindle-shaped. Hemangiopericytomas sometimes appear in whorls, which distinguishes them from other soft tissue sarcomas such as fibrosarcomas, neurofibrosarcomas, fibromas, schwannomas, myxosarcomas, and myxomas.

Lipoma (Color Figure 14)

Lipomas are very common tumors in dogs but are rarely seen in cats. When a fine-needle aspiration sample is placed on a slide, the sample is oily and fails to dry on the slide. The sample will often rinse off the slide with alcohol. Adipocytes will appear to range from very large cells that are fully distended with fat to collapsed cells with lacy cytoplasm.

Osteosarcoma (Color Figure 24)

Osteosarcomas may have sufficient distinguishable cytologic characteristics to allow the practitioner to make a tentative diagnosis based on fine-needle aspiration cytology, especially when combined with the history, physical examination, and radiographs. These tumors often occur in the metaphyses of long bones. Cytologically, the tumor may be composed primarily of osteoblasts that vary dramatically in size, but they usually are quite large. The cells are often spindle-shaped and have abundant foamy basophilic cytoplasm that surrounds a variably sized nucleus, with coarse chromatin and variable numbers of nuclei. Some of these cells have an eosinophilic substance within the cytoplasm that occasionally may be noted extracellularly as an osteoid matrix. Normal osteoblasts may be seen in conjunction with the malignant cells.

REFERENCES

1. Rebar AH: *Handbook of Veterinary Cytology.* Ralston Purina, St Louis, MO, 1977.
2. Wellman ML: The cytologic diagnosis of neoplasia. *Vet Clin North Am Small Anim Pract* 20:919–938, 1990.
3. MacWilliams PS: Cytologic techniques in cancer diagnosis, in Withrow SJ, MacEwen EG (eds): *Clinical Veterinary Oncology.* Philadelphia, JB Lippincott, 1989, pp 41–52.

CLINICAL BRIEFING: SAFE HANDLING OF CHEMOTHERAPEUTIC AGENTS

Use of a vertical laminar air flow hood is recommended for all drug handling

Risk	Recommendation
Absorption via skin or mucous membranes	Wear latex gloves; protective eyewear; and a disposable gown with long, cuffed sleeves
Inhalation	Wear a respirator-type or high-dust mask
Aerosol formation when reconstituting or removing liquid chemotherapy	Use a hydrophobic filter (chemotherapy "pin")
Metabolites or drug (e.g., cisplatin) in urine	Wear latex gloves when handling waste
Self-inoculation when recapping needles	Do not recap needles
Other precautions: wash hands frequently; do not allow food in work area	

The use of chemotherapeutic agents is rapidly expanding as the benefits of these anti-cancer drugs become more apparent. With increased use, however, there is increased risk of exposure during drug preparation and administration. All chemotherapeutic agents are potentially toxic, most are mutagenic or teratogenic, and at least some are proven carcinogens. Reliable information regarding the amount of drug exposure needed for any of these effects is difficult to obtain; however, some toxicities have been seen in people who prepare and administer chemotherapy for human patients.[1,2]

Exposure to cytotoxic agents can occur in three ways:
- inhalation due to aerosolization during mixing and/or administration of the drug
- absorption of the drug through the skin
- ingestion through contact with contaminated food or cigarettes

Common clinical examples of situations where exposure may occur include:
- withdrawal of a needle from a pressurized drug vial
- transferral of drugs between various containers
- opening of glass ampules
- expulsion of air from drug-filled syringes
- failure of equipment or improperly set up equipment
- exposure to excreta from patients that have received certain cytotoxic drugs
- crushing or breaking tablets of cytotoxic drugs

Safe drug handling certainly is possible in veterinary practice. Owing to the relatively low volume of chemotherapy delivered by most practitioners, the

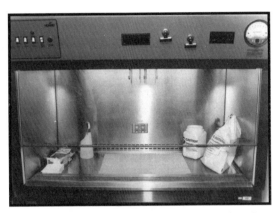

Figure 2-1: Whenever possible, a biological safety cabinet should be used. Latex gloves and a nonpermeable gown should be worn when preparing chemotherapeutic agents.

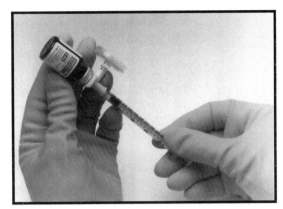

Figure 2-2: Hydrophobic filters (chemo-pins) are essential to prevent aerosolization of cytotoxic agents during preparation. Note that the side vent is filtered for protection from the accidental escape of the drug.

risk of exposure is low. However, everyone who prepares or administers antineoplastic drugs should have routine health examinations. Women of child-bearing age should exercise extreme caution when handling cytotoxic agents. Pregnant women should not handle antineoplastic drugs.

Antineoplastic agents should be stored according to the manufacturer's directions. Drugs that require refrigeration should be stored in a separate refrigerator away from other medications and foodstuffs. If a reconstituted drug is stored, the vial should be placed in a "ziplock-style" bag, which should be labelled with the date of reconstitution.

The ideal way to prepare cytotoxic agents is in a biological safety cabinet, specifically, a Class II, type A vertical laminar air flow cabinet exhausted outside the facility (Figure 2-1). It is impractical for most veterinary practices to own such a hood, but many of the safety principles involved in drug handling and reconstitution are the same regardless of whether a hood is used. If a hood is not available, other pieces of equipment can help provide a safe environment in which to prepare chemotherapeutic agents. All drug preparation should be done in a low-traffic area, away from doorways, windows, or any place there may be

a draft. Eating, drinking, and smoking should not take place in the drug preparation area. The same equipment used to prepare chemotherapy in a biological safety hood also should be used when a hood is not available. Specifically, a disposable plastic-backed pad or liner should be used. Gloves and a gown should be worn, as should a dust and mist respirator and goggles. Using chemotherapy dispensing pins ("chemo-pins") or hydrophobic filters (Figure 2-2) further reduces the risk of exposure to injectable drugs being prepared. Drugs are prepared in exactly the same manner as in the hood, and all materials must be disposed of properly. The following information is provided for those who are involved in the day-to-day technical aspects of chemotherapy preparation and administration. The reader is advised to read this section for information that can reduce the risks inherent in handling these drugs.

PREPARING CHEMOTHERAPY, WITH OR WITHOUT A VERTICAL LAMINAR AIR FLOW HOOD

The biological safety cabinet or hood should be serviced routinely and certified by a qualified person at least yearly. It should be operated according to the manufacturer's directions and specifications and in accordance with OSHA requirements. The hood blower should be on at all times unless it is used infrequently (1–2 times a week).

Some materials should always be kept in the hood. These include a plastic-lined absorbent pad to wipe up any leaks and spills, which should be changed when the cabinet is cleaned or when it is contaminated with any drug, a stack of gauze squares, and alcohol-soaked cotton balls or swabs. A large, plastic ziplock-style bag should be available for chemotherapy waste, and a puncture-proof container is needed for all contaminated sharps.

All materials needed for drug preparation should be placed in the hood before starting any work. All outer packages should be discarded outside the hood to prevent accumulation of debris in the hood. Before reconstituting a drug, recommendations for the diluent should be verified. For most chemotherapy drugs, 0.9% saline or sterile water is used; however, for some drugs (e.g., carboplatin), a solution of 5% dextrose in water is required.

When preparing cytotoxic agents, a gown with long sleeves, closed cuffs, and a closed front should be worn. The gown should be made of a disposable fabric that has low permeability. Latex gloves should be pulled over the cuffs of the gown to protect the skin from exposure to the drug. Vinyl gloves are not recommended because they are more permeable and therefore more likely to allow contamination of the skin. When preparing drugs in a vertical laminar air flow hood, wearing goggles or a mask is not necessary; however, they should be worn when preparing drugs without a hood. The use of a dust and mist respirator or a mask with a filter to prevent inhalation of aerosolized drugs is recommended. A conventional surgery mask does not have such a filter. Finally, wearing goggles is advisable.

The arms should always be held up above the vents when under the hood. Resting the arms on the bottom of the hood will disrupt the airflow, which increases the risk of contamination. All work should

be performed in the middle of the hood, because airflow diminishes toward the sides of the hood.

Chemo-pins, which are recommended for injectable drugs, prevent aerosolization of the drug and prevent pressure from building in the vials when reconstituting drugs. Luer-lok® syringes (Figures 2-3 and 2-4) are recommended because they prevent the syringe from separating from the chemo-pin or needle. Luer-lok® syringes are somewhat of a hindrance when using a butterfly catheter for drug administration because these syringes take longer to screw on and off. This delay may allow drug to leak back when changing syringes unless the tubing is clamped or an injection port is used.

To prepare injectable drugs, the first step is removing the plastic lid from the vial and wiping the top of the vial with an alcohol swab. All procedures should be done as aseptically as possible. The chemo-pin is then inserted into the vial. The vial is kept upright while the syringe is attached to the chemo-pin and twisted tight. When reconstituting a drug, diluent is slowly pushed into the vial, and the bottle is gently shaken. A Luer-lok® syringe can be left attached while mixing. If not using a Luer-lok® syringe, the syringe should be removed from the vial and the cap for the chemo-pin replaced before mixing. Next, the vial is turned upside down, and the drug is aspirated into the syringe slowly, to avoid excess air bubbles. When the correct amount has been retrieved, any air or any excess drug should be pushed back into the vial. The vial should then be turned upright and put down. The next step is to wrap a gauze square around the top of the pin and syringe and gently pull the syringe from the pin. The gauze will trap any drug that leaks or aerosolizes. A covered needle should be placed on the syringe and a cap placed on the chemo-pin. The labelled syringe should then be put into a plastic ziplock bag. The chemo-pin is left attached to the vial to allow access for multiple doses if the remaining drug is to be stored.

If chemo-pins are not available, the diluent must be slowly added to the drug directly through the needle and the displaced air allowed to escape back into

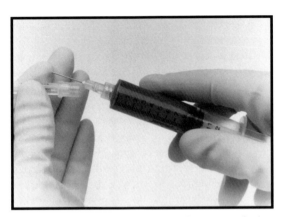

Figure 2-3: *To prevent puncturing the operator and risking unnecessary exposure to cytotoxic agents, avoid replacing needle covers after use. Note the use of the Luer-lok® syringe to reduce the risk of accidental needle detachment and leakage of the drug.*

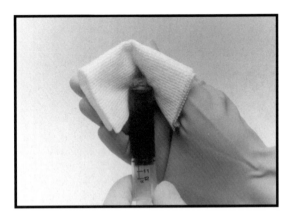

Figure 2-4: *If air bubbles are to be expelled from a syringe containing a cytotoxic drug, alcohol moistened gauze should be used to prevent aerosolization. This is particularly important if a vertical laminar air flow hood is not available. Latex gloves and Luer-lok® syringes should be used at all times.*

the syringe to avoid excess pressure in the vial. Once the drug has been reconstituted and the correct dose retrieved, a gauze square should be wrapped around the top of the vial and the needle. Then, the needle should be slowly pulled out of the vial. Any air bubbles that are present should be injected into an alcohol-soaked cotton ball and discarded in the appropriate waste container (Figure 2-4). The cap should be *carefully* placed on the needle and the syringe put into a ziplock bag and labelled. As a general rule, needles should not be recapped (see Figure 2-3), although this is sometimes unavoidable.

It is extremely important to label all chemotherapeutic drugs. All syringes, fluid bags, pill bottles, and so forth must have a chemotherapy label that lists the drug name and dose. The drug vial should be put into a ziplock bag to be stored in a refrigerator, or it can be discarded according to storage instructions. Every drug has a package insert that states the expiration date and storage conditions.

All nonsharp materials used in drug preparation should be placed into a large, ziplock bag, and all sharps must be placed in a puncture-proof container stored in the hood. Once everything is discarded and

all vials and syringes are inside the ziplock bags, gloves should be removed while still under the hood. The gloves should be rolled off. Care must be taken to avoid touching the outside of the glove. The gloves are then placed in the large ziplock bag.

Bags with syringes and/or vials should be placed outside the hood before removing the gown and other safety equipment. If not using a hood, all bags containing drug should be sealed before removing protective gear. If protective garments are contaminated during drug preparation, they should be discarded and replaced immediately. Thorough hand washing following drug preparation is strongly recommended to remove any potential chemotherapeutic drug residues. A large, clearly labelled barrel or chemotherapy waste container should be kept in the drug preparation area for full ziplock waste bags from the hood, all contaminated safety equipment (e.g., gowns, gloves, masks, etc.), and any other contaminated materials (e.g., gauze squares, cotton balls, etc.).

When preparing a drug that is to be delivered by intravenous drip infusion, it is a good idea to prime the administration set by filling the fluid lines with diluent from the bag before adding the chemothera-

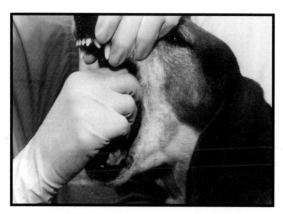

Figure 2-5: Owners or health care professionals should wear latex gloves when administering oral medication, such as cyclophosphamide, to prevent exposure to the cytotoxic drug.

peutic agent to the bag. This reduces the risk of exposure when connecting the dripset to the patient. Once reconstituted, the drug should be slowly injected into the bag. Once the drug is injected, a gauze square can be wrapped around the injection port and the needle withdrawn. This helps to prevent aerosolization of drug. The fluid that contains the drug should be stored in a labelled, sealable bag until it is administered. Again, materials should be discarded appropriately.

Some chemotherapy agents are prepared for oral administration. When preparing pills, nonporous latex gloves are strongly recommended. Cytotoxic powder has been documented as far as 12 inches away from where tablets are crushed or split; therefore, drugs are best dispensed in whole tablet amounts only. Some drugs that are to be administered orally may be prepared as an elixir for dosing of small quantities (rather than splitting tablets). In situations in which crushing or splitting pills cannot be avoided, and especially if a safety hood is not available, a gown, goggles, and respirator mask are mandatory. The preparation surface must be well cleaned after such use. Oral medications should be placed in clearly labelled containers with a warning label for dispensing to owners. Owners who are administering these oral agents should wear latex

gloves (Figure 2-5) and should return empty vials for proper disposal by the veterinarian.

Intralesional injections that consist of a cytotoxic agent mixed with a vehicle such as bovine collagen matrix or sterile sesame oil, which acts to slowly release drug into the tumor, have been recommended for some localized cancers. Preparation of these mixtures is performed in the biological safety cabinet as for other drugs, but two Luer-lok® syringes, one containing the cytotoxic agent and one containing the vehicle, should be prepared. Each agent should be placed into a syringe that is of sufficient volume to contain both liquids when combined. The next step is to attach the syringes to a three-way stopcock; then, the two liquids can be rapidly mixed between the syringes to create an oily emulsion. The syringe that now contains all of the mixture should be detached after covering the attachment with a gauze swab to prevent aerosolization, then a needle is attached. The remaining syringe and stopcock should be discarded as contaminated waste. It is preferable to mix multiple small volumes of drug in this way rather than as one large volume, because separation of drug from vehicle may occur rapidly, thereby reducing the efficacy of the treatment. For this reason, it is recommended that the drug-vehicle mixture be administered soon after preparation. If a delay is encountered, remixing of the drug with vehicle can be achieved with a new syringe and three-way stopcock; however, if outside the hood, gloves, mask, goggles, and a gown must be worn. It may be wise to mix inside a ziplock bag. The needle on used syringes should not be recapped. All materials should be disposed of as contaminated waste.

REFERENCES

1. OSHA Work Practice Guidelines for Personnel: *Dealing with Cytotoxic Drugs.* OSHA Instructional Publication 8-1.1, Washington DC, Office of Occupational Medicine, 1986.
2. Falck K, Grohn P, Sorsa M, et al: Mutagenicity in urine of nurses handling cytotoxic drugs. *Lancet* 1:1250–1255, 1979.

CLINICAL BRIEFING: METHODS OF DRUG ADMINISTRATION

Most drugs are dosed on a body surface area (m²) basis

Methods of Administration	Drug Example
Intravenous	
Butterfly catheter	Vincristine and vinblastine
Over-the-needle catheter	Doxorubicin and actinomycin D
Indwelling catheter	Cisplatin
Intramuscular	L-asparaginase
Oral	Cyclophosphamide, chlorambucil, and melphalan
Intracavitary	Cisplatin
Intralesional	Cisplatin and 5-fluorouracil

There are many routes by which to administer chemotherapeutic agents: intravenously, intramuscularly, intracavitarily, subcutaneously, intralesionally, and orally. Less commonly used routes in veterinary medicine include intrathecal and intraarterial administration. Regardless of the route of administration, latex gloves should be worn when handling cytotoxic agents. Wearing a gown and mask is recommended to minimize the risk of exposure.

DOSING

Almost all doses for chemotherapeutic drugs are calculated using the body surface area (BSA) in square meters (m²).[1-4] Recent studies have shown this method of dosing may not be ideal for all *veterinary* patients, especially the smallest animals, in which increased toxicity may be observed.[4] Until a better dosing scheme is developed, however, most chemotherapeutic agents should still be dosed on a m² basis.

To determine the BSA in m² of an animal, its weight in pounds is divided by 2.2. This yields the weight in kilograms. Next, the kilogram weight should be found on the conversion table of weight-to-body surface area (see Table 2-1). If a conversion table is not available, the following formula can be used to calculate the m²:

DOGS

$$m^2 = \frac{10.1 \times (weight\ in\ grams)^{2/3}}{10^4}$$

CATS

$$m^2 = \frac{10.0 \times (weight\ in\ grams)^{2/3}}{10^4}$$

To determine the dose of a drug (in this case, vincristine), multiply the dosage (0.75 mg/m²) by the patient's body surface area (m²).

Example: 40-lb dog to receive vincristine at a dose of 0.75 mg/m².
1) 40 ÷ 2.2 = 16.8 kg
2) 16.8 kg = 0.66 m² (from Table 2-1, page 67)
3) 0.66 m² × 0.75 mg/m² = 0.50 mg vincristine

The concentration of vincristine = 1 mg/ml; therefore, the dog will receive *0.50* ml of vincristine.

$$\frac{0.50 \; mg \; vincristine}{1 \; mg/ml} = 0.50 \; ml$$

Before handling any chemotherapeutic agent, the concentration is checked. For example, doxorubicin, as well as some other drugs, has a concentration of 2 mg/ml, so it is necessary to divide the milligrams by 2 to determine how many milliliters of these drugs to administer.

Many chemotherapy agents are myelosuppressive; therefore, a complete blood count (CBC) must be obtained before administering any chemotherapy. If the neutrophil count is <3000/µl, the drug should not be given, and the CBC should be rechecked in 3 to 4 days. Also, a CBC should be taken 7 days after administering any drug that has the potential to cause myelosuppression, such as doxorubicin or cyclophosphamide, as 7 days is the neutrophil nadir for most drugs (see drug tables in the following section for individual variation). If the neutrophil count is below 1500/µl at 7 days after treatment, the dose of the drug should be reduced by 25%.

Example: Seven days after receiving 250 mg/m² of cyclophosphamide, a cat has a neutrophil count of 1020/µl. All subsequent doses of cyclophosphamide should be given at a dose of 187.5 mg/m². If a subsequent neutrophil count is 1500/µl or greater, this new dose is continued; however, if it is <1500/µl, the dose is *again* reduced by 25% (to 140.5 mg/m² in this case).

Before giving cisplatin, a biochemical profile to include BUN, creatinine, and phosphorus should be performed, because this drug is a potent nephrotoxin. If the dog is azotemic or has poor urine concentrating ability, cisplatin should not be administered.

INTRAVENOUS CHEMOTHERAPY ADMINISTRATION

Most chemotherapeutic agents are administered intravenously. This usually is done using one of the following:
1. a butterfly catheter,
2. an over-the-needle catheter, or
3. a through-the-needle intracatheter (such as used for central venous access).

Peripheral vessels are preferred for intravenous drug administration owing to the ease of monitoring for extravasation of drug. Regardless of the type of catheter used for administration, certain preparatory steps should be taken. The leg to be used should be clipped at the site of injection and prepared using aseptic technique. When a drug is known to be a vesicant, an indwelling catheter should be used, particularly if the drug is not being administered as a bolus.

Drugs should not be administered after an "unclean" venipuncture (i.e., when the vein is entered more than once). If this occurs, another leg should be used. If it is the only available leg, it is advisable to wait for clotting to occur before trying proximal to the site of the previous attempt. A second venipuncture

> **KEY POINT:**
>
> *If the neutrophil count is <3000/µl, the drug should not be given and the CBC should be checked again in 3 to 4 days. A CBC should be taken 7 days after administering any drug that has the potential to cause myelosuppression to ensure the neutrophil count is above 1500/µl.*

should never be attempted distal to the site of a failed attempt. It is a good idea to alternate the veins used for administration to allow them to recover from previous administrations.

It is important to ensure that the catheter is patent before any drug is administered. If there is any doubt, it is best to use another leg. The catheter should be flushed with saline (minimum of 12 ml) to determine patency and should also be flushed after *each* drug administration (i.e., if two drugs are to be given, the catheter should be flushed between administrations). Only nonheparinized 0.9% saline is recommended for use with chemotherapeutic drug administrations, because heparin causes precipitates to form when mixed with some drugs, such as doxorubicin.

The catheter and leg should be monitored constantly during drug administration to note any extravasation that may occur. If the catheter is to be secured, it is best to use one piece of tape that does not obstruct visualization of the injection site, the area surrounding the injection site, or the leg proximal to the injection site.

It is important to check whether there is a specific rate at which to administer a drug to minimize toxicity. For example, undiluted doxorubicin should be given at a rate of 1 ml per minute, whereas vincristine can be given as a bolus. Alternatively, the dose of doxorubicin can be placed in 150 ml of 0.9% NaCl and administered over 30 minutes. The drug should be injected slowly and evenly to prevent excessive pressure to the vein and leakage of drug around the needle or catheter.

After administering the drug and after each flush, a piece of gauze or an alcohol-soaked cotton ball should be placed with a gloved hand over the needle as it is withdrawn from the injection port or over the catheter as it is removed from the vein. This minimizes aerosolization of drug. All of the drug should be flushed through the catheter after administration without re-aspirating the catheter. Re-aspirating at this time dilutes the drug in the flush and causes diluted drug to be left in the catheter. A cotton ball can be taped over the insertion site after catheter removal, and pressure is then applied for at least several minutes.

All materials should be discarded into appropriate chemotherapy waste containers. The syringes and needles should be placed in a puncture-proof, leak-proof container, which must be clearly marked as hazardous or chemotherapy waste. It is important to wash the hands thoroughly after every drug administration.

Butterfly Catheter (Figure 2-6)

Generally, a butterfly catheter is recommended when administering a small amount of drug (3 ml or less) and when the drug can be given quickly. When using a butterfly catheter, it is best to have all the materials organized and readily available (within arm's reach) before starting. There should be two to three syringes of 12 ml of nonheparinized 0.9% saline flushes available, the labelled drug, an alcohol swab, the butterfly catheter, and a pressure bandage. It is best to place the labelled syringes on a pad or a plastic bag and line them up in order of use. The needles should be removed, or the caps loosened, to help the administration proceed as swiftly and smoothly as possible.

> **KEY POINT:**
>
> *Dosages should always be double-checked. Care should be taken with drugs for which milligrams do not equal milliliters (e.g., doxorubicin, which is 2 mg/ml). Chemotherapeutic drugs can be toxic enough at the correct dose! If there is a question about anything, stop! Do not proceed until all questions are answered.*
>
> *It is impossible to be too careful with chemotherapeutic agents.*

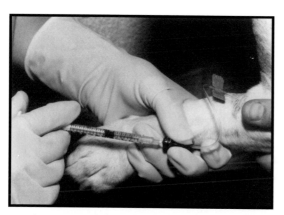

Figure 2-6: Butterfly catheters are ideal for administering small volumes of drugs, such as vincristine intravenously. Care should be taken to ensure that the catheter is patent to prevent extravasation.

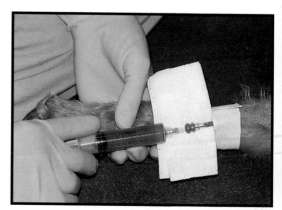

Figure 2-7: Intravenous over-the-needle catheters are ideal for administering slow bolus infusions of drugs such as doxorubicin intravenously. The area of the injection site, the injection port, and the leg above the injection site should be clearly visible to the administrator so that any extravasation or leakage can be attended to promptly.

When all of the drug has been delivered, the syringe should be detached and a saline flush attached quickly to avoid letting any drug leak back out. When delivering a very small amount of drug (e.g., vincristine administered to a cat), a small amount of leakage during this step can result in loss of a substantial portion of the dose. The following methods can be used to reduce leakage:

- It is helpful to produce an air bubble at the bottom of the syringe containing the drug so that air, rather than drug, will leak out (i.e., at the end farthest from the needle).
- The tubing of the catheter can be clamped or kinked while changing syringes. This technique is cumbersome and may dislodge the catheter.
- A three-way stopcock may be helpful.
- Butterfly catheters with an injection port "inbuilt" (Butterfly® INJ 25 × ³/₄; 3″ tubing, Abbott Laboratories, North Chicago, IL) are easier to use as it is not necessary to detach syringes during administration, and an injection technique as for an over-the-needle catheter is used.

Intravenous Over-the-Needle Catheter
(Figure 2-7)

Generally, drugs are given through intravenous over-the-needle catheters (e.g., Abbotcath®-T; Teflon IV catheter, Abbott Laboratories, North Chicago, IL) as a bolus (but over a period of minutes) or for drugs that are in a volume greater than 3 ml. Over-the-needle catheters should be used for doxorubicin administration, in which a slow rate of delivery is important to prevent an anaphylactoid reaction. It is preferable to place the catheter while wearing latex gloves; however, the catheter may be placed before drugs are prepared as long as patency is again confirmed before administration.

For over-the-needle catheter administration, long, clear male adapter plugs allow for better viewing of the flashback of blood and the drug being administered. In addition, these plugs allow the administrator to determine when all of the drug has been flushed out of the catheter at the final stages of the procedure.

Once the catheter has been placed, a 4 × 4 gauze square should be folded in half and slipped under the injection cap. This will absorb any drug that may leak out of the injection cap during administration. Needles should be inserted as *far as possible* into the adaptor plug to allow for easier flushing of residual drug after injection.

Continuous Intravenous Infusion

When administering drugs over a long period (6 to 48 hours) (e.g., cisplatin or cytosine arabinoside), an indwelling catheter should be used.[4] The catheter site and all connections in the intravenous line should be monitored frequently for patency and leakage. The patient must be prevented from chewing or disconnecting the intravenous line.

During long periods of drug administration, disposal of contaminated waste, particularly urine, becomes important. When the patient or any waste is handled, latex gloves should be worn, and a gown, goggles, and mask may reduce the risk of exposure to excreted active metabolites. A metabolic cage is preferred for such chemotherapeutic administrations; however, in the absence of such a cage, frequently walking the patient (dogs) in an area where urine will not remain exposed (i.e., grass or dirt) is recommended. Cages or excreta should not be hosed, because this aerosolizes drug and distributes it more widely. All waste should be discarded as contaminated material.

When using the 4- or 6-hour cisplatin protocol, it is best to use an over-the-needle (18- to 20-ga) catheter because of the high volume of fluids infused per hour. An infusion pump is also recommended to ensure that the correct amount of fluid is administered.

When administering doxorubicin and cisplatin together, the doxorubicin can be given during the prediuresis period through an injection port on the IV line. Gloves should be worn, and a gauze square should be held underneath the syringe to catch any drug that may leak through the port.

INTRAMUSCULAR OR INTRALESIONAL CHEMOTHERAPY ADMINISTRATION

Intramuscular injections are administered in the normal fashion, but latex gloves should be worn. L-asparaginase can cause an anaphylactic reaction if given intravenously; therefore, the syringe must be checked for blood to ensure that a vessel has not been entered inadvertently before injecting the drug. Preferred sites of injection include well-muscled areas, such as the caudal thigh region or lumbar musculature. Intralesional chemotherapy also should be administered while wearing latex gloves, and it is important to watch the area carefully for any leakage of chemotherapeutic agent. If leakage occurs, the area should be swabbed and cleaned with soap and water, and the cleaning materials disposed of as hazardous waste.

ORAL CHEMOTHERAPY ADMINISTRATION

Wearing latex gloves is necessary when administering pills. The patient is given the pills in the normal fashion. If owners are to administer oral chemotherapy, they must be instructed to wear disposable protective gloves and wash their hands after administration.

INTRACAVITARY CHEMOTHERAPY ADMINISTRATION

Some chemotherapeutic agents (e.g., cisplatin) can be administered into body cavities, either intrathoracically or intra-abdominally.[1,4] Both the administrator and the restrainer should wear gloves. As with intravenous administration, the IV line needs to be primed *before* the drug is added to the bag.

For thoracic administration, the patient is placed in lateral recumbency and the injection site is aseptically prepared. The right side is preferred. The area of the cardiac notch provides the least risk of lung puncture. The area is infiltrated with lidocaine, and a 14-ga rigid plastic intravenous cannula (e.g., Argyle® Medicut®; Sherwood Medical Industries, St. Louis, MO) is inserted between the ribs and flushed with a minimum of 12 ml of saline to ensure a patent pathway. If there is resistance to the flush or if the animal appears uncomfortable or coughs, the cannula should be removed and a new cannula inserted. For abdominal administration, the patient is placed in dorsal recumbency and a midline site caudal to the umbilicus is used. Allowing the patient to urinate before administration reduces the risk of bladder puncture, and the site should be caudal enough to avoid the spleen. The site is aseptically prepared, and the catheter should be placed as for thoracic administration. Once the patency is determined, the fluid line is attached and the drug is administered.

The fluid should flow fairly easily into the cavity. If the fluid drip slows or is only intermittent, the cannula can be adjusted slightly. The area should be monitored constantly to make sure the fluid is not going subcutaneously. Once the bag is empty, the IV line should be turned off. Then, a piece of gauze should be wrapped around the cannula and the cannula is slowly pulled out. At this point, the restrainer should hold a gauze square over the site and apply pressure to stop any bleeding and/or leakage that may occur. Finally, the patient should be walked for a few minutes to allow the drug to distribute over the entire cavity. All materials must be discarded as contaminated waste.

REFERENCES

1. Chabner BA: Principles of cancer therapy, in Wyngaarden JB, Smith LH (eds): *Cecil Textbook of Medicine.* Philadelphia, WB Saunders, 1982, p 1032.
2. Madewell BR, Theilen GH: Chemotherapy, in Theilen GH, Madewell B (eds): *Veterinary Cancer Medicine.* Philadelphia, Lea & Febiger, 1979, pp 157–183.
3. Madewell BR: Adverse effects of chemotherapy, in Kirk RW (ed): *Current Veterinary Therapy IIX.* Philadelphia, WB Saunders, 1983, p 419.
4. Ogilvie GK: Principles of oncology, in Morgan RV (ed): *Handbook of Small Animal Internal Medicine.* Philadelphia, Churchill & Livingston, 1992, pp 799–812.

CLINICAL BRIEFING: CHEMOTHERAPY— PROPERTIES, USES, AND PATIENT MANAGEMENT

Alkylating Agents

Common Drugs	Potential Toxicoses	Reported Indications
Cyclophosphamide	Bone marrow suppression-alopecia-gastrointestinal toxicity (BAG); rarely, sterile hemorrhagic cystitis	Lymphoma, sarcomas, and mammary adenocarcinoma
Chlorambucil	BAG and cerebellar toxicity	Chronic lymphocytic leukemia and lymphoma
Melphalan	BAG	Multiple myeloma
Thiotepa	BAG	Transitional cell carcinoma

Antimetabolites

Common Drugs	Potential Toxicoses	Reported Indications
Cytosine Arabinoside	BAG	Lymphoma, leukemia
Methotrexate	BAG	Lymphoma

Antibiotics

Common Drugs	Potential Toxicoses	Reported Indications
Doxorubicin	BAG; unique colitis; cardiomyopathy; perivascular slough; allergic reaction during administration; rarely, renal failure	Lymphoma; sarcomas, including hemangiosarcoma; thyroid carcinoma, mammary adenocarcinoma, and mesothelioma
Mitoxantrone	BAG	Lymphoma, mammary adenocarcinoma, and squamous cell carcinoma
Actinomycin D	BAG and perivascular slough	Lymphoma

Enzymes

Common Drugs	Potential Toxicoses	Reported Indications
L-asparaginase	Anaphylaxis, disseminated intravascular coagulopathy, pancreatitis, and pain on injection	Lymphoma

Vinca Alkaloids

Common Drugs	Potential Toxicoses	Reported Indications
Vincristine	AG, peripheral neuropathy, and perivascular slough	Lymphoma, sarcomas, mast cell tumor, transmissible venereal tumor, and thrombocytopenia
Vinblastine	BAG, peripheral neuropathy, and perivascular slough	Lymphoma and mast cell tumor

Hormones

Common Drugs	Potential Toxicoses	Reported Indications
Prednisone	Iatrogenic Cushing's syndrome	Lymphoma and mast cell tumor

Miscellaneous Agents

Common Drugs	Potential Toxicoses	Reported Indications
Cisplatin	BAG with bimodal nadir; potent emetic shortly at or after administration; nephrotoxicity; rarely, neuropathy, including ototoxicity	Osteosarcoma, transitional cell carcinoma, mesothelioma, testicular and ovarian neoplasia, squamous cell carcinoma, nasal adenocarcinoma, and thyroid carcinoma
Carboplatin	BAG; neuropathy; nephrotoxicity; rarely, emesis	Osteosarcoma and squamous cell carcinoma
Paclitaxel	BAG; diluent Cremophor EL causes acute allergic reaction upon administration	Lymphoma and mammary adenocarcinoma
Piroxicam	GI ulceration and nephrotoxicity	Transitional cell carcinoma, squamous cell carcinoma, and pain relief

BAG=bone marrow suppression, alopecia, and gastrointestinal toxicity, AG=alopecia and gastrointestinal toxicity.

Advances in the treatment of tumors in animals with chemotherapy are continually being made. Before treating neoplastic disorders with anticancer drugs, an understanding of the principles of chemotherapy is essential. The following is a review of some of the principles and properties of chemotherapeutic agents and the subsequent management of animals that are treated with these drugs.

GENERAL PRINCIPLES OF CANCER THERAPY

A therapeutic strategy should be clearly defined for each patient with cancer. Before therapy is instituted, the patient should be fully evaluated and stabilized, and the tumor should be identified histologically and staged to determine the extent of disease. Before the owner and veterinarian decide on a drug or combination of drugs for the treatment of a malignant condition, awareness of the following is important:

- The owner and veterinarian should be aware of the potential benefits and toxicoses associated with the administration of chemotherapeutic agents. Both parties should be willing to handle any toxicoses that occur in a timely manner.
- The owner and the veterinarian must be willing to arrange to have the patient treated on an appropriate schedule for maximum efficacy. Before initiating a treatment protocol, both sides must be committed to meet the treatment guidelines.
- The owner must be made aware of the expenses associated with the treatment of a malignancy with chemotherapeutic agents. Fortunately, many chemotherapeutic agents are becoming available as generic products at a fraction of the cost of the patented parent drug.

Chemotherapeutic agents are used for *remission induction* and for *intensification* or *consolidation* and *maintenance therapy*. *Remission* is attained when all clinical evidence of tumors has disappeared. *Intensification* is accomplished when a chemotherapeutic agent with a different mechanism of action is introduced after a remission is obtained to kill any resistant tumor cells. *Consolidation* is the phase of treatment when different drugs are administered after remission is attained to improve response by reducing the microscopic tumor burden. *Maintenance therapy* is the administration of drugs to keep the patient in remission. Consolidation and maintenance therapies are more important for the treatment of hematopoietic tumors than for solid tumors. Chemotherapeutic agents also can be used as *adjuvant therapy* following another treatment modality to delay recurrence and increase survival time. *Neoadjuvant therapy* is used to decrease the bulk of primary tumors with chemotherapy before surgery or radiation. The beneficial effects of chemotherapy are inversely proportional to the amount of tumor to be treated; therefore, whenever anticancer drugs are not being used as adjuvants, the tumor should be reduced to its smallest volume and number of cells before chemotherapy is initiated.

To use chemotherapeutic agents to their fullest advantage, the clinician should be knowledgeable about indications for the use of drugs, dosage, timing, resistance, and toxicity. Chemotherapy should be considered for patients with malignancies, such as leukemia, lymphoma, multiple myeloma, and other hematopoietic tumors or with highly malignant tumors that metastasize rapidly. Recent studies reported beneficial results when animals with mammary neoplasia, thyroid carcinoma, squamous cell carcinoma, osteosarcoma, transmissible venereal tumor, hemangiosarcoma, and other sarcomas are treated with antitumor compounds.[1–9]

DRUGS

Compared to multiple-drug regimens, single-drug treatment regimens are less toxic and less expensive. Disadvantages of single-drug regi-

KEY POINT:

The most effective dose of chemotherapeutic agents is often very close to the toxic dose.

mens include decreased efficacy and the development of tumor resistance. Multiple-drug treatment protocols generally are more effective, and tumor resistance develops more slowly than with single-drug treatment regimens. Multiple-drug protocols tend to be more costly and toxic than single-agent protocols.

Dosage

The objective is to use the dose that combines minimal toxicity with maximal effectiveness. The most effective dose of chemotherapeutic agents often is very close to the toxic dose. In addition, a given dose of drug kills a constant fraction of cells regardless of the number of cells present at the start of therapy. Doses of chemotherapeutic agents are often given on the basis of body surface area (BSA) in square meters (m^2). Two notable exceptions to the dosing of chemotherapeutic agents on a m^2 basis are melphalan and doxorubicin. Recently, these two drugs have been shown to be best dosed on a mg/kg basis because they are neither excreted nor metabolized in a complex fashion. All other antineoplastic agents seem to be metabolized or excreted in a complex fashion and should be dosed on a m^2 basis. Table 2-1 is a conversion chart from weight to body surface area.

Dosing can depend on many factors, including the ability of the animal to metabolize and eliminate chemotherapeutic agents. Table 2-2 reviews some of the conditions in which dosages may need to be changed depending on the way a drug is metabolized.

Timing

The timing of administration of antitumor drugs is critical. Unlike many tumor cells, normal cells have repair mechanisms that are able to correct cellular damage. Therefore, cytotoxic drugs must be given at proper intervals to allow the tumor cells to die while normal cells recover. Improper timing of the drug dose results in excess toxicity or lack of antitumor activity.

Resistance

In contrast to normal cells, most tumor cells

TABLE 2-1

Conversion table to convert body weight (kg) to body surface area (m^2) for dogs and cats. Most chemotherapeutic agents are dosed on a body surface area basis.

kg	m^2	kg	m^2
0.5	0.06	26.0	0.88
1.0	0.10	27.0	0.90
2.0	0.15	28.0	0.92
3.0	0.20	29.0	0.94
4.0	0.25	30.0	0.96
5.0	0.29	31.0	0.99
6.0	0.33	32.0	1.01
7.0	0.36	33.0	1.03
8.0	0.40	34.0	1.05
9.0	0.43	35.0	1.07
10.0	0.46	36.0	1.09
11.0	0.49	37.0	1.11
12.0	0.52	38.0	1.13
13.0	0.55	39.0	1.15
14.0	0.58	40.0	1.17
15.0	0.60	41.0	1.19
16.0	0.63	42.0	1.21
17.0	0.66	43.0	1.23
18.0	0.69	44.0	1.25
19.0	0.71	45.0	1.26
20.0	0.74	46.0	1.28
21.0	0.76	47.0	1.30
22.0	0.78	48.0	1.32
23.0	0.81	49.0	1.34
24.0	0.83	50.0	1.36
25.0	0.85	51.0	1.38

TABLE 2-2
Possible effect of organ dysfunction on dosing of select chemotherapeutic agents

Drug	Critical Organ	Dose Modifications
Doxorubicin Vincristine Vinblastine	Liver	Initial dose reductions of as much as 50% when bilirubin is >1.5 mg/100 ml
Carboplatin	Kidney	Dose reduction is directly proportional to creatinine clearance
Bleomycin	Kidney	Decrease initial dose by as much as 50%–75% if creatinine clearance is <25 ml/min/m^2
Cyclophosphamide	Kidney, Liver	Decrease initial dose by as much as 50%–75% if creatinine clearance is <25 ml/min/m^2; because the liver is necessary to activate the drug, liver disease may warrant dose modification
Cisplatin	Kidney	Do not use with clinically evident renal failure; use caution in animals with any renal problems
Methotrexate	Kidney	Dose reduction is directly proportional to creatinine clearance

develop resistance to antitumor medicine. Resistance is one of the limiting factors in tumor chemotherapy. This resistance results from an acquired or induced phenomenon known as multiple drug resistance (MDR). Multiple drug resistance is caused by a cell membrane protein that literally pumps out cellular toxins, such as chemotherapeutic agents. Anticancer drugs, such as doxorubicin and taxol, are eliminated from the cell by this membrane pump even though they have different molecular structures. Drugs such as verapamil, quinine, and tamoxifen may block this protein, making MDR-mediated drug resistance reversible. In contrast, there seems to be little cross-resistance between alkylating agents (e.g., cyclophosphamide, chlorambucil, and melphalan). Resistance to other drugs, such as the enzyme L-asparaginase, is induced when antibodies are formed to the drug, which causes a rapid destruction of the substance after it is administered.

KEY POINT:

The response to chemotherapy is inversely proportional to the amount of tumor present. In addition, the success of therapy is directly related to the proper use of appropriate doses and timing of therapy.

Toxicity

Several chemotherapeutic agents and their toxicities are noted in the Clinical Briefing. Most chemotherapeutic agents kill or damage rapidly dividing cells. The most clinically important toxicoses include *b*one marrow suppression, *a*lopecia, and *g*astrointestinal toxicity (a "B.A.G." of adverse effects, or BAG). Methods of identifying and treating some of the more common side effects follow.

Bone Marrow Toxicity (Table 2-3, Figure 2-8)

Many antitumor drugs cause a

TABLE 2-3
Myelosuppressive potential of some commonly used chemotherapeutic agents in veterinary medicine

Highly Myelosuppressive	Moderately Myelosuppressive	Mildly Myelosuppressive
Doxorubicin	Melphalan	L-asparaginase[*]
Vinblastine	Chlorambucil	Vincristine[*]
Cyclophosphamide	5-fluorouracil	Bleomycin
Actinomycin D	Methotrexate	Corticosteroids

*Myelosuppression can occur if these two drugs are administered concurrently.

decrease in the number of blood cells days to weeks after administration. Neutropenia and thrombocytopenia are the early signs of bone marrow suppression. Anemia may develop later because red blood cells have a longer life span. Clinical signs may include those related to sepsis, petechial and ecchymotic hemorrhages, pallor, and weakness. Many animals do quite well with low white blood cell and platelet counts; therefore, only patients that exhibit clinical signs should be treated. The treatment of clinically significant bone marrow toxicity includes using aseptic techniques when placing indwelling devices (such as catheters), minimizing trauma, and controlling any bleeding with prolonged application of direct pressure or cold packs. If the animal develops a fever or becomes septic, the urine, blood, and, if indicated, any material obtained with a transtracheal aspirate should be cultured. The affected animal should be treated with appropriate bactericidal antibiotics (e.g., cephalosporins, trimethoprim-sulfa, or gentamicin); supported with fluids, warmth, and nutritional therapy; and transfused as needed with individual cell lines or

> **KEY POINT:**
>
> *Resistance of the tumor to chemotherapy develops with each passing day. Use chemotherapeutic agents at appropriate doses and schedules from the very beginning to minimize resistance to chemotherapeutic agents.*

fresh whole blood collected in plastic containers. The availability of recombinant human granulocyte-colony-stimulating factor now makes it possible to treat this serious condition by boosting endogenous production of neutrophils. Recombinant human erythropoietin is useful in treating animals with nonregenerative anemia secondary to chemotherapy or the underlying malignancy. Caution is advised when using recombinant human products, because antibodies can develop to these foreign proteins in approximately 2 weeks and occasionally may react with the patient's own hematopoietic growth factors. The drug(s) that induced the bone marrow suppression should be discontinued until the blood counts have recovered; subsequently, this myelosuppressive drug should be administered at a reduced dose (e.g., decrease cyclophosphamide dose by 25%).

Alopecia

Alopecia is an uncommon complication of chemotherapy. Dogs with constantly growing haircoats (e.g., poodles, Old English sheepdogs, schnauzers, etc.) are more likely to develop alopecia. Cats can lose their

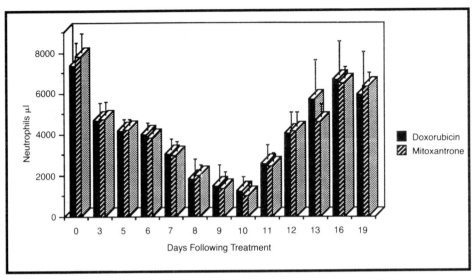

Figure 2-8: *The neutrophil counts from dogs that have received doxorubicin (30 mg/m² IV) and mitoxantrone (5 mg/m² IV) decreased to their lowest level approximately 10 days after each drug was given. (From Ogilvie GK, Moore AS: Mitoxantrone chemotherapy in veterinary medicine, in Kirk RW (ed):* Current Veterinary Therapy. *XI. Philadelphia, WB Saunders, 1992, pp 399–401; with permission.)*

whiskers or may develop a generalized alopecia, but this is much less common than in dogs.

Gastrointestinal Toxicity

The clinical signs of this relatively common side effect include vomiting, anorexia, and diarrhea. The treatment includes antiemetics (e.g., metoclopramide and chlorpromazine); motility modifiers (e.g., diphenoxylate); protectants and absorbants (e.g., Pepto-Bismol®); and broad-spectrum antibiotics, if indicated. In addition, support with fluids, warmth, and nutritional therapy should be provided. Some clinicians dispense metoclopramide to the owners to initiate therapy at home if nausea and vomiting are noted. Because colitis is a significant prob-

lem secondary to doxorubicin therapy, sulfasalazine may be dispensed with instructions to initiate this drug if signs of colitis (fresh blood and mucus in the stool) are noted.

Allergic Reactions

Signs of L-asparaginase hypersensitivity include urticaria, vomiting, diarrhea, hypotension, and loss of consciousness soon after administration. Animals with doxorubicin-induced allergic reactions develop cutaneous hyperemia, intense pruritus, head shaking, and vomiting during administration. These reactions can be reduced substantially by slowing the rate of infusion so that, for example, a medium-sized dog is given the entire dose in approximately 20 to 30 minutes. (Note: Some vet-

KEY POINT:

Anaphylaxis caused by the administration of L-asparaginase can be reduced substantially if the drug is administered intramuscularly rather than intravenously or intraperitoneally.

erinarians continue to give doxorubicin despite cutaneous reactions. The signs abate soon after the drug is administered.) Other drugs that can induce allergic reaction include bleomycin, cytosine arabinoside, and procarbazine. Etoposide (VP-16) and taxol both induce dramatic cutaneous reactions and hypotension during administration secondary to the vehicle that keeps each drug in solution. The treatment for allergic reactions includes discontinuing drug administration and giving epinephrine, diphenhydramine, and glucocorticoids for acute allergic reactions. Premedication with diphenhydramine, cimetidine, and glucocorticoids may prevent or reduce allergic reactions to doxorubicin, taxol, or etoposide.

Cardiac Toxicity

Doxorubicin has been known to induce a dose-dependent dilated (congestive) cardiomyopathy and transient dysrhythmias during administration in dogs. To reduce the number of drug-induced cardiomyopathies, some oncologists limit the cumulative dose of doxorubicin to 180 to 240 mg/m^2 (6 to 8 treatments) during the dog's lifetime. Anecdotally, breeds that are predisposed to doxorubicin-induced cardiomyopathy include Doberman pinschers, boxers, and giant breeds such as Great Danes. In these breeds, a pretreatment echocardiogram and an electrocardiogram should be performed to eliminate those dogs with pre-existing cardiac disease. Routine echocardiograms and electrocardiograms should be performed on dogs given doxorubicin at dosages greater than 180 mg/m^2. In addition, pretreatment with a drug called ICRF 187 has been shown to reduce or minimize doxorubicin-induced cardiotoxicity in dogs and humans. The treatment for dysrhythmias includes stopping infusion of the drug and the use of antiarrhythmic agents, if indicated. Dox-

KEY POINT:

Doxorubicin may cause cardiomyopathy. Therefore, dogs with pre-existing cardiac disease should be treated with extreme caution.

orubicin use should be discontinued if cardiomyopathy is detected. In addition, milrinone or digoxin, diuretics, a low-salt diet, and vasodilators may be employed as standard medical supportive care for congestive heart failure.

Cystitis

Cyclophosphamide is known to induce a sterile chemical cystitis. Clinical signs include stranguria, hematuria, and dysuria. Treatment of this problem includes substituting another alkylating agent (e.g., chlorambucil) for the cyclophosphamide to prevent exacerbation of the condition. Palliative therapy with intravesicular installation of dilute 1% formalin or dilute dimethylsulfoxide (DMSO) (20 ml of a 25% solution instilled for 20 minutes) may be beneficial in severe cases. In each case, urine should be collected for culture and sensitivity, as secondary infections are common. Appropriate antibiotics may be used if cystitis becomes septic. The risk of developing cystitis can be reduced by administering the drug in the morning (allowing maximum opportunity to urinate during the day), encouraging fluid intake (salting food, etc.), and, if in a combination protocol that includes prednisone, administering cyclophosphamide at the same time as the glucocorticoid because of the tendency of steroids to induce polydipsia and secondary polyuria.

Neurotoxicity

Vincristine, 5-fluorouracil, and cisplatin are reported to cause neurotoxicity in animals. The neuropathy associated with vincristine presents as a peripheral neuropathy, whereas 5-fluorouracil has been shown to cause severe seizures and disorientation in dogs and cats. Because neurologic signs are sufficiently severe in cats, 5-fluorouracil is contraindicated in that species. Rarely does cisplatin cause deafness.

Local Dermatologic Toxicity

Doxorubicin, actinomycin D, vincristine, and vinblastine have been known to cause a severe localized cellulitis if they are extravasated. These extravasation reactions[2] are discussed in the Extravasation of Chemotherapeutic Agents chapter in the Oncologic Emergencies section. Briefly, the treatment for this problem includes stopping the injection, aspirating the drug and 5 ml of blood back into the syringe, and then withdrawing the syringe. For doxorubicin, vincristine, and vinblastine perivascular injections, it may be helpful to infiltrate the area with 4 to 6 ml of 8.4% sodium bicarbonate and approximately 8 mg of dexamethasone and then apply warm compresses. For deep, ulcerative lesions, aggressive surgical debridement and skin grafts may be necessary.

Pulmonary Toxicity

Bleomycin and cisplatin have been associated with the development of pulmonary toxicoses. Bleomycin can induce a severe pulmonary fibrosis. Even in very low doses, cisplatin may induce a severe, often fatal pulmonary edema and pleural effusion in cats; therefore, cisplatin is contraindicated in this species.

SPECIFIC DRUGS USED IN VETERINARY CHEMOTHERAPY

Drugs used in chemotherapy can be classified as alkylating agents, antimetabolites, antibiotics, enzymes, plant alkaloids, nitrosoureas, and synthetic anticancer drugs. Note that under cost, the range is from $/$$$$ to $$$$/$$$$, with $$$$/$$$$ being the most expensive.

Alkylating Agents

Alkylating agents, such as cyclophosphamide, chlorambucil, and melphalan, are cell-cycle nonspecific drugs that act by cross-linking DNA.

KEY POINT:

Any chemotherapeutic agent that is administered intravenously should be given through a "first stick" patent catheter to prevent extravasation of the drug.

CYCLOPHOSPHAMIDE *(Trade name: Cytoxan, Endoxan, Neosar)*

Supplier: Bristol-Meyers, Elkins-Sinn Inc., Adria Labs, Wyeth-Aherst Labs

Generic available: No

Dose supplied: 25- and 50-mg tablets; 100-mg, 200-mg, 500-mg, 1-g and 2-g vials

Dosage: 50 mg/m^2 PO daily in morning, 3 to 4 days/week; 250 mg/m^2 every 3 weeks orally

Route of administration: Orally in morning; IV over 20 to 30 minutes. May be mixed with saline for IV administration. Shake IV drug well; allow to stand for 10 to 15 minutes so crystals dissolve completely.

Storage: Vials of unreconstituted drug can be stored at room temperature. After reconstitution, the solution should be used within 24 hours if stored at room temperature or within 6 days if refrigerated.

Cost: $/$$$$

Mechanism of action: Alkylating agent; prevents cell division by cross-linking strands of DNA.

Metabolism: The drug requires in vivo activation by enzymes (phosphamidase) in the liver and serum. Cyclophosphamide and its metabolites are excreted by the kidney. Dosage of cyclophosphamide should be reduced if serum creatinine levels are greater than 2 mg/dl.

Toxicity: Vomiting occurs frequently with IV administration and usually begins 6 hours after administration of the drug. Oral administration may reduce the incidence of vomiting.

Leukopenia may be the dose-limiting toxicity. The nadir is 7 to 14 days. Recovery is in 7 to 10 days after the nadir. Thrombocytopenia usually is not a problem. Sterile chemical cystitis may occur in some dogs treated with IV and oral cyclophosphamide. This is believed to result from chemical irritation of the bladder by metabolites of cyclophosphamide and has been associated with development of bladder tumors in dogs and humans. The risk of this complication can be reduced by maintaining high fluid intake (salting food), frequent urination, morning administration, and concurrent use of corticosteroids. If cyclophosphamide-induced hemorrhagic cystitis occurs, use of the drug should be discontinued indefinitely.

Note: Cyclophosphamide is one of the most common and effective antineoplastic agents used in veterinary medicine. This drug is effective for the treatment of lymphoma, soft tissue sarcomas (when combined with vincristine and doxorubicin), feline mammary neoplasia (when combined with doxorubicin), and other sarcomas.

CHLORAMBUCIL *(Trade name: Leukeran)*

Supplier: Burroughs Wellcome
Generic available: No
Dose supplied: 2-mg tablets
Dosage: 0.1 mg/kg daily, 6–8 mg/m² daily
Route of administration: Orally
Storage: Store at room temperature.
Cost: $$/$$$$
Mechanism of action: Alkylating agent similar to nitrogen mustard.
Metabolism: The drug is well absorbed from the gastrointestinal (GI) tract, but information on metabolism is incomplete.
Toxicity: Toxicity can include bone marrow suppression, alopecia, and GI signs. In the original toxicity studies performed by the National Cancer Institute, cerebellar toxicity was the dose-limiting toxicity in dosages exceeding 8 mg/m² orally daily.
Note: Chlorambucil is used for treatment of lymphoma (especially when substituted for cyclophosphamide in those patients with an induced sterile hemorrhagic cystitis) and chronic lymphocytic leukemia. Remissions of longer than 1 year often have been reported in patients with chronic lymphocytic leukemia treated with chlorambucil.

MELPHALAN *(Trade name: Alkeran)*

Supplier: Burroughs Wellcome
Generic available: No
Dose supplied: 2-mg tablets, 500-mg vial
Dosage: 0.1 mg/kg daily for 10 days, then 0.05 mg/kg/day; 2 mg/m² daily, administered for 7 to 10 days, then no therapy for 2 to 3 weeks
Route of administration: Orally or IV
Storage: Store at room temperature; injectable must be used within 60 minutes of reconstitution.
Cost: $$/$$$$
Mechanism of action: Alkylating agent; cytotoxic action produced by cross-linking of DNA.
Metabolism: Absorption from GI tract; erratic metabolism.
Toxicity: Myelosuppression can be marked. Recovery may take up to 4 weeks. IV product may cause severe slough if injected perivascularly.
Note: Melphalan has been used for several years to treat multiple myeloma (also known as plasma cell myeloma). Remissions exceeding 1 year frequently have been reported. Melphalan has been used with limited success to treat oral malignant melanoma, macroglobulinemia, and polycythemia.

N.N', N" TRIETHYLENETHIOPHOSPHORAMIDE
(Trade Name: Thiotepa)

Supplier: Lederle
Generic available: No
Dose supplied: 15-mg vial
Dosage: Maximum systemic dosage 9 mg/m². Bladder instillation: 30 mg/m² once every 3 to 4 weeks; remove after 1 hour.
Route of administration: For intravesicular administration into bladder, 5 to 10 mg powder diluted in 30 ml of 0.9% NaCl. For systemic administration, give IM or SQ. Drug may be administered into the pleural or abdominal cavity. Maximum systemic dose is 9 mg/m².
Storage: Refrigerate the vial until use. The reconstituted solution is stable at 4°C for 5 days.
Cost: $$/$$$$
Mechanism of action: Alkylating agent; multiple cross-linking of DNA.

Metabolism: The metabolism of this drug is unknown. Twenty percent of the dose introduced into the bladder for topical treatment is absorbed systemically.

Toxicity: Myelosuppression is the dose-limiting toxicity. Leukopenia and thrombocytopenia reach their nadir at 7 to 28 days.

Note: Thiotepa has been used to treat transitional cell carcinoma of the bladder (intravesicularly) and malignant pleural or peritoneal effusions (intracavitary).

BUSULFAN (*Trade name: Myleran*)

Supplier: Burroughs Wellcome

Generic available: No

Dose supplied: 2-mg tablets

Dosage: 2 mg/m^2 daily

Route of administration: Orally

Storage: Store at room temperature.

Cost: $/$$$$

Mechanism of action: Alkylating agent

Metabolism: The drug is well absorbed orally. Metabolites are excreted in the urine.

Toxicity: Myelosuppression is the major toxicity. Thrombocytopenia may be particularly dangerous. Prolonged bone marrow supression may occur. Pulmonary fibrosis has been reported in humans.

Note: Busulfan has been reported to be effective for the treatment of chronic myelogenous leukemia and polycythemia.

HYDROXYUREA (*Trade name: Hydrea*)

Supplier: Immunex

Generic available: No

Dose supplied: 500-mg capsules

Dosage: 80 mg/kg every 3 days. Capsule can be mixed in water and administered immediately to the patient if it is unable to swallow capsules.

Route of administration: Orally

Storage: Store at room temperature.

Cost: $/$$$$

Mechanism of action: Inhibits DNA synthesis.

Metabolism: The drug is rapidly absorbed from the GI tract and excreted in the urine.

Toxicity: Myelosuppression is often rapid and marked; thus, frequent monitoring of white blood cells (WBCs) for dose adjustment is required.

Note: Hydroxyurea has been used to treat chronic myelogenous leukemia and polycythemia.

Antimetabolites

Antimetabolites act by interfering with biosynthesis of nucleic acids by substituting them for normal metabolites and inhibiting normal enzymatic reactions. The dose of each drug differs with different protocols.

METHOTREXATE (*Trade name: Rheumatrex*)

Supplier: Lederle, Astra, Mylan

Generic available: No

Dose supplied: 2.5-mg tablets; 5-mg, 20-mg, 50-mg, 100-mg, 200-mg, 250-mg, and 1-g vials for injection

Dosage: 2.5 mg/m^2 daily

Route of administration: Orally, IV, IM, or SQ

Storage: Store at room temperature.

Cost: $/$$$$

Mechanism of action: Antimetabolite; inhibits the conversion of folic acid to tetrahydrofolic acid by binding to the enzyme dihydrofolate reductase, which inhibits synthesis of thymidine and purines that are essential for DNA synthesis.

Metabolism: A large percentage of the drug is excreted in the urine unchanged. The drug is bound to serum albumin, so simultaneous administration of drugs that displace the methotrexate from the plasma protein (i.e., sulfa drugs, aspirin, chloramphenicol, phenytoin, and tetracycline) should be avoided to prevent excessive toxicity. Daily dosage should be divided by serum creatinine level if above 2 mg/dl. The drug must be protected from light. Vials may be frozen.

Toxicity: Vomiting occurs frequently but may be prevented by premedication with antiemetics. The nadir of myelosuppression is at 6 to 9 days.

Note: Methotrexate has been used in combination with other drugs to treat lymphoma and osteosarcoma. Methotrexate, a folic acid-inhibitor, can be given at a very high dose and then reversed ("rescued") with leucovorin.

6-MERCAPTOPURINE *(Trade name: Purinethol, 6MP)*

Supplier: Burroughs Wellcome
Generic available: No
Dose supplied: 50-mg tablets
Dosage: 50 mg/m² daily
Route of administration: Orally
Storage: Store at room temperature.
Cost: $$/$$$$
Mechanism of action: Purine antimetabolite; inhibits nucleotide synthesis required for RNA and DNA synthesis.
Metabolism: The drug is metabolized by the liver and also is degraded by the enzyme xanthine oxidase. Xanthine oxidase is the enzyme inhibited by allopurinol, so concurrent use of other drugs that use this enzyme necessitates a 75% dosage reduction.
Toxicity: Myelosuppression is the major toxicity.
Note: 6-mercaptopurine has been suggested as a treatment for leukemia and lymphoma. Results are varied.

5-FLUOROURACIL *(Trade name: 5-FU, Efudex cream, Fluoroplex topical, Fluorouracil injection)*

Supplier: Roche, Allergan Herbert
Generic available: No
Dose supplied: 500-mg, 5-g ampules or vials; 1% or 2% topical ointment or solution
Dosage: 5–10 mg/kg weekly IV
Route of administration: IV push; topical
Storage: Store at room temperature; protect from light.
Cost: $/$$$$
Mechanism of action: Pyrimidine antimetabolite; blocks methylation reaction of deoxyuridylic acid to thymidylic acid, interfering with synthesis of DNA and, to a lesser extent, RNA.

Metabolism: The drug is metabolized by the liver and partially excreted by the kidneys.
Toxicity: This drug is extremely neurotoxic in cats; therefore, it is contraindicated in that species. Myelosuppression (neutropenia and thrombocytopenia) reaches a nadir in 9 to 14 days.
Note: This drug has had limited use in veterinary medicine because of its neurotoxicity. It reportedly is effective for the treatment of tumors of the GI tract. 5-FU is available as a topical cream and has been used to treat superficial malignancies, including cutaneous lymphoma and squamous cell carcinoma, with varying results.

CYTOSINE ARABINOSIDE, CYTARABINE *(Trade name: Cytosar-U)*

Supplier: Upjohn
Generic available: No
Dose supplied: 100-mg, 500-mg, 1-g, and 2-g vials
Dosage: 100 mg/m² daily IV continuous infusion for 4 days; if no toxicity, increase to 150 mg/m² daily for 4 days OR 10 mg/m² SQ daily.
Route of administration: IV, SQ. If administered IV, infuse via a volutrol over 10 to 20 minutes or as continuous infusion over 48 to 96 hours.
Storage: Store at room temperature. The reconstituted solution is stable at room temperature for 48 hours. Discard any solution in which a slight haze develops.
Cost: $/$$$$
Mechanism of action: Antimetabolite. Pyrimidine analogue; inhibits DNA synthesis.
Metabolism: The drug is activated and inactivated by liver enzymes.
Toxicity: Myelosuppression is the major toxicity. Leukopenia and thrombocytopenia frequently occur and apparently are related to the dose and frequency of administration. They reach a nadir at 7 to 14 days. Fever and thrombophlebitis are rarely seen.
Note: This drug has been used alone or in combination with other drugs to treat lymphoreticular neoplasms and myeloproliferative disorders. It has

been administered intrathecally to treat lymphoma of the CNS.

Antibiotics

Antibiotics form stable complexes (intercalate) with DNA and therefore inhibit DNA or RNA synthesis. Examples of antibiotics used in chemotherapy include doxorubicin, bleomycin, and actinomycin D.

DOXORUBICIN *(Trade name: Adriamycin, Doxorubicin, Rubex)*

Supplier: Adria Labs, Astra, Cetus Oncology, Immunex

Generic available: Yes

Dose supplied: 10-mg, 20-mg, 50-mg, 150-mg, and 200-mg vials

Dosage: Dogs: 30 mg/m^2; cats and very small dogs: 1 mg/kg IV every 3 weeks, total cumulative dosage of ≤180–240 mg/m^2.

Route of administration: Dilute with sodium chloride (250 ml) and administer IV over 30 minutes or give undiluted drug at a rate of 1 ml/minute IV. (*Do not* heparinize because this will cause precipitation.)

Storage: Store at room temperature. Reconstituted solution is stable for months if refrigerated. Avoid storing with needles with aluminum hubs.

Cost: Generic: $$/$$$$

Mechanism of action: Antitumor antibiotic; inhibits DNA and RNA synthesis.

Metabolism: The drug is metabolized predominantly by the liver. Approximately 50% of the drug is excreted in the bile. In animals with bilirubin levels above 2, the dose should be reduced 50% to reduce toxicity. The drug is also excreted in the urine and causes a red color in the urine for up to 2 days after administration.

Toxicity: Leukopenia and thrombocytopenia have a nadir at 7 to 10 days. Cardiotoxicity seems to be the most severe and dose-limiting toxicity. The cardiomyopathy produced by doxorubicin results in irreversible congestive heart failure. Based on limited experience, dogs apparently are more sensitive to these effects than cats and humans, and a cumulative dose of more than 180 to 240 mg/m^2 should not be exceeded without cardiac monitoring. Extravasation will cause severe tissue necrosis. Doxorubicin also causes a unique hemorrhagic colitis in dogs 2 to 4 days after administration. The drug has been reported to cause a unique renal toxicity in cats and dogs. Allergic reactions occur occasionally. They may be eliminated by slowing the infusion or by pretreating with antihistamines. Severe hair loss is seen in about half the dogs. Breeds such as poodles and Old English sheepdogs are the most severely affected.

Note: Doxorubicin is used to treat lymphoma, thyroid carcinomas, sarcomas, and mammary neoplasia. This antineoplastic agent seems to have a broad spectrum of activity against a variety of tumors.

MITOXANTRONE *(Trade name: Novantrone)*

Supplier: Lederle

Generic available: No

Dose supplied: 20-mg, 25-mg, and 30-mg multidose vial

Dosage: Dogs: 6 mg/m^2 IV every 3 weeks; cats: 6.5 mg/m^2 IV every 3 weeks administered over at least 3 minutes.

Route of administration: IV

Storage: Store at room temperature. The drug is incompatible with heparin. Do not freeze.

Cost: $$$/$$$$

Mechanism of action: Intercalates DNA; inhibits DNA and RNA synthesis.

Metabolism: Liver

Toxicity: Bone marrow suppression, GI toxicity, and alopecia. Unlike doxorubicin, this drug does not readily cause allergic reactions, cardiomyopathy, cardiac arrhythmias, colitis, and tissue damage at the site of extravasation. It is more myelosuppressive than doxorubicin and can cause alopecia and GI disturbances.

Note: Mitoxantrone is moderately effective for the

treatment of lymphoma, squamous cell carcinoma, transitional cell carcinoma, mammary gland tumors, and a number of other neoplastic conditions.

IDARUBICIN *(Trade name: Idamycin)*
Supplier: Adria Labs
Generic available: No
Dose supplied: 2-mg tablets; 5-mg and 10-mg vials
Dosage: 2 mg per cat
Route of administration: Orally, IV
Storage: Store at room temperature. Injectable form stable for 7 days if refrigerated. Incompatible with heparin.
Cost: $$$$/$$$$
Mechanism of action: Antitumor antibiotic; inhibits DNA and RNA synthesis.
Metabolism: The drug is metabolized predominantly by the liver.
Toxicity: The drug causes bone marrow suppression, GI disturbances, and whisker loss in cats.
Note: Orally administered idarubicin has been shown to be effective for the treatment of lymphoma in cats.

BLEOMYCIN *(Trade name: Blenoxane)*
Supplier: Bristol-Myers Oncology
Generic available: No
Dose supplied: 15-unit vial (1 unit = 1 mg)
Dosage: 0.3–0.5 units/kg weekly IM or SQ to an accumulated dosage of 125–200 mg/m². IV push over at least 10 minutes.
Route of administration: IM, SQ. May cause pain at injection site. IV administration should be slow (1 unit/min).
Storage: Store for 24 hours at room temperature. Drug can be stored for 1 to 2 months if refrigerated and for 2 years if frozen. This drug should not be used with heparin.
Cost: $$$$/$$$$
Mechanism of action: Antitumor antibiotic; inhibits DNA synthesis and, to a lesser extent, RNA and protein synthesis.
Metabolism: The drug is rapidly excreted by the kid-

ney. If renal failure occurs, dose should be reduced by dividing calculated dose by serum creatinine level.
Toxicity: Pulmonary fibrosis has been reported in dogs and humans and seems to be dose-related. A maximum cumulative dose of 200 mg/m² is recommended. In addition, allergic reactions in the form of a fever have been reported (1mg = 1 unit).
Note: Bleomycin has been suggested as a treatment for squamous cell carcinoma. Bleomycin currently is cost-prohibitive for most cases.

ACTINOMYCIN D *(Trade Name: Dactinomycin)*
Supplier: Merck, Sharp and Dohme
Generic available: No
Dose supplied: 0.5-mg vials
Dosage: 0.5–0.9 mg/m² IV slow infusion (20 minutes) every 3 weeks.
Route of administration: IV. May cause pain at injection site. IV administration should be slow (over a minimum of 20 minutes).
Storage: Use within 24 hours of reconstitution because of the absence of preservatives.
Cost: $/$$$$
Mechanism of action: Antitumor antibiotic that inhibits DNA synthesis and, to a lesser extent, RNA and protein synthesis.
Metabolism: Excreted by the liver.
Toxicity: Bone marrow suppression, GI toxicity, alopecia, and extravasation reaction can occur with this drug.
Note: This drug has been used to treat lymphoma and sarcomas in dogs.

Enzymes
The enzyme most commonly used in veterinary and human medicine is L-asparaginase.

L-ASPARAGINASE *(Trade name: Elspar)*
Supplier: Merck, Sharp and Dohme
Generic available: No
Dose supplied: 10,000-unit vials
Dosage: 10,000 units/m²

Route of administration: IM

Storage: Refrigerate. Reconstituted drug may be active for up to 7 days. Do not use if cloudy.

Cost: $$/$$$$

Mechanism of action: Enzyme; inhibits protein synthesis by depriving tumor cells of the amino acid, asparagine.

Metabolism: Not completely understood.

Toxicity: Allergic and anaphylactic reactions are seen, especially after several doses have been given. If administered IM, the incidence of anaphylaxis is minimal. If the drug is administered IV, the potential for inducing an acute anaphylactic reaction is high. Pretreatment with antihistamines and steroids may reduce reactions. If anaphylaxis occurs, L-asparaginase should be discontinued indefinitely. Other toxicities include fever and vomiting, which occur shortly after administration of the drug. The drug has been associated with acute pancreatitis.

Note: The drug is used to treat lymphoma and lymphoblastic leukemia and may be combined with other antineoplastic agents. Asparaginase does not induce a sustained remission when used alone to treat lymphoma.

Hormones

Hormones are believed to interfere with the cellular receptors that stimulate growth. The most common example of hormones used to treat cancer are the corticosteroids used to treat lymphoma and mast cell tumors.

PREDNISONE (*Trade name: Many available*)

Supplier: Many available

Generic available: Yes

Dose supplied: 5-mg, 10-mg, 20-mg, 50-mg tablets; 1 mg/ml syrup; injectable

Dosage: 30–40 mg/m^2 daily or every other day; 1 mg/kg daily for 4 weeks; 1 mg/kg every other day thereafter.

Route of administration: Orally, IV

Storage: Store at room temperature.

Cost: $/$$$$

Mechanism of action: Binds to cytoplasmic receptor sites, which then interact with DNA and prevent cell division.

Metabolism: This drug is metabolized by the liver and excreted in the urine. Prednisone is activated by the liver to its active form, prednisolone. Severe liver disease, however, does not significantly affect activation.

Toxicity: Polydipsia and polyuria are the major side effects. Long-term use may be associated with the development of alopecia and other signs of iatrogenic Cushing's syndrome.

Note: Active in the treatment of lymphoma and mast cell tumors. Prednisone does not induce a sustained remission when used alone to treat lymphoma.

Plant Alkaloids

Plant alkaloids bind to the microtubules to prevent the normal formation and function of the mitotic spindle, thus arresting the cell division in metaphase. Examples of alkaloids used in chemotherapy include vincristine and vinblastine.

VINCRISTINE (*Trade name: Oncovin*)

Supplier: Lilly, Lypho-med, Pasadena Research, Quad

Generic available: Yes

Dose supplied: 1-mg, 2-mg, and 5-mg vials; hyporets (disposable syringes: 1 and 2 mg/ml)

Dosage: 0.5–0.75 mg/m^2 weekly

Route of administration: Administer through a patent IV catheter; follow by adequate saline flush (10 ml). Protect from light until immediately before injection.

Storage: Refrigerate

Cost: Generic $/$$$$

Mechanism of action: Plant alkaloid. Causes metaphase arrest by binding to microtubular protein used in formation of mitotic spindle.

Metabolism: The drug is rapidly cleared from the plasma and excreted in the bile. Dosage should be reduced by 50% in animals with bilirubin levels greater than 2 mg/dl.

Toxicity: The drug can cause neurotoxicity and resultant paresthesia, constipation, and paralytic ileus. Anorexia in treated cats may be due to ileus. This drug is a potent irritant that can cause severe tissue irritation and necrosis if extravasated. If extravasation occurs, apply warm compresses immediately and infiltrate with saline. Myelosuppression is rare unless the drug is given in combination with L-asparaginase. Vincristine causes a marked increase in peripheral platelet count in animals with adequate megakaryocytes.

Note: Vincristine is most commonly used to treat lymphoma, transmissible venereal tumors (TVTs), and mast cell tumors. It is the drug of choice for TVTs, for which it results in a greater than 90% cure rate with an average of 3.3 doses.

VINBLASTINE (*Trade name: Velban; Sterile vinblastine sulfate USP*)

Supplier: Lilly, Cetus Oncology

Generic available: Yes

Dose supplied: 10-mg vial

Dosage: 2 mg/m^2

Route of administration: Potent irritant, avoid extravasation. Administer through a patent IV catheter. Follow by adequate saline flush (10 ml).

Storage: Refrigerated reconstituted drug is stable for 30 days. Protect from light.

Cost: Generic $/$$$$

Mechanism of action: Plant alkaloid. Causes metaphase arrest by binding to microtubular protein used in the formation of the mitotic spindle.

Metabolism: The drug is rapidly cleared from the plasma and is excreted in the bile. A 50% decrease in dose is recommended in animals with bilirubin levels over 2 mg/dl.

Toxicity: Unlike vincristine, this drug may cause severe bone marrow suppression. The WBC nadir occurs 4 to 7 days after administration. Neurotoxicity and mild peripheral neuropathies occur but

are less severe than with vincristine. Extravasation can cause severe tissue irritation and necrosis. If extravasation occurs, immediately pack with ice and infuse with saline.

Note: Vinblastine is used to treat lymphoma and mastocytoma.

Miscellaneous

CISPLATIN (CIS-DIAMMINEDICHLOROPLATINUM II)

(*Trade name: Platinol*)

Supplier: Bristol-Meyers Oncology

Generic available: No, soon

Dose supplied: 10-mg, 50-mg, and 100-mg vials

Dosage: 50–70 mg/m^2 every 3 weeks. Hydration schedules essential; (e.g., pretreat with fluids 3 hours, 25 ml/kg/hr; cisplatin IV 20 min followed by 1 hour of fluids [25 ml/kg/hr]). 10-mg vial: add 10 ml of sterile water. Aluminum causes precipitation; therefore, do not use aluminum needles.

Route of administration: Intravenous, intracavitary, and intralesional administration. There are several accepted IV administration schedules (see Appendix).

Storage: Dry powder is stable at room temperature for 2 years. The reconstituted solution is stable for 20 hours at room temperature. The reconstituted solution should not be refrigerated, because a precipitate will form.

Cost: $$$/$$$$

Mechanism of action: Similar to alkylating agents and to other heavy metals. Binds to DNA and causes cross-linkage.

Metabolism: Rapidly distributed to liver, intestine, kidneys; less than 10% is in the plasma after 1 hour. Fifty percent of the administered dose is excreted in urine in 24 to 48 hours. Dosage should be reduced if serum creatinine level is greater than normal.

Toxicity: Small dogs are more likely to develop toxicity than large dogs. Nephrotoxicity is common. It may be avoidable with adequate hydration or mannitol diuresis and careful monitoring. The nephrotoxicity is irreversible and cumulative. This necessitates careful assessment of kidney function prior to each administration. All animals should receive hydration and diuresis prior to cisplatin therapy. Nausea and vomiting within 1 hour of administration may be severe. Treatment with butorphanol (0.4 mg/kg IM immediately following cisplatin treatment) may decrease the probability of emesis. Myelosuppression is moderate to severe. The bimodal nadir occurs at days 6 and 15 after administration.

Note: Cisplatin is effective for the treatment of osteosarcoma, squamous cell carcinoma, bladder tumors, ovarian carcinoma, and mesotheliomas.

CARBOPLATIN *(Trade name: Paraplatin)*
Supplier: Bristol-Meyers Oncology
Generic available: No
Dose supplied: 50-mg, 150-mg, and 450-mg vials
Dosage: Dogs: 300 mg/m^2 every 3 weeks; cats: 150 mg/m^2 every 3 weeks (investigational).
Route of administration: IV; must be diluted with 5% dextrose in water.
Storage: Dry powder is stable at room temperature for 2 years. Once reconstituted, stable at room temperature for 8 hours.
Cost: $$$$/$$$$
Mechanism of action: Similar to alkylating agents and other heavy metals. Binds to DNA and causes cross-linkage.
Metabolism: Metabolized by the liver and kidney.
Toxicity: Myelosuppression is the most significant toxicity. Unlike cisplatin, nephrotoxicity and emesis are rare toxicities.
Note: Carboplatin is a relatively new chemotherapeutic agent that has a spectrum of activity similar to cisplatin.

PACLITAXEL *(Trade name: Taxol)*
Supplier: Bristol-Meyers Oncology
Generic available: No
Dose supplied: 50-mg/5-ml vials
Dosage: Dogs (investigational): 170 mg/m^2 every 3 weeks; cats and small dogs: 5 mg/kg.

Route of administration: IV. Must dilute with 0.9% NaCl to a concentration of 0.6 to 0.7 mg/ml. Prepare in a glass; administer through a 0.22-μm in-line filter using non-PVC tubing. Pretreat with corticosteroids, diphenhydramine, and H$_2$ receptor antagonists.
Storage: Refrigerate vials before use. Once reconstituted, stable at room temperature for 24 hours.
Cost: $$$$/$$$$
Mechanism of action: Inhibits microtubule disassembly.
Metabolism: Metabolized by the liver and kidney.
Toxicity: Myelosuppression and anaphylactoid reactions are the most significant toxicities.
Note: Taxol is a relatively new chemotherapeutic agent. Studies are underway to define its usefulness in veterinary medicine.

PIROXICAM *(Trade name: Feldene)*
Supplier: Many, including Pfizer, URL
Generic available: Yes
Dose supplied: 10-mg and 20-mg capsules
Dosage: Dogs: 0.3 mg/kg daily for 4 days, then every 48 hours
Route of administration: Orally. Avoid other GI irritants and nephrotoxins.
Storage: Store at room temperature.
Cost: $$/$$$$
Mechanism of action: Unknown; possible biological response modifier.
Metabolism: Metabolized by the liver and kidney.
Toxicity: Nephrotoxicity and GI irritation.
Note: Feldene® is a nonsteroidal anti-inflammatory agent that has been shown to cause measurable regression in transitional cell carcinoma of the urinary bladder and of squamous cell carcinoma in dogs.

ETRETINATE *(Trade name: Tegison)*
Supplier: Roche
Generic available: No
Dose supplied: 10-mg and 25-mg capsules
Dosage: Dogs: 2 to 3 mg/kg TID

Route of administration: Orally
Storage: Store at room temperature.
Cost: $$$/$$$$
Mechanism of action: Differentiating agent
Metabolism: Metabolized by the liver and kidney.
Toxicity: Hepatotoxicity, nephrotoxicity, and the development of hypertriglyceridemia and keratoconjunctivitis sicca are the primary toxicities.
Note: Etretinate is valuable for the treatment of premalignant squamous cell lesions of the skin.

APPLIED CHEMOTHERAPY

As noted earlier, there are many benefits to multiple-drug treatment protocols. They generally are more effective, and tumor resistance generally develops more slowly than with single-drug treatment regimens. Disadvantages of multiple antineoplastic agents include increased cost and toxicity. Cures attributable to chemotherapy were not seen in human medicine until effective combinations were employed. Whenever drugs are used in combination, several important points must be kept in mind:

- Each drug in a combination must be effective when used alone to treat a specific malignancy.

- Drugs with overlapping toxicities should be avoided to prevent unacceptable toxicity unless they are arranged in a protocol to prevent superimposition of their toxicoses.

- Drugs should be used with an intermittent treatment schedule for maximum efficacy.

- Combined chemotherapeutics are most effective when they have different mechanisms of action and act at different stages of the cell cycle.

The following are examples of commonly used combination protocols for neoplastic conditions in veterinary medicine.

MELPHALAN AND PREDNISONE PROTOCOL FOR MULTIPLE MYELOMA

Melphalan is administered at 2 mg/m^2 daily PO for 10 days. It is then withheld for 10 days, and then given PO for 10 more days. The cycle is continued. Prednisone is given at 40 mg/m^2 daily PO for 10 days, then 40 mg/m^2 is given every other day.

A CBC is taken at the beginning and end of each 10-day course of melphalan.

Day	Melphalan	Prednisone	CBC
1	•	•	•
2	•	•	
3	•	•	
4	•	•	
5	•	•	
6	•	•	
7	•	•	
8	•	•	
9	•	•	
10	•	•	•
11			
12		•	
13			
14		•	
15			
16		•	
17			
18		•	
19			
20		•	
21	•		•
22	•	•	
23	•		
24	•	•	
25	•		
26	•	•	
	⇓	⇓	⇓

DOXORUBICIN AND CISPLATIN: PROTOCOL 1[8]

Doxorubicin is administered at 30 mg/m^2 IV. Cisplatin is given at 60 mg/m^2 IV.

Day	Doxorubicin	Cisplatin
1	•	
21		•
41	•	
61		•

DOXORUBICIN AND CISPLATIN: PROTOCOL 2

1) Pretreatment fluid diuresis (4 hours)
   (18.3 ml/kg/hr, 0.9% NaCl) _____ ml/hr

2) Doxorubicin treatment:
   Dose: 17.5 mg/m^2 _____ mg _____ ml
   (Given as IV bolus over 20 minutes)

3) Cisplatin infusion (20 minutes)
   Dose: 60–70 mg/m^2 IV
   Rate = 18.3 ml/kg/hr _____ ml/hr

4) Posttreatment antiemetic
   (Butorphanol, 0.4 mg/kg IM)
   _____ mg _____ ml

5) Posttreatment diuresis (2 hours)
   (18.3 ml/kg/hr, 0.9% NaCl) _____ ml/hr

V.A.C. PROTOCOL

(vincristine, Adriamycin® [doxorubicin], cyclophosphamide [Cytoxan®])

Doxorubicin is administered at 30 mg/m^2 IV to dogs and 25 mg/m^2 IV to cats. Cyclophosphamide (Cytoxan®) is given at 50 mg/m^2 PO. The dose for vincristine is 0.75 mg/m^2 IV.

Day	Doxorubicin*	Cytoxan®	Vincristine	CBC
1	•			•
3		•		
4		•		
5		•		
6		•		
7			•	•
14			•	
21	•			•
24		•		
25		•		
26		•		
27		•		
28			•	
35			•	
42	•			•
45		•		
46		•		
47		•		
48		•		
49			•	
56			•	
63	•			•
66		•		
67		•		
68		•		
69		•		
70			•	•
77			•	

REPEAT CYCLE EVERY 21 DAYS (Doxorubicin on day 0, 21, 42, etc., followed by the rest of the protocol as shown above.)

*If the neutrophil count is <1500/µl on day 7 of a cycle, the dose of doxorubicin should be reduced by 25%. Doxorubicin should be given only if the pretreatment CBC shows a neutrophil count >3000/µl.

DOXORUBICIN AND CYCLOPHOSPHAMIDE PROTOCOL[9]

The dose for doxorubicin is 30 mg/m^2 IV for dogs and 25 mg/m^2 IV for cats. Cyclophosphamide is given at 50 mg/m^2 PO each day for 4 consecutive days.

Day	Doxorubicin*	Cyclophosphamide	CBC
1	•		•
3		•	
4		•	
5		•	
6		•	
7			•
21	•		•
23		•	
24		•	
25		•	
26		•	
27			•
42	•		•
43		•	
44		•	
45		•	
46		•	
47			•
	⇓	⇓	⇓

*If the neutrophil count is <1500/µl on day 7 of a cycle, the dose of doxorubicin should be reduced by 25%. Doxorubicin should be given only if the pretreatment CBC shows a neutrophil count >3000/µl.

REFERENCES

1. Chabner BA: Principles of cancer therapy, in Wyngaarden JB, Smith LH (eds): *Cecil Textbook of Medicine.* Philadelphia, WB Saunders, 1982, p 1032.
2. Ogilvie GK: Principles of oncology, in Morgan RV (ed): *Handbook of Small Animal Internal Medicine.* Philadelphia, Churchill Livingston, 1992, pp 799–812.
3. MacEwen EG, Rosenthal RC: Approach to treatment of cancer patients, in Ettinger SJ (ed): *Textbook of Veterinary Internal Medicine.* Philadelphia, WB Saunders, 1989, pp 527–546.
4. Rosenthal RC: Chemotherapy, in Slatter D (ed): *Textbook of Small Animal Surgery,* ed 2. Philadelphia, WB Saunders, 1993, pp 2067–2074.
5. Moore AS: Recent advances in chemotherapy for nonlymphoid malignant neoplasms. *Compend Contin Educ Pract Vet* 15:1039–1052, 1993.
6. Vail DM: Recent advances in chemotherapy for lymphoma of dogs and cats. *Compend Contin Educ Pract Vet* 15:1031–1037, 1993.
7. O'Brien MG, Straw RC, Withrow SJ: Recent advances in the treatment of canine appendicular osteosarcoma. *Compend Contin Educ Pract Vet* 15:939–947, 1993.
8. Mauldin GN, Metus RE, Withrow SJ, et al: Canine osteosarcoma. Treatment by amputation versus amputation and adjuvant chemotherapy using doxorubicin and cisplatin. *J Vet Intern Med* 2:177–180, 1988.
9. Jeglum KA, DeGuzman E, Young KM, et al: Chemotherapy of advanced mammary adenocarcinoma in 14 cats. *JAVMA* 187(2):157–160, 1985.

APPENDIX
Toxicities of Some Commercially Available Anticancer Drugs and Hormones
(Dose-limiting effects are italicized)

Drug	Acute Toxicity	Delayed Toxicity
Asparaginase	*Anaphylaxis* or hypersensitivity (less likely if given IM), nausea and vomiting, fever, chills, abdominal pain, and hyperglycemia leading to coma	CNS depression or hyperexcitability, acute hemorrhagic pancreatitis, coagulation defects, thrombosis, renal damage, and hepatic damage
Bleomycin	*Nausea and vomiting, fever,* anaphylaxis, and other allergic reactions	*Pneumonitis and pulmonary fibrosis,* rash, and alopecia
Busulfan	*Nausea and vomiting* and rare diarrhea	*Bone marrow suppression,* pulmonary infiltrates and fibrosis, hyperpigmentation, alopecia, and leukemia
Cisplatin	*Nausea and vomiting,* anaphylactic reactions, fever, hemolytic–uremic syndrome, and pulmonary edema (cats); never use systemically in cats	*Renal damage,* bone marrow suppression, ototoxicity, hemolysis, hypomagnesemia, and peripheral neuropathy
Carmustine	*Nausea and vomiting* and local phlebitis	*Leukopenia and thrombocytopenia* (may be prolonged), pulmonary fibrosis (may be irreversible), renal damage, and reversible liver damage
Chlorambucil	*Bone marrow suppression,* pulmonary infiltrates and fibrosis, leukemia, hepatic toxicity, and hallucinations	
Cyclophosphamide	*Nausea and vomiting* and Type I (anaphylactoid) hypersensitivity	*Bone marrow suppression,* hemorrhagic cystitis, bladder fibrosis and cancer, sterility may be temporary, pulmonary infiltrates and fibrosis, hyponatremia, leukemia, and alopecia
Cytarabine HCl	*Nausea and vomiting,* diarrhea, and anaphylaxis	*Bone marrow suppression,* oral ulceration, hepatic damage, and fever
Dacarbazine	*Nausea and vomiting,* diarrhea, anaphylaxis, and pain on administration	*Bone marrow suppression,* renal impairment, hepatic necrosis, photosensitivity, and alopecia
Dactinomycin	*Nausea and vomiting,* diarrhea, local reaction and phlebitis, and anaphylactoid reaction	*Stomatitis, oral ulceration, bone marrow suppression,* alopecia, folliculitis, and dermatitis in previously irradiated areas

APPENDIX (continued)

Drug	Acute Toxicity	Delayed Toxicity
Daunorubicin	*Nausea and vomiting,* diarrhea, severe local tissue damage and necrosis on extravasation, transient ECG changes, and anaphylactoid reaction	*Bone marrow suppression, cardiotoxicity* (may be irreversible), *alopecia,* anorexia, diarrhea, and fever and chills
Doxorubicin	*Nausea and vomiting,* severe local tissue damage and necrosis on extravasation, diarrhea and colitis, transient ECG changes, ventricular arrhythmia, anaphylactoid reaction, and urticaria and pruritus after 1 injection	*Bone marrow suppression, cardiotoxicity,* stomatitis, anorexia, diarrhea, fever, renal damage (cats), and alopecia
Etoposide VP16-213	*Nausea and vomiting, profound hypotension, anaphylaxis, cutaneous reactions,* diarrhea, and fever	*Bone marrow suppression,* peripheral neuropathy, allergic reactions, hepatic damage, and alopecia
Floxuridine	*Nausea and vomiting,* and diarrhea	*Oral and GI ulcers, bone marrow suppression,* alopecia, and dermatitis
Fluorouracil	*Nausea and vomiting,* diarrhea and hypersensitivity reaction; never use in cats	*Oral and GI ulcers, bone marrow suppression,* neurologic defects, and alopecia
Hydroxyurea	*Nausea and vomiting*	*Bone marrow suppression,* stomatitis, dysuria, and alopecia
Lomustine	*Nausea and vomiting*	*Delayed* (4 to 6 weeks) *leukopenia and thrombocytopenia* (may be prolonged), transient elevation of transaminase activity, neurological reactions, and pulmonary fibrosis
Mechlorethamine	*Nausea and vomiting* and local reaction and phlebitis	*Bone marrow suppression,* diarrhea, oral ulcers, pulmonary infiltrates and fibrosis, leukemia, and alopecia
Melphalan	Mild nausea and hypersensitivity reactions	*Bone marrow suppression* (especially platelets), pulmonary infiltrates and fibrosis, and leukemia
Methotrexate	*Nausea and vomiting,* diarrhea, fever, and anaphylaxis	*Oral and GI ulcers; bone marrow suppression;* hepatic toxicity, including cirrhosis and acute hepatic necrosis; renal toxicity; pulmonary infiltrates and fibrosis; alopecia; depigmentation; and encephalopathy and anaphylactoid reactions with high doses

APPENDIX (continued)

Drug	*Acute Toxicity*	*Delayed Toxicity*
Mercaptopurine	*Nausea and vomiting* and diarrhea	*Bone marrow suppression; cholestasis and, rarely, hepatic necrosis; oral and intestinal ulcers;* and pancreatitis
Mitotane	*Nausea and vomiting* and diarrhea	*Adrenal insufficiency, CNS depression*, rash, albuminuria, and hypertension
Mitoxantrone	*Nausea and vomiting*	*Bone marrow suppression*
Thiotepa	*Nausea and vomiting* and local pain	*Bone marrow suppression*, pulmonary infiltrates and fibrosis, and leukemia
Vinblastine sulfate	*Nausea and vomiting* and local reaction and phlebitis with extravasation	*Bone marrow suppression*, stomatitis, loss of deep tendon reflexes, jaw pain, muscle pain, paralytic ileus, inappropriate ADH secretion, and alopecia
Vincristine	Local slough with extravasation	*Peripheral neuropathy*, mild bone marrow suppression, constipation, paralytic ileus, inappropriate ADH secretion, hepatic damage, jaw pain, seizures, and alopecia

Adapted from Ogilvie GK: Principles of oncology, in Morgan RV (ed): *Handbook of Small Animal Internal Medicine.* Philadelphia, Churchill Livingston, 1992, pp 799–812; with permission.

CLINICAL BRIEFING: RADIATION THERAPY— PROPERTIES, USES, AND PATIENT MANAGEMENT

Types	*Teletherapy:* External beam radiation therapy delivered by orthovoltage or megavoltage machines *Brachytherapy:* Placement of radioactive substances within or around malignant cells *Systemic Therapy:* Administration of radioactive substances that preferentially localize within specific tissues in the body
Possible Tissues Injured and Possible Therapy	*Skin:* Clean with mild soap and water; prevent self-mutilation. Other possible treatments include vitamin E and hydrogen peroxide/saline lavages as well as selected systemic therapy. Ear canals can be treated with DMSO and/or steroid-containing ear medication *Oral Cavity, Pharynx:* Consider palatable food and gastrostomy tube feeding early; oral rinses with saline or tea. Lidocaine viscous solution may help animals that experience pain when swallowing *Colon, Rectum:* Low-residue diet with a stool softener may alleviate painful defecation. Steroid enemas and a high-fiber diet may be helpful for nonresponsive colitis *Eye:* Artificial tears for keratoconjunctivitis sicca and steroid ophthalmic solution or ointment for selected nonerosive conditions after fluoroscein staining *Bone:* Bone sequestra should be removed
Selected Indications	Local control of oral tumors; nasal tumors; soft tissue sarcomas; mast cell tumors; brain tumors; thyroid tumors, including thyroid adenomas in cats; and some malignant effusions. Can be palliative for primary or metastatic bone disease

Radiation therapy has been used for decades in veterinary and human oncology. The equipment only recently became readily available to large segments of the veterinary profession, primarily through referral centers. Radiation therapy is effective for controlling a wide range of tumors in domesticated animals. Dosages range from 30 to 60 Gray (Gy), delivered in 9 to 30 treatments over 3 to 6 weeks.[1-22] This treatment modality is used alone or in combination with other cancer therapies, including surgery, chemotherapy, and hyperthermia. Radiation therapy is a local treatment; therefore, extreme care should be taken to ensure that the animal is staged properly to delineate the extent of the neoplastic process. Consultation with an oncologist is essential to determine whether a particular patient with a malignancy is likely to benefit from radiation therapy. Before the practitioner can understand the potential benefits and risks of radiation therapy, a brief review of the properties and uses of radiation therapy is warranted.

TELETHERAPY, BRACHYTHERAPY, AND SYSTEMIC RADIATION THERAPY

Teletherapy

The delivery of radiation therapy from a machine to the patient is called *teletherapy* or *external beam radiation therapy*. In veterinary medicine, external beam radiation therapy primarily is delivered by linear accelerators, radioactive cobalt (^{60}Co) or cesium (^{137}Cs) source units, or orthovoltage radiation therapy machines.

Megavoltage radiation produced either by a linear accelerator or a ^{60}Co source machine is preferred for the treatment of many neoplastic conditions (Figure 2-9). Megavoltage radiation has excellent penetrating capability and is able to reach deep-seated tumors while minimizing injury to overlying tissues. If megavoltage radiation therapy is used to treat superficial tumors, the energy must be slowed down by using a sheet of tissue-equivalent material called *bolus*, which is placed over the tumor. This allows most of the energy to be deposited more superficially on the tumor itself. Alternatively, electron beams produced by a linear accelerator can be used to treat superficial tumors, because electrons do not penetrate to deep tissues.

Orthovoltage radiation therapy, on the other hand, is not suitable for tumors lying deep within the body, because the radiation produced by orthovoltage machines does not penetrate effectively more than a few centimeters. Orthovoltage, however, is valuable for treating superficial tumors and tumors within air-filled cavities, such as nasal tumors. Orthovoltage radiation therapy units deposit maximum doses to the skin surface, which can result in injury to those tissues.

Brachytherapy

Radiation therapy is administered not only from external sources of energy, but also from implanted radiation sources within or around the tumor itself in a radiation therapy procedure termed *brachytherapy*. Brachytherapy is performed by delivering very

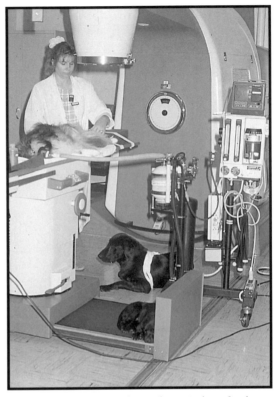

Figure 2-9: *Megavoltage radiation is the preferred treatment for many neoplastic conditions. This linear accelerator, like all other megavoltage radiation therapy units, has excellent penetrating capability and is able to reach deep-seated tumors while minimizing injury to overlying tissues.*

high dosages of radiation to very localized sites within the body. One technique involves implanting "seeds" or "straws" of radioactive materials within the tumor. Radioactive sources also can be administered into body cavities. Sources vary depending on the tissue to be implanted (e.g., cesium or radium for intracavitary placement and iridium for interstitial implants). Interstitial brachytherapy sources often are implanted in a removable package (e.g., silastic tubing) and are removed once the calculated dose has been delivered. Brachytherapy is very effec-

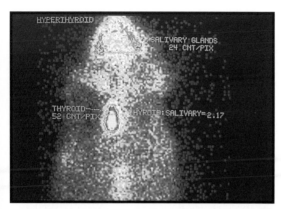

Figure 2-10: Hyperthyroidism is effectively treated with ^{131}I administered intravenously or orally. Prior to ^{131}I therapy, another radioactive material, technetium-99m, is used to determine the extent of disease. In hyperthyroid cats, technetium-99m is taken up by the abnormal thyroid gland to a much greater extent than the salivary gland.

tive for delivering extremely high doses very specifically to a local site, and normal tissue damage usually is restricted to surrounding tissues. In part, this is because the radiation particles do not usually penetrate far in tissues in this type of therapy. The amount of normal tissue injured is directly proportional to the energy of the radiation implanted or delivered to a specific site.

Systemic Therapy

Radioactive materials injected systemically are very useful for treating hyperthyroidism in cats (^{131}I) and some dogs and for selected bone tumors in dogs (Figure 2-10). The radioactive material is designed to be selectively taken up by, or incorporated in, the tissue to be treated. Many oncology centers around the world use this form of therapy. Recently, radioactive material has been linked to monoclonal antibodies that "seek out" specific tumor tissues.

TREATMENT METHODS

Delivering the proper doses of radiation therapy specifically to a tumor while minimizing normal tis-

sue damage requires the skills of highly trained individuals. In addition, specific imaging is required to delineate the extent of the tumor. Computerized treatment planning is essential to clearly delineate a safe and effective treatment method.

External beam radiation therapy can be delivered to the tumor with maximum efficacy while minimizing injury to surrounding normal tissues by using radiation planning. Radiation planning, which is usually done in combination with computerized tomography (CT), uses computer technology and lead wedges to distribute the dose evenly throughout the tumor while minimizing normal tissue injury and maximizing tumor control. Whenever external beam radiation therapy is delivered, the adverse effects of radiation therapy can be minimized by expanding the time the radiation dosage is delivered (i.e., 6 weeks versus 3 weeks), increasing the number of doses in which this energy is delivered to the patient, and delivering the radiation through several different portals while using lead "wedges" to distribute the energy evenly. Delivering radiation therapy daily (Monday through Friday) for 3 weeks is generally less toxic to normal tissues than delivering the same total dosage of energy on a twice-weekly basis over the same 3-week period.

Treatment planning precisely prescribes the best way to administer radiation therapy to control the tumor while minimizing any unnecessary morbidity to the patient. After the treatment plan has been devised, a dosage is prescribed and least toxic method of administering the energy is determined. The dosage generally is limited by the tolerance of nearby normal tissues. The goal is to have less than 5% of the patient experiencing significant toxicity. External beam radiation therapy is delivered frequently over several weeks; therefore, the animal must be positioned in the same position for each treatment. The skin can be tattooed or other methods may be used to ensure the patient is placed in the exact same position each time it is treated. Owing to the number of treatments, short-acting induction agents such as propofol are preferred prior to endotracheal intubation and isoflurane anesthesia.

FACTORS THAT INFLUENCE TUMOR CONTROL

The beneficial effect of radiation therapy depends on the modulation of at least four factors that affect irradiated cells: repair, repopulation, redistribution, and reoxygenation.

Repair

Both normal cells and tumor cells repair themselves within a few hours of irradiation, and repair from radiation injury apparently is approximately equal in normal and malignant cells. Inhibiting this repair mechanism can enhance the beneficial effects of radiation therapy on the tumor.

Repopulation

Repopulation involves the replacement of cells killed by radiation therapy with the progeny of surviving cells through cell multiplication. Both normal and malignant tissues are capable of recovering from radiation therapy in this way. The repopulation of cells differs depending on the tissue from which they originate, which explains why some tissues are more sensitive to radiation than others. Drugs or methods that reduce repopulation can enhance tumor control.

Redistribution

Redistribution of cells throughout all phases of the cell cycle (e.g., M, S, G_1, G_2, G_0) occurs after a dose of radiation therapy. Because radiation therapy is most effective in G_1 and G_2 phases, the beneficial effects of radiation therapy can be enhanced by administering treatments when the majority of cells are in these phases of the cell cycle. Fractionation of radiation therapy takes advantage of this pheonomenon.

Reoxygenation

During reoxygenation, the tumor or normal tissues re-establish an oxygen source. This is very important because hypoxic tumor cells are known to be radioresistant. Therefore, any method such as the use of drugs that enhance oxygenation and also can increase the oxygenation of tumor cells can heighten the effect of radiation therapy.

ADVERSE EFFECTS AND PATIENT MANAGEMENT[21,23]

Radiation therapy is a local treatment; therefore, side effects are confined to the area being treated. The only exception to this is when the entire body is irradiated, as with bone marrow transplantation, which is an uncommon procedure in veterinary medicine. It is important to educate the client about this localized effect regarding the way in which different tissues will respond to radiation therapy and the timing of the appearance of adverse effects.

Skin

The skin is often injured in external beam radiation therapy, particularly with orthovoltage sources (Figures 2-11 and 2-12). Acute reactions that generally appear toward the end of radiation therapy include erythema, dry desquamation with pruritus, and moist desquamation. The best treatment for these cutaneous injuries involves cleansing the area with mild soap and water, if symptomatic. A Water-Pic® or hydropulsion with a 60-ml syringe may help clean the lesion. If self-mutilation is a problem, an Elizabethan collar, side bars, or bandages should be employed. Non-petroleum-based vitamin E ointments have been used. Although controversial, some suggest that pets with severe pruritus or

> **KEY POINT:**
>
> *Generally, the acute effects of radiation therapy start toward the end of the treatment period, may actually worsen substantially 1 to 3 weeks after treatment is discontinued, and may last for several weeks. Late effects may occur 6 months to years after the end of treatment.*

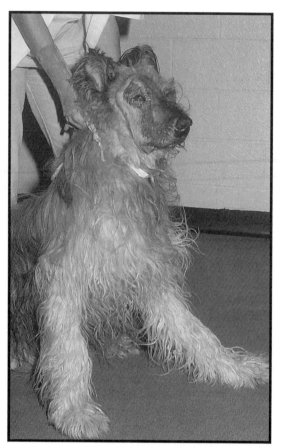

Figure 2-11: Acute reactions generally appear toward the end of radiation therapy; they include erythema, dry desquamation with pruritus, and moist desquamation. This dog was treated with radiation therapy for a nasal tumor. Acute adverse effects started in the third week of radiation therapy and worsened to this point 2 weeks later. Generally, the best treatment for these cutaneous injuries includes cleansing the area with mild soap and water, if symptomatic. A Water-Pic® or hydropulsion with a 60-ml syringe may help clean the lesion. If self-mutilation is a problem, an Elizabethan collar, side bars, or bandages should be employed. This patient recovered uneventfully.

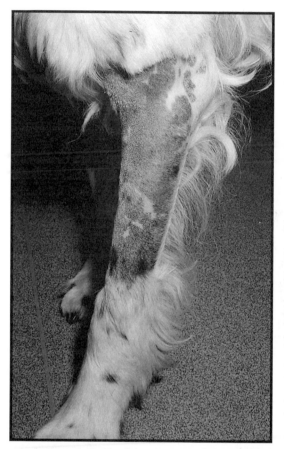

Figure 2-12: These lesions demonstrate the hyperpigmentation and alopecia that can occur months to years after the completion of the radiation therapy. The lesions on this dog occurred weeks to months after a fibrosarcoma was treated with megavoltage radiation therapy.

moist desquamation may benefit from cleansing the area with a 1:1 solution of hydrogen peroxide and normal saline and may require treatment with a top-ical or oral corticosteroid. If a topical corticosteroid is used, a non-petroleum–based product is recommended. Combining cleansing with a wetting solution such as Cara-klenz® with subsequent application of aloe vera gel extract (Carrington Dermal Wound Gel®) has been suggested. Telfa pads should be used whenever the area needs to be covered. Occasionally, a patient may develop a pruritic rash that originates

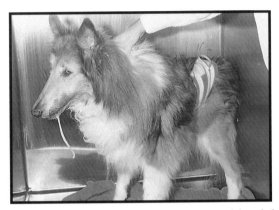

Figure 2-13: Profuse salivation may occur toward the end of radiation therapy and may persist for several weeks after the treatment is completed. The saliva is thick and tenacious and is associated with bad breath and a significant oral mucositis. The mucositis can be profound enough to cause anorexia and weight loss. A gastrostomy tube can allow enteral feeding to maintain a good plane of nutrition, which enhances quality of life and decreases morbidity and mortality.

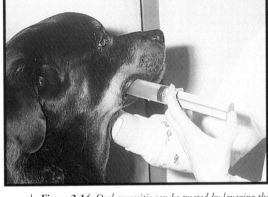

Figure 2-14: Oral mucositis can be treated by lavaging the mouth frequently with a variety of liquids, including tea. The tea contains astringents and can decrease oral discomfort, decrease the bacterial count in the mouth, and reduce the viscosity of the saliva. This improves quality of life and reduces morbidity and mortality.

from the area of treatment and spreads to areas outside the treatment field. Systemic antihistamines, such as diphenhydramine, or topical corticosteroids may be indicated for these patients. Other adverse effects that can occur at higher doses include hyperpigmentation or hypopigmentation; telangiectasia; ulceration; and fibrosis, which, if extensive, can be quite painful. Debilitating late skin changes, which are extremely rare, can be repaired with reconstructive techniques using well-vascularized tissue.

Oral Cavity and Pharynx

Damage to the oral cavity and pharynx is very common in dogs and cats that receive radiation therapy for nasal and oral tumors (Figures 2-13 and 2-14). This area can be very frustrating to treat, because radiation-induced oral mucositis may result in anorexia and secondary debilitation. Placing a gastrostomy tube before initiating radiation therapy is recommended in any animal that does not have a good plane of nutrition and any time that the oral cavity is to be included in the radiation therapy field (e.g., oral squamous cell carcinoma in older cats) Oral mucositis and anorexia are common in the acute phase of radiation therapy, and xerostomia and dental caries may be seen in the chronic phase. Occasionally, bone necrosis of the mandible or maxilla may be noted as a late injury. Because oral damage can be so debilitating, care should be taken to ensure that all necessary dental work is completed prior to the start of radiation therapy. During treatment, owners may want to rinse their pet's mouth out with a solution of salt and water (1 teaspoon in 1 quart of water). Some recommend adding Maalox® to this saltwater solution to coat the mouth. Cool tea solutions can be used to lavage the mouth 3 to 6 times per day (Figure 2-14), which may reduce the discomfort of the oral cavity and freshen the breath. If the patient experiences pain when swallowing, 5 to 15 ml of 2% lidocaine (xylocaine viscous solution) may be squirted into the mouths of dogs (this should never be done in cats because of the potential for lidocaine toxicity in this species) several times a day.

Because oral and nasal damage from radiation therapy may reduce smell and taste sensations, more palatable, warmed, aromatic foods should be prescribed. Increasing the amount of liquids given may help overcome xerostomia brought on by salivary gland radiation. Artificial saliva preparations, such as a mixture of sorbitol, sodium, carboxymethyl cellulose, and methylparaben (Salivart®) may be beneficial in these patients. Mucositis usually resolves within 21 days after radiation therapy is completed.

Colon and Rectum

Occasionally, the colon and rectum are in the area of radiation. Irritation to the colon and rectum can be manifested by bleeding, tenesmus, and pain. A low-residue diet and a stool softener may provide relief. Steroid enemas (e.g., Proctofoam®) may be beneficial in select patients. Whenever the anus and perianal areas are injured by radiation therapy, the area should be kept clean using soap and water and dried thoroughly.

Eye

The eye often is in the field of radiation therapy in dogs and cats with nasal tumors (Figure 2-15). The lens of the eye is considered sensitive to relatively low doses of radiation therapy, which can result in cataract formation months to years after radiation therapy is complete. In addition, retinal hemorrhages may result in blindness. Conjunctivitis or keratoconjunctivitis sicca may occur acutely, and it is important to monitor tear production in animals during and after therapy. For keratoconjunctivitis sicca, artificial tear preparations may be beneficial. It is important to confirm that no corneal ulcers are present before prescribing steroid-containing ophthalmic ointments.

Hematology

If a significant amount of the bone marrow is included in the radiation therapy field, bone marrow suppression may occur. In addition, all lymphocytes that pass through the radiation field are lysed.

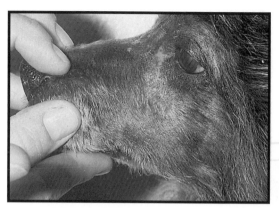

Figure 2-15: The eye often is in the field of radiation therapy for dogs and cats with tumors of the head. The lens of the eye generally is considered sensitive to relatively low doses of radiation therapy, which can result in cataract formation months to years after radiation therapy is complete. Conjunctivitis or keratoconjunctivitis sicca also may occur. This dog was treated for a nasal tumor 3 months ago. Note the alopecia and change in skin color. This patient developed conjunctivitis that resolved 3 weeks after radiation therapy was complete.

Bone

If bone is included in the radiation therapy field, bone sequestrum due to necrosis may result. This is a late effect that occurs many months to years after therapy. Removal of the sequestrum is indicated in such cases. Whenever brachytherapy is used to deliver radiotherapy to very localized areas, radiation from these local sources can damage surrounding structures, including bone.

Miscellaneous Sites

Other areas that can be damaged include the esophagus, stomach, small intestine, and liver. The endocrine system, including the pituitary gland and thyroid, may be injured whenever radiation therapy to the head and neck is performed. Lung radiation can result in radiation pneumonitis at relatively low radiation doses, which can cause decreased respiratory tidal volume. When the heart is included in the radiation therapy field, pericarditis and resultant pericardial effusion may be identified 4 to 6 months after radiation therapy is complete. A pericardectomy may be necessary to treat these animals. Whenever the urinary bladder is in the radiation therapy field, high single doses of radiation, such as those used in intraoperative radiation therapy, can result in severe fibrosis and lack of elasticity. Fibrosis also may occur as a late effect of fractionated external beam radiation therapy. Cranial radiation therapy occasionally results in headache, nausea, vomiting, and papilledema. Steroid therapy generally is indicated for these patients and should be considered during and after treatment. The most severe effect of radiation therapy to the brain includes brain necrosis, which can result in severe neurologic problems.

CLINICAL USE OF RADIATION THERAPY TO CONTROL MALIGNANT DISEASE

Radiation therapy is effective for the treatment of oral, nasal, rectal, perianal, and anal tumors; soft tissue sarcomas; mast cell tumors; osteosarcoma; lymphoproliferative disorders; malignant melanoma; and tumors of the central nervous system (CNS) in veterinary patients. The variability in response to radiation therapy of these various tumor types depends on the amount of radiation therapy delivered, the method by which radiation therapy is given, and the course and scheduling of radiation therapy. With the increased availability of megavoltage radiation therapy, computerized treatment planning, and the delineation of the extent of the disease by CT and MRI, the beneficial effects of radiation therapy are bound to increase substantially. The future of radiation therapy will be tied into the use of radiobiologic and tumor biology information to enhance the beneficial effects of radiation therapy. In addition, the combination of radiation therapy with surgery, hyperthermia, and chemotherapy may result in substantial improvement in the efficacy of this treatment modality.

Oral Tumors

The most common oral tumors in dogs are squamous cell carcinoma, malignant melanoma, fibrosar-

coma, and epulides. In cats, squamous cell carcinoma and fibrosarcoma predominate. Radiation therapy is effective for local control of many of these oral tumors.

Epulides in Dogs

Acanthomatous epulis is the most radioresponsive of all the epulides. Acanthomatous epulis differs from other epulides in that this tumor frequently invades bone. Permanent tumor control was reported in 36 of 39 dogs with acanthomatous epulides treated with orthovoltage radiation therapy.[6] Therefore, the treatment of choice for acanthomatous epulides can be either aggressive surgical resection (e.g., mandibulectomy) or radiation therapy.

Squamous Cell Carcinoma in Dogs

Squamous cell carcinomas of the oral and pharyngeal area are reported to have a moderate to good response to radiation therapy. Response rates of approximately 70% have been reported.[1] The amount of radiation therapy needed to control 50% of all carcinomas in dogs for 1 year was reported to be 38 Gy, whereas 75% of the tumors were controlled with 45 Gy.[2] In this aforementioned study, tumor control was defined as lack of any clinical evidence of any malignancy 1 year after therapy. Orthovoltage also is effective for the treatment of nontonsillar carcinomas. The disease-free interval has been reported to be 12 months for maxillary squamous cell carcinomas, 3.4 months for mandibular squamous cell carcinomas, and 1.8 months for squamous cell carcinomas of the tongue.[3] Dogs with oral squamous cell carcinomas had longer survival times following treatment if the tumor was small or occurred rostral to the second premolar tooth. Median survival times range from 12 to 20 months.

Oral Fibrosarcomas in Dogs

Fibrosarcomas occur commonly in the oral cavities of dogs; but they are unlikely to metastasize. Oral fibrosarcomas are considered to be less radioresponsive than epulides and squamous cell carcinomas. Approximately 50% tumor control at 1 year has been reported with radiation therapy.[4]

Melanomas in Dogs

Traditionally, melanomas have been considered to be radioresistant. Recent research suggests that melanomas may be one of the few tumors for which large-dose fractions are necessary to cause death of tumor cells. Therefore, high dose per fraction schedules may be warranted with malignant melanomas. Oral melanomas have a high metastatic rate, especially when the tumor is large, restricting the beneficial results of radiation therapy for this tumor.

Oral Tumors in Cats

Oral squamous cell carcinomas in cats generally are considered resistant to the effects of radiation therapy. Control rates of 10% to 20% at 1 year have been reported by one investigator.[7] Others have better results treating oral squamous cell carcinomas with a combination of radiation therapy and mitoxantrone chemotherapy for which the median survival time was 6 months, as compared to 2 months with any other treatment modality. For this treatment combination, a dose of nearly 60 Gy was delivered to the tumor.[9] Oral fibrosarcomas of cats are believed to be relatively refractory to the effects of radiation therapy.

Squamous Cell Carcinoma of Nonoral Sites

Tonsillar squamous cell carcinomas typically have a poor response to therapy, primarily because of the high metastatic rate. In a study involving eight dogs with tonsillar carcinomas, median survival time was 110 days when radiotherapy was combined with surgical excision.[11] Another study used orthovoltage radiation therapy, cisplatin, and doxorubicin to treat tonsillar squamous cell carcinomas; the median disease-free interval was 240 days, and median survival was approximately 300 days in 6 dogs.[10] Squamous cell carcinoma of the nasal planum in dogs has been reported to be refractory to the beneficial effects of radiotherapy.[12] Seventy percent of cats with dermal squamous cell carcinomas, however, have been reported to respond to this treatment modality.[7] The reason for this difference in response rate among species is unknown.

Nasal Tumors
Nasal Tumors in Dogs

There is little doubt that radiation therapy is the treatment of choice for dogs with nasal tumors. There is much variation within the literature regarding response to therapy. Surgical cytoreduction followed by orthovoltage radiation therapy offers the best prognosis; median survival time is up to 23 months.[12] Megavoltage radiation therapy generally results in control rates of nearly 1 year.[14] The prognostic factors that may influence response to therapy include tumor histology, clinical stage, tumor size, the type of radiation therapy, and the dose of energy delivered, as well as whether surgery was performed prior to radiation therapy.[15]

Nasal Tumors in Cats

Although nasal tumors are much less common in cats than in dogs, they apparently respond better to radiation therapy. In a recent study, nine cats with nasal tumors were treated with surgery prior to radiation therapy and subsequent orthovoltage treatment. This treatment resulted in mean and median survival times of 27.9 and 20.8 months, respectively.[16] Radiation therapy of intranasal lymphoma in cats can result in control times exceeding 500 days.[16] Therefore, nasal tumors are effectively treated with radiation therapy in cats, and the response to therapy depends on the histologic type of tumor.

Soft Tissue Sarcomas

Soft tissue sarcomas are challenging neoplastic conditions that frequently recur after incomplete surgical excision. In part, this is because these tumors have many "fingers" that extend out into surrounding tissues. Often, the tumor is excised only around

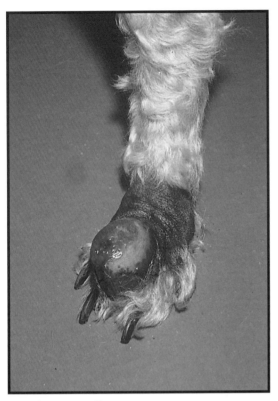

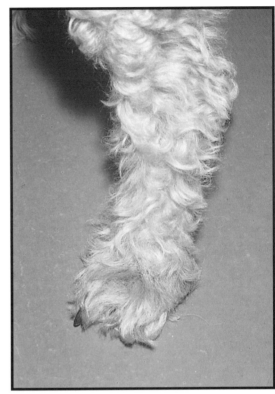

Figure 2-16A

Figure 2-16B

Figure 2-16: *This dog had a soft tissue sarcoma of the distal extremity that was treated with radiation therapy. Radiation therapy is an ideal alternative for the treatment of tumors that cannot be completely excised. The tumor was quite large prior to therapy (A). The mass was not palpable 2 months after therapy was completed (B).*

the area that can be palpated, which ensures that disease will recur. Radiation therapy frequently is used to prevent recurrence of incompletely excised tumors. In addition, radiation therapy seems to be effective for treating gross evidence of malignant soft tissue sarcomas (Figure 2-16). For example, two studies reported that 50% of dogs with soft tissue sarcomas have their disease controlled at 1 year after receiving radiation therapy dosages ranging from 45 Gy to 50 Gy delivered in 10 fractions.[4,17] Predictably, smaller tumors respond better to radiation therapy; 75% of such

tumors were controlled at 1 year when treated with 52 Gy of radiation therapy. When radiation therapy was used to treat soft tissue sarcomas after incomplete surgical excision, a 1- and 2-year disease-free interval of 60% and 41%, respectively, was reported.[18] Forelimb hemangiopericytomas tended to respond to treatment better than hindlimb hemangiopericytomas. Currently, if complete excision cannot be attained, debulking down to the level of microscopic disease followed by radiation therapy is the recommended treatment for all soft tissue sarcomas.

Mast Cell Tumors

Mast cell tumors have been shown to respond well to radiation therapy. The most significant problem of mast cell tumors is that they may not be localized. Most anaplastic mast cell tumors tend to have distant metastatic disease, which can result in poor survival times even though the local tumor can be controlled with radiation therapy. Therefore, before treating mast cell tumors with radiation therapy, a complete staging procedure must be performed. In one study, 85 dogs with mast cell tumors were treated with radiation therapy after surgical excision or after the tumor recurred following surgery.[20] The clinical stage and location of the malignant mast cell tumor affected the disease-free interval. Dogs with local disease that has been incompletely resected had a significantly longer disease-free interval than did dogs with any other stage. Regrowth occurred sooner in mast cell tumors on the trunk than in tumors on the legs. Recently, ^{60}Co radiation of incompletely excised grade II (moderately anaplastic, see the Mast Cell Tumors chapter) mast cell tumors resulted in a control rate of greater than 80% after 5 years.

Brain Tumors

Sixty-five dogs treated with radiation therapy for brain tumors at Colorado State University had a median survival time of 13.5 months. This radiotherapy was delivered to animals with and without surgical removal of the tumor. Meningiomas and hypophyseal macroadenomas were the most radioresponsive; however, responses were seen in dogs with other types of malignant disease.[21]

Other Tumors

Thyroid adenomas or adenomatous hyperplasia are treated effectively with ^{131}I with a high probability (>80%) of permanent control of this condition. Owing to the non-uniform uptake of ^{131}I, thyroid tumors in dogs are not treated as successfully with this modality.

Rectal, colonic, bladder, and prostate tumors have been treated successfully with radiation therapy. In each case, the extent of the disease must be clearly defined and the animal appropriately staged with at least abdominal radiography or ultrasonography, hemogram, biochemical profile, and urinalysis. When radiation therapy is delivered to these particular sites, problems such as dysuria, colitis, and prostatitis must be expected. Whenever possible, radiation therapy should be combined with other treatment modalities to enhance their beneficial effects.

Palliative Therapy

Radiation therapy can be given to alleviate the pain and discomfort of a wide variety of malignancies, especially those that involve bone. Palliative radiation therapy of osteosarcoma is a logical and often effective mode of improving quality of life for patients in which surgical removal or amputation is not an option.

KEY POINT:

The best tumor control for all malignancies is achieved if radiation is used early in the course of disease rather than after multiple surgeries owing to the difficulty in identifying the extent of disease in patients that have undergone multiple surgical procedures.

REFERENCES

1. Dewhirst MW, Sim DA, Sapareto S, et al: Importance of minimum tumor temperature in determining early and long term response of spontaneous canine and feline tumors to heat and radiation. *Cancer Res* 44:43–50, 1984.
2. Gillette EL, McChesney SL, Dewhirst MS, et al: Response of canine oral carcinomas to heat and radiation. *Int J Rad Oncol Biol Phys* 13:1861–1867, 1987.
3. Evans SM, Shofer F: Canine oral nontonsillar squamous cell carcinoma. Prognostic factors for recurrence and survival following orthovoltage radiation therapy. *Vet Radiol* 29: 133–137, 1988.

4. McChesney SL, Withrow SJ, Gillette EL, et al: Radiotherapy of soft tissue sarcomas in dogs. *JAVMA* 194:60–63, 1989.

5. Overgaard J, Vondermaase H, Overgaard M, et al: A randomized study comparing two high dose per fraction radiation schedules in recurrent or metastatic malignant melanoma. *Int J Rad Oncol Biol Phys* 11: 1837–1839, 1985.

6. Thrall DE: Orthovoltage radiotherapy of acanthomatous epulides in 39 dogs. *JAVMA* 184:826–829, 1984.

7. Turrel JM: Radiation and hyperthermia, in Holzworth J (ed): *Diseases of the Cat: Medicine and Surgery.* Philadelphia, WB Saunders, 1987, pp 606–619.

8. Hutson CA, Willamer CC, Walder EJ, et al: Treatment of mandibular squamous cell carcinoma in cats by use of mandibulectomy and radiotherapy: Seven cases (1987–1989). *JAVMA* 201:777–781, 1992.

9. Ogilvie GK, Moore AS, Obradovich JE, et al: Toxicoses and efficacy associated with the administration of mitoxantrone to cats with malignant tumors. *JAVMA* 11:1839–1844, 1993.

10. Brooks WMB, Matus RE, Leifer CE, et al: Chemotherapy vs chemotherapy post-radiotherapy in the treatment of tonsillar squamous cell carcinoma in the dog. *J Vet Intern Med* 2:206–211, 1988.

11. MacMillan R, Withrow SJ, Gillette EL: Surgery and regional irradiation for treatment of canine tonsillar squamous cell carcinoma: Retrospective review of eight cases. *JAAHA* 18:311–314, 1982.

12. Thrall DE, Adams WM: Radiotherapy of squamous cell carcinoma of the canine nasal plane. *Vet Radiol* 23: 193–196, 1982.

13. Thrall DE, Harvey CE: Radiotherapy of malignant nasal tumors in 21 dogs. *JAVMA* 183:663–666, 1983.

14. McEntee MC, Thrall DE, Page RL, et al: A retrospective study of 27 dogs with intranasal neoplasms treated with radiation therapy. *Vet Radiol* 32:135–139, 1991.

15. Evans SM, Goldschmidt M, McKee LJ, et al: Prognostic factors in survival after radiotherapy for intranasal neoplasms in dogs - 70 cases (1974–1985). *JAVMA* 194:1460–1463, 1989.

16. Evans SM, Hendrick M: Radiotherapy of feline nasal tumors: A retrospective study of 9 cats. *Vet Radiol* 30:128–132, 1989.

17. McChesney SL, Gillette EL, Dewhirst MW, et al: Influence of WR 2721 on radiation responsive canine soft tissue sarcomas. *Int J Rad Oncol Biol Phys* 12:1957–1963, 1986.

18. Evans SM: Canine hemangiopericytoma: A retrospective analysis of response to surgery and orthovoltage radiation. *Vet Radiol* 28:13–16, 1987.

19. Atwater SW, LaRue SM, Powers BE: Adjuvant radiotherapy of soft tissue sarcomas in dogs. *Proc Vet Canc Soc.*41–42, 1992.

20. Turrel JM, Kitchell BE, Miller LM, et al: Prognostic factors for radiation treatment of mast cell tumors in 85 dogs. *JAVMA* 193:936–940, 1988.

21. LaRue SM, Gillette EL: Recent advances in radiation oncology. *Compend Contin Educ Pract Vet* 15:795–805, 1993.

22. Elmslie RE, Ogilvie GK, LaRue, et al: Radiotherapy with and without chemotherapy for localized lymphoma in 10 cats. *Vet Radiol* 32:277–280, 1991.

23. Savage DE: Principles of radiation oncology, in Rosenthal S, Casignan JR, Smith BD (eds): *Medical Care of the Cancer Patient*, ed 2. Philadelphia, WB Saunders, 1989, pp 27–39.

CLINICAL BRIEFING: BIOLOGICAL RESPONSE MODIFIERS— PROPERTIES, USES, AND PATIENT MANAGEMENT	
Definition	Agents that reconstitute or enhance the immune system to fight the malignancy using endogenous biological processes
Categories	BCG, L-MTP-PE, acemannan, levamisole, cimetidine, TNF, IL-2, and monoclonal antibodies
Efficacy	Lymphoma; melanoma; mastocytoma; osteosarcoma; soft tissue sarcomas, including fibrosarcoma; and hemangiosarcoma

Biological response modifiers (BRMs) are rapidly becoming an important modality for the treatment of cancer in humans and animals. In this type of therapy, the immune system is reconstituted or enhanced to fight the malignancy using endogenous biological processes. This can be done with a wide variety of substances, including biological products, chemicals, lymphokines, cytokines, hematopoietic growth factors, antibodies, and vaccines.[1-3] A few of the substances used as biological response modifiers are listed in Table 2-4.

This chapter focuses on agents that are likely to be of clinical use by the veterinary practitioner now or in the near future. These include bacillus Calmette-Guerin (BCG), liposome-encapsulated muramyl-tripeptide-phosphatidylethanolamine (L-MTP-PE), acemannan, levamisole, cimetidine, tumor necrosis factor (TNF), interleukin-2 (IL-2), and monoclonal antibodies. Hematopoietic growth factors, also considered by some as BRMs, are covered in a separate chapter.

NONSPECIFIC IMMUNOMODULATORS

Biologic agents (e.g., BCG and L-MTP-PE) and chemical immunopotentiators (e.g., levamisole and cimetidine) are categorized as active nonspecific immunotherapeutic agents. These agents actively stimulate the immune system to respond to a wide variety of substances that may harm the body, including cancer.[1-3]

BCG has been evaluated extensively in a variety of neoplastic diseases in humans and animals.[1-3] The active subunit of BCG is muramyl dipeptide, which is a potent macrophage activator that also has been used therapeutically.[4] Recently, BCG has been described as an effective agent for the treatment of some early cases of transitional cell carcinomas of the bladder in humans. The therapeutic utility of this substance is being investigated in veterinary medicine.

Several recent studies have shown that L-MTP-PE has potent antitumor properties.[5,6] L-MTP-PE is a nonspecific activator of monocytes and macrophages that results in anticancer effects. In one randomized, double-blind study involving dogs with osteosarcoma, those that received L-MTP-PE after amputation had a median survival time of 7.4 months, whereas those dogs that had an amputation and empty liposomes (control) had a median survival time of 3 months.[5] Although this study clearly showed that L-MTP-PE was very important for increasing survival time, 70% of the dogs developed metastatic disease, which

TABLE 2-4
Substances used as biological response modifiers

General Category	Biological Response Modifier
Nonspecific Immunomodulators	BCG
	Corynebacterium parvum
	Staphage lysate
	L-MTP-PE
	Levamisole
	Cimetidine
	Acemannan
Lymphokines/Monokines	Interleukin-1
	Interleukin-2
	Interferon
	Tumor necrosis factor
Adoptive Cellular Therapy	Lymphokine-activated killer cells
	Tumor-infiltrating lymphocytes
Antibody Therapy	Antibody directed to lymphoma cells
Growth Factors	Granulocyte colony-stimulating factor
	Granulocyte-macrophage colony-stimulating factor
	Macrophage colony-stimulating factor

prompted the initiation of the second double-blind, randomized study. In this second study, 40 dogs with osteosarcoma of the extremity without evidence of metastatic disease were treated with amputation followed by four doses of cisplatin (70 mg/m^2 IV every 28 days).[6] They were randomized to receive L-MTP-PE or empty liposomes. Of 14 dogs in the placebo group, 13 died of metastases; median survival time was 10 months, and median disease-free interval was 7.6 months. The dogs that received L-MTP-PE had a median survival time of 14.6 months and a median disease-free interval of 12 months; eight of the 11 dogs developed metastases. These studies clearly

show that L-MTP-PE is an important BRM. Studies are underway to determine whether L-MTP-PE is effective for the treatment of other neoplastic disorders in dogs and cats.

Acemannan, an extract from the aloe vera plant, is a nonspecific immunostimulator that has been shown to be taken up by macrophages, which enhances the release of interferon, interleukin 1-α, tumor necrosis factor, and prostaglandin E$_2$.[1] It has direct immunostimulatory effects and, apparently, direct antiviral activity against HIV-1. The commercially available product has been reported to delay the development of clinical signs in cats infected with feline leukemia virus. Acemannan has been promoted to have antitumor properties against fibrosarcoma in dogs and cats.[7] There is some controversy about this effect. This polymer is the only BRM that is approved for commercial use as an antitumor agent for treatment of solid tumors in veterinary medicine.

Levamisole is an imidazole compound that has immunorestorative properties.[8–10] Three veterinary studies have been performed involving this particular agent. In one study evaluating 73 cases of feline mammary tumors, cats were randomized after surgery to receive levamisole or a placebo.[9] No significant difference in survival time between the two groups was found in this study. A second study evaluated 144 dogs with mammary neoplasia.[8] In this study, there was no difference in survival between dogs that received levamisole and those that were treated with a placebo after surgery. Finally, 154 dogs with lymphoma were divided into two groups.[10] The first group received chemotherapy and levamisole, and the second group received chemotherapy and a placebo. No significant difference was noted in the remission times or survival times in these groups. Recently, levamisole has been shown to be beneficial for the treatment of colon carcinoma in humans. Additional studies in veterinary medicine will be needed to explore the potential benefit of this agent in veterinary medicine.

Cimetidine is an H_2-receptor antagonist that potentiates the immune system.[1,11] As a single agent, it has been shown to alter the activity level of suppressor cells. Some studies have shown that cimetidine is synergistic with interferon in the treatment of oral malignant melanoma in humans. One recent study demonstrated that this drug is effective in treating cutaneous malignant melanomas in horses.[11] The therapeutic value of this drug in small animal medicine has not been defined.

CYTOKINES

Cytokines are soluble mediators secreted by a variety of cell types that regulate several aspects of the immune system.[1–3] Biotechnology has resulted in the development of production methods to provide healthcare professionals with large quantities of cytokines for therapeutic uses. TNF and IL-2 are examples of these therapeutic cytokines.

TNF is secreted from macrophages in response to a number of substances, including lipopolysaccharides. TNF results in the death of tumor cells by a variety of mechanisms, such as by causing changes on the cell membrane that result in the development of cytopathic pores and by inhibiting protein and RNA synthesis. TNF-α combined with IL-2 results in positive responses in dogs with oral malignant melanoma and cutaneous mastocytoma.[12] IL-2 also may be effective used alone or with cytokines other than TNF to treat specific malignancies.

SPECIFIC MONOCLONAL ANTIBODIES

Specific monoclonal antibodies developed against tumor-specific or tumor-associated transformation antigens may prove to be an important therapeutic modality.[1,13,14] These monoclonal antibodies can be used for therapeutics and diagnostics. Using hybridomas, large quantities of monoclonal antibodies can be developed to a wide variety of malignant cells. These antibodies can be used to mediate antitumor cytotoxicity through either complement-mediated cytotoxicity or through antibody dependent cellular cytotoxicity. In addition, the antibodies can be "tagged" with a radioactive material to identify the presence of malignancies within the body.

The only monoclonal antibody approved and marketed for the treatment of cancer in humans or animals is CL/MAb 231 (Synbiotics Corporation, San Diego, California), which recognizes canine lymphoma cells.[13,14] It mediates antibody-dependent cellular cytotoxicity against a canine lymphoma cell line and has been reported to prolong remission duration when used in combination with chemotherapy in dogs with lymphoma.[14] The median survival time of dogs treated with the monoclonal antibody and chemotherapy was 591 days, as compared to historical controls, which had a median survival time of 189 days. Additional studies are needed to further understand the clinical utility of this treatment modality.

REFERENCES

1. MacEwen EG, Helfand SC: Recent advances in the biologic therapy of cancer. *Compend Contin Educ Pract Vet* 15:909–922, 1993.
2. Elmslie RE, Dow SW, Ogilvie GK: Interleukins: Biological properties and therapeutic potential. *J Vet Intern Med* 5:283–293, 1991.
3. MacEwen EG: Approaches to cancer therapy using biological response modifiers. *Vet Clin North Am Small Anim Pract* 15:667–688, 1985.
4. Meyer JA, Dueland RT, Rosenthal RC, et al: Canine osteogenic sarcoma treated by amputation and MER. *Cancer* 49:1613–1616, 1982.
5. MacEwen EG, Kurzman ID, Rosenthal RC, et al: Therapy for osteosarcoma in dogs with intravenous injection of liposome-encapsulated muramyl tripeptide. *J Natl Cancer Inst* 81:935–938, 1989.
6. Sheets MA, Unger BA, Giggleman GF, et al: Studies of the effect of acemannan on retrovirus infections: Clinical stabilization of feline leukemia virus-infected cats. *Mol Biother* 3:41–45, 1991.
7. Harris C, Pierce K, King G, et al: Efficacy of acemannan in treatment of canine and feline spontaneous neoplasms. *Mol Biother* 3:207–213, 1991.
8. MacEwen EG, Harvey HJ, Patnaik AK, et al: Evaluation of effect of levamisole after surgery on canine mammary cancer. *J Biol Response Mod* 4:418–426, 1985.
9. MacEwen EG, Hayes AA, Mooney S, et al: Evaluation of effect of levamisole on feline mammary cancer. *J Biol Response Mod* 5:541–546, 1984.
10. MacEwen EG, Hayes AA, Mooney S, et al: Levamisole as adjuvant to chemotherapy for canine lymphosarcoma. *J Biol Response Mod* 4:427–433, 1985.
11. Goetz T, Ogilvie GK: Cimetidine for the treatment of malignant melanoma in 3 horses. *JAVMA* 196:449–452, 1990.
12. Moore AS, Theilen GH, Newell AD, et al: Preclinical study of sequential tumor necrosis factor and interleukin-2 in the treatment of spontaneous canine neoplasms. *Cancer Res* 51:233–238, 1991.
13. Rosales C, Jeglum AK, Obrocka M, et al: Cytolytic activity of murine anti-dog lymphoma monoclonal antibodies with canine effector cells and complement. *Cell Immunol* 115:420–428, 1988.
14. Jeglum AK: Monoclonal antibody treatment of canine lymphoma. *Proc East States Vet Conf*: 222–223, 1992.

CLINICAL BRIEFING: SURGICAL ONCOLOGY—PROPERTIES, USES, AND PATIENT MANAGEMENT

Cancer Prevention	Education and preventative surgery (ovariohysterectomy and orchiectomy)
Diagnosis	Perform carefully premeditated biopsy procedures using the following: aspiration, needle, incisional, and excisional biopsy procedures. In each case, the biopsy should be performed in close consultation with the surgeon who will perform the definitive surgery
Definitive Treatment	The surgical plan should include therapy for the primary tumor, and if indicated, residual and metastatic disease
Palliation	Therapy for pain relief
Rehabilitation	Reconstructive techniques allow rapid return to normal function

Surgery is the oldest form of cancer therapy in human and veterinary medicine and has been responsible for the cure of more patients than any other treatment modality available in biomedical sciences. This great success is mainly due to the development of new surgical techniques and a greater understanding of the biologic behavior of malignancies.[1–4] Development of new adjunctive treatments, such as chemotherapy, radiation therapy, and biologic response modifiers, has enhanced the control of microscopic disease and prompted surgeons to reassess the type of surgery necessary. Despite advances in these fields, the surgeon has an important role in the prevention, diagnosis, definitive treatment, palliation, and rehabilitation of the veterinary cancer patient. The surgeon who treats cancer must have an understanding of the biologic behavior of individual malignancies and must have a strong command of the principles of surgical oncology as well as the aforementioned modalities.

ROLES FOR SURGERY
Prevention of Cancer

The surgeon must take a leading role in the education of the public regarding simple surgical procedures such as ovariohysterectomy and orchiectomy for the prevention of malignant diseases.[1–3] It has been clearly shown that spaying dogs prior to the first heat reduces the probability of developing malignant and benign mammary tumors to almost zero.[4] Similarly, early spaying apparently reduces the risk of mammary neoplasia in cats. In addition, castration of male dogs results in a dramatic reduction in such tumors as perianal adenomas and testicular neoplasia, particularly in cryptorchid dogs.[4] Therefore, surgery is important for the prevention of cancer in small animal cancer patients.

Diagnosis of Cancer

The surgical oncologist plays an important role in staging and determining the extent of malignant disease in the veterinary cancer patient.[1–4] Although a tentative diagnosis often may be made based on the clinical appearance of a tumor, surgical biopsy is always required to make a definitive diagnosis. The methods that the surgeon can use to diagnose the malignant condition or the extent of this disease are[1–4] aspiration biopsy, needle biopsy, incisional biopsy, and excisional biopsy. It is exceedingly important to know the histologic diagnosis of a malignancy prior to most definitive procedures. For example, knowing whether a tumor is a benign lipoma or a malignant mast cell tumor is extremely important. This is because even though they have the same outward appearance, the latter requires an extensive surgical resection and additional diagnostic procedures to determine the extent of disease (i.e., bone marrow aspiration/biopsy, abdominal and chest radiographs, lymph node aspiration/biopsy or aspirate, and a buffy coat smear). In contrast, a lipoma may not need to be removed; if it does, it may require only a simple resection.

The following principles should be kept in mind when a surgical biopsy is performed[1–4]:

1. Needle tracts or biopsy incisions should be placed with careful thought so that the entire biopsy tract can be removed when the definitive surgical procedure is performed. When a diagnostic biopsy is performed by a person who is unlikely to perform the definitive surgery, the surgeon who will perform the definitive procedure should be consulted.

2. Extreme care should be taken to not contaminate surrounding tissues or tissue planes during the biopsy procedure. For example, care must be taken to avoid the formation of a hematoma, because the hematoma might spread cancer cells as it dissects between fascial planes, which would require a more extensive definitive resection. When multiple biopsy specimens are taken from different sites, care should be taken to change instruments so that tumor cells are not transplanted from one site to another by the surgeon.

3. Biopsy techniques should be carefully selected to allow the acquisition of sufficient tissue to make a histopathologic diagnosis. Additionally, tissues should be prepared in such a manner as to allow adequate evaluation of the tissue by different procedures, such as electron microscopy, immunohistochemistry, and histopathology. Taking multiple biopsy specimens increases the likelihood of an accurate diagnosis if an excisional biopsy is not being planned.

4. The biopsy specimen should be handled with extreme care to prevent crushing, artifact, or alteration of the orientation of the tissue specimen. Specimens should be sufficiently small and placed in enough preservative to allow complete fixation (a good rule is 1 part tissue to 10 parts formalin). Using inked margins or sutures may give the pathologist information regarding orientation of biopsy tissue within the body.

5. The surgeon should have an acute awareness of the biologic behavior of malignant conditions to ensure that all possible sites of metastases are evaluated. Additionally, the surgeon should consider further adjunctive therapy (e.g., place radiopaque clips during biopsy and staging if radiation therapy is being considered).

Treatment of Cancer

Surgical treatment of cancer can be divided into six areas: the definitive surgical treatment for primary cancer, surgery to reduce the bulk of residual disease, surgical resection of metastatic disease, surgery for treatment of emergencies, surgery for palliation, and surgery for reconstruction and rehabilitation.

Surgery for Primary Cancer

This is the most common use of surgery for the veterinary cancer patient. The surgeon must consider all options and alternatives when planning a definitive procedure. For example, a relatively conservative surgery may result in a 90% cure rate for cutaneous melanoma.[4] A mast cell tumor or a soft tissue sarcoma, however, must be treated with a wide surgical excision that should extend at least one fascial layer below the detectable margins of the tumor. Therefore, it is important to know the specific tumor type being treated and the biological behavior of the tumor so that the client can be educated about the prognosis and "dose" of surgery that is necessary for a satisfactory outcome. Finally, other options such as radiation therapy should be considered as alternatives that may be offered to the client either instead of, or as an adjunct to, surgery.

Surgery for Residual Disease

It is important to integrate other treatment modalities, such as radiation therapy and chemotherapy, with surgery and to formulate a treatment plan that includes surgery that will provide maximum benefit for the patient.[1-3] For example, resection of a soft tissue sarcoma in the distal extremity may result in significant morbidity if the tumor is completely resected, whereas if the tumor is removed until only microscopic disease remains and the surgical field is irradiated postoperatively, there is usually minimal morbidity and a very good probability for 1 to 2 years of tumor control.[4] "Debulking" surgery alone is rarely an acceptable form of therapy, and cytoreductive surgery should not be used inappropriately to reduce the bulk of the tumor without anticipating another effective modality to control residual disease.[1] Except in cases of palliative surgery, there is no role for cytoreductive surgery when there are other effective therapies for the treatment of that malignant disease.

KEY POINT:

Whenever considering surgery for a neoplastic process, the following questions should be asked:

1. What am I treating?

2. What is the biologic behavior?

3. Is a cure possible?

4. What "surgical dose" should be used?

5. What are my alternatives?

(Courtesy of SJ Withrow, DVM, surgical oncologist, Colorado State University, 1994.)

Surgery for Metastatic Disease

One of the best examples of the use of surgery for metastatic disease is for metastatic osteosarcoma to the lung.[4] In patients in which the primary tumor has been controlled for many months to years, in patients in which the metastatic lesion is growing very slowly, and in those with only a few metastatic lesions, metastasectomy has resulted in substantial long-term control. Therefore, resection of metastases should be considered in select cases when it is obvious that the malignant disease is not progressing rapidly and that the metastatic disease is restricted to a single site that is amenable to surgical excision. In most instances, however, surgery has a little role except for palliation of bulky disease once a tumor has metastasized.

Surgery for Oncologic Emergencies

The most common applications for oncologic surgery in an emergency setting include the treatment of hemorrhage, perforation, drainage of abscesses, or obstruction of organs.[1-3] An example of the treatment of hemorrhage is ligation of the carotid in dogs with nasal tumors on the ipsilateral side of the malignancy, which can reduce the chance for fatal episodes of epistaxis. Another example is the removal of a bleeding abdominal tumor, such as a ruptured splenic hemangiosarcoma. Intestinal resection and anastomosis to treat a perforated malignancy of the GI tract can be lifesaving.

Palliation

When a tumor or its metastasis results in significant discomfort for the veterinary cancer patient, surgery can be employed to improve or maintain the quality of life.[1-4] In these patients, surgery should be used only if the owner is clearly aware that this procedure will not be curative. An example may be amputation of an extremity in a dog with osteosarcoma that also has pulmonary metastatic disease. If the osteosarcoma of the extremity is causing substantial morbidity, amputation can improve quality of life by reducing pain, although the overall survival time may not be substantially increased with that procedure.

Surgery for Reconstruction and Rehabilitation

Very wide resection of a malignancy is now possible as a result of the development of plastic surgical techniques, including free flap and microvascular anastomotic methods. These techniques can be used to rehabilitate areas that have been irradiated and where substantial tissue injury is noted.

REFERENCES

1. Rosenberg SA: Principles of surgical oncology, in DeVita VT, Helman S, Rosenberg SA (eds): *Cancer Principles and Practice of Oncology*, ed 4. Philadelphia, JB Lippincott, 1993, pp 238–247.
2. Merrick HW: Principles of surgery in cancer management, in Skeel RT (ed): *Handbook of Cancer Chemotherapy*, ed 3. Boston, Little, Brown & Co, 1991, pp 27–31.
3. Langmuir VK, Schwartz SI, Patterson WB: Principles of surgical oncology, in Rubin P (ed): *Clinical Oncology: A Multidisciplinary Approach for Physicians and Students*, ed 7. Philadelphia, WB Saunders, 1993, pp 41–50.
4. Withrow SJ: Surgical oncology, in Withrow SJ, MacEwen EG (eds): *Clinical Veterinary Oncology*. Philadelphia, JB Lippincott, 1989, pp 58–62.

CLINICAL BRIEFING: HYPERTHERMIA AND CRYOTHERAPY— PROPERTIES, USES, AND PATIENT MANAGEMENT

Equipment	*Hyperthermia:* In practice, local hyperthermia generally is applied with a handheld radiofrequency device; whole-body hyperthermia is not practical for the average clinical practice *Cryotherapy:* Liquid nitrogen units use a probe or spray applicator; nitrous oxide comes from standard tanks and is applied via probes
Indications	*Local Hyperthermia:* Most effective for the treatment of localized tumors in combination with radiation therapy or chemotherapy; handheld hyperthermia devices are effective for the treatment of small (<1.0 cm diameter), benign, and malignant superficial tumors *Cryotherapy:* Used for the treatment of small (<1.0 cm diameter), benign, and malignant superficial tumors of areas such as the eyelid, perianal region, oral cavity, or skin

Hyperthermia and cryotherapy have been used for decades for the treatment of neoplastic conditions in veterinary medicine. Hyperthermia can be delivered by whole body hyperthermia units that raise the body temperature of the entire animal to approximately 42°C. In private practice, local hyperthermia techniques are more practical for increasing tissue temperatures regionally, which kills tumor cells without causing burns. Hyperthermia alone is of limited efficacy for the treatment of malignant conditions; it is most effective when used with chemotherapy, radiation therapy, or surgery.

Cryotherapy is the use of very cold temperatures to kill tumor cells. Initially, cryotherapy was used to treat a wide variety and sizes of malignant and non-malignant tumors. Currently, it is used most effectively to treat very small, select tumors. Because this treatment modality is fast, relatively inexpensive, and can be employed with only local anesthesia, it remains a standard treatment for a variety of localized small malignancies in veterinary medicine.

HYPERTHERMIA
Equipment

Whole-body hyperthermia can be achieved by raising core body temperatures to 41.8°C to 42.0°C using various energy sources, including a radiant heat device (Figure 2-17), as well as by extracorporeal heating techniques. Although whole-body hyperthermia is only available in specific research institutions, it generally results in a more uniform temperature increase within tumor tissues compared to local treatment techniques, in which areas of extreme heat and of relatively normal temperatures may reduce the efficacy of hyperthermia.

Local hyperthermia techniques involve the use of either external or internal heating sources. External hyperthermia uses either microwaves, ultrasound (Figure 2-18), or radiofrequency (Figure 2-19) energy sources to deposit energy within the tissue from an external applicator. Microwaves and radiofrequency methods deposit adequate energy approximately 3 to 4 cm in depth. Ultrasonographic hyperthermia units can penetrate from 6 to 14 cm. Radiofrequency and microwave energy

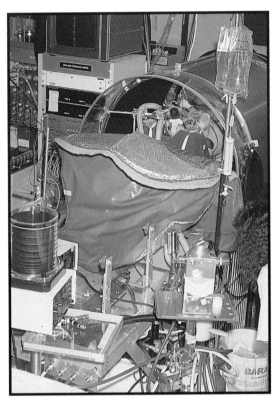

Figure 2-17: *Whole-body hyperthermia can involve the use of a radiant heat device. The patient is placed under general anesthesia, chemically paralyzed to ablate any panting during heating, and then placed in a semi-enclosed chamber during intensive physiologic monitoring. Whole-body hyperthermia (42°C) is used in conjunction with radiation and chemotherapy to control malignancies.*

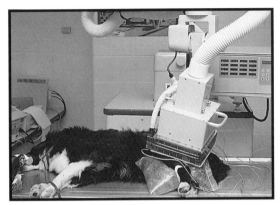

Figure 2-18: *Computer-controlled multisector ultrasound hyperthermia devices are effective at providing uniform heating to a relatively large localized area. Although the equipment used in this type of local hyperthermia is much more effective than handheld devices, it is expensive and relatively complex to operate.*

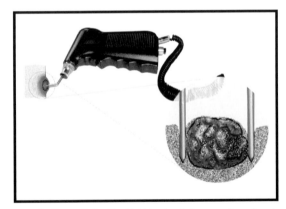

Figure 2-19: *Handheld local radiofrequency hyperthermia unit. Lidocaine is first injected around the lesion to be treated so that a biopsy specimen can be obtained. In this case, a handheld radiofrequency hyperthermia unit is used so that the applicator tips are placed at either side of the lesion. Because this lesion is suspected to be >0.2 cm below the skin surface, the invasive radiofrequency tips are placed through the skin, down to the level of the deepest portion of the tumor. The lesion is heated at least twice; the applicator probes are used again if nearby tissue is to be treated. The tumor and a surrounding "cuff" of normal tissue should reach therapeutic temperatures (>42°C).*

sources also can be inserted directly into the tissues to be heated for interstitial hyperthermia.

General Technique

Whole-body hyperthermia is a complicated technique that involves intensive measurement of a wide variety of physiologic parameters during the treatment (Figure 2-17). Very few academic centers use whole-body hyperthermia because of the cost and labor-intensive need for specific monitoring.

Handheld radiofrequency hyperthermia units are commonly used in some small animal practices. A general description of this methodology is as follows (Figure 2-19):

1. Ideally, the lesion to be treated should be smaller than 1 cm in diameter.
2. Local anesthesia (1–3 ml of lidocaine) is injected around the lesion to be treated.
3. After a biopsy specimen is obtained, radiofrequency tips are placed at either side of the lesion. If the lesion is suspected to be >0.2 cm below the skin surface, invasive radiofrequency tips are placed through the skin and down to the level of the deepest portion of the tumor.
4. The lesion is heated at least twice with subsequent replacement of the applicator probes if nearby tissue is to be treated. It is important to remember that the tumor and a surrounding "cuff" of normal tissue should reach therapeutic temperatures (>42°C).
5. The area heated will become indurated and somewhat painful the first 24 to 48 hours after therapy. A scab may form and later fall off, revealing a bed of granulation tissue. The lesion gradually gets smaller, leaving a small, hairless area or an area where the hair and skin are a different color.

Clinical Application

Several studies in animals have shown efficacy of local hyperthermia when combined with radiation therapy.[1,2] Dogs with oral and facial sarcomas have been reported to have a 1-year tumor control rate of 50%. Gillette and colleagues observed that the efficacy of radiation therapy could be enhanced by using local hyperthermia in animals with squamous cell carcinoma.[3] A group at Purdue University showed that hyperthermia was synergistic with radiation therapy in treating dogs with hemangiopericytoma.[4] In a randomized study, Dewhirst and colleagues evaluated long-term tumor control when radiation therapy was combined with hyperthermia for the treatment of a variety of malignant conditions.[5] The overall probability for complete response and local control 2 years after treatment was significantly better in patients treated with hyperthermia plus radiation therapy compared to those treated with radiation therapy alone.[4,5]

A variety of anecdotal reports have documented that hyperthermia and chemotherapy (thermochemotherapy) is effective for the treatment of malignancies in dogs. One study of local hyperthermia with intralesional chemotherapy reported tumor response in five of ten pets with solid tumors.[6] In a randomized study that compared use of doxorubicin to doxorubicin plus whole body hyperthermia in dogs with lymphoma, the median duration of the first remission was not different in any treatment group, although there was a trend favoring the combined modality.[7]

CRYOTHERAPY[8]
Equipment

Equipment for cryotherapy most often uses liquid nitrogen or nitrous oxide. Liquid nitrogen evaporates slowly and requires careful monitoring. Nitrous oxide uses the same type of tank used for anesthetic purposes, and the gas does not evaporate between uses, unlike liquid nitrogen. The cost for procedures of the two cryogens is similar. Nitrous oxide is effective for lesions smaller than 1 cm in diameter. It cannot be used for spray applicators and has limited depth of penetration. Liquid nitrogen is much more effective for larger lesions or for lesions with a rich blood supply that need to be frozen faster or that would be better treated with a spray applicator. Regardless of the

KEY POINT:

When cryotherapy and hyperthermia are used, margins of normal tissue around the tumor and the tumor itself must be frozen or heated to appropriate temperatures to result in adequate tumor control.

cryogen used, temperature-monitoring devices, such as thermocouple needles, should be used to ensure that the tumor is frozen to critical temperatures (–20°C).

General Technique

1. Cryotherapy should be restricted to tumors of the skin and other external areas that are <1.0 cm in diameter.
2. Local anesthesia (1–3 ml 2% lidocaine) is injected around the area to be frozen.
3. The surrounding hair is parted or minimally clipped and cleaned.
4. The tumor is debrided and the tissue submitted for histopathology.
5. The tissue can be coagulated with silver nitrate or a caustic agent, or a pursestring suture can be applied to reduce bleeding at the site to be frozen. Blood flow should be restricted whenever possible to decrease the rate of warming and increase the rate of freezing.
6. Each tumor should have at least two rapid freezes and slow thaws. When a probe is used, it should be approximately the same size as the lesion. Warm probes are applied to a warm, moist tumor surface. When the freezing is initiated, the tumor freezes to the applicator and is maintained in that position throughout the freezing period, which can last from seconds to several minutes.
7. Once the first iceball forms and adequate temperatures (<–20°C) are reached at the peripheral margins of the tissue surrounding the tumor, the freezing is discontinued, and the probe is allowed to thaw until it detaches from the lesion. The entire lesion is allowed to thaw, whereupon a second and, possibly, a third freezing are initiated. Liquid nitrogen can be used as a spray, especially for larger tumors (Figure 2-20).
8. After the treatment, the owner should be warned that a scab will form at the site of freezing and that the scab will fall off in approximately 10 to 21 days, exposing a pink bed of epithelium or granulation tissue. This area will contract and epithe-

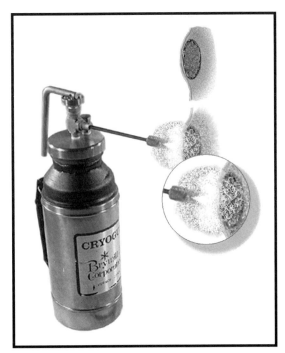

Figure 2-20: *Liquid nitrogen cryotherapy. After the area is prepared and local anesthesia is injected around the area to be frozen, the tumor is debrided, and the tissue is submitted for histopathology. If necessary, the remaining tissue is coagulated with silver nitrate or cauterized, or a pursestring suture can be applied to reduce bleeding at the site to be frozen. When possible, blood flow should be temporarily restricted to decrease the rate of cooling and increase the rate of freezing. Each tumor should undergo at least two rapid freezes and slow thaws using either a probe or spray. In this figure, a liquid nitrogen container and spray nozzle are used to form an iceball. Adequate temperatures (<–20°C) are reached at the peripheral margins of the tissue surrounding the tumor. Once the freezing is discontinued, the entire lesion is allowed to thaw, whereupon a second and, possibly, a third freezing is initiated.*

lialize, leaving a small, hairless area. The hair around the area being frozen may change color, which must be mentioned to the owner. If bone is frozen, it may need to be debrided 2 to 3 months after the freezing episode. General hygiene is all that is required for the freezing site.

Clinical Application

Cryotherapy has been used for decades to control localized tumors successfully in humans and animals. Best results occur with small (<1.0 cm), localized tumors that are benign histologically. The following is a brief description of some of the sites successfully treated with cryotherapy.

Eyelid

Benign tumors of the eyelid, such as meibomian gland adenomas, papillomas, and melanomas, generally are treated very effectively with cryotherapy. The tumor should be submitted for histopathology prior to freezing. Recurrence rates are less than 5% if the tumor is adequately frozen and is smaller than 1 cm in diameter.[9]

Perianal Tumors

Perianal adenomas are effectively treated with cryotherapy, especially when combined with castration. When combined with castration, recurrence rates generally are less than 5%.[10]

Oral Tumors

Cryotherapy is effective in treating very small lesions of the oral cavity that invade bone, especially benign lesions such as epulides. After freezing, the tissue sloughs rapidly as a result of abrasion within the oral cavity. A superficial area of dead bone may be exposed and become necrotic. If a sequestrum forms, it must be removed.[11]

Skin Tumors

Benign skin tumors, especially in dogs, are commonly treated with cryotherapy.[12] For example, cutaneous melanomas, sebaceous adenomas, and papillomas smaller than 1 cm in diameter can be frozen with excellent response. As a general rule, tumors larger than 1 cm in diameter should be treated by other therapeutic modalities.

REFERENCES

1. Dewhirst MW, Page RL, Thrall DE: Hyperthermia, in Withrow SJ, MacEwen EG (eds): *Clinical Veterinary Oncology.* Philadelphia. JB Lippincott, 1989, pp 113–123.
2. Brewer WG, Turrel JM: Radiotherapy and hyperthermia in the treatment of fibrosarcoma in the dog. *JAVMA* 18:146–150, 1982.
3. Gillette EL, McChesney SL, Dewhirst MW, Scott RJ: Response of canine oral carcinomas to heat and radiation. *Int J Rad Oncol Biol Phys* 13:1861–1867, 1987.
4. Richardson RC, Anderson VL, Voorhees WD, et al: Irradiation-hyperthermia in canine hemangiopericytomas. Large animal model for therapeutic response. *J Natl Canc Instit* 73:1187–1194, 1984.
5. Dewhirst MW: The utility of thermal dose as a predictor of tumor and normal tissue responses to combined radiation and hyperthermia. *Cancer Res* 44:4772S–4780S, 1984.
6. Theon AP, Madewell BR, Moore AS, et al: Localized thermo-cisplatin therapy. A pilot study in spontaneous canine and feline tumors. *Int J Hyperthermia* 7:881–892, 1991.
7. Page RL, Macy DW, Ogilvie GK, et al: Phase III evaluation of doxorubicin and whole body hyperthermia in dogs with lymphoma. *Int J Hyperthermia* 8:187–197, 1992.
8. Withrow SJ: Cryosurgery, in Withrow SJ, MacEwen EG (eds): *Clinical Veterinary Oncology.* Philadelphia, JB Lippincott, 1989, pp 106–112.
9. Roberts SM, Severin GA, Lavach JD: Prevalence and treatment of palpebral neoplasms in the dog: 200 cases (1975–1983). *JAVMA* 189:1355–1359, 1986.
10. Liska WD, Withrow SJ: Cryosurgical treatment of perianal gland adenomas in the dog. *JAAHA* 14:457–463, 1978.
11. Harvey HJ: Cryosurgery of oral tumors in dogs and cats. *Vet Clin North Am Small Anim Pract* 10:821–830, 1980.
12. Krahwinkel DJ, Jr: Cryosurgical treatment of skin diseases. *Vet Clin North Am Small Anim Pract* 10:787–801, 1980.

CLINICAL BRIEFING: TREATMENT OF PAIN

General Concepts of Pain Management	Analgesics should be used preventatively for maximum benefit; compassionate care, gentle handling, and a comfortable environment, accompanied by local and systemic analgesics, are ideal to minimize discomfort
Mild Pain	See General Concepts; consider aspirin and other NSAIDs
Moderate Pain	See General Concepts; consider aspirin and other NSAIDs with or without opiate analgesics; changing the route of administration (e.g., oral to IV) may be beneficial
Severe Pain	See General Concepts; opiate analgesics should be combined (if needed) with local analgesia, epidural analgesia, sustained-release patches, and palliative procedures (e.g., radiation therapy and surgery); maximize blood levels with systemic administration

Comprehensive management of pain involves careful evaluation and treatment of each patient.[1-6] To maximize quality of life, response to therapy, and survival time for the patient, adequate pain control must be the highest goal for the veterinary practitioner. Pain control in veterinary medicine has come into the forefront of attention only recently, primarily because of the inappropriate attitudes of clinicians, lack of knowledge about analgesic medications, and lack of skill in assessing pain and appropriate therapeutic methods.[2,3] In many cases, analgesics have been withheld because of fear of adverse side effects of these drugs and because very little research exists demonstrating the beneficial effects of pain relief in veterinary patients. Despite this, pain relief is and must be a priority of the veterinary caregiver.

MECHANISM OF CANCER PAIN

The most common mechanism of cancer pain is associated with tumor invasion and subsequent tissue damage that causes activation of pain receptors.[1,6]

Therapy also can be associated with the induction of pain. For example, although surgery and radiation therapy may relieve pain and suffering, they can cause significant discomfort from tissue and nerve damage. Alkaloids, such as vincristine and vinblastine, can produce polyneuropathy that has been noted to be painful in human cancer patients.

The types of cancer pain include visceral, inflammatory, and somatic pain; neuritis; and neuropathic pain.[1-6]

Visceral Pain

Human patients describe this type of pain as dull, deep, constant, aching pain. Visceral pain is also poorly defined and, when significant in human patients, often responds best to narcotic and nonnarcotic analgesics.

Inflammatory and Somatic Pain

Frequently described, this pain is well localized, constant, and aching.[6] Common sources of this type of pain include bone metastases; tissue damage; and musculoskeletal, dental, and integumental pain.

Neuritic Pain

Inflammation of nerves or nerve roots causes neuritic pain and can present as part of a paraneoplastic syndrome or as a direct effect of tumor compression. Humans describe it as a constant, dull, aching pain that may have periods of burning "shock-like" sensations.

Neuropathic Pain

This type of pain is the result of a damaged segment of the nervous system that normally transmits pain stimuli. It arises from metabolic, immunologic, or direct physical effects on the nervous system. Neuropathic pain is difficult to control with standard analgesics.

GENERAL CONCEPTS OF PAIN THERAPY (Figure 2-21)

Recent research has demonstrated that once pain is elicited, the pain response is magnified. Whenever possible, therefore, preventative therapy is preferable to suppression of established pain. Premeditated, judicious use of analgesics is likely to increase patient comfort, decrease need for hospitalization and its expense, and reduce the amount of pain medication used to achieve the same level of comfort.[3,6]

The management of pain begins with high-quality, compassionate care. Careful nursing with gentle handling and provision of an environment that is comfortable and relaxing is of great benefit to the patient. Local anesthesia should be employed whenever possible to alleviate local discomfort. Systemic analgesia should be used whenever there is a possibility that discomfort is not localized or alleviated by local analgesia.

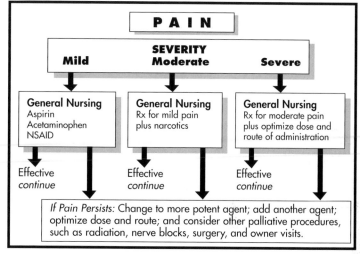

Figure 2-21: *General approach for the treatment of pain. Pretreatment of discomfort and pain generally requires fewer analgesics at a lower dosage and results in a better quality of life.*

Mild Pain[1,3,6]

The treatment of mild pain with regular doses of such nonsteroidal anti-inflammatory drugs (NSAIDs) as aspirin or acetaminophen (dogs only!) may be quite effective. Although efficacious, these analgesics are not perceived by owners as having a significant analgesic effect and therefore may be dismissed as useful drugs. Because they work peripherally, these drugs do not cause CNS toxicity and can cause GI upset.

Moderate and Severe Pain

Moderate pain can be treated with NSAIDs, such as aspirin, acetaminophen, or piroxicam; however, these frequently fail to meet the needs of the patient. Opiate analgesic agents are often used for relief of moderate pain because they have peripheral as well as central analgesic effects. If moderate to severe pain is not relieved with either NSAIDs or opiate analgesics when these drugs are given individually, then combining analgesics for pain relief can certainly be considered; however, additive toxicity must be monitored. If this is not effective, then adjuvant therapy for the malignancy itself may be indicated. For exam-

TABLE 2-5
Select analgesics in dogs and cats[2-5]

Drug	Dose (mg/kg)	Route	Dose Interval (hr)
Morphine	0.05–0.4 (dog)	IV	1–4
	0.2–1.0 (dog)	IM, SQ	2–6
	0.05–0.2 (cat)	IM, SQ	2–6
Oxymorphone	0.02–0.1 (dog)	IV	2–4
	0.02–0.05 (cat)	IV	2–4
	0.05–0.2 (dog)	IM, SQ	2–6
	0.05–0.1 (cat)	IM, SQ	2–6
Butorphanol	0.2–1.0 (dog)	IV, IM, SQ	1–4
	0.1–0.4 (cat)	IV, IM, SQ	1–4
Aspirin	10 (dog)	PO	8–12
	10 (cat)	PO	48
Piroxicam	0.3 (dog)	PO	48

ple, radiation therapy to sites of bone pain may be of profound benefit. In addition, administration of analgesics by another route—for example, switching from subcutaneous to intravenous administration—may be effective. In some cases, sustained-release fentanyl patches may be helpful. Fentanyl patches are applied to the skin to slowly release the analgesic over 72 hours. Nerve blocks or other surgical procedures to alleviate discomfort can be employed.

ANALGESIC AGENTS
(Table 2-5)
Nonsteroidal Anti-Inflammatory Agents
Aspirin
Aspirin (acetylsalicylic acid) is a commonly used analgesic with antipyretic and anti-inflammatory effects. Aspirin increases bleeding time by decreasing platelet aggregation. This increased bleeding time may complicate surgery and may cause gastric irritation and bleeding. Feeding at the time of the administration of aspirin seems to decrease gastric irritation. Aspirin is most effective for the treatment of musculoskeletal discomfort. The recommended dose for dogs is 10 mg/kg every 8 to 12 hours.[2,3,5] The recommended oral dose for cats is 10 mg/kg once every 48 hours.[2,3,5]

Phenylbutazone
Although it is rarely used in small animal medicine, phenylbutazone has analgesic and antipyretic effects

> **KEY POINT:**
>
> *Aspirin should be used with extreme caution in cats because the half-life is substantially prolonged in this species, especially in young and old cats.*

as well as anti-inflammatory properties. Extreme care is necessary when using this drug because it can cause renal necrosis, gastric irritation, and increased bleeding times by decreasing platelet aggregation. The authors do not recommend the use of phenylbutazone for pain relief in dogs, and its use is contraindicated in cats.

Acetaminophen

Acetaminophen has analgesic and antipyretic properties. This drug causes less gastric irritation than does aspirin. Cats have a poorly developed hepatic glutathione-dependent enzyme system, which can result in development of a toxic metabolite (N-acetylbenzoquinoneimine) that covalently bonds to liver proteins and causes hepatic necrosis. Therefore, acetaminophen may be effective for mild pain in dogs, but its use is contraindicated in cats.

Ibuprofen

Ibuprofen is not commonly used in veterinary medicine because of potential serious adverse effects that include acute renal failure, bleeding gastric ulcers, and oral ulcers. A dose of 10 mg/kg every 24 to 48 hours has been employed by some clinicians for use in dogs.[2,3,5]

Piroxicam

Piroxicam is a relatively new and potent NSAID that is probably a more effective analgesic than the aforementioned drugs. The most common adverse effects associated with piroxicam therapy include gastric ulceration and renal damage. The drug should be used with caution in dogs. Its use has not yet been evaluated in cats. The dose for dogs is 0.3 mg/kg daily for 4 days, then 0.3 mg/kg every other day thereafter.

Local Anesthetics

Local anesthetics and analgesics are effective for relief of mild pain. Lidocaine hydrochloride blocks sodium ion channels along the axons. This stops the conduction of action potentials and therefore reduces the perception of pain. Intercostal nerve blocks are effective for reducing postsurgical pain associated with thoracotomy.

Epidural Analgesics

Epidural bupivacaine hydrochloride can induce analgesia that lasts from 4 to 6 hours with some inhibition of motor function. Epidural administration of morphine can provide central analgesia for hours. It is currently being explored for use in dogs with hindlimb and, in some cases, forelimb amputation.

Opioids
Morphine

Morphine is a natural opioid agonist. When administered to dogs, it may produce initial excitement manifested by panting, salivation, nausea, vomiting, urination, defecation, and hypotension. These arise from activation of the chemoreceptor trigger zone, vagal stimulation, and histamine release. Initial excitement may be succeeded by CNS depression, constipation, urine retention, bradycardia, respiratory depression, and hypothermia. Recommended dosages in dogs are 0.2 to 1.0 mg/kg IM or SQ every 2 to 6 hours and 0.05 to 0.4 mg/kg IV every 1 to 4 hours.[2,3,6] Compared to dogs, cats are more resistant to stimulation of the chemoreceptor trigger zone. Analgesia and CNS depression are noted when the drug is given to cats at a dose of 0.05 to 0.2 mg/kg IM or SQ every 2 to 6 hours.[2,3,6] Dosages approaching 1 mg/kg can induce marked hyperexcitability, aggression, and stimulation of the chemoreceptor trigger zone in cats.

Oxymorphone

Oxymorphone is a semisynthetic opioid agonist that is approximately 10 times more potent than morphine in its analgesic properties, although its adverse effects on the respiratory, cardiovascular, and GI systems are less pronounced. In dogs, the drug is used at 0.05 to 0.2 mg/kg (maximum dose, 1.5 mg)

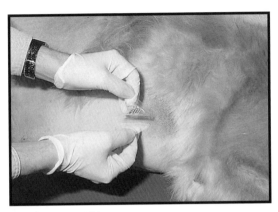

Figure 2-22A

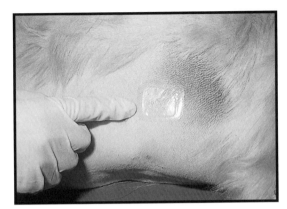

Figure 2-22B

Figure 2-22: *The backing of the transdermal fentanyl patch is removed (A). The patch is then placed in a flat, hairless area of skin where it is unlikely to be removed by the patient (B). Latex rubber gloves should be worn whenever the patches are handled. The patches are capable of delivering the analgesic over a 72-hour period. Because therapeutic blood levels of the analgesic are not attained for 12 to 24 hours in dogs, patches may be most effective when used prior to surgery or other painful procedures.*

IM or SQ; in cats, the drug is given by the same routes at a dose of 0.05 to 0.1 mg/kg.[2,3,6] Lower doses are used for IV administration. Oxymorphone provides 2 to 6 hours of analgesia.

Butorphanol

Butorphanol is a synthetic opioid agonist/antagonist that is preferable to morphine and oxymorphone in that it is not a scheduled drug. It has five times the analgesic potency of morphine with a duration of analgesia of approximately 1 to 4 hours. Adverse effects such as nausea and vomiting are rare, but the drug can induce sedation in dogs and cats. The recommended dose in dogs is 0.2 to 1.0 mg/kg IV, IM, or SQ. In cats, the recommended dose is 0.1 to 0.4 mg/kg IV, IM, or SQ.[2,3,6]

New Advances in Pain Relief

Fentanyl-impregnated transdermal patches reliably release a controlled amount of fentanyl over a 72-hour period (Figure 2-22).[6] Two sizes of patches are available that are capable of releasing fentanyl at a rate of 2.5 or 5.0 µg/hr. Both sizes are adequate for treating a 10- to 20-kg dog, depending on the severity of the discomfort. Patches that release fentanyl sustain adequate blood levels of the analgesic for 72 hours. Therapeutic levels are not attained for 12 to 24 hours. It seems that the patches may be used with caution in cats; absorption and resultant blood levels are not as predictable as in dogs.

A transdermal patch system that contains analgesics provides constant pain relief over the dosing period and obviates the need for constant reevaluation of schedules and dosing. The disadvantages of fentanyl patches include a slow onset of action, difficulty in application so that the patient will not remove it, and persistence of drug levels despite removal of the patch.

Other methods of administering analgesics are available for specific conditions. For example, rectal sup-

> **KEY POINT:**
>
> *A transdermal patch system that contains analgesics provides constant pain relief over the dosing period and obviates the need for constant reevaluation of schedules and dosing.*

positories that contain morphine or oxymorphone are available to control pain in animals that cannot take drugs orally.

In some cases, the patient's attitude may preclude adequate pain management. Therapeutic trials of benzodiazepines (e.g., diazepam) and tranquilizers (e.g., acepromazine) to relax the patient may be of substantial benefit. Surgical procedures such as amputation for tumor-associated fractures or radiation therapy to sites of bone pain due to a malignant disease may be indicated.

REFERENCES

1. Patt RB, Loughner JE: Management of pain in the cancer patient, in Rosenthal S, Carignan JR, Smith BD (eds): *Medical Care of the Cancer Patient*, ed 2. Philadelphia, WB Saunders, 1993, pp 255–264.
2. Pascoe PJ: Patient aftercare, in Slatter D (ed): *Textbook of Small Animal Surgery*, ed 2. Philadelphia, WB Saunders, 1993, pp 230–240.
3. Hansen B: Analgesics in cardiac, surgical and intensive care patients, in Kirk RW, Bonagura JD (eds): *Current Veterinary Therapy XI: Small Animal Practice*. Philadelphia, WB Saunders, 1992, pp 82–87.
4. Potthoff A, Carithers RW: Pain analgesia in dogs and cats. *Compend Contin Educ Pract Vet* 11:887–898, 1989.
5. Kelly MJ: Pain (general, back, extremities, abdomen), in Ettinger SJ (ed): *Textbook of Veterinary Internal Medicine: Diseases of the Dog and Cat*, ed 3. Philadelphia, WB Saunders, 1989, pp 18–22.
6. Weintraub M, Rubio A: Cancer pain, in Skeel RJ (ed): *Handbook of Cancer Chemotherapy*, ed 3. Boston, Little, Brown & Co, 1991, pp 474–492.

CLINICAL BRIEFING: TREATMENT OF EMESIS

Emetic Potential	Emesis is rarely associated with chemotherapy; cisplatin is an exception. Small dogs are at greater risk of vomiting than larger dogs when given this drug. Emesis primarily originates from the chemoreceptor trigger zone and the emetic center
Self-Limiting Vomiting	*Therapy:* Correct underlying cause; do not feed by mouth until vomiting ceases for 12–24 hours; initiate small amounts of water, then bland low-fat diet; monitor hydration and electrolytes
Life-Threatening Vomiting	*Therapy:* Follow same protocol as for self-limiting vomiting except administer IV fluids (maintenance needs + hydration deficits + losses) and correct electrolyte and pH abnormalities (e.g., serum potassium); in addition, give antiemetics (e.g., metoclopramide, butorphanol, or ondansetron) parenterally
Prevention	Patients at high risk for vomiting or those that are given drugs that are powerful inducers of emetics (e.g., cisplatin) may benefit from pretreatment with antiemetics

Nausea and vomiting are common problems associated with the presence of a primary tumor or metastatic disease.[1-3] They also can result from cancer therapy and may reduce the quality of life of veterinary cancer patients.[1-5] Vomiting can lead to life-threatening problems, such as dehydration and metabolic imbalance, and wound dehiscence may occur following increased abdominal pressure. In addition, owners often get the impression that their pet is experiencing unnecessary toxicities, which may result in abandonment of life-saving treatment and lead to subsequent euthanasia. Management of nausea and vomiting is important to improve the quality of life for the patient, which subsequently can enhance response to therapy and increase survival time.

MECHANISM OF VOMITING

The presence of a tumor can result in problems, such as physical obstruction of the intestinal tract and vomiting. Surgical resection of the tumor is the only solution to this clinical problem. Chemotherapeutic agents differ both in emetic potential and in the length of time after administration that they cause emesis.[1-5] Unlike humans, animals rarely exhibit any evidence of nausea and vomiting at or shortly after the time drugs are administered, with the exception of dogs that receive cisplatin chemotherapy.[2-5] The emetic potential of all of these drugs depends on the sensitivity of each patient as well as on the route of administration and the dosage. Drugs associated with low, moderate, and relatively high probabilities of vomiting are listed in Table 2-6.

Cisplatin may induce vomiting within 1 to 6 hours, whereas cyclophosphamide may induce vomiting 4 to 12 hours after treatment. Doxorubicin may induce vomiting in a few patients 4 to 6 hours after

TABLE 2-6
Chemotherapeutic agents with a low, moderate, and high probability of inducing nausea or vomiting in dogs or cats at or following administration of the drug

Low	Moderate	High
L-asparaginase	Carboplatin	Cisplatin
Bleomycin	Cyclophosphamide	Dacarbazine
Chlorambucil	Cytosine arabinoside	Nitrogen
Tamoxifen	Daunorubicin	mustard
Vincristine	Doxorubicin	
Vinblastine	Etoposide	
Steroids	5-fluorouracil	
Mitoxantrone	Procarbazine	
	Methotrexate	

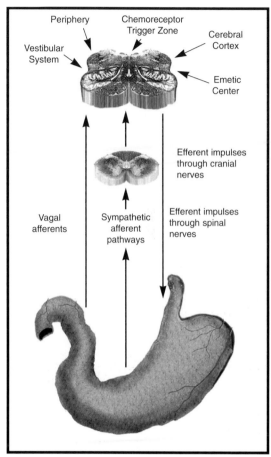

Figure 2-23: *Vomiting results from a complex array of central and peripheral components that are common targets for therapy with antiemetics. Pharmacologic intervention through any one or all of the impulse pathways is important for eliminating vomiting in the cancer patient.*

treatment. All of these chemotherapeutic agents can induce vomiting 3 to 5 days after treatment because of damage to the GI tract.

The mechanism of chemotherapy-induced vomiting is complex (Figure 2-23). The emetic center in the medulla coordinates vomiting and receives input from at least four sources: the chemoreceptor trigger zone (CTZ), peripheral receptors, the cerebral cortex, and the vestibular apparatus. The vestibular apparatus probably does not influence cancer or chemotherapy-associated vomiting. The CTZ is located in the fourth ventricle of the medulla. It is activated solely by chemical stimuli and plays an important role in chemotherapy-induced nausea and vomiting. Peripheral receptors can be triggered either directly by chemotherapeutic agents or indirectly by substances released by their effects on other sites; these impulses arrive at the emetic center via the vagus nerve and other autonomic nerve afferents. Input from higher cognitive centers, a common source of vomiting in humans, is rarely identified in animals. Pharmaco-logic intervention through any one or all of these pathways is important for eliminating vomiting in the cancer patient.

GENERAL CONCEPTS OF EMESIS THERAPY (Figure 2-24)

Most chemotherapeutic agents are unlikely to induce vomiting in animals shortly after administra-

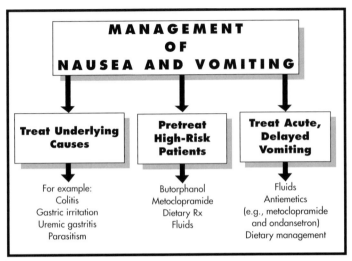

MANAGEMENT
OF
NAUSEA AND VOMITING

Treat Underlying Causes	Pretreat High-Risk Patients	Treat Acute, Delayed Vomiting
For example: Colitis Gastric irritation Uremic gastritis Parasitism	Butorphanol Metoclopramide Dietary Rx Fluids	Fluids Antiemetics (e.g., metoclopramide and ondansetron) Dietary management

Figure 2-24: *General scheme for the treatment of nausea and vomiting in the veterinary cancer patient. Impulses are transmitted by both vagal and sympathetic afferents to the emetic center of the medulla. Appropriate motor reactions are then initiated to cause vomiting. The act of vomiting is initiated by motor impulses through several cranial nerves to the upper GI tract and through the spinal nerves to the diaphragm and abdominal muscles.[2]*

tion.[2-5] Cisplatin is associated with vomiting within a few hours after treatment,[4,5] but this usually is brief and self-limiting. Moore and colleagues[5] demonstrated that butorphanol administered intramuscularly (0.4 mg/kg) at the end of cisplatin infusion was effective for reducing cisplatin chemotherapy-induced vomiting from an incidence of 90% to less than 20%. Another study[4] demonstrated that when vomiting occurred, it was almost always in smaller dogs. If an animal vomited after the first dose of cisplatin, that animal was much more likely than other patients to vomit subsequently.

SELF-LIMITING VOMITING[1-3]

An underlying cause for acute, potentially self-limiting vomiting should be identified and corrected whenever possible. Animals with self-limiting vomiting should be given nothing by mouth until vomiting ceases for at least 12 to 24 hours. Subsequently, very small amounts of water (e.g., ice cubes) followed by a bland

diet can be offered every 2 to 4 hours. Once the animal is able to take in food without vomiting, it can be slowly returned to a normal diet. During this transition period, the food should be soft in consistency, low in fat, and high in carbohydrates. Fat is a complex nutrient that is difficult to digest and therefore may induce diarrhea; compared to carbohydrates, fat can delay gastric emptying. Animals with minimal dehydration can receive fluids subcutaneously; however, intravenous therapy is preferred for significantly dehydrated patients. Many dogs and cats improve dramatically shortly after the administration of intravenous fluids. Potassium supplementation should be provided if hypokalemia is identified (Table 2-7).

LIFE-THREATENING VOMITING[1-3,5]

Specific treatment, including fluid therapy, should be administered to patients that are severely dehydrated (8% to 12% of normal hydration). Deficits in fluid and electrolytes secondary to dehydration should be replaced during the first 24 hours. Approximately 66 ml/kg/day of maintenance

TABLE 2-7
Intravenous potassium supplementation to correct hypokalemia

Serum Potassium (mEq/L)	KCl Added to Each Liter of Fluid (mEq)	Maximum Rate of Infusion (ml/kg/hr)
<2	80	6
2.1–2.5	60	8
2.6–3.0	40	12
3.1–3.5	28	16

TABLE 2-8
Selected antiemetics for use in dogs and cats

Generic Name	Product	Dosage for Dogs and Cats
Chlorpromazine	Thorazine®	0.5 mg/kg q 6–8 hours IM, SQ (dogs, cats)
Prochlorperazine	Compazine®	0.1–0.5 mg/kg q 6–8 hours IM, SQ (dogs, cats) 1.0 mg/kg q 8 hours rectally (dogs)
Diphenhydramine	Benadryl®	2.0–4.0 mg/kg q 8 hours PO (dogs, cats)
Butorphanol	Torbugesic®	0.4 mg/kg q 8 hours IM (dogs, cats)
Dimenhydrinate	Dramamine®	8 mg/kg q 8 hours PO (dogs, cats)
Trimethobenzamide	Tigan®	3 mg/kg q 8 hours IM (dogs)
Prochlorperazine	Darbazine®	0.5–0.8 mg/kg q 12 hours, IM, SQ (dogs, cats)
Metoclopramide	Reglan®	1–2 mg/kg constant rate infusion IV over 24 hours (dogs, cats)
Haloperidol	Haldol®	110 µg/kg q 4 days (dogs, investigational)
Pimozide	Orap®	100 µg/kg q 6 days (dogs, investigational)
Ondansetron	Zofran®	0.1 mg/kg IV 15 minutes before and 4 hours after chemotherapy (dogs, investigational)
Dexamethasone	Many available	1–3 mg IV (dogs, investigational)

fluids should be administered. Continued losses, such as from vomiting and diarrhea, should be estimated and replaced. As noted previously, potassium chloride (KCl) should be supplemented in the fluids if hypokalemia is identified. Potassium should not be administered at a rate greater than 0.5 mEq/kg/hr because this may cause cardiac arrest and death. The patient should be monitored for fluid overload using the following parameters: body weight, capillary refill time, skin turgor, chest auscultation, packed cell volume, total solids, and central venous pressure. If vomiting is not likely to subside in a short period, antiemetics

KEY POINT:

Special attention should be focused on pretreating smaller patients, especially those that have vomited after a previous dosage of cisplatin, by administering drugs such as butorphanol.

should be employed. If vomiting is caused by chemotherapeutic agents, pretreatment with antiemetics is indicated for all future administrations.

ANTIEMETIC AGENTS
(Table 2-8)
Metoclopramide[1–3]

In veterinary medicine, metoclopramide is one of the most commonly administered antiemetics. Its antiemetic effect is both central and peripheral. Centrally, metoclopramide is a dopamine antagonist that blocks the chemoreceptor trigger zone and prevents emesis. Peripherally, metoclopramide increases the tone of the caudal esophageal sphincter and increases gastric antral contractions by relaxing the pylorus and duodenum. Metoclopramide can be given to dogs and cats at a dosage of 0.2 to 0.4 mg/kg IM or SQ every 8 hours, or at dosages of 1 to 2 mg/kg as a constant rate infusion over a 24-hour period by an intravenous pump.

Phenothiazines[1-3]

Phenothiazines (e.g., chlorpromazine and prochlorperazine) are commonly used as antiemetics for mild chemotherapy-induced nausea; they block the chemoreceptor trigger zone of the emetic center. In human medicine, phenothiazines generally are not effective for reducing efferent gastrointestinal irritation. These drugs can induce vasodilation and therefore should not be used in dehydrated patients or in those with poor cardiac output. In addition, phenothiazines can induce mild depression and make patient monitoring difficult. All phenothiazines can cause seizures in predisposed animals. Chlorpromazine can be administered at 0.5 mg/kg IM or SQ every 6 to 8 hours; prochlorperazine can be dosed at 0.1 to 0.5 mg/kg IM or SQ every 6 to 8 hours. A suppository form (Compazine®, SmithKline Beecham) is available for use in select patients.

Narcotic Analgesics

Butorphanol (0.4 mg/kg IM) has been shown to reduce the prevalence of vomiting in response to the administration of cisplatin. The drug also has analgesic properties. For best results, butorphanol should be administered intramuscularly at the end of the cisplatin infusion.

Antihistamines

Antihistamines (e.g., diphenhydramine, dimenhydrinate, and trimethobenzamide) are another class of antiemetics. They block input from the vestibular sys-

> **KEY POINT:**
>
> *Metoclopramide should not be administered if a gastrointestinal obstruction is identified or suspected.*

tem and work against motion-induced vomiting. Diphenhydramine can be administered at 2 to 4 mg/kg every 8 hours PO; it can cause mild sedation.

Dopamine Antagonists and Diphenylbutylpiperidine[1-3]

Haloperidol is another dopamine antagonist that blocks the chemoreceptor trigger zone and can prevent vomiting for up to 4 days in dogs at a dose of 110 µg/kg. Pimozide, a long-acting diphenylbutylpiperidine, can protect dogs from drug-induced vomiting for up to 6 days when given at a dose of 100 µg/kg. Clinical experience with these two drugs is minimal.

Serotonin Antagonists[1-3]

Drugs that inhibit the 5-HT-3 (5-hydroxytryptamine) receptor constitute an entirely new and effective class of antiemetics. Ondansetron (Zofran®) is currently available, and similar agents are being explored for use in human and veterinary cancer patients. Serotonin antagonists are effective for reducing cisplatin-induced vomiting. They are less toxic than metoclopramide. Ondansetron and other serotonin antagonists are very expensive, but their cost is expected to decline in the future. (For dosage, see Table 2-8.)

Corticosteroids[1-3]

Dexamethasone has been shown to have antiemetic activity. Its mechanism is unknown. Side effects are few except in patients with diabetes or gastric ulcers. Relatively small (1–3 mg) IV doses of dexamethasone are effective in humans; an appropriate dosage in dogs and cats is not known at this time.

REFERENCES

1. Morrow GR: Management of nausea in the cancer patient, in Rosenthal S, Carignan JR, Smith BD (eds): *Medical Care of the Cancer Patient*, ed 2. Philadelphia,

WB Saunders, 1993, pp 565–571.

2. Tams TR: Vomiting, regurgitation and dysphagia, in Ettinger SJ (ed): *Textbook of Veterinary Internal Medicine: Diseases of the Dog and Cat*, ed 3. Philadelphia, WB Saunders, 1989, pp 27–32.

3. Leib MS: Acute vomiting: A diagnostic approach and systematic management, in Kirk RW, Bonagura JD (eds): *Current Veterinary Therapy. XI.* Philadelphia, WB Saunders, 1992, pp 583–587.

4. Ogilvie GK, Moore AS, Curtis CR: Cisplatin-induced emesis in the dog with malignant neoplasia: 115 cases (1984–1987). *JAVMA* 195:1399–1403, 1989.

5. Moore AS, Rand WM, Berg J, L'Heureux DA: A randomized evaluation of butorphanol and cyproheptadine for prevention of cisplatin-induced vomiting in the dog. *JAVMA* 205:441–443, 1994.

CLINICAL BRIEFING: NUTRITIONAL SUPPORT

Enteral Feeding

General	Enteral routes are preferred whenever possible. Consider diets that are relatively low in simple carbohydrates and moderate in fats; omega-3 fatty acids may be valuable. Diets should provide adequate amounts of highly bioavailable proteins. Adequate fiber is essential for general health. Energy requirements must be determined on an individual basis but may not be higher in a cancer patient than in a normal animal, even during recovery from surgery
Oral Feeding	Best enteral route. Enhance intake by providing highly palatable foods. Warm foods to just below body temperature and consider appetite stimulants, such as benzodiazepine derivatives, cyproheptadine, and megestrol acetate. Consider other routes when weight loss approaches 10%
Nasogastric Tube Feeding	Excellent for short-term feeding. Use liquid nutrient solutions to meet all nutrient needs
Gastrostomy Tube Feeding	Excellent for long-term feeding in patients that are not vomiting and have functional GI tracts. Use blenderized foods to meet nutrient needs
Jejunostomy Tube Feeding	Excellent choice to bypass the upper GI tract. Use liquid nutrient solutions. The use of a pump or frequent small feedings by syringe is required

Parenteral Feeding

General	Excellent choice whenever enteral feeding is not possible. An infusion pump, specially designed nutrients, absolute dedication to aseptic technique, and a separate indwelling catheter are needed

Recently, a great deal of information has been published on the nutritional management of the veterinary cancer patient.[1-11] The routine use of nutrient delivery systems, such as nasogastric, gastrostomy, and jejunostomy tubes as well as parenteral feeding techniques, has increased substantially in veterinary medicine. This has resulted in a better quality of life and better response to therapy for animals that receive this type of care. The results of recent research suggest that many tumor-bearing animals need not only special methods for delivering nutrients but also specific types of fluid and nutrient support. This is because many animals with cancer have dramatic and often unique alterations in metabolism; these changes in metabolism are collectively known as cancer cachexia (see the chapter on Cancer Cachexia).

Cancer cachexia is a complex paraneoplastic syndrome of progressive involuntary weight loss that occurs even in the face of adequate nutritional intake. The importance of this syndrome cannot be overstated. For example, humans with cancer cachexia have a decreased quality of life, decreased response to treatment, and a shortened survival time compared to patients who have similar diseases but do not exhibit clinical or biochemical signs associated with this condition. Understanding the metabolic alterations in pets with cancer is essential to provide adequate nutritional support to these patients.

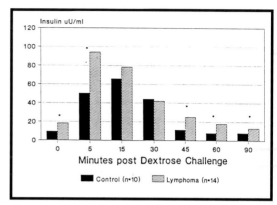

Figure 2-25: *Serum insulin concentrations in dogs with and without lymphoma before and after IV administration of 500 mg/kg dextrose. Asterisks (*) indicate values from dogs with lymphoma that differ significantly (P <0.001) from control dogs at the same time. (From Vail DM, Ogilvie GK, Wheeler SL, et al. Alterations in carbohydrate metabolism in canine lymphoma. J Vet Intern Med 4:8–14, 1990; with permission.)*

METABOLIC ALTERATIONS IN CANCER CACHEXIA

The abnormalities in carbohydrate, protein, and lipid metabolism in animals and humans with cancer cachexia can lead to serious debilitation and death unless addressed by appropriate therapy. These abnormalities are seen not only in animals with overt signs of cachexia but also in those with asymptomatic disease.

Carbohydrate Metabolism

Perhaps the most dramatic metabolic disturbances in animals with cancer occur in carbohydrate metabolism.[1-4] Abnormalities have been documented in peripheral glucose disposal, hepatic gluconeogenesis, and whole body glucose oxidation and turnover.

The normal animal utilizes glucose through aerobic metabolism, resulting in the production of large quantities of ATP for future use. Cancer cells possess all the enzymes necessary to carry out glucose metabolism aerobically, but, for obscure reasons, the tumor preferentially metabolizes glucose by anaerobic glycolysis, forming lactate as an end product, which must be converted by the host into a usable form. This conversion requires energy. The result is that the tumor gains energy while the host has a dramatic energy loss. This is of profound clinical importance and is a reason for therapeutic intervention.

Recent research has documented that dogs with lymphoma and a wide variety of malignant diseases have significant alterations in carbohydrate metabolism:

- Dogs with a wide variety of malignant conditions have elevated resting insulin and lactate levels compared to control animals (Figures 2-25 and 2-26).
- Insulin and lactate levels of dogs with cancer increase above levels compared to control dogs in response to a glucose and diet tolerance test (Figure 2-25 and 2-26).
- Elevated lactate and glucose levels do not improve after dogs with cancer are rendered free of disease

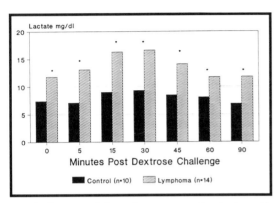

Figure 2-26: *Serum lactate concentrations in dogs with and without lymphoma before and after IV administration of 500 mg/kg dextrose. Asterisks (*) indicate values from dogs with lymphoma that differ significantly (P <0.001) from control dogs at the same time. (From Vail DM, Ogilvie GK, Wheeler SL, et al. Alterations in carbohydrate metabolism in canine lymphoma. J Vet Intern Med 4:8–14, 1990; with permission.)*

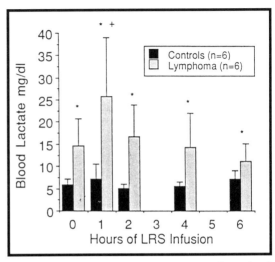

Figure 2-27: *Blood lactate concentrations in dogs with and without lymphoma before and during IV infusion of lactated Ringer's solution. Asterisks (*) indicate values from dogs with lymphoma that differ significantly (P <0.05) from controls at the same time. Plus sign (+) indicates values that differ significantly (P <0.05) from preinfusion baseline values within the same test group. (From Vail DM, Ogilvie GK, Fettman MJ, et al. Exacerbation of hyperlactatemia by infusion of lactated Ringer's solution in dogs with lymphoma. J Vet Intern Med 4:228–232, 1990; with permission.)*

with chemotherapy and surgery (Figure 2-27). This suggests that the malignancy causes a fundamental change in metabolism that persists after all clinical evidence of cancer is eliminated.

- Elevated lactate levels can result in inefficient Cori cycle activity to convert lactate back to glucose; this results in a net energy loss by the patient.
- The administration of lactate-containing parenteral fluids such as lactated Ringer's solution has been shown to increase lactate levels in dogs with lymphoma, suggesting that these types of fluids may place an additional energy burden on the host.

Protein and Lipid Metabolism

A recent report documented that dogs with cancer have alterations in protein metabolism that are very similar to those observed in humans and laboratory animals.[1] There was a significant decrease in a wide variety of amino acids, suggesting that a high-quality, highly bioavailable protein source would be beneficial to the animal and to the tumor.

The net results of these alterations in protein metabolism are of great clinical significance.[1–4] For example, alterations in many important bodily functions, such as immune response, GI function, and surgical healing, have been identified. Meeting amino acid needs may be of significant benefit to the cancer patient.

Serum lipid profiles were performed in dogs with lymphoma before and after they were put into remission with chemotherapy. These profiles were compared to those of normal dogs before and after they were given the same anticancer drug.[8]

- The dogs with cancer had significantly lower levels of high-density lipoproteins. The total triglyceride levels and very low-density triglycerides of untreated dogs with lymphoma were significantly higher than untreated control dogs.

- Following a total of five doses of chemotherapy, the total cholesterol level increased in dogs with lymphoma but decreased in treated control dogs.
- All other parameters remained unchanged after doxorubicin therapy, suggesting that lipid abnormalities do not improve significantly even after a clinical remission is obtained.

Abnormalities in lipid metabolism have been linked to a number of clinical problems, including immunosuppression, which correlates with decreased survival in affected humans.[1-4] The clinical impact of the abnormalities in lipid metabolism may be lessened with dietary therapy. In contrast to carbohydrates and proteins, some tumor cells have difficulty using lipid as a fuel source, but host tissues continue to oxidize lipids for energy. This has led to the hypothesis that diets relatively high in fat may be beneficial for animals with cancer compared to diets that are high in simple carbohydrates, assuming that the protein content, caloric density, and palatability remain constant. A recently completed study suggested that a high-carbohydrate, low-fat diet did induce elevated lactate and insulin levels compared to a diet relatively high in fat and low in carbohydrates. There was some suggestion that the high-fat diet may result in a higher probability of going into remission with chemotherapy as well as a longer survival time. The kind of fat in the diet, rather than the amount, may be the important factor. For example, omega-3 fatty acids have been shown experimentally to have many beneficial properties.[12-14]

- Omega-3 fatty acids, arginine, and RNA improve the immune system, metabolic status, and clinical outcome of human cancer patients.
- When used alone, omega-3 fatty acids improve the immune system and decrease the time for wound healing, duration of hospitalization, and complication rate in humans with GI cancer.

- Omega-3 fatty acids inhibit tumorigenesis and cancer spread in animal models.
- Essential fatty acids that contain omega-3 fatty acids reduce radiation-induced damage to skin. This seems to be specific for normal, not malignant, cells.
- Eicosapentaenoic acid not only has antitumor effects but also anticachectic effects, in part because there is decreased protein degradation without an effect on protein synthesis.

In a study recently completed at Colorado State University, hyperlactatemia was reversed and eliminated in dogs with lymphoma by dietary supplementation with omega-3 fatty acids. Further studies are essential to determine whether dogs with other malignancies will benefit from this effect. Similarly, it is essential to determine whether diets supplemented with omega-3 improve quality of life and response to therapy.

Many nutrients other than omega-3 fatty acids have been suggested to have anticancer properties. For example, antioxidants, such as vitamins C, E, and A, have anticancer effects. Selenium, vitamin K_3, arginine, glutamine, and garlic have been shown to be beneficial in some experimental settings. Further research is essential to define the value, if any, of these nutrients in veterinary cancer therapy.

Nutritional and Water Needs

Our knowledge of the nutrient and water needs of dogs and cats is primarily based on work done many years ago or extrapolated from research completed on rodents or humans. The majority of data concerning energy and water requirements in dogs and cats may be overestimates.[9,10] For example, it has been determined that the resting energy expenditure, which is an estimate of the nutrient and water needs of normal dogs, is *lower* than data previously published.[10] In addition, one study showed that dogs with lymphoma or dogs that have undergone surgery for various problems have resting energy requirements that are *lower* than normal animals.[9] This is in stark contrast to publications that suggest that cancer and surgery result in dramatic increases in the nutrient and water requirements of animals. This is of critical value for practicing veterinarians in attempting to meet the nutrient and fluid needs of normal and ill veterinary patients. This also may be of great importance for pet owners.

NUTRITIONAL SUPPORT FOR CANCER PATIENTS

The ideal way of treating cancer cachexia is to eliminate the underlying neoplastic condition. Unfortunately, this is not possible for many veterinary patients. Therefore, dietary therapy has been examined as a modality to reverse or eliminate cancer cachexia. Investigators have demonstrated concern about the possibility of increasing tumor growth by enhancing the nutritional status of the host. Several studies have failed to show this correlation. The benefits that have been shown with dietary support include weight gain and increased response to and tolerance of radiation, surgery, and chemotherapy. Other factors that have been shown to improve with nutritional support include thymic weight, immune responsiveness, and immunoglobulin and complement levels as well as the phagocytic ability of white blood cells.[1-4]

Rodents and humans with cancer that consume diets that contain 30% to 50% of nonprotein calories as fat have increased nitrogen and energy balance as well as increased weight gain.[1-4] In addition, this type of diet results in slower tumor growth and decreases in both glucose intolerance and fat loss. Glucose-containing fluids may result in increased lactate production, which may cause an energy drain on the host. In addition, as noted earlier, diets containing omega-3 fatty acids have been shown to decrease lactate concentrations in dogs with lymphoma. Although the

> **KEY POINT:**
>
> *The energy needs of animals with cancer usually are not higher than the needs of normal animals. Similarly, recent research has shown that the energy needs do not increase after major or minor surgery.*

ideal dietary formulation for dogs and cats is not known, these facts may serve as guides for future research in this area. The following are general guidelines for dietary therapy for veterinary patients with cancer.

Parenteral Nutrition

Parenteral nutrition should be considered for animals with cancer whenever enteral feeding is not feasible. Parenteral feeding does require some specialized equipment such as pumps, but the procedure can safely be carried out in private practice.

Administration and Complications

In veterinary medicine, parenteral nutrients are generally administered through a dedicated single-lumen polyurethane catheter or a more expensive multilumen catheter.[1-4] It is essential to ensure that the catheter remains sterile to reduce the incidence of catheter-induced sepsis. One method of keeping the catheter port clean is to place a sealable plastic bag over the end. Most veterinary centers that administer parenteral nutrients use intravenous pumps to ensure a constant rate of infusion. The rate of infusion is simplified if lipid is used to provide a percentage of nonprotein calories, because dextrose-containing fluids need to be gradually increased over several days.

With proper technique and patient care, problems associated with the administration of parenteral nutrition are relatively uncommon. Complications can result from destruction or occlusion of the catheter or tubing and pump failure; however, the most serious complication is related to catheter- or solution-related sepsis, which can be avoided by using aseptic technique. Other complications include metabolic and electrolyte abnormalities, including lactic acidosis. Mildly elevated serum urea nitrogen levels and hyperglycemia with glucosuria occasionally occur in dogs and cats receiving parenteral nutrient therapy. Hypokalemia is perhaps the most common related electrolyte disturbance, but it is easily corrected with additional supplementation.

Calculating Contents and Volumes

Although recent research may suggest that animals with cancer do not have increased requirements, the determination of the amount of parenteral solution for the dog is relatively straightforward.[1-4]

Energy Requirements

- The basal energy requirement (BER, in Kcal/day) is calculated by multiplying 70 by the animal's weight in $kg^{0.75}$ and then multiplying by a factor to derive the illness energy requirement (IER).
- The standard dogma states that for normal dogs that are at rest in a cage, the BER is multiplied by 1.25. For dogs that have undergone recent surgery or that are recovering from trauma, the BER is multiplied by 1.2 to 1.6. For dogs that are septic or have major burns, the BER is multiplied by 1.5 to 2.0.
- The IER (Kcal/day as nonprotein calories) has not been determined for dogs with cancer but is reported to be quite high, even in animals without sepsis, burns, trauma, or surgery. Our work[9,10] suggests that energy requirement in dogs with cancer may not exceed those of normal dogs. Until this is confirmed, it may be better to overestimate, rather than underestimate, nutrient requirements of the cancer patient.

Protein Requirements

- The protein requirement for dogs is 4 g/kg/day for normal dogs and 6 g/kg/day for dogs that have heavy protein losses. Dogs with renal or hepatic failure may have a reduced protein requirement of 1.5 g/kg/day. Utilization of amino acids in cancer patients is significantly altered compared to patients without cancer.
- The volumes of nutrient solutions to be administered to each patient depends on their content. For example, to calculate the amount of an 8.5% amino acid solution required for a 24-hour period, the amount of protein (mg) required for the animal patient for 1 day is divided by 85 mg/ml to determine the volume of the amino acid solution to administer.

Lipid and Carbohydrate Requirements

- Most authors recommend giving 40% to 60% of the nonprotein calories as lipid; the remainder of nonprotein calories are given as dextrose. Therefore, because a 20% lipid solution has 2 Kcal/ml, 40% to 60% of the IER is divided by 2 Kcal/ml to yield the volume of the lipid solution to administer. Lipemic patients should not be given lipid-containing solutions.
- To determine the volume of a 50% dextrose solution to be administered (1.7 Kcal/ml), divide 40% to 60% of IER by 1.7 Kcal/ml. Because the volume of the dextrose-containing fluids should be increased gradually, half of this calculated volume should be administered on the first day and gradually increased to the full amount over the next day or two.

Enteral Nutrition

As a general rule, mature dogs and cats with functional GI tracts that have a history of inadequate nutritional intake for 5 to 7 days or that have lost at least 10% of their body weight over a 1- to 2-week period are

> **KEY POINT:**
>
> *Although the ideal "cancer diet" is not known, a diet composed of relatively low amounts of simple carbohydrates, modest amounts of fats (especially omega-3 fatty acids), and adequate amounts of highly bioavailable proteins may be beneficial.*

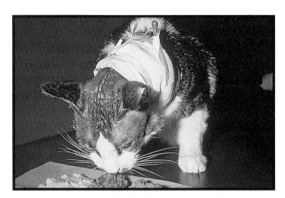

Figure 2-28: *All methods to encourage food consumption, including feeding a variety of highly palatable aromatic foods, warming the food to just below body temperature, and chemical stimulants, should be tried before starting enteral support. The optimum pharmacologic agent for use in the veterinary cancer patient is unknown; however, megestrol acetate has been shown to result in substantial weight gain in humans with cancer.*

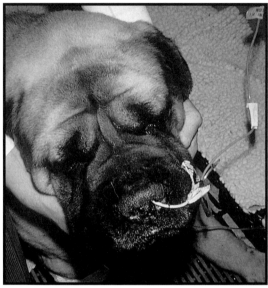

Figure 2-29: *Nasogastric tube feeding is one of the most common methods used for short-term nutritional support of dogs and cats. The use of small-bore silastic or polyurethane catheters has minimized complications associated with this delivery system. Lidocaine is instilled into the nasal cavity, and the tube is lubricated and passed to the level of the thirteenth rib in dogs and the ninth rib in cats. In dogs, permanent adhesive or a suture should be used to secure the tube to the side of the face that is ipsilateral to the intubated nostril.*

candidates for enteral nutritional therapy. All methods to encourage food consumption should be attempted (Figure 2-28). These include warming the food to just below body temperature; providing a selection of palatable, aromatic foods; and providing comfortable, stress-free surroundings. When these simple procedures fail, such chemical stimulants as benzodiazepine derivatives (e.g., diazepam and oxazepam) and antiserotonin agents (cyproheptadine and pizotifen) can be used. Cyproheptadine (2–4 mg daily or twice daily PO) generally is effective in stimulating appetite in cats, as are megestrol acetate (2.5 mg daily for 4 days, then every 2–3 days thereafter) and diazepam (0.05–0.5 mg/kg IV). Dogs may respond to megestrol acetate administration. Dogs and cats may have improved appetite when metoclopramide is given orally to decrease nausea associated with chemotherapy or surgery. When all the aforementioned fails, enteral nutritional support, designed to deliver nutrients to the GI tract by various methods, should be considered because it is practical, cost-effective, physiologic, and safe.[1–4]

> **KEY POINT:**
>
> *Enteral feeding should be used whenever possible: if the gut works, use it!*

Routes of Enteral Feeding

Nasogastric Tubes. In the eighteenth century, Hunter was the first to use nasogastric tubes for feeding; it is still the most common method used today.[1–4] The use of small-bore, silastic or polyurethane catheters has minimized complications associated with this delivery system. The procedure is simple to perform (Figure 2-29).

1. Tranquilization is sometimes re-

quired during placement of the tube, especially in cats. To decrease any discomfort associated with the initial placement of the catheter, lidocaine is instilled into the nasal cavity with the nose pointed up. It may be helpful to place a finger on the septum and push the animal's nose back parallel to the long axis of the head, thereby straightening the nasal passageway.

2. The tube is lubricated and passed to the level of the thirteenth rib in dogs and the ninth rib in cats.

3. After the tube has been properly placed, it should be secured. In cats, the tube should be bent dorsally over the bridge of the nose and secured to the frontal region of the head with a permanent adhesive (Superglue®, Loctite Corp, Cleveland, OH). A suture may be used to further secure the tube in place. In dogs, the permanent adhesive should be used to secure the tube to the side of the face that is ipsilateral to the intubated nostril. Care should be taken to prevent any contact with whiskers.

4. An Elizabethan collar should always be used to prevent the patient from removing the tube.

Gastrostomy Tubes. Gastrostomy tubes are used frequently in veterinary practice for animals that need nutritional support for more than 7 days.[1-4] These tubes can be placed surgically or with endoscopic guidance. A 5-ml balloon-tipped urethral catheter (e.g., Foley Catheter, Bardex, Murray Hill, NJ) can be placed surgically, as can a mushroom-tipped Pezzer proportionate head urologic catheter (Bard Urological Catheter, Bard Urological Division, Covingtion, GA). For smaller dogs and cats, an 18- to 24-Fr catheter is used; larger dogs require a 26- to 30-Fr tube. The procedure is as follows:

1. Prior to placement of the tube, the left paracostal area just below the paravertebral epaxial musculature is clipped and prepared for surgery. A 2- to 3-cm incision is made just caudal to the last rib through the skin and subcutaneous tissue to allow blunt dissection through the musculature into the abdominal cavity.

2. The stomach is inflated through a tube that is placed down the esophagus to allow the surgeon to easily locate the stomach through the opening in the abdominal wall. Stay sutures are placed to allow a temporary fixation of the stomach against the abdominal wall; these stay sutures are used later to help close the muscular wall.

3. Two concentric pursestring sutures of 2-0 nonabsorbable nylon suture are then placed deep in the stomach wall; the first pursestring is deep to the second to allow a two-layered closure.

4. The feeding tube is placed into the lumen of the stomach through a stab incision in the middle of the pursestring sutures. The tip of the catheter generally is clipped off to allow easy introduction of food through the tube and into the stomach.

5. Once the tube is in place, the balloon is inflated with water if the balloon-tipped catheter is used; the Pezzer-tipped catheter has an expanded head that flattens and then returns to its normal shape when a stylet is extended and then removed in the catheter lumen during placement through the stab incision into the stomach.

6. With the tube in place, the pursestrings are tied to cause the stomach to invert in the region adjacent to the tube. The free ends of the pursestrings are then used to close the lateral abdominal musculature and subcutaneous tissue.

7. The skin is closed before the tube is secured to the abdominal skin by sutures. To prevent the animal from removing the tube, an abdominal wrap and an Elizabethan collar are recommended.

Feeding can begin soon after the animal has recovered from anesthesia. The tube should be checked daily to ensure proper placement. In addition, the tube should be flushed with warm water after each feeding to maintain patency. After 7 to 10 days, an adhesion will form, allowing the tube to be removed or replaced as needed. The fistula generally heals within a week after the tube is removed permanently.

The percutaneous placement of a gastrostomy tube

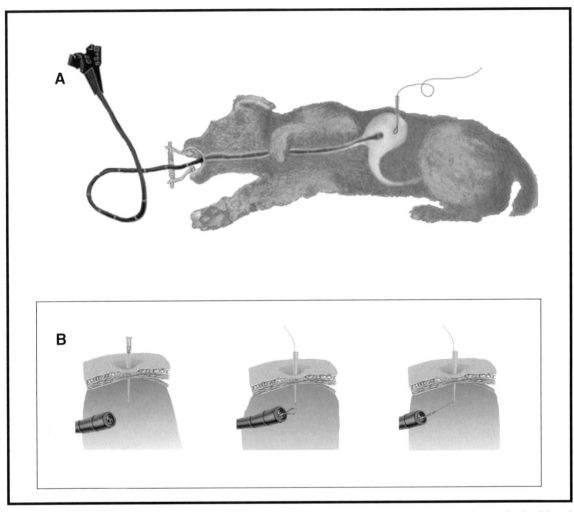

Figure 2-30: *Gastrostomy tube placement. Note that an endoscope is used to insufflate the stomach so that a catheter can be placed through the skin and into the stomach to facilitate the passage of nylon suture into the stomach (**A**). The endoscope is then used to grasp the suture, which is then pulled through the esophagus and out of the mouth (**B**).*

by endoscopic guidance is quick, safe, and effective.[1-4] In this procedure (Figures 2-30 and 2-31), a specialized 20-Fr tube (e.g., Dubhoff PEG, Biosearch, Summerville, NJ; Bard Urological Catheter, Bard Urological Division, Covingtion, GA) is used in both dogs and cats.

1. The first step is to clip and surgically prepare the area of skin outlined previously, and then distend the stomach with air from an endoscope that is placed into the stomach.
2. Once the stomach is distended to the point that it is in apposition with the body wall, a finger is used

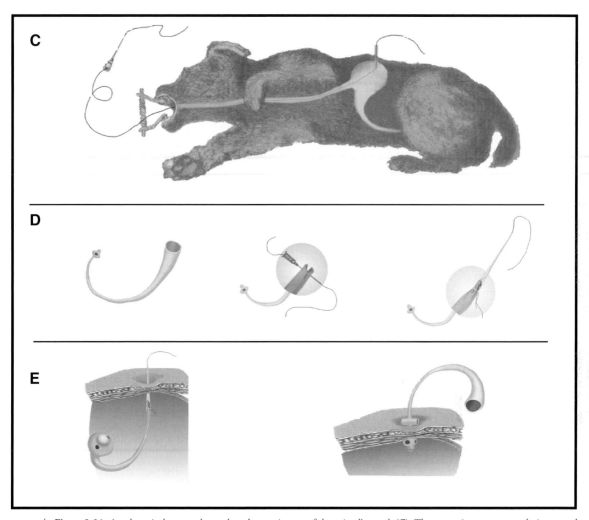

Figure 2-31: *A catheter is then passed over the nylon coming out of the animal's mouth (**C**). The pezzer tip gastrostomy tube is prepared (**D**) by cutting a "V" out of both sides of the open end of the tube. A needle is used to pass the nylon suture coming out of the mouth through the end of the tube, where a knot is securely fastened. The tube is then stretched and forced into the end of the catheter. The catheter–tube combination is pulled with the nylon suture down the esophagus, into the stomach, and through the abdominal wall (**E**), where a "bumper" is placed down the tube and against the body wall.*

to depress an area just caudal to the last left rib below the transverse processes of the lumbar vertebrae. This area of depression is then located by the person viewing the stomach lining by endoscopy.
3. A polyvinylchloride (PVC) over-the-needle IV catheter is placed through the skin and into the stomach in the area previously located by the endoscopist. The stylet is removed to allow the introduction of the first portion of a 5-foot-long piece of 8-lb test weight nylon filament or suture.

4. The piece of nylon is grabbed by a biopsy snare passed through the endoscope. The endoscope and the attached nylon are pulled up the esophagus and out the oral cavity so that the piece of nylon extends through the body wall and out of the mouth of the animal.

5. The end of the gastrostomy tube opposite the mushroom tip is trimmed so that it has a pointed end that will fit inside another PVC catheter, after the stylet is removed and discarded. This second PVC IV catheter is then placed over the nylon suture so that the narrow end points toward the stomach. The free end of the nylon that has just been pulled out of the animal's mouth is sutured to the end of the tube and is tied securely.

6. The catheter–tube combination is pulled firmly but slowly from the end of the suture located outside the abdominal wall until the pointed end of the IV catheter comes down the esophagus and out the abdominal wall.

7. The tube is grasped and pulled until the mushroom tip is adjacent to the stomach wall, as viewed by endoscopy.

8. To prevent slippage, the middle of a 3- to 4-inch piece of tubing is pierced completely through both sides and passed over the feeding tube so that it is adjacent to the body wall. This bumper or retainer is then glued or sutured securely in place. The tube is capped and bandaged in place.

An Elizabethan collar is almost always required to prevent the animal from removing the tube. To remove the tube once it has been in place for 7 to 10 days, the tube just below the bumper is severed to allow the "mushroom" tip to fall into the stomach. This piece may need to be removed by endoscopy in all but very large dogs.

Needle Catheter Jejunostomy Tubes. Needle catheter jejunostomy tubes should be considered for dogs and cats with functional lower intestinal tracts that will not tolerate nasogastric or gastrostomy tube feeding.[1-4] This method is especially valuable in cancer

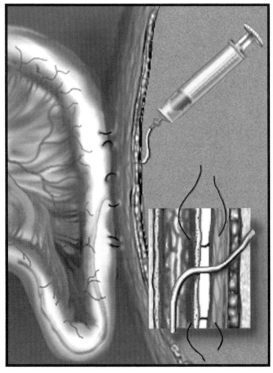

Figure 2-32: A jejunostomy tube is surgically placed through a stab incision in the antimesenteric side of the jejunum. The other end of the tube is then placed through the abdominal wall, whereupon the jejunum is securely sutured to the abdominal wall. Jejunostomy tubes are ideal for supporting cancer patients with alterations in the upper GI tract.

patients that have had surgery to the upper GI tract. The procedure is as follows (Figure 2-32):

1. The distal duodenum or proximal jejunum is located and isolated by surgery. A pursestring suture of 3-0 nonabsorbable suture is placed in the antimesenteric boarder of the isolated piece of bowel.

2. A 12-ga needle is placed from the serosa located at the center of the area encircled by the pursestring suture, subserosally 2 to 3 cm through the wall of the intestine, into the lumen of the loop of bow-

el. Alternatively, a stab incision can be made into the same location of the bowel using a number 11 surgical blade.

3. A 5-Fr nasogastric infant feeding tube is passed through the hypodermic needle or the stab incision to an area down the bowel, 20 to 30 cm from the enterostomy site.

4. If a needle was used, it is then removed.

5. The pursestring is tightened and secured around the tube.

6. The free end of the feeding tube is passed from the serosal surface of the abdominal wall out of the skin through a second hypodermic needle.

7. The loop of bowel with the enterostomy site is secured to the abdominal wall with four sutures that are later cut after the tube is removed in 7 to 10 days, when feeding is complete.

As with gastrostomy tubes, complications with this method include peritonitis, diarrhea, and cramping.

Enteral Feeding Methods

The type of nutrients to be used depends largely on the enteral tube that is used and on the status of the patient.[1-4] Blended canned pet foods may be adequate for feeding by gastrostomy tubes, and human enteral feeding products are easily administered though nasogastric and jejunostomy tubes. In any case, feeding usually is not started until 24 hours after the tube is placed. Once feeding is started, the amount of nutrients is gradually increased over several days and is administered frequently in small amounts, which allows the animal to adapt to this method of feeding. Continuous feeding may reduce the risk of vomiting caused by overloading the GI tract. Regardless, the tube should be aspirated 3 to 4 times a day to ensure there is not excessive residual volume in the GI tract. The tube should be flushed periodically with warm water to prevent clogging.

Calculating Contents and Volumes

Calculation of the nutritional requirements for enteral feeding is essentially the same as for parenteral feeding noted earlier.[1-4] The illness energy requirement (IER) for the animal with cancer is calculated. It should be kept in mind that some patients have a very high energy expenditure that may exceed those seen in animals that have infections, sepsis, or burns. Other research suggest that the energy needs of most cancer patients do *not* exceed that of a healthy animal. Dogs and cats with renal or hepatic insufficiency should not be given high protein loads (< 3 g/100 Kcal in dogs; <4 g/100 Kcal in cats). Because most high-quality pet foods can be put through a blender to form a gruel that can be passed through a large feeding tube, the IER of the animal is divided by the caloric density of the canned pet food to determine the amount of food to feed. The same calculation can be done with human enteral feeding products; the volume fed may need to be increased if the enteral feeding product is diluted to ensure it is approximately iso-osmolar before administration.

REFERENCES

1. Ogilvie GK, Vail DM: Nutrition and cancer: Recent developments. *Vet Clin North Am Small Anim Pract* 20:1–29, 1990.

2. Ogilvie GK: Paraneoplastic syndromes, in Withrow SJ, MacEwen EG (eds): *Clinical Veterinary Oncology.* Philadelphia, JB Lippincott, 1989, pp 29–35.

3. Vail DM, Ogilvie GK, Wheeler SL: Metabolic alterations in patients with cancer cachexia. *Compend Contin Educ Pract Vet* 12:381–395, 1990.

4. Ogilvie GK: Metabolic alterations and nutritional therapy for the veterinary cancer patient. *Compend Contin Educ Pract Vet* 15:925–937, 1993.

5. Ogilvie GK, Vail DM, Wheeler SJ, et al: Effect of chemotherapy and remission on carbohydrate metabolism in dogs with lymphoma. *Cancer Res* 69:233–238, 1992.

6. Vail DM, Ogilvie GK, Fettman MJ, et al: Exacerbation of hyperlactatemia by infusion of lactated Ringer's solution in dogs with lymphoma. *J Vet Intern Med* 4:228–332, 1990.

7. Vail DM, Ogilvie GK, Wheeler SL, et al: Alterations in carbohydrate metabolism in canine lymphoma. *J Vet Intern Med* 4:8–14, 1990.

8. Ogilvie GK, Ford RD, Vail DM: Alterations in

lipoprotein profiles in dogs with lymphoma. *J Vet Intern Med* 8:62–66, 1994.

9. Ogilvie GK, Walters LM, Fettman MJ, et al: Energy expenditure in dogs with lymphoma fed two specialized diets. *Cancer* 71:3146–3152, 1993.

10. Walters LM, Ogilvie GK, Fettman MJ, et al: Repeatability of energy expenditure measurements in normal dogs by indirect calorimetry. *Am J Vet Res* 54:1881–1885, 1993.

11. Ogilvie GK, Vail DM: Unique metabolic alterations associated with cancer cachexia in the dog, in Kirk RW (ed): *Current Veterinary Therapy. XI.* Philadelphia, WB Saunders, 1992, pp 433–438.

12. Daly JM, Lieberman M, Goldfine J, et al: Enteral nutrition with supplemental arginine, RNA and omega-3 fatty acids: A prospective clinical trial. Abstract, 15th Clinical Congress, American Society for Parenteral and Enteral Nutrition, *J Paren Enteral Nutr* 15:19S–27S, 1991

13. Lowell JA, Parnes HL, Blackburn GL: Dietary immunomodulation: Beneficial effects on carcinogenesis and tumor growth. *Crit Care Med* 18:S145–S148, 1990.

14. Beck SA, Smith KL, Tisdale MJ: Anticachectic and antitumor effect of eicosapentaenoic acid and its effect on protein turnover. *Cancer Res* 51:6089–6093, 1991.

CLINICAL BRIEFING: TRANSFUSION SUPPORT

Enteral Feeding

Blood Donor Characteristics	*Dogs:* Group A negative donors are compatible with Group A negative and Group A positive recipients; major cross-match recommended after the first transfusion *Cats:* Most recipients in the United States are Group A positive and should receive A positive blood; Group B recipients must be given B negative blood; Group AB blood is rare
Indications	Clinically significant acute blood loss, hemolytic anemia, nonregenerative anemia, thrombocytopenia, DIC, and hypoproteinemia
Complications	Clinical signs from incompatible blood: Hemolysis, hyperthermia, tachycardia, tachypnea, vomiting, collapse, urticaria and angioneurotic edema, and CNS alterations; discontinue transfusion

Transfusions are frequently needed for veterinary cancer patients because of a variety of problems, including blood loss from the primary tumor, disseminated intravascular coagulation (DIC), clinical syndromes associated with the hypocoagulable state of malignancy, and other hematologic abnormalities.[1-3] In general, transfusions and administration of specific blood components should be given only when specifically indicated.

SEROLOGY
Dogs[1] (Table 2-9)

The most clinically important canine antigens include dog erythrocyte antigen DEA 1.1 and DEA 1.2. Approximately 60% of dogs have one of these two blood antigens. These dogs are considered Group A positive; all others dogs are considered Group A negative. Clini-

cally significant antibodies against Group A antigens do not exist naturally but can develop after exposure to Group A positive blood. Therefore, a patient that has received an A-positive blood transfusion should be assumed to have developed antibodies and is at high risk for a "transfusion reaction."

Dogs that have received previous transfusions should be cross-matched using only a major cross-match (e.g., testing the donor red blood cells against the recipient's plasma), because this allows determination of incompatibility in a cost-effective manner. Donor plasma should not have antibodies to the recipient's red blood cells unless the donor has been previously transfused.

Cats[2] (Table 2-10)

All feline blood donors should be grouped. Most recipients in the United States have Group A blood; there-

> ### KEY POINT:
>
> *All canine blood donors should be Group A negative unless donor and recipient are both Group A positive.*

fore, most donors should have Group A blood. Group B donors are less common and rarely required in a clinical setting. It is ideal to have a Group B donor available for situations in which a recipient with Group B blood is identified in need of blood. This is much more likely to occur in Australia, where Group B blood predominates. Prior to a first transfusion, cats should have their blood group determined to provide a safely matched transfusion. In emergencies, the clinician should remember that Group A is the most common group, Group B varies in frequency among breeds, and Group AB is extremely rare.

TABLE 2-9
Canine transfusions[1]

Blood Groups:		
Recipient	Donor	Clinical Results
A+	A+	Compatible: no problems
A–	A–	Compatible: no problems
A–	A+	Compatible unless antibodies to DEA 1.1 or 1.2 (i.e., previously transfused)
A+	A–	Compatible: no problems

COMPONENT THERAPY

Blood components should be administered when clinically indicated to dogs and cats. Whole blood or packed red blood cells may be administered immediately or may be stored for up to 21 days (Figures 2-33 and 2-34). Fresh frozen plasma has adequate levels of clotting factors for up to 1 year. Frozen plasma stored for more than 1 year may have a diminished amount of clotting factors V, VII, VIII, and von Willebrand's factor. Dog blood can be drawn into human unit bags that hold approximately 450 ml of blood and 50 ml of anticoagulant. The plasma can be decanted after settling has occurred to provide packed cells (Figure 2-33). In cats, a unit typically is defined as 50 ml, which is the maximum amount that can be drawn safely from the average adult cat.

INDICATIONS FOR TRANSFUSION THERAPY[1-3]
Hemorrhage

Although there is a theoretical advantage to transfusing fresh whole blood, packed red blood cells can be administered with excellent results. Canine red blood cells stored for more than 2 weeks can have a depletion in 2,3 DPG (diphosphoglycerate), which may decrease red blood cell oxygen-carrying capacity. When blood loss is chronic, transfusion should be performed to keep the hematocrit levels above 15%

TABLE 2-10
Feline transfusions[2]

Blood Groups:			
Recipient	Donor	RBC Half-life	Clinical Results
A	A	32.8 ± 3.1 days	Compatible: no problems
B	B	34.4 ± 2.8 days	Compatible: no problems
A	B	2.1 ± 0.2 days	Not compatible: mild problems
B	A	1.3 ± 2.3 hours	Not compatible: severe problems

in dogs and above 10% in cats, when possible. In acute and chronic blood loss, the patient's response to transfusion should be just as important a determinant as the hematocrit level or amount to be transfused. Dogs and cats with acute blood loss are less tolerant of low hematocrit values, whereas those that have a gradual reduction in red blood cell numbers are able to adapt to extremely low red blood cell numbers, especially cats.

Hemolytic Anemia

Immune-mediated hemolytic anemia may require the administration of red blood cells, even if this results in lysis of some of the transfused blood. Primary therapy with glucocorticoids, azathioprine, and cyclosporine is often essential to treat the underlying disease. The blood group of dogs and cats with hemolytic anemia frequently cannot be determined adequately because of the presence of

> ### KEY POINT:
>
> *Because most feline recipients in the United States have Group A blood, Group A blood generally is the safest to use for transfusions. If the donor is known to have Group B blood, then blood from this cat should only be given to a Group B recipient.*

antibodies. Frequent evaluation of packed cell volume is essential.

Nonregenerative Anemia

Nonregenerative anemia can be relatively mild and often requires no transfusion. In some cases, however, nonregenerative anemia can be severe enough to require either fresh whole blood, when platelets are needed, or packed red blood cells. In addition, recombinant erythropoietin may be of value; however, antibodies directed to erythropoietin, which may cross-react with the animal's own erythropoietin, are a possible complication.

Thrombocytopenia

Platelet counts greater than $30,000/\mu l$ to $40,000/\mu l$ are rarely associated with bleeding disorders. Indeed, a very gradual reduction in platelet counts can result in patients that appear healthy but have only 2000 to 3000 platelets/μl, especially when the platelets are relatively "young," as in

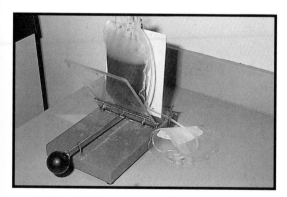

Figure 2-33A

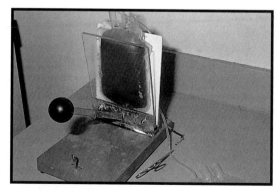

Figure 2-33B

Figure 2-33: Fresh whole blood is placed into a device (A) that squeezes the blood from the bottom of the bag (B), allowing the plasma to be decanted, through a tube already in place, into a separate bag. The process results in packed red blood cells and plasma that can be used for specific clinical settings. This procedure also is used to harvest platelet-rich plasma, which is located at, or just above, the interface between red blood cells and plasma from a unit of blood that has been centrifuged.

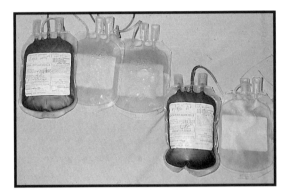

Figure 2-34: The interconnected bags in the upper left are packed red blood cells, platelet-rich plasma, and plasma that is ready to be administered to the patient. The interconnected bags on the lower right are packed red blood cells and plasma. The self-contained interconnected system allows separation of blood components without outside contamination. One unit (450 ml) of whole blood is equivalent to 270 ml of packed red blood cells. Whole blood or packed red blood cells may be administered immediately or stored for up to 21 days. Alternatively, fresh frozen plasma can be stored and used effectively for 1 year or more.

immune-mediated thrombocytopenia. Recently released platelets have much greater function than older ones. Platelet transfusion is recommended only for dogs or cats that exhibit clinical signs. Platelet-rich plasma may be considered in these patients; however, the circulating half-life of platelets may be only minutes, especially when immune-mediated conditions exist. One unit per 20 kg of platelet-rich plasma or fresh whole blood should be administered every hour until an adequate platelet count is reached. During this time, vincristine (0.5 mg/m^2 IV as a single dose or every 1–3 weeks) can be administered to induce a premature release of platelets from the bone marrow. The platelet count usually increases 3 to 5 days after vincristine administration. This is especially valuable in immune-mediated thrombocytopenia, because vincristine not only directly increases platelet numbers, but is also taken up by platelets, where it is cytotoxic to phagocytic cells.

Disseminated Intravascular Coagulation

Disseminated intravascular coagulation (DIC) can result in severe bleeding and consumption of clotting factors and platelets. In affected patients, approximately 1 U/20 kg of fresh frozen plasma can be given and repeated as needed to maintain prothrombin and partial thromboplastin time to 1 to 1.5 times the normal bleeding time. Heparin use is controversial; however, if given in conjunction with plasma, it may be of benefit. In patients in which all cell lines (red blood cells and platelets) are decreased, fresh whole blood can be used (also see the Oncologic Emergencies section).

Hypoproteinemia

Plasma transfusions can be valuable in patients that have decreased albumin levels. Increase in plasma proteins can be slower than expected after protein administration, because only 40% of the body albumin is in the intravascular space, whereas 60% resides within the interstitial space. Thus, administration of fresh frozen plasma must not only increase albumin within the circulating space but also within interstitial spaces, which may require multiple units and repeated plasma administration. Obviously, the administration of fresh frozen plasma from various donors can result in development of antibodies. Although their circulating half-life can be quite short, colloidal solutions, such as dextrans or hetastarch, may be more useful in these patients. Approximately 6 units of plasma are needed to raise the albumin of a 32-kg dog from 1.8 g/dl to 3 g/dl.

AMOUNT TO TRANSFUSE

Animals with significant acute blood loss should first be treated for shock with crystalloid solutions. Hypertonic saline is useful in selected patients. Packed red blood cells can be given with crystalloid fluids or whole blood may be used. As a general rule, one unit of packed red blood cells is administered per 20 kg of patient, with close adjustments to maintain the hematocrit values above 15%. Dogs that require whole blood for either acute or chronic anemias should be transfused using the general guideline below:

General Rule: Amount to Transfuse

$$\text{ml donor} = [(2.2 \times \text{wt}_{kg}) \times (40_{dog} \text{ or } 30_{cat})] \times$$

$$\frac{(PCV_{desired} - PCV_{recipient})}{PCV_{donor}}$$

Note: 2.2 ml of whole blood/kg or 1 ml/kg of packed red blood cells raises PCV 1% (transfused whole blood has a PCV of 40%).

General Rule: Rate of Transfusion

Dogs: 0.25 ml/kg/30 minutes or faster (22 ml/kg/day) with close patient monitoring

Cats: 40 ml/30 minutes with close patient monitoring

COMPLICATIONS OF TRANSFUSIONS[1-3]

Hemolysis is probably the most serious adverse effect of transfusion; however, it is relatively rare. Signs of an acute hemolytic reaction include elevated temperature, increased heart and respiration rate, and tremors, followed by vomiting and collapse. When this occurs, transfusion should be stopped and the patient's plasma should be checked for hemoglobinemia. Crystalloid fluids should be initiated, and urine output should be monitored and preserved. Delayed hemolysis may occur in some patients. Fever that develops during transfusion can indicate either bacterial contamination of the blood or association with leukocyte antigens that elevate endogenous pyrogens.

This elevation in body temperature is more common in cats than in dogs. Allergic reactions may manifest as urticaria and angioneurotic edema. If these occur, the transfusion should be discontinued and glucocorticoids should be administered. When large volumes of blood are administered, volume overload can occur; therefore, the patient's circulating volume should be monitored (e.g., central venous pressure and body weight) and treated appropriately (e.g., fluid restrictions and furosemide). Citrate toxicity is a possible complication of stored whole blood transfusion and can cause an acute decrease in serum ionized calcium, especially in dogs with liver disease. Hypocalcemia results in muscle tremors, facial twitches, and seizures. Intravenous calcium gluconate and cessation of transfusion is the treatment of choice. Rarely, blood ammonia levels can rise and cause associated clinical signs, such as mental dullness or seizures, particularly in animals with compromised liver function. This usually occurs in patients that received blood that has been stored for a prolonged period and is usually associated with packed red blood cells. Treatment for this condition is the same as for hepatoencephalopathy.

REFERENCES

1. Stone MS, Cotter SM: Practical guidelines for transfusion therapy, in Kirk RW, Bonagura JD (eds): *Current Veterinary Therapy XI.* Philadelphia, WB Saunders, 1992, pp 479–485.
2. Giger U: The feline AB blood group system and incompatibility reactions, in Kirk RW, Bonagura JD (eds): *Current Veterinary Therapy XI.* Philadelphia, WB Saunders, 1992, pp 470–474.
3. Smith MR: Disorders of hemostasis in transfusion therapy, in Skeel RT (ed): *Handbook of Cancer Chemotherapy,* ed 3. Boston, Little, Brown & Co, 1991, pp 449–458.

CLINICAL BRIEFING: HEMATOPOIETIC GROWTH FACTOR SUPPORT

Recombinant Erythropoietin	*Indications:* Anemia caused by inadequate production of red blood cells from normal bone marrow; especially effective when endogenous production of erythropoietin is low. Patients with anemia caused by chronic renal failure, anemia of chronic malignant disease, chemotherapy, or radiation therapy *Complications:* Erythrocytosis is a rare complication; antibodies can develop to human recombinant erythropoietin, rendering this therapy ineffective
Recombinant Granulocyte Colony-Stimulating Factor (G-CSF)	*Indications:* Neutropenia caused by inadequate production from the bone marrow. Canine recombinant G-CSF is effective for treating most neutropenias; response is directly proportional to the number of granulocyte precursors present and inversely proportional to the amount of endogenous G-CSF production. Canine recombinant G-CSF is effective for long-term therapy in dogs and cats *Contraindications:* Neutrophilia can occur but is rarely a clinical problem; antibodies can develop to human recombinant G-CSF, rendering this therapy ineffective
Recombinant Granulocyte-Macrophage Colony-Stimulating Factor (GM-CSF)	*Indications:* Neutropenia caused by inadequate production from the bone marrow. Canine recombinant GM-CSF is effective for treating neutropenia from most causes; response is directly proportional to the number of granulocyte precursors present and inversely proportional to the amount of endogenous GM-CSF production. Canine recombinant GM-CSF is effective for long-term therapy in dogs *Contraindications:* Neutrophilia and monocytosis can occur but are rarely clinical problems; antibodies can develop to human recombinant GM-CSF, rendering this therapy ineffective

Hematopoietic growth factors have the potential for long-term improvement of animal health.[1,2] The most clinically useful growth factors are erythropoietin, granulocyte colony-stimulating factor (G-CSF), and granulocyte-macrophage colony-stimulating factor (GM-CSF). Studies have been performed in dogs using interleukin-3 (IL-3) and a fusion protein called pIXY 321.

ERYTHROPOIETIN

Human recombinant erythropoietin has been used experimentally in dogs with chronic renal failure and has produced some beneficial results.[3] Recombinant erythropoietin has been demonstrated to improve quality of life in human cancer patients who have anemia of chronic disease due to their malignancies or due to chemotherapy and radiation

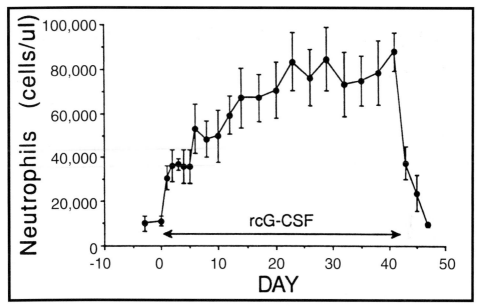

Figure 2-35: *Mean neutrophil counts (± standard deviation) of five normal cats treated with recombinant canine granulocyte colony-stimulating factor (rcG-CSF). Administration of rcG-CSF began on day 0 and ended on day 42 (arrow). Neutrophil counts returned to pretreatment values within 5 days of discontinuing rcG-CSF. (From Obradovich JA, Ogilvie GK, Stadler-Morris S, et al: Evaluation of canine recombinant granulocyte colony-stimulating factor in the cat. J Vet Intern Med 7:65–69, 1993; with permission.)*

therapy. Similar results have been seen in dogs and cats with cancer. Treated dogs seem to have improved attitude and quality of life as well as increased numbers of circulating red blood cells. Potential secondary effects of human recombinant erythropoietin include systemic hypertension, iron deficiency, hyperkalemia, polycythemia, and the development of antibodies to the recombinant protein in approximately 30% of patients weeks to months after treatment is initiated.

Human recombinant erythropoietin can be administered to dogs and cats at a dosage of 75 to 100 U/kg/day for 5 to 7 days SQ, followed by the same dosage given 2 to 3 times a week until the hematocrit approaches the desired level. Erythropoietin can be administered weekly thereafter. Hemotocrit levels should be monitored, and if antibodies develop and result in a rapid decrease in the number of red blood cells, erythropoietin therapy should be discontinued.

GRANULOCYTE COLONY-STIMULATING FACTOR

Recombinant human and canine granulocyte colony-stimulating factor (G-CSF) have been produced in large quantities through recombinant technology using *Eschericha coli* bacteria. Most work done with G-CSF has shown that the cytokine is lineage-specific, acting primarily on committed granulocytic precursors to increase neutrophil phagocytosis, superoxide generation, and antibody-dependent cellular cytotoxicity.

- A dose-dependent increase in neutrophil and monocyte counts occurs when canine recombinant G-CSF (rcG-CSF) is given subcutaneously to normal

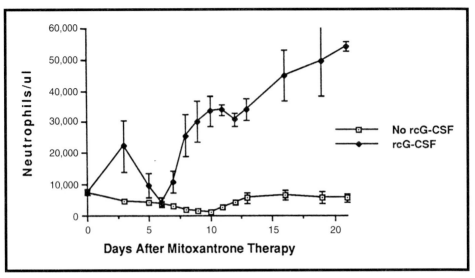

Figure 2-36: *Mean neutrophil counts (± standard deviation) from two groups of five normal dogs that received mitoxantrone (5 mg/m² IV) on day 0. Administration of rcG-CSF began on day 1 and ended on day 20 in one of the two groups of dogs designated with closed diamonds. (From Ogilvie GK, Obradovich JA, Cooper MF: The use of recombinant colony-stimulating factor to decrease myelosuppression associated with the administration of mitoxantrone in the dog.* J Vet Intern Med *6:44–47, 1992; with permission.)*

dogs at dosages ranging from 3 to 25 µg/kg/day.[3]
- The only toxicity noted has been occasional, mild irritation at the injection site.

A study was recently completed evaluating the changes in neutrophil counts when rcG-CSF was administered at a dose of 5 µg/kg/day to a group of healthy dogs.[4] At that dosage, mean neutrophil counts increased significantly to 26,330/µl within 24 hours after the first injection of rcG-CSF. The neutrophils reached a maximum of 72,125/µl by day 19. The neutrophil counts remained in this range until the cytokine therapy was discontinued. Blood counts returned to normal within 5 days after discontinuing treatment. Re-initiation of G-CSF treatment resulted in a more rapid, dramatic increase in neutrophil numbers. Long-term (>30 days) use of human recombinant G-CSF (rhG-CSF) in dogs has been shown to induce significant decreases in neutrophil counts, presumably caused by antibody formation to the for-

eign rhG-CSF.[5] Therefore, if rhG-CSF is to be used in dogs, it should be used on a short-term basis. Our studies suggest that long-term treatment with rcG-CSF does not induce antibody formation in dogs.

We have found that rhG-CSF induces a short-term increase in the number of neutrophils in normal cats.[6] After approximately 14 days, the number of neutrophils and their precursors decreases significantly, presumably because rhG-CSF is sufficiently different from the cat's own native G-CSF to induce antibody formation. Canine recombinant G-CSF increases neutrophils in normal cats to approximately 30,000/µl within 24 hours after initiation of therapy (Figure 2-35).[7] The neutrophil counts continue to rise, reaching approximately 67,000/µl on day 14, and then remain within a range of 67,000/µl to 88,000/µl for 42 days. As in dogs, once rcG-CSF administration was discontinued, neutrophil counts returned to pretreatment levels within 5 days. Occasional irritation at the injection site was the only toxicity noted. Apparently, rcG-CSF is sufficiently homologous to feline G-CSF so that antibody formation does not result.

One of the most promising areas of clinical application of G-CSF is in the prevention and treatment of chemotherapy- and radiation-induced cytopenias. We recently showed that rcG-CSF is effective in significantly reducing the myelosuppression associated with mitoxantrone chemotherapy in dogs (Figure 2-36). The dose-limiting toxicity associated with mitoxantrone therapy in dogs is myelosuppression. In our study, ten healthy dogs were given intravenous mitoxantrone at a dose of 5 mg/m^2 body surface area.[8] Recombinant canine G-CSF was administered to five of these dogs at a dose of 5 µg/kg/day SQ for 20 days starting 24 hours after the chemotherapy was administered. The median neutrophil counts dropped below normal (<3000/µl) for 2 days in dogs that received rcG-CSF and dropped for 5 days in dogs that only received mitoxantrone. Four of five dogs that were not treated with rcG-CSF, but none of the dogs receiving rcG-CSF developed serious neutropenia (<1500/µl). The neutrophil counts were significantly higher in the dogs treated with rcG-CSF at all times evaluated except prior to the administration of the cytokine and mitoxantrone and on the sixth day of therapy. Therefore, rcG-CSF seems to be safe and effective for preventing chemotherapy-induced myelosuppression in dogs.

Clinical trials of rhG-CSF and GM-CSF in gray collies and humans with cyclic neutropenia have successfully increased neutrophil counts and decreased clinical signs associated with prolonged myelosuppression.[5] Daily treatment is essential to maintain the increased neutrophil counts. Chronic use of rhG-CSF resulted in autoantibody formation in the studies investigating cyclic neutropenia in dogs.

GRANULOCYTE-MACROPHAGE COLONY-STIMULATING FACTOR

Granulocyte-macrophage colony-stimulating factor (GM-CSF)is a glycoprotein that is produced by a number of different tissues in the body, including T lymphocytes, monocytes, endothelial cells, and fibroblasts. As its name implies, GM-CSF stimulates the production of granulocytes and macrophages and acts in concert with erythropoietin and IL-3 to stimulate erythroid precursors. This cytokine also acts along with IL-3 to regulate thrombopoiesis. This stimulator of multilineage and committed progenitors also increases the function of mature granulocytes, monocytes, macrophages, and eosinophils. More specifically, the cell-killing activity of neutrophils is enhanced by inhibiting migration of these cells, increasing chemotaxis, adhesion, phagocytosis, and superoxide generation; therefore, GM-CSF increases tumoricidal cytotoxicity.

The use of GM-CSF in clinical medicine has the potential for being at least as profound and widespread as that of G-CSF. Recently, canine GM-CSF was shown to be effective for increasing granulocyte counts in dogs. We have used recombinant human GM-CSF in dogs with chemotherapy-induced myelosuppression with variable results. One reason that GM-CSF may not have had as profound an effect as G-CSF in dogs is because of variable sequence homology between the recombinant products and the native GM-CSF of dogs. This has been shown in various species; for example, there is only a 57% sequence homology between human and murine GM-CSF and up to 75% homology between human and murine G-CSF.

In an attempt to overcome this problem, the use of nonspecific inducers of hematopoietic growth factors have been explored. For example, Imuvert® (Cell Technolo-

> **KEY POINT:**
>
> *Long-term use of recombinant human hematopoietic growth factors may result in antibody formation that can cross-react with the patient's own factors ("autoantibodies").*

gies, Inc, Boulder CO), a biological response modifier composed of ribosomes and other subcomponents of *Serratia marcescens*, is known to induce a variety of cytokines, including IL-1, IL-2, and GM-CSF. Imuvert® decreased the duration and severity of doxorubicin chemotherapy-induced myelosuppression in Imuvert®-treated dogs compared to controls.[9] The mechanism of action of this biological response modifier in dogs is unknown; endogenous G-CSF as determined by ELISA methodology did not increase in response to administration of Imuvert.

Like G-CSF, GM-CSF has been shown to decrease the duration and severity of chemotherapy- and radiation-induced neutropenia in humans and laboratory animals. Because GM-CSF affects several cell lines, a variety of disease states can be treated with this growth factor. Diseases linked with leukopenia-associated acquired immune deficiency syndrome (AIDS); bone marrow failure states, such as myelodysplasia; and aplastic anemia as well as chronic and acute bacterial infections have been shown to be substantially improved with GM-CSF therapy. GM-CSF may be superior to G-CSF for rapid recovery from bone marrow transplantation. GM-CSF can stimulate some leukemic cells and therefore may be of value for forcing cells into the cell cycle, thus making them more susceptible to cell cycle-specific drugs. Some hypothesize that GM-CSF, like G-CSF, may force leukemic cells to differentiate and die.

IL-3

Like GM-CSF, IL-3 affects multipotential marrow progenitors; however, IL-3 seems to have activity at an earlier stage than does GM-CSF. Humans with myelodysplasia and aplastic anemia treated with IL-3 showed dramatic increases in granulocytes, platelets, and red blood cells. Unlike G-CSF and GM-CSF therapy, responses to IL-3 do not occur until the fourth week after the start of treatment. Some investigators have shown that IL-3 can be used to decrease chemotherapy induced myelosuppression. Sequential administration of IL-3 and GM-CSF has been shown

to cause a marked increase in white cells, including myeloid lineages and platelets; the effect was clearly additive. We have used human recombinant IL-3 in dogs without significant changes in any cell line.

pIXY 321

A recently completed study demonstrated that human recombinant IL-3, GM-CSF, and a fusion protein of these cytokines, called pIXY 321, did not significantly increase platelets, neutrophils, monocytes, or red blood cells in normal dogs.[10] This was unfortunate, because these multilineage growth factors have the potential to treat a wide variety of bone marrow disorders in veterinary medicine.

REFERENCES

1. Elmslie RE, Dow SW, Ogilvie GK: Interleukins: Biological properties and therapeutic potential. *J Vet Intern Med* 5:283–293, 1991.
2. Obradovich JE, Ogilvie GK: Evaluation of recombinant canine granulocyte colony-stimulating factor as an inducer of granulopoiesis. *J Vet Intern Med* 5:75–79, 1991.
3. Cowgill LD: Clinical experience and use of recombinant human erythropoietin in uremic dogs and cats. *Proc 9th ACVIM Forum*:147–149, 1991.
4. Obradovich JE, Ogilvie GL, Cooper MF, et al: Effect of increasing dosages of canine recombinant granulocyte colony-stimulating factor on neutrophil counts in normal dogs. *Proc Vet Cancer Soc 10th Annu Conf*:5, 1990.
5. Lorthrup CD Jr, Warren DJ, Souza LM, et al: Correction of canine cyclic hematopoiesis with recombinant human granulocyte colony-stimulating factor. *Blood* 72:1324–1334, 1988.
6. Fulton R, Gasper PW, Ogilvie GK, et al: Effect of recombinant human granulocyte colony-stimulating factor on hematopoiesis in normal cats. *Exp Hematol* 19:759–767, 1991.
7. Obradovich JE, Ogilvie GK, Stadler-Morris S, et al: Evaluation of canine recombinant granulocyte colony-stimulating factor in the cat. *J Vet Intern Med* 7:65–69, 1993.
8. Ogilvie GK, Obradovich JE, Cooper MF, et al: The use of recombinant canine granulocyte colony-stimulating factor to decrease myelosuppression associated with with the administration of mitoxantrone in the dog. *J Vet Intern Med* 6:44–47, 1992.

9. Ogilvie GK, Elmslie RE, Pearson F: The use of a biological extract of *Serratia marcescens* to decrease myelosuppression associated with doxorubicin-induced myelosuppression in the dog. *Am J Vet Res* 53:1787–1790, 1992.

10. Ciekot PE, Ogilvie GK, Fettman MJ, et al: Evaluation of GM-CSF, IL-3, and GM-CSF/IL-3 fusion protein (pIXY 321) as multilineage colony stimulating factors in the dog [Abstr]. *Vet Cancer 11th Ann Conf* 41–43, 1991.

CLINICAL BRIEFING: NEUTROPENIA, SEPSIS, AND THROMBOCYTOPENIA

Neutropenia and Sepsis

Diagnosis	*History:* Acute decompensation, anorexia, and collapse, usually 5–7 days after receiving myelosuppressive chemotherapy *Clinical Signs:* Pyrexia, brick-red mucous membranes, tachycardia, rapid capillary refill (hyperdynamic shock) or pale mucous membranes, decreased capillary refill time, and evidence of decreased cardiac output (hypodynamic shock) *Diagnostics:* Evidence of neutropenia; multi-organ failure; hypoglycemia; positive cultures of blood, urine, pulmonary airways, or other tissues; and metabolic acidosis
Therapy	Treat the underlying cause Restore tissue perfusion with fluids and stabilize cardiovascular system Correct acid–base balance, electrolyte imbalances, and hypoglycemia Initiate parenteral bactericidal antibiotic therapy Consider hematopoietic growth factor support, transfusions of fresh whole blood, or, in rare conditions, granulocyte transfusions

Thrombocytopenia

Diagnosis	*History:* Bleeding without due cause *Clinical Signs:* Evidence of bleeding after minimal trauma, petechial and ecchymotic hemorrhages, hematuria, and hemarthrosis *Diagnostics:* Complete blood and platelet counts and bone marrow aspirates; consider antimegakaryocyte antibody and platelet factor III tests as well as coagulation screening tests (APTT, OSPT, fibrinogen, and FDPs)
Therapy	Treat the underlying cause Minimize activity and enforce rest Correct secondary conditions (e.g., treat DIC and drug-induced myelosuppression) Consider vincristine therapy to cause premature release of platelets, transfusion with platelet-rich plasma, and epsilon aminocaproic acid

NEUTROPENIA AND SEPSIS

In humans, sepsis is the most common cause of death in cancer patients, exceeding all other causes combined.[1-7] Neutropenia secondary to malignancy or as a result of the myelosuppressive effects of chemotherapy is a common predisposing factor for

TABLE 3-1
Myelosuppressive effects of chemotherapeutic agents used in veterinary medicine

Highly Myelosuppressive	Moderately Myelosuppressive	Mildly Myelosuppressive
Doxorubicin	Melphalan	L-asparaginase
Vinblastine	Chlorambucil	Vincristine
Cyclophosphamide	5-fluorouracil	Bleomycin
Actinomycin D	Methotrexate	Corticosteroids

development of sepsis in dogs and cats. Septic shock is the state of circulatory collapse that occurs secondary to overwhelming sepsis and/or endotoxemia. This syndrome frequently is fatal; the mortality rate is 40% to 90%. The profound systemic effects of septic shock include cardiovascular effects, such as vasoconstriction leading to multi-organ failure; cardiac dysfunction, in part from lactic acidosis; and increased vascular permeability, leading to hyperviscosity and hypovolemia. Other systemic effects include liver dysfunction from splanchnic vascular pooling and tissue ischemia; acute renal failure; neutropenia; thrombocytopenia and coagulopathies; severe gastrointestinal (GI) damage; and a variety of metabolic effects, such as decreased insulin release and an initial hyperglycemia followed by hypoglycemia. In short, septic shock leads to multi-organ failure and alterations in metabolism that in part result from hyperlactatemia and energy-inefficient "futile cycling."

The bacteria that most commonly cause morbidity and mortality in veterinary cancer patients arise from the animal's own flora.[8] Prolonged hospitalization and antibiotic use result in susceptibility to resistant strains of organisms. The most important thing a clinician can do for the septic veterinary cancer patient is to identify the source and type of bacterial infection and initiate therapy with broad-spectrum antibiotics. The increasing risk for fungal infections is an emerging problem in human oncology and will probably be recognized soon in veterinary medicine. Therefore, antifungal drugs are likely to be used more often in the future.

Predisposing Factors

The most common factors that predispose patients to infections are granulocytopenia, cellular immune dysfunction, humoral immune dysfunction, splenectomy, the presence of indwelling vascular catheters, prolonged hospitalization, poor nutrition, neurologic dysfunction, and the effects of the cancer itself.[1-8] These problems must be avoided or recognized and corrected early.

Granulocytopenia may result from bone marrow destruction caused by leukemia or lymphoma or from the myelosuppressive effects of chemotherapy. The myelosuppressive effects of chemotherapeutic agents can be categorized as high, moderate, or mild (Table 3-1). These drugs cause a nadir (lowest part of the white blood cell count) at different times after administration (Table 3-2).

Infection early in the course of granulocytopenia typically is caused by endogenous bacteria that are relatively nonresistant. Frequent acquisition of blood samples greatly increases the risk of infection in cancerous animals. Other sites of entry of organisms include the skin, oral cavity, colon, and perianal area. The gram-negative bacteria most commonly associated

KEY POINT:

The incidence of sepsis increases significantly when the neutrophil count drops to less than 1000 to 1500/μl.

TABLE 3-2
Myelosuppressive drugs associated with the development of pyrexia and sepsis at different times after treatment

Delayed Myelosuppression (3–4 Weeks)	Mid-Range Myelosuppression (7–10 Days)	Early Myelosuppression (<7 Days)
Carmustine (BCNU)	Cyclophosphamide	Taxol
Lomustine (CCNU)	Doxorubicin	
Mitomycin C	Mitoxantrone	

with infection of patients with granulocytopenia are *Escherichia coli*, *Klebsiella pneumoniae*, *Pseudomonas*, and Enterobacteriaceae.[1-8] The most common gram-positive bacteria include *Staphylococcus epidermatidis* and *Staphylococcus aureus*. The increase in the prevalence of infection with gram-positive bacteria possibly may result from the chronic use of venous catheters. The incidence of *Candida* and *Aspergillus* fungal infection is rising in humans and is likely to become a problem with aggressive use of antibiotics in animals.

Defects in cellular immunity also cause sepsis in veterinary cancer patients. Cellular immune dysfunction may result from an underlying cause or from antineoplastic agents and corticosteroids. Lymphoma has been associated with cellular immune dysfunction in humans. Cellular immune dysfunction results in a variety of bacterial and mycobacterial as well as fungal and viral infections.

Humoral immune dysfunction is also associated with increased prevalence of sepsis in human cancer patients and may cause similar problems in veterinary cancer patients. Agammaglobulinemic or hypogammaglobulinemic animals are susceptible to infections because they lack opsonizing antibodies to common encapsulated pyrogenic bacteria. Many of these patients also have dysfunctional complement activity. Multiple myeloma or chronic lymphocytic leukemia are common neoplasms associated with humoral immune dysfunction. Splenectomized human cancer patients are at higher risk of sepsis, most likely because of inefficient

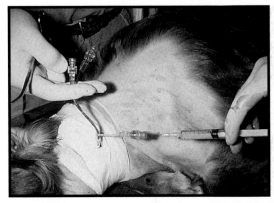

Figure 3-1: *Sepsis secondary to any indwelling catheter, especially one that has been in place for several days, is a serious problem in neutropenic animals. Strict aseptic technique should be adhered to when handling catheters, especially multilumen catheters.*

removal of nonopsonized bacteria. Splenectomized animals may also be susceptible to overwhelming sepsis when infected with a strain of encapsulated bacteria against which they have never made antibodies.

Indwelling vascular catheters have been associated with increased prevalence of sepsis (Figure 3-1). The longer a catheter is in place, the higher the probability for infection; this is especially true in neutropenic patients. The risk of catheter-induced sepsis can be minimized by using aseptic technique and by placing a new catheter in a new site every 2 to 3 days as well as monitoring the local area for phlebitis. Other contributing factors include prolonged hospitalization, malnutrition, and neurologic dysfunction. Patients that are nonambulatory for any reason are at increased risk of sepsis.

Diagnosis

The diagnosis of septic shock begins with the physical examination, which may reveal hyperdynamic septic shock. Brick-red mucous membranes, tachycardia, and short capillary refill times are the hallmarks of hyperdynamic shock.[1–6] These signs may be followed by gastrointestinal signs, altered mentation, decreased capillary refill time, and a decrease in blood pressure. End-stage signs (e.g., hypothermia, mucous membrane pallor, marked mental depression, bloody diarrhea, and signs of multi-organ failure) reflect a hypodynamic state. Thrombocytopenia and neutropenia are often identified during the course of septic shock. Hyperglycemia is an early finding that often is followed by hypoglycemia. Although bacterial cultures may be deceptively negative, a positive culture is common. Metabolic acidosis is commonly identified.

The absence of circulating neutrophils results in a urinalysis without pyuria and chest radiographs that are normal because of lack of a neutrophilic infiltrate, which is responsible for many of the radiographic changes associated with pneumonia. Therefore, any suspicious sites should be cultured (Figure 3-2). Two, and preferably four, sets of blood cultures (aerobic and anaerobic) should be acquired. The timing of the sampling is controversial; however, sampling every 20 to 30 minutes prior to antibiotic therapy may be adequate. At least 5 ml of blood should be injected into appropriate culture containers. If central venous catheters are present, cultures of the port should be obtained. Ideally, culture bottles that contain an antibiotic binding resin or other antibiotic binding substance should

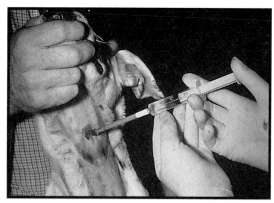

Figure 3-2: *Septic cancer patients with severe neutropenia may have bacterial pneumonia without any radiographic abnormalities owing to the lack of inflammatory cells. Therefore, any septic, neutropenic animal that is coughing or that has abnormal lung auscultation should have a transtracheal wash for cytology and bacterial culture and sensitivity testing.*

be included with each culture from patients on antibiotics. A cystocentesis specimen for urine culture and analysis should be acquired in each case after the patient has been evaluated to ensure that there are at least 60,000 platelets/µl. When neurologic signs are present, a cerebrospinal fluid (CSF) tap should be obtained and cultured appropriately. Cerebrospinal fluid should always be sent for Gram's staining, bacterial culture, cell count and differential, and glucose and protein determination. A cryptococcal antigen titer or India ink preparation should be performed in suspect cases. Acid-fast stains and culture usually are not necessary. For animals with diarrhea, appropriate cultures should be done for *Clostridium* species, including appropriate assays for endotoxin. In addition, chest radiographs should be taken when a site for infection is not obvious. Ultrasonography, especially echocardiography, should be considered to identify the presence of

> **KEY POINT:**
>
> *When laboratory and clinical data from a neutropenic animal are evaluated, the clinician must remember that many results may be surprisingly normal, even in the face of overt sepsis.*

valvular endocarditis. Invasive tests that should be performed to identify specific sites of infection include bronchoscopy (when pulmonary disease is suspected); skin biopsy (if deep cutaneous infection is identified); and bone marrow biopsy, percutaneous liver biopsy, or exploratory laparotomy in select cases. In addition, a complete blood count (CBC), biochemical profile, and urinalysis should be performed on each patient.

Treatment[1-8]

Treatment for the septic, neutropenic animal is primarily directed at restoring adequate tissue perfusion, improving the alterations in metabolism, and controlling systemic infection. Standard therapy includes crystalloid solutions and antibiotics. Although the use of hypertonic solutions for the treatment of shock is being investigated, lactated Ringer's solution is cited in most veterinary texts as "the first line of therapy." The initial infusion rate for critical animals is 70 to 90 ml/kg IV for 1 hour, then 10 to 12 ml/kg/hour thereafter. The fluid rate should then be adjusted to meet the needs of each patient as directed by monitoring body weight, heart and respiratory rates, central venous pressure, ongoing losses (e.g., vomiting and diarrhea), and urine output.

Lactate-containing fluids may be contraindicated, because septic animals are already hyperlactatemic and engage in futile cycling throughout the course of septic shock; septic animals with cancer are even more likely to be detrimentally affected by lactate-containing fluids. The administration of lactate-containing fluids to hypermetabolic patients that are septic (which will likely further enhance lactate levels and futile cycling) may further tax this energy-consuming system and result in further debilitation of the cancer patient. Therefore, 0.9% NaCl or a balanced electrolyte crystalloid solution should be used. Dextrose should be included in fluids when systemic hypoglycemia is identified during constant patient monitoring. In states of severe cardiovascular shock, 70 to 90 ml/kg crystalloid fluids that contain 2.5% to 5% dextrose for the first hour followed by up to 10 ml/kg per hour thereafter is recommended. When

fluids are administered at this rate, the patient must be monitored closely and the rate of fluid administration must be changed to meet the needs of the animal.

Asymptomatic animals with fewer than 1000 to 1500 neutrophils/μl should be started on antibiotics as prophylaxis. Trimethoprim-sulfa (7.5 mg/kg BID PO) is often recommended for prophylactic therapy in the neutropenic animal. Neutropenic animals in septic shock should be started on intravenous fluids and antibiotic therapy as soon as samples for bacterial cultures are acquired (Tables 3-3 and 3-4). Reevaluation of an empiric antibiotic regimen is mandatory when the identity and sensitivity pattern of the bacteria becomes available. For gram-negative infections, two antibiotics that are effective against the isolated organism are often recommended. Gram-positive infections generally are treated with a single, appropriate antibiotic. When infection is caused by a catheter, the infected indwelling device is removed, and long-term antibiotic therapy is initiated. In humans, approximately 70% to 80% of these types of patients are cured. Myelosuppressive chemotherapeutics should be withheld until the patient has recovered.

Other specific therapy can include granulocyte transfusions; however, controlled trials have not shown these transfusions to be beneficial. In addition, transfusion reactions and allosensitizations to specific antigens of the granulocytes can occur and increased prevalence of severe pulmonary reactions may be noted. Canine recombinant granulocyte-colony stimulating factor (rcG-CSF, 5 μg/kg/day SQ) and canine recombinant granulocyte macrophage-colony stimulating factor (rcGM-CSF, 10 μg/kg/day SQ) have been associated with an increased prevalence of myeloid recovery in dogs and cats with neutropenia. These hematopoietic growth factors increase cell numbers and enhance neutrophil function, but they are not yet available commercially. Human recombinant G-CSF and GM-CSF are commercially available, but long-term use may induce antibody formation to the protein. Of the two human recombinant proteins, rhG-CSF induces the most profound increase in the number of canine and feline

TABLE 3-3
Approach to the febrile, neutropenic patient[1-10]

Approach	Action
Identify the site of infection	Perform complete physical examination
	Acquire complete blood and platelet count, biochemical profile, and urinalysis
	Acquire 2–4 blood cultures, cystocentesis for culture and sensitivity, chest radiographs, and transtracheal wash for culture and sensitivity
	If indicated, culture and sensitivity testing for CSF, catheters, joint fluid, and feces
Initiate supportive care	Establish indwelling intravenous catheter aseptically and initiate fluid therapy; for shock: 70–90 ml/kg for the first hour followed by 10–12 ml/kg/hr; adjust as needed thereafter
	Withhold chemotherapeutic agents
Initiate intravenous antibiotic therapy after cultures	If aminoglycosides are contraindicated (e.g., dehydration and renal disease)
	— Cefoxitin (22 mg/kg TID)
	If aminoglycosides not contraindicated
	— Cefoxitin (22 mg/kg TID) and gentamicin (2–3 mg/kg TID over 30 minutes)
	Monitor for nephrotoxicity
	Granulocyte-colony stimulating factor, if available (5 µg/kg/day SQ)
Redefine antibiotic therapy based on culture and sensitivity results	Monitor fever and neutrophil count
Discharge for home care (neutrophils >1500/µl and afebrile)	Appropriate antibiotic therapy (e.g., trimethoprim-sulfa 7.5 mg/kg BID PO)
Consider dose reduction with next chemotherapy (e.g., decrease by 25%)	

neutrophils before development of antibodies is noted. Tumor necrosis factor antiserum, antibody to tumor necrosis factor, interleukin and interferon therapy, pooled immunoglobulin preparations, and monoclonal antibodies to neutralize endotoxin may be future treatments of choice.

Sepsis can be prevented by altering environment and by using surveillance cultures. Typical environmental manipulations include washing hands between handling each patient and wearing protective gloves. This may prevent carrying infections from patient to patient and from veterinarian to animal. Foods, objects, or specific materials (e.g., rectal thermometers) may harbor bacteria. Prophylactic antibiotic therapy is recommended by some but may result in increased bacterial resistance, especially in areas of high antibiotic use, such as university hospitals. In humans, the most common prophylactic antibiotic therapy includes the use of non-

TABLE 3-4
Antibiotics used to treat patients with septic cancer

Antibiotic	Potential Toxicoses
Gram-Negative Bacteria	
Gentamicin (1–3 mg/kg IV TID)	Nephrotoxicity, especially when pre-existing renal damage is present; ototoxicity. Ensure adequate hydration and check frequently for renal damage during use
Cephalothin (20–30 mg/kg IV QID)	Phlebitis, muscle pain after IV or IM administration; rare prevalence of nephrotoxicity
Cefoxitin (22 mg/kg IV TID)	Phlebitis; discomfort with rapid IV injection; rare prevalence of nephrotoxicity
Gram-Positive Bacteria	
Na or K penicillin (25,000 units/kg IV QID)	Allergy to penicillin can cause anaphylaxis, hives, fever, and pain; neurologic signs may occur with rapid infusion
Cephalothin (20–30 mg/kg IV QID)	See above
Cefoxitin (22 mg/kg IV TID)	See above
Anaerobic Bacteria	
Metronidazole (15 mg/kg IV or IM TID)	Anorexia, vomiting, and neurologic signs
Cefoxitin (22 mg/kg IV TID)	See above

absorbable agents, quinolones, trimethoprim-sulfamethoxazole, antifungal drugs, antiviral drugs, and antiparasitics. Immunization with appropriate viral vaccines may be of value but must be initiated prior to starting therapy with chemotherapeutic agents.

THROMBOCYTOPENIA

A decreased platelet count is most commonly caused by the cytotoxic effects of chemotherapeutic agents, bone marrow infiltration by a malignant process, or secondary to a consumption coagulopathy. If a chemotherapeutic agent induces bone marrow suppression that results in cytopenia, thrombocytopenia usually occurs a few days after neutropenia and before a decrease in red blood cell numbers.

Predisposing Factors

Thrombocytopenia can occur in any cancer patient that receives myelosuppressive chemotherapeutic agents. Drugs such as vincristine, bleomycin, and prednisone do not cause as significant a thrombocytopenia as do myelosuppressive agents (e.g., doxorubicin). Compared to other myelosuppressive drugs, cyclophosphamide induces less suppression in platelet numbers. Dogs and cats with bone marrow infiltration by a malignant process are more sensitive to the cytotoxic effects of chemotherapeutic agents that can result in thrombocytopenia. Other conditions that affect the bone marrow (e.g., ehrlichiosis and estrogen toxicity from exogenous supplementation or from a productive testicular tumor) are likely to make the marrow more sensitive to cytotoxic agents. Tumors that are frequently associated with coagulopathies (e.g., hemangiosarcoma and thyroid carcinoma) may cause a consumptive thrombocytopenia. In addition, hypersplenism and chronic bleeding of any cause can result in a decrease in the number of platelets.

Diagnosis

Clinical signs include, but are not limited to, bleeding diatheses, melena, and weakness. The blood loss can occur into any organ and result in multisystemic abnormalities. An acute decline in the number of platelets may result in the development of clinical signs at higher platelet counts than if the decline in platelets is much slower. Diagnosis is confirmed by obtaining platelet counts and by examining bone marrow aspirate or biopsy specimens. Bone marrow evaluation is essential and helps the clinician determine whether decreased production is the problem. Clotting profiles (e.g., activated partial thromboplastin time, one-step prothrombin time [OSPT], and fibrin degradation products [FDP]) may help determine if the thrombocytopenia is from a coagulopathy, such as disseminated intravascular coagulopathy (DIC).

Therapy

Thrombocytopenia-related clinical signs can be exacerbated when drugs that affect platelet function are administered during the time of overt or impending thrombocytopenia. Therefore, aspirin and aspirin-like drugs should be withheld from patients with thrombocytopenia.

Obviously, animals with thrombocytopenia should be kept quiet. In academic or large private practice settings, platelet transfusions can be administered to specific animals that are, or have a high likelihood of, bleeding uncontrollably. The amount of random donor platelet transfusion is generally about 3 units/m² body surface area or 0.1 U/kg body weight.[8,9] Admin-

> **KEY POINT:**
>
> *Clinical evidence of bleeding is likely when the platelet count is below 20,000/µl.*

istering each unit with 30 to 60 ml of plasma per each unit of platelets is recommended. In animals with acute bleeding that is not responsive to other treatments or procedures, hemostatic, epsilon aminocaproic acid (Amicar®) can be given IV or PO (250 mg/m² QID).[9] Vincristine (0.5 mg/m² body surface area) can be administered IV to induce premature release of platelets from megakaryocytes.[8] Platelet counts increase 4 days after vincristine is given.

REFERENCES

1. Goodwin JK, Schaer M: Septic shock. *Vet Clin North Am Small Anim Pract* 19:1239–1258, 1989.
2. Haskins SC: Shock, in Kirk RW (ed): *Current Veterinary Therapy VIII*, Philadelphia, WB Saunders, 1983, pp 2–27.
3. Kirk RW, Bistner SI: Shock, in *Handbook of Veterinary Procedures Emergency Treatment*, ed 4. Philadelphia, WB Saunders, 1985, pp 59–68.
4. Parker MM, Parrillo JE: Septic shock, hemodynamics and pathogenesis. *JAMA* 250:2324–2230, 1983.
5. Hardie EM, Rawlings CA: Septic shock. *Compend Contin Educ Pract Vet* 5:369–373, 1983.
6. Wolfsheimer KJ: Fluid therapy in the critically ill patient. *Vet Clin North Am Small Anim Pract* 19:361–378, 1989.
7. Lazarus HM, Creger RJ, Gerson SL: Infectious emergencies in oncology patients. *Semin Oncol* 6:543–560, 1989.
8. Couto CG: Management of complications of cancer chemotherapy. *Vet Clin North Am Small Anim Pract* 4:1037–1053, 1990.
9. Woodlock TJ: Oncologic emergencies, in Rosenthal S, Carignan JR, Smith BD (eds): *Medical Care of the Cancer Patient*, ed 2. Philadelphia, WB Saunders, 1993, pp 236–246.
10. Hughes WT: Infectious Diseases Society of America: Guidelines for the use of antimicrobial agents in neutropenic patients with unexplained fever. *J Infect Dis* 161: 381–390, 1990.

CLINICAL BRIEFING: ACUTE TUMOR LYSIS SYNDROME	
Diagnosis	*History:* Acute decompensation, anorexia, and collapse after chemotherapy for chemoresponsive tumor *Clinical Signs:* Pale mucous membranes, decreased capillary refill time, evidence of decreased cardiac output (hypodynamic shock), arrhythmias, vomiting, diarrhea, and evidence of lysis of tumor *Diagnostics:* Evidence of multi-organ failure, metabolic acidosis, hyperkalemia, hyperphosphatemia, and azotemia
Therapy	Prevention is essential Restore tissue perfusion with fluids and stabilize cardiovascular system Correct acid–base balance, electrolyte imbalances, and azotemia

ACUTE TUMOR LYSIS SYNDROME

Acute tumor lysis syndrome (ATLS) (Figure 3-3) is a condition of acute collapse that may lead to death soon after administration of a chemotherapeutic agent to an animal with a chemosensitive tumor.[1–3] In humans, ATLS has been documented in patients with lymphoma, leukemia, and small-cell lung cancer; in dogs, it has been associated with lymphoma and leukemia. Acute tumor lysis syndrome can occur after effective chemotherapy in animals with rapidly growing, bulky, chemosensitive tumors. Patients often present with a history of acute decompensation over a short period, sometimes to the point of imminent death. Rapid diagnosis and therapy are essential to reduce mortality.

Predisposing Factors

In humans and animals, rapid tumor lysis may cause an acute release of intracellular phosphate and potassium. This release of electrolytes causes hypocalcemia, hyperkalemia, and hyperphosphatemia. In human patients who undergo ATLS, hyperuricemia is also seen. As noted earlier, ATLS is most common in lymphoma or leukemia patients, partly because the intracellular concentration of phosphorus in human lymphoma and leukemic cells is 4 to 6 times higher than in normal cells.[1] Acute tumor lysis syn-

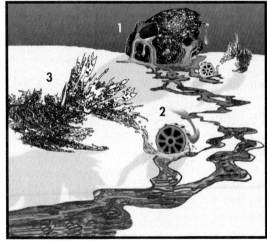

Figure 3-3: *Illustration of the acute tumor lysis syndrome, in which the chemoresponsive cancer cells (1) lyse rapidly after therapy, releasing potassium and phosphorus into the systemic circulation. The phosphorus combines with the calcium (2) to cause the precipitation of calcium into soft tissues (3). The result is acute decompensation of the cancer patient, hyperkalemia, hyperphosphatemia, and secondary hypocalcemia as noted on a biochemical profile.*

drome is most common in animals with some degree of volume contraction and a large tumor mass that responds rapidly to cytolytic therapy. In addition, septic animals or animals with extensive neoplastic

TABLE 3-5
Therapy for the patient with ATLS

Problem	Approach
Acute decompensation (hours to days after therapy for a chemoresponsive tumor)	**Evaluate the patient.** Determine whether tumor is responding rapidly. Perform complete physical examination to evaluate for systemic disease, hydration status, cardiac output, etc. Rule in or out neutropenia, sepsis, coagulopathies, organ failure with a hemogram, biochemical profile, urinalysis, blood cultures, etc.
Initiate specific support	**Treat for shock, provide daily fluid needs, correct dehydration, correct electrolyte abnormalities, and compensate for external fluid losses.** Consider nonlactate-containing fluids. In ATLS, 0.9% NaCl may be ideal until hyperkalemia and hyperphosphatemia are corrected. Daily fluid needs are approximately 66 ml/kg. Fluids can be administered during acute shock or shock-like states at a rate of 70–90 ml/kg for the first hour, followed by 10 ml/kg/hr with very close patient monitoring to adjust fluid rate as needed. If hypocalcemia secondary to hyperphosphatemia causes clinically significant clinical signs (rare), exogenous parenteral calcium supplementation may be indicated.
Monitor patient	**Monitor hydration, electrolytes, and renal and cardiovascular function.** Rate of fluid administration must be "fine tuned" based on hydration, cardiovascular, renal, and electrolyte status.
Delay additional chemotherapy	**Withhold additional chemotherapy pending patient recovery.**

disease that infiltrates the parenchyma are predisposed to ATLS. Veterinary patients at highest risk are volume-contracted dogs with stage IV or V lymphoma that are treated with chemotherapy and that undergo very rapid remission; therefore, this condition may be identified within 48 hours after the first treatment.

Diagnosis

To reduce morbidity and mortality, rapid diagnosis and therapy for ATLS is essential. Animals with ATLS may show cardiovascular collapse, vomiting, diarrhea, and ensuing shock. The hyperkalemia may result in bradycardia and diminished P-wave amplitude and spiked T-waves on an electrocardiogram. Biochemical analysis of blood may confirm the presence of hypocalcemia, hyperkalemia, and hyperphosphatemia. Hyperuricemia (seen in humans with ATLS) has not been identified in dogs or cats. In the presence of elevated serum phosphate levels, hypocalcemia develops as a result of calcium and phosphate precipitation. Without effective treatment, renal failure may occur in this syndrome; therefore, the blood urea nitrogen (BUN) and creatinine concentrations should be monitored closely.

> **KEY POINT:**
>
> *Patients with acute tumor lysis syndrome often present with a history of acute decompensation, sometimes to the point of imminent death (within hours).*[1–3]

Treatment

Treatment is primarily preventive. Because the kidneys are the main source of electrolyte excretion, metabolic abnormalities may be exacerbated in animals with renal dysfunction. Identification of these patients and correction of any volume depletion or azotemia may reduce the risk of ATLS, and chemotherapy should be delayed until metabolic disturbances, such as azotemia, are corrected. If ATLS is identified, the animal should be treated with aggressive crystalloid fluid therapy (Table 3-5). Further chemotherapy should be withheld until the animal is clinically normal and all biochemical parameters are within normal limits.

REFERENCES

1. Marcus SL, Einzig AI: Acute tumor lysis syndrome: Prevention and management, in Dutcher JP, Wiernik PH (eds): *Handbook of Hematologic and Oncologic Emergencies.* New York, Plenum Press, 1987, pp 9–15.
2. Woodlock TJ: Oncologic emergencies, in Rosenthal S, Carignan JR, Smith BD (eds): *Medical Care of the Cancer Patient,* ed 2. Philadelphia, WB Saunders, 1993, pp 236–246.
3. Couto CG: Management of complications of cancer chemotherapy. *Vet Clin North Am Small Anim Pract* 4:1037–1053, 1990.

CLINICAL BRIEFING: DISSEMINATED INTRAVASCULAR COAGULATION	
Diagnosis	*History:* Acute decompensation, anorexia, collapse, and inappropriate bleeding from any site *Clinical Signs:* Pale mucous membranes; decreased capillary refill time; evidence of decreased cardiac output due to blood loss or thrombosis; bleeding from any part of the body, including venipuncture sites; dyspnea from blood loss or pulmonary thrombosis *Diagnostics:* Evidence of blood loss, multi-organ failure, or coagulopathies based on abnormal PT, APTT, FDPs, ACT, fibrinogen, antithrombin III and platelet counts, and metabolic acidosis
Therapy	Treat the underlying cause Restore tissue perfusion with fluids; stabilize the cardiovascular system Correct acid–base and electrolyte imbalances Blood component therapy, including plasma for clotting factors Heparin therapy may be of value if thrombosis predominates

DISSEMINATED INTRAVASCULAR COAGULATION

Disorders of hemostasis are a common cause of morbidity and mortality in veterinary and human cancer patients[1-4] and can be loosely categorized as follows:
1. Disseminated intravascular coagulopathy (DIC)
2. Malignancy-associated fibrinolysis
3. Platelet abnormalities
4. Clinical syndrome of the hypercoagulable state of malignancy
5. Chemotherapy-associated (e.g., L-asparaginase) thromboembolism

Disseminated intravascular coagulation is a consumptive coagulopathy that often results in a life-threatening condition. Disseminated intravascular coagulopathy has been associated with the above parameters 2 through 5 and occurs with many malignancies. The malignancy sometimes induces DIC when clotting factors are activated by tumor-induced procoagulants or when the tumor directly or indirectly stimulates platelet aggregation. The resultant formation of clots in the circulation consumes clotting factors and platelets, which leads to widespread bleeding. In addition, deposition of fibrin throughout the body may result in concurrent microangiopathic hemolytic anemia. To reduce morbidity and mortality, DIC must be identified and treated early.

Predisposing Factors

Disseminated intravascular coagulopathy occurs with a wide variety of malignant conditions, including hemangiosarcoma, lymphoma, thyroid carcinoma, and inflammatory carcinoma. Treatment with chemotherapeutic agents or surgery or concurrent infection may induce or exacerbate DIC. Renal failure and loss of low molecular weight coagulation factors through glomeruli may increase the risk of coagulation abnormalities. Thrombosis with or without DIC has been identified in dogs with hyperadrenocorticism and in dogs that have been treated with high doses of glucocorticoids. The syndrome is more common in dogs than in cats.

TABLE 3-6
Clinical and laboratory parameters used to diagnose DIC

Tests/Observations	Acute DIC	Chronic DIC
Clinical signs	Clinically evident coagulopathies	Few clinical signs evident
Onset and duration	Rapid onset and quick progression	Insidious and prolonged
PT, APTT, and ACT	Prolonged	Normal to slightly decreased
Platelets	Decreased	Often normal
FDP	Very high	High
Fibrinogen	Decreased to normal	Normal
Antithrombin III	Reduced	Normal
Prognosis	Grave	Good

Diagnosis

Clinical signs supportive of a diagnosis of DIC include, but are not limited to, oozing from venipuncture sites, nosebleeds, oral bleeding, melena, ecchymoses and petechial hemorrhages anywhere on the body, and hematuria.[1-4] Widespread thrombosis can cause multi-organ failure that may result in a variety of clinical signs, such as acute renal failure and acute onset of respiratory distress. Laboratory abnormalities associated with DIC vary depending on the organs involved and whether the DIC is acute or chronic; the chronic form of DIC is rarely associated with clinical signs. In addition, red blood cell fragmentation may result from microangiopathic events that occur in this syndrome. Diagnosis is based on clinical findings and an elevated prothrombin time (PT), activated partial thromboplastin time (APTT), thrombocytopenia, prolonged activated coagulation time (ACT), decreased antithrombin III (AT-III) concentrations, hypofibrinogenemia, and increased fibrin degradation products (Table 3-6). There are many causes for DIC-associated abnormalities.[1-4] Decreased platelet count can be caused by bone marrow failure, increased platelet consumption, or splenic pooling of platelets. Prolonged PT may result from lack of one or more of the following clotting factors: VII, X, V, II (prothrombin), and I (fibrinogen). Increased APTT time may be cause by a deficiency in one or more of the following clotting fac-

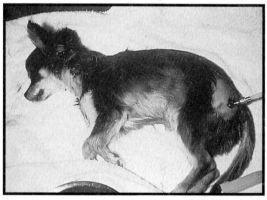

Figure 3-4: *Whenever venous access is not possible in tiny animals, fluids or blood component therapy can be administered through a bone marrow needle placed into the bone marrow cavity of any long bone. Blood and fluids are absorbed rapidly when administered in this way.*

tors: XII, XI, IX, VIII, X, V, II, and I. Heparin and oral anticoagulant therapy prolongs the APTT. Low fibrinogen levels are associated with decreased production or increased consumption of this protein.

Treatment[1-4]

The most important therapy for DIC is treatment of the underlying cause. Fluid therapy is essential to correct volume contraction and to reduce the possibility of ensuing renal failure and acid–base abnormalities (Figure 3-4). Increased body weight, heart and respiratory rates, and central venous pressure may suggest volume overload. Volume overload is especially threatening in patients that are anuric secondary to acute renal shutdown.

Specific treatment for DIC is controversial. Few data exist that document efficacy of treatment modalities. In animals with severe bleeding diatheses, fresh blood or plasma with clotting factors and platelets may be useful for replacing components of the blood that are consumed (Figure 3-4). If thrombosis seems to be the most clinically evident problem, then heparin therapy may reduce the formation of thrombi. The amount of heparin to be used is controversial. One method is to administer heparin by intermittent subcutaneous or intravenous dosages or by constant rate infusion to prolong the APTT by 1.5 to 2 times. Another method is to use "mini dose" heparin therapy (5 to 10 IU/kg/hr by constant rate infusion or 75 IU/kg every 8 hours SQ). Alternatively, 10 IU/kg SQ daily can be used.

Chemotherapeutic agents, including prednisone, should be withheld in patients with coagulopathies

> ## KEY POINT:
>
> *Because the effect of heparin often is directly related to the amount of antithrombin III present, administration of fresh plasma or whole blood may enhance the efficacy of heparin.*

until all evidence of DIC is eliminated and the patient has recovered completely.

Animals in acute DIC have a poor prognosis; therefore, identifying patients at high risk and initiating prophylactic treatment is of great value. Routine monitoring of ACTs and platelet counts can identify animals that are in the early phases of DIC.

REFERENCES

1. Couto CG: Management of complications of cancer chemotherapy. *Vet Clin North Am Small Anim Pract* 4:1037–1053, 1990.
2. Smith MR: Disorders of hemostasis and transfusion therapy, in Skeel RT (ed): *Handbook of Cancer Chemotherapy*, ed 3. Boston, Little, Brown & Co, 1991, pp 449–459.
3. Parry BW: Laboratory evaluation of hemorrhagic coagulopathies in small animal practice. *Vet Clin North Am Small Anim Pract* 4:729–742, 1989.
4. Woodlock TJ: Oncologic emergencies, in Rosenthal S, Carignan JR, Smith BD (eds): *Medical Care of the Cancer Patient,* ed 2. Philadelphia, WB Saunders, 1993, pp 236–246.

CLINICAL BRIEFING: CENTRAL NERVOUS SYSTEM

Brain Herniation

Diagnosis	*History:* History relating to acute neurologic decompensation *Clinical Signs:* Altered mentation, progressive drowsiness, altered pupil size and function, altered respiration, extensor rigidity, disconjugate eye movements, and arrhythmias *Diagnostics:* CT, MRI, nuclear imaging of brain, and electroencephalogram
Treatment	Control respiration Decrease intracranial pressure with mannitol, glucocorticoids, and surgical decompression in rare cases Treat the underlying cause

Seizures

Diagnosis	*History:* The seizure is preceded by an aura and followed by a postictal period *Clinical Signs:* The seizure is characterized as partial, simple partial, complex partial, generalized, or generalized nonconvulsive *Diagnostics:* Metabolic and traumatic causes should be eliminated immediately and other causes evaluated upon recovery via CBC, biochemical profile, urinalysis, radiographs, fasting blood glucose, CSF analysis, and brain imaging methods
Treatment	Evaluate patient and treat metabolic causes, if identified (glucose and calcium) Stop the seizures with diazepam or phenobarbital, if indicated Stabilize metabolic abnormalities Monitor and treat appropriately during recovery

Spinal Cord Compression

Diagnosis	*History:* History compatible with acute upper or lower neurologic decompensation *Clinical Signs:* Back pain, root signature, weakness, muscle atrophy, conscious proprioceptive deficits, altered spinal reflexes, and upper or lower motor neuron damage *Diagnostics:* Myelogram, CT, CSF analysis, spinal decompression and biopsy; in cats, consider FeLV test and bone marrow aspirate to rule out lymphoma
Treatment	Corticosteroids Spinal decompression Treat the underlying cause with chemotherapy, surgery, or radiation therapy

The most common central nervous system (CNS) emergencies are cerebral herniation, seizures, and epidural spinal cord compression.[1-5] Other CNS emergencies are bacterial meningitis and other acute infections that may be associated with tumor- or drug-induced neutropenia. Infectious conditions of the CNS are reviewed in the section on neutropenia and sepsis.

BRAIN HERNIATION
Predisposing Factors
Brain herniation can be caused by a wide variety of primary or secondary malignancies of the brain or by intracerebral hemorrhage and intradural hematoma, brain abscess, and acute hydrocephalus. Regardless of the cause, diagnosis must be made swiftly and therapy initiated without hesitation to prevent irreparable neurologic damage or death.

Clinical Signs
Brain herniation is characterized by any CNS abnormality, including progressive drowsiness, small reactive pupils, periodic respirations (Cheyne-Stokes), and, in the most severe cases, bilateral extensor rigidity.[2,4] As the herniation evolves, hyperventilation, disconjugate eye movements, pupillary fixation, and abnormal motor postures can be noted. The "brain–heart syndrome" may be evident if the brain stem is compressed.

Diagnosis
The diagnosis and decision to treat are based primarily on the presence of relatively rapidly developing abnormal neurologic signs. Because the decision to withhold therapy may result in death or severe neurologic abnormalities that persist for the remainder of a pet's life, treatment should be initiated immediately or concurrently with diagnostic methods, such as computerized tomography (CT), mag-

---

KEY POINT:

In the "brain–heart syndrome," the clinician may be distracted by the occurrence of bizarre arrhythmias that are actually caused by compression of the cardiac control center and centers of the brain that regulate autonomic control of the heart.

---

netic resonance imaging (MRI), nuclear scans, and, if available, an electroencephalogram. A CSF tap at the cisterna magna may actually cause or exacerbate brain herniation; therefore, this procedure should not be used if increased intracranial pressure is suspected.

Treatment
The goals are to prevent further herniation and to treat existing herniation and the underlying cause.[2,4] Intubation and control of respiration may be required when hyperventilation produces cerebral vasoconstriction, decreased blood volume, and decreased intracranial pressure. Mannitol (1–2 g/kg QID IV slowly) can reduce brain water content, reduce brain volume, and decrease intracranial pressure rapidly. Steroids (e.g., dexamethasone $NaPO_4$ [2 mg/kg IV once, followed by 0.25 mg/kg QID IV]) can be administered acutely but may take hours to have full effect. Recent work suggests that hydrocortisone (10–50 mg/kg IV) given at the time of brain trauma may be beneficial.[2,4] In rare cases, surgical decompression may be beneficial. Once treatment is underway, plain and contrast CT or other imaging techniques may help identify the cause of decompensation in the neurologic patient.

SEIZURES
Predisposing Factors
A variety of metastatic and nonmetastatic conditions can cause seizures in veterinary cancer patients. Vascular disorders, such as intracerebral hemorrhage, subdural hematomas, and thrombosis of the CNS vessels, may be associated with seizures. Hypoglycemia secondary to insulinoma or hepatic tumor may induce CNS abnormalities.[1,2,4,5] Several chemotherapeutic agents and radiosensitizers are reported to cause seizures (e.g., cisplatin, mitoxantrone, 5-fluorouracil, and vincristine).[3,4]

Clinical Presentation

Seizures may appear clinically as one of the following: partial (focal or local), simple partial (symmetric and rarely associated with loss of consciousness), complex partial (alterations in consciousness plus complex behavior), generalized seizures (involuntary, uncontrolled motor activity), and generalized non-convulsive seizures (loss of consciousness with lack of spontaneous motor activity and transient collapse).[1,2] There is generally an aura or period of behavioral change before each type of seizure, followed by ictus or the actual clinical seizure, and finally a postictal period that lasts for approximately 30 minutes, during which the animal exhibits abnormal behavior that may include weakness and blindness. If malignancy is associated with the condition, the seizures generally get progressively worse over time because of the enlarging intracranial mass or because of progressive worsening of hypoglycemia in insulin-producing tumors.

Diagnosis

The diagnosis generally is evident from the historical or physical findings. In an emergency situation (often associated with an animal in status epilepticus), a definitive diagnosis is made after the patient is stabilized. A diagnosis is generally made with imaging techniques that include skull radiographs, CT, nuclear imaging, or MRI of the brain. If a neoplasm is suspected, a complete staging scheme must be initiated as soon as the animal is stable. This should include a complete history, complete physical and neurologic examinations, CBC, biochemical profile, urinalysis, chest and abdominal radiographs, fasting (>24 hours) blood glucose and insulin levels, a CSF tap if the animal is not at risk for brain herniation, and an electroencephalogram, if available.

Treatment

Caution should be used when handling the seizuring patient (Figure 3-5). The general schema for a seizuring patient is noted in Table 3-7; Table 3-8 lists anticonvulsants used in acute situations to treat seizuring cats and dogs. If a seizure is in progress,

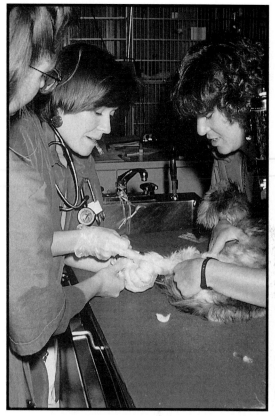

Figure 3-5: *Seizuring animals can be difficult to handle. Firm yet gentle restraint is used while assessing patients, acquiring venous access, obtaining blood samples before therapy, and administering appropriate therapy.*

diazepam should be administered intravenously. Respiration should be monitored and, when necessary, intubation and ventilation should be considered. In these patients, phenobarbital can be given via a loading dose, which is followed by a maintenance dose. Phenobarbital therapy also may be valuable when a single seizure is expected to continue or if clusters of seizures occur within a short period.

SPINAL CORD COMPRESSION
Predisposing Factors

Many malignancy-induced spinal cord compressions in veterinary cancer patients are extradural.[3,6]

TABLE 3-7
Emergency procedures for status epilepticus[1-5]

General Principle	Specific Details
Evaluate the patient	Brief history and physical examination
	If possible, place indwelling catheter
	If possible, acquire blood samples; immediately determine glucose and calcium levels while therapy is continued
Stop the seizures	Administer diazepam IV (2.5–15.0 mg, depending on size of patient)
	Test dosages or definitive therapy for hypoglycemia (e.g., 0.5 g dextrose as a 25% solution given IV over 5 minutes); if hypocalcemia is present, specific therapy for that should be initiated (e.g., 1.0–1.5 ml/kg of 10% calcium gluconate solution)
	If necessary, repeat diazepam bolus every 10 minutes for 3 dosages
	If diazepam is inadequate for seizure control, administer phenobarbital or pentobarbital intravenously (see Table 3-8); pentobarbital is less effective for controlling seizures but has a more rapid onset of action compared to phenobarbital
	Acid–base status, ability to ventilate, body temperature, electrolyte balance, and hydration status are monitored and treated appropriately
Monitor during recovery from seizures	Phenobarbital may be administered (0.5 mg/kg TID IM) to reduce seizures; monitor blood levels. When seizures are controlled and the patient is able to swallow, oral phenobarbital therapy should be continued
Initiate definitive diagnostics	CBC, biochemical profile and fasting blood glucose and insulin measurement, CSF tap, CT or MRI of the brain (if indicated), and electroencephalogram (if available)

This is especially true in cats with posterior paresis, which probably results from an extradural lymphoma. These cats are almost always young, FeLV-positive, and have lymphoma in the bone marrow.[6]

Diagnosis

Clinical signs include back pain, a root signature, paresis, or paralysis.[6] Significant spinal cord compression may occur before clinical signs are evident because of slow progression of the tumor and compensation of the nervous tissue. In some cases, such as with neurofibrosarcomas, lower motor neuron signs (e.g., muscle atrophy, weakness, and lack of spinal reflexes) may precede clinical signs that are referable to the spinal cord.

The importance of early diagnosis cannot be overemphasized. When spinal cord compression is identified, immediate action must be taken to ensure

TABLE 3-8
Anticonvulsants used in an acute situation to treat seizuring dogs and cats[1,2,4,5]

Anticonvulsant	Recommended Dosages, General Indications, and Precautions
Phenobarbital	**Dogs:** 5–16 mg/kg/day divided BID–TID; drug of choice for long-term seizure control; half-life: 40 hours
	Cats: 2.2–4.4 mg/kg/day divided BID–TID; drug of choice for long-term seizure control; half-life: 40 hours
	(Grand mal seizures and partial seizures; this drug is most effective in delaying progressive activity known as kindling; monitor for sedation, ataxia, polydipsia, and polyuria; these adverse effects usually abate with time)
Primidone	**Dogs:** 15–80 mg/kg/day divided BID; not as effective as phenobarbital for emergency therapy; this drug is metabolized down to phenobarbital, which has a half-life of 40 hours
	(Metabolized down to metabolites, including phenobarbital; expensive; grand mal seizures, partial seizures, and status epilepticus; most effective in delaying progressive activity known as kindling; monitor for sedation, ataxia, polydipsia, polyuria, and personality trait changes; these adverse effects usually abate with time; hepatotoxicity)
Phenytoin	**Dogs:** Generally not recommended for emergency therapy
	Cats: Generally not recommended for emergency therapy
Diazepam	**Dogs:** 5–15 mg TID; half-life: 2–4 hours
	Cats: 2.5–5 mg TID; half-life: 15–20 hours
	(Grand mal seizures and status epilepticus; monitor for sedation)

that the underlying cause is specifically diagnosed and treated. Diagnosis is based on clinical findings, which include back pain, spinal tenderness, a root signature, abnormal findings on CT or contrast myelogram, and bone scans via scintigraphy. Extradural lymphoma is one of the most common causes of posterior paresis in cats that have no evidence of trauma and good femoral pulses. Most of these cats can be diagnosed by first determining whether they are FeLV positive and have lymphoma based on the diagnosis of lymphoma from a bone marrow aspirate. In many animals with spinal cord compression, a diagnosis can be made by performing a surgical spinal cord decompression and biopsy.

Treatment[3,4,6]

The optimal treatment for epidural spinal cord compression caused by metastatic disease is debated in human medicine. Corticosteroids (i.e., prednisone, 2 mg/kg BID initially) and radiotherapy are the mainstays of therapy for most patients that have solid tumors of the spinal cord. Cats with lymphoma are treated effectively with chemotherapy (e.g., cyclophosphamide, prednisone, or vincristine) and/or radiation therapy to the area of compression. Steroids reduce spinal cord edema and may be beneficial when administered before and during radiation treatment. Surgical intervention is indicated if tissue diagnosis is required, if the cause of the spinal cord compression is uncertain, if relapse occurs in the area of prior irradiation, if spinal instability is present, or if radiation therapy and steroid treatment fail.

REFERENCES

1. Fenner WR: Seizures, narcolepsy and cataplexy, in Birchard SJ, Sherding RG (eds): *Saunders Manual of Small Animal Practice.* Philadelphia, WB Saunders, 1993, pp 1147–1156.
2. Fenner WR: Diseases of the brain, in Birchard SJ, Sherding RG (eds): *Saunders Manual of Small Animal Practice.* Philadelphia, WB Saunders, 1993, pp 1126–1146.
3. Couto CG: Management of complications of cancer chemotherapy. *Vet Clin North Am Small Anim Pract* 4:1037–1053, 1990.
4. Woodlock TJ: Oncologic emergencies, in Rosenthal S, Carignan JR, Smith BD (eds): *Medical Care of the Cancer Patient,* ed 2. Philadelphia, WB Saunders, 1993, pp 236–246.
5. Bunch SE: Anticonvulsant drug therapy in companion animals, in Kirk RW (ed): *Current Veterinary Therapy IX, Small Animal Practice.* Philadelphia, WB Saunders, 1986, pp 836–844.
6. Luttgen PJ: Spinal cord disorders, in Birchard SJ, Sherding RG (eds): *Saunders Manual of Small Animal Practice.* Philadelphia, WB Saunders, 1993, pp 1157–1164.

CLINICAL BRIEFING: METABOLIC EMERGENCIES— HYPERCALCEMIA, HYPONATREMIA, AND HYPOGLYCEMIA

Emergency Due to Hypercalcemia

Diagnosis	*History:* Acute history of polyuria, polydipsia, severe dehydration, vomiting secondary to renal failure, coma, seizures, and death *Clinical Signs:* Vomiting, bradycardia, skeletal muscle weakness, depression, stupor, coma, and seizures *Diagnostics:* Hypercalcemia and secondary renal damage; the underlying cause for this electrolyte abnormality can be identified with a CBC, biochemical profile, urinalysis, ionized calcium, bone marrow aspirate, radiographs, ACTH stimulation, and (if indicated) parathyroid hormone or parathyroid hormone-related peptide concentrations
Treatment	Treat the underlying cause while initiating diagnostics and therapy Rehydration with a saline diuresis is essential to stabilize the patient and decrease serum calcium concentrations; furosemide may be valuable to decrease calcium in a well-hydrated animal; consider prednisone only after a diagnosis of the underlying cause has been made In refractory cases, consider salmon calcitonin, biphosphonates, gallium nitrate, and mithramycin

Syndrome of Inappropriate Secretion of Antidiuretic Hormone (SIADH)

Diagnosis	*History:* Anorexia, muscle stiffness leading to confusion or unresponsive state, and history of recent administration of drug that may cause hyponatremia or SIADH *Clinical Signs:* Nausea and neurologic signs progressing to coma and death *Diagnostics:* Biochemical profile to include serum sodium, fractional excretion of sodium, urinalysis, serum osmolality, and adrenal and thyroid function tests
Treatment	Treat the underlying cause while initiating supportive, symptomatic therapy Judicious water restriction Demeclocycline and furosemide Lithium carbonate, phenytoin, and hypertonic saline in refractory cases

Emergency Due to Hypoglycemia	
Diagnosis	*History:* Weakness, confusion, seizures, and coma *Clinical Signs:* CNS abnormalities, including weakness, seizures, and coma *Diagnostics:* CBC, biochemical profile, urinalysis, fasting blood glucose and insulin levels, radiographs, abdominal ultrasonography, and (when stable) exploratory surgery and biopsy
Treatment	Treat the underlying cause while initiating supportive, symptomatic therapy Glucose infusion, prednisone, diazoxide + hydrochlorothiazide Propranolol may be useful in refractory cases

HYPERCALCEMIA

Hypercalcemia is the most common metabolic emergency in oncology.[1-6] Lymphoma is the leading cause of hypercalcemia in dogs. Other causes include apocrine gland anal sac adenocarcinoma, mammary adenocarcinoma, and primary hyperparathyroidism. Parathyroid carcinomas or adenomas are a rare malignancy associated with intractable hypercalcemia caused by elevated parathyroid hormone levels. A parathyroid hormone-related peptide (PTH-rp) is most commonly associated with hypercalcemia in dogs. Although it has been suggested that bone metastasis can be associated with hypercalcemia, this is rare in veterinary medicine.

Clinical Presentation

The oncologic emergency secondary to hypercalcemia of malignancy revolves around clinical signs associated with a decreased ADH sensitivity of the distal convoluted tubules and collecting ducts as well as the vasoconstrictive properties of calcium that result in decreased renal blood flow and a reduced glomerular filtration rate.[1-4] The epithelium undergoes degenerative changes, necrosis, and calcification. The aforementioned physiologic and pathologic changes result in progressive renal disease, noted clinically as polyuria and polydipsia, followed by vomiting, hyposthenuria, and dehydration. Calcium also may affect the gastrointestinal, cardiovascular, and neurologic systems directly and cause anorexia, vomiting, constipation, bradycardia, hypertension, skeletal muscle weakness, depression, stupor, coma, and seizures.

Diagnosis

Other diagnostic differentials that must be considered in animals presented for true hypercalcemia (Ca^{++} >12 mg/dl) include laboratory error, error in interpretation (e.g., young, growing dogs), hyperproteinemia from dehydration, acute renal failure, vitamin D and calcium toxicosis, granulomatous disorders, nonneoplastic disorders of bone, hypoadrenocorticism, true hyperparathyroidism, and chronic disuse osteoporosis.[2,5,6]

It is important to interpret calcium levels in relation to serum albumin and blood pH. A correction formula that takes the albumin into account is:

adjusted calcium (mg/dl) = [calcium (mg/dl) – albumin (g/dl)] + 3.5

Acidosis results in an increase in the free, ionized fraction of calcium and can magnify the observed clinical signs associated with hypocalcemia.

> **KEY POINT:**
>
> *The most common cause of confirmed hypercalcemia in dogs is anterior mediastinal lymphoma.*

Serial serum calcium, electrolytes, BUN, and creatinine levels should be measured in all hypercalcemic patients. Elevated immunoreactive PTH levels in association with hyperphosphatemia may suggest ectopic hormone production. Patients with multiple myeloma may have elevated calcium levels secondary to abnormal calcium binding to a paraprotein without an elevation in ionized calcium, and malnourished patients with hypoalbuminemia may have symptoms of hypercalcemia with normal serum calcium levels.

Treatment[2,5,6]

Treatment of an emergency secondary to hypercalcemia depends on the severity of the clinical signs and the presence of renal disease. This almost always entails the use of intravenous saline in volumes that exceed daily maintenance (>132 ml/kg$^{0.75}$/day or approximately >66 ml/kg/day, plus exogenous losses from vomiting and diarrhea, plus replacement fluids for dehydration). Potassium depletion should be prevented by addition of potassium chloride to fluids based on serum potassium levels (Table 3-9).

The rate of potassium administered intravenously should not exceed 0.05 mEq/kg/hr. In addition, patients should be watched carefully for signs consistent with overhydration and congestive heart failure and effective antitumor therapy should be initiated as soon as possible. Thiazide diuretics or vitamins A and D (which may elevate calcium levels) should never be used with these patients. Furosemide (1–4 mg/kg BID, IV or PO) and intravenous biphosphonates (e.g., etidronate and disodium palmidroate) may be used in addition to saline diuresis. Intravenous biphosphonates have rapid hypocalcemic effects by inhibiting osteoclast activity. Gallium nitrate produces concentration-dependent reduction in osteolytic response to PTH and certain other types of lymphokines that cause hypercalcemia. In humans, gallium nitrate is infused at doses of approximately 100 mg/m^2 daily for 5 consecutive days and results in successful reduction of high calcium levels in 86% of the patients.[7,8]

Mithramycin, a chemotherapeutic agent that decreases bone reabsorption by reducing osteoclast

TABLE 3-9
Intravenous potassium supplementation to correct hypokalemia

Serum Potassium (mEq/L)	KCl Added to Each Liter of Fluids (mEq)	Maximum Rate of Infusion (ml/kg/hr)
<2.0	80	6
2.1–2.5	60	8
2.6–3.0	40	12
3.1–3.5	28	16

number and activity, has been shown to be effective in humans. Because mithramycin is a sclerosing agent, it must be given as a bolus through a newly placed intravenous line. If extravasation occurs, ulceration and fibrosis will develop. Mithramycin (25 µg/kg IV once or twice weekly) is rarely used but is effective for reducing calcium levels in dogs. Salmon calcitonin (4–8 MRC units/kg SQ) also can be used in refractory patients; when administered at approximately 40 units/kg, it may result in hypocalcemia for several days. Calcitonin inhibits bone reabsorption, which causes a decrease in serum calcium levels within hours of administration. Corticosteroids are effective for treatment of hypercalcemia. Corticosteroids block bone reabsorption caused by osteoclast-activating factor, increase urinary calcium excretion, inhibit vitamin D metabolism, and increase calcium absorption after long-term use. To be effective, high doses are generally required for several days. Steroids should not be used until tissue diagnosis is made, primarily because lymphomas are the primary cause of malignancy-associated hypercalcemia.

Most patients are effectively treated with hydration, mobilization, antitumor therapy, and treatment with hypocalcemic-inducing agents, such as mithramycin, calcitonin, or corticosteroids. Serum calcium should be monitored at least twice weekly.

HYPONATREMIA

An emergency condition relating to the syndrome of inappropriate antidiuretic hormone secretion (SIADH) is a rare but important cause of true hyponatremia in the cancer patient.[6–8] As the name implies, SIADH is the presence of excessive quantities of antidiuretic hormone secondary to a malignancy. In SIADH, animals have a low plasma osmolality despite inappropriate urine concentration (high sodium). Because this situation also can occur in renal disease, hypothyroidism, and adrenal insufficiency, these disorders must be excluded to confirm the diagnosis of SIADH.

Predisposing Factors

The condition may be caused by a malignancy or a drug that results in renal activation or enhanced release of antidiuretic hormone. SIADH has been identified in dogs with lymphoma. Drugs in veterinary medicine that can cause this condition include chlorpropamide, vincristine, vinblastine, cyclophosphamide, opiates, thiazide diuretics, barbiturates, isoproterenol, mannitol, morphine, and diuretics. Steroids that are abruptly withdrawn may also cause SIADH.[6–8]

When hyponatremia develops rapidly or sodium falls below 115 mg/dl, patients may develop mental status abnormalities, confusion, or coma. Serum and urine electrolytes, osmolality, and creatinine levels should be measured in suspect cases.

Diagnosis

In SIADH, there is inappropriate sodium concentration in the urine for the level of hyponatremia in the serum. Therefore, urine osmolality is greater than plasma osmolality, but the urine specific gravity is never maximally dilute. The urea nitrogen values in the serum are usually low because of volume expansion. Hypophosphatemia may be noted. Adrenal and thyroid function should be normal.

Treatment

In an emergency setting, initial treatment should be directed at resolution of the hyponatremia. Fluids should be restricted to ensure that the patient receives only the amount needed to maintain normal hydration and to keep serum sodium concentration within normal levels. In emergencies, demeclocycline may correct hyponatremia by reducing ADH stimulus for free water reabsorption at the collecting ducts. The most common side effect of demeclocycline is nausea and vomiting. Lithium carbonate and phenytoin have some use in treating SIADH. Hypertonic sodium chloride (3%–5%) can be used in an emergency situation; however, if not used carefully, this treatment may result in fluid and circulatory overload. Furosemide can be used concurrently with hypertonic saline to reduce the volume overload. It should be noted that rapid correction of hyponatremia may lead to neurologic damage. The following formula may help to determine approximate amounts of sodium to administer for hyponatremia correction[9]:

Na for replacement (mEq) = (desired serum sodium [mEq/L] – observed serum sodium [mEq/L]) × body weight (kg) × 0.6

HYPOGLYCEMIA

Predisposing Factors

Fasting hypoglycemia in the face of hyperinsulinemia occurs most commonly with insulinomas; however, other tumors of the liver (e.g., hepatomas and carcinomas) have also been associated with this condition.[6–11] Liver disease (including glycogen storage diseases and sepsis) may mimic hypoglycemia of malignancy. In addition, because red blood cells can metabolize glucose rapidly, delay in separating red blood cells from the serum may lead to spurious results.

Clinical Signs

Before presenting with seizures, coma, and impending death, most animals have a history of exhibiting signs of fatigue, weakness, dizziness, and confusion associated with paroxysmal lowering of the blood glucose levels. Neurologic signs of hypoglycemia may mimic other CNS abnormalities, such as brain tumors, brain trauma, meningitis, or metabolic encephalopathy.

Insulin-producing tumors can be diagnosed by

identifying elevated insulin levels in association with low blood glucose concentrations. In some cases, the identification of malignancy-associated hypoglycemia may require periodic sampling during a 72-hour fast.[10] The diagnosis is made when the blood glucose is dramatically reduced, but insulin levels are elevated. Although controversial, the amended insulin:glucose ratio has been advocated as a method to help diagnose insulin-producing tumors in domesticated animals[11]:

$$\frac{\text{serum insulin } (\mu U/ml \times 100)}{\text{serum glucose } (mg/dl) - 30} = \begin{array}{l}\text{amended insulin:} \\ \text{glucose ratio}\end{array}$$

Values above 30 suggest a diagnosis of an insulinoma or other insulin-producing tumors.

Treatment[6–11]

In an emergency setting, medical management is often necessary before, during, and after definitive therapy, especially for insulinomas, which have a high metastatic rate. Glucose-containing fluids (2.5%–5% dextrose in 0.9% NaCl or other isotonic crystalloid solution) should be administered to meet fluid requirement needs and to maintain blood glucose concentrations within acceptable limits. It should be noted, however, that the administration of glucose may trigger the tumor to release more insulin; therefore, a constant infusion of glucose to maintain normal serum glucose levels is preferred to intermittent high-dose bolusing.

Prednisone (0.5–2.0 mg/kg divided BID PO) is often effective in elevating blood glucose levels by inducing hepatic gluconeogenesis and decreasing peripheral utilization of glucose. Diazoxide (10–40 mg/kg divided BID PO) may be effective in elevating blood glucose levels by directly inhibiting pancreatic insulin secretion and glucose uptake by tissues, enhancing epinephrine-induced glycogenolysis, and increasing the rate of mobilization of free fatty acids. Diazoxide's hyperglycemic effects can be potentiated by concurrent administration of hydrochlorothiazide (2–4 mg/kg daily BID PO). Propranolol (0.2–1.0 mg/kg TID PO), a β-adrenergic blocking agent, may also be effective in increasing blood glucose levels by inhibition of insulin release through the blockade of β-adrenergic receptors at the level of the pancreatic β cell, inhibition of insulin release by membrane stabilization, and alteration of peripheral insulin receptor affinity. Combined surgical and medical management of pancreatic tumors has been associated with remission periods of 1 or more years. Once a patient's condition is stable, surgical extirpation may be the best treatment for a tumor that causes hypoglycemia. Because many tumors (including insulinomas) that induce hypoglycemia as a paraneoplastic syndrome are malignant, surgery often is not curative. A partial pancreatectomy may be indicated for insulinomas; iatrogenic pancreatitis and diabetes mellitus are recognized complications.

KEY POINT:

Whenever possible, treat an animal with significant hypoglycemia with a constant infusion of dextrose-containing fluids. A seizuring animal with hypoglycemia (<60 mg/dl) should be treated with 0.5 g dextrose/kg administered IV slowly over 3 to 5 minutes. Repeat doses may be needed.

REFERENCES

1. Besarb A, Caro JF: Mechanisms of hypercalcemia in malignancy. *Cancer* 41:2276–2285, 1978.
2. Meuten DJ: Hypercalcemia. *Vet Clin North Am Small Anim Pract* 14:891–899, 1984.
3. Weir EC, Burtis WJ, Morris CA, et al: Isolation of a 16,000-dalton parathyroid hormone-like protein from two animal tumors causing humoral hypercalcemia of malignancy. *Endocrinology* 123:2744–2755, 1988.
4. Weir EC, Nordin RW, Matus RE, et al: Humoral hypercalcemia of malignancy in canine lymphosarcoma. *Endocrinology* 122:602–610, 1988.
5. Kruger JM, Osborne CA, Polzin DJ: Treatment of hypercalcemia, in Kirk RW (ed): *Current Veterinary Therapy IX.* Philadelphia, WB Saunders, 1986, pp 75–90.
6. Lowitz BB: Paraneoplastic syndromes, in Haskell CM (ed): *Cancer Treat-*

ment, ed 3. Philadelphia, WB Saunders, 1990, pp 841–849.

7. Glover DJ, Glick JH: Oncologic emergencies and special complications, in Calabrese P, Schein PJ, Rosenberg SA (eds): *Medical Oncology: Basic Principles and Clinical Management of Cancer*. New York, MacMillan, 1985, pp 1261–1326.

8. Felds ALA, Jese RG, Bergaagel DE: Metabolic emergencies, in DeVita VT, Hellman S, Rosenberg SA (eds): *Cancer Principles and Practice of Oncology*. Philadelphia, JB Lippincott, 1985, pp 1874–1876.

9. Franco-Saenz R: Endocrine syndromes, in Skeel RT (ed): *Handbook of Cancer Chemotherapy*, Boston, Little, Brown & Co, 1991, pp 379–404.

10. Leifer CE, Peterson ME, Matus RE, Patnaik AK: Hypoglycemia associated with nonislet cell tumors in 13 dogs. *JAVMA* 186:53–62, 1985.

11. Giger U, Gorman NT: Acute complications of cancer and cancer therapy, in Gorman NT (ed): *Oncology*. New York, Churchill Livingstone, 1986, pp 147–168.

CLINICAL BRIEFING: CHEMOTHERAPY- OR RADIATION-INDUCED CONGESTIVE HEART FAILURE

Congestive Heart Failure

Diagnosis	*History:* Acute decompensation, anorexia, lethargy, dyspnea, collapse, and exercise intolerance *Clinical Signs:* Pale mucous membranes; decreased capillary refill time; evidence of decreased cardiac output, such as poor femoral and jugular pulses, pulmonary edema, hepatomegaly and splenomegaly, and ascites *Diagnostics:* Document myocardial failure and secondary heart failure by evaluating central venous pressure, chest and abdominal radiographs, electrocardiography, fluid analysis (if indicated), and echocardiography
Therapy	Eliminate the underlying cause Initiate enforced rest Enhance oxygenation and reduce effusion and/or edema with thoracocentesis and diuretics Increase contractility with digoxin or dobutamine Reduce afterload with enalapril, captopril, or hydralazine Control arrhythmias

---

CONGESTIVE HEART FAILURE

Cardiac disease secondary to anthracycline or anthracycline-like drugs is a common problem that can become life-threatening. Doxorubicin is the anthracycline most commonly associated with the development of such cardiac diseases as arrhythmias or dilatative cardiomyopathy. Cardiomyopathy may occur in response to the administration of any number of dosages of doxorubicin, but the risk of developing this cardiac condition increases significantly in dogs that receive a total cumulative dosage exceeding 240 mg/m^2.[1,2] The risk in cats is still unknown; however, histologic abnormalities have been found in asymptomatic cats that were given doxorubicin at total cumulative doses ranging from 130 to 320 mg/m^2.[2]

Radiation can induce cardiomyopathy if the heart is in the radiation therapy field and if sufficiently high dosages are used.[3] Histologic and clinically significant pericardial effusion develops approximately 3 months after a 3-week radiation treatment schedule is completed. Radiation can induce a thinning of the myocardium and development of significant amounts of fibrosis 1 year after treatment.

Predisposing Factors

Doxorubicin-induced cardiac disease may occur more frequently in animals with pre-existing cardiac disease and in those that cannot metabolize or eliminate the drug adequately after administration. Similarly, rapid infusion of the drug, which establishes very high serum concentrations, may increase the prevalence of cardiac disease. Therefore, increased time for infusion of a dosage of doxorubicin may reduce the prevalence of acute and chronic cardiac disease.

Diagnosis

In a recent study,[4] 32 of 175 dogs treated with doxorubicin developed clinically evident cardiac disease. Thirty-one dogs had electrocardiographic abnormalities, including arrhythmias (i.e., atrial premature complexes, atrial fibrillation, paroxysmal atrial and sinus tachycardia, ventricular arrhythmias, bundle branch blocks, and atrioventricular dissociation) and nonspecific alterations in R wave, ST segment, or QRS duration. Seven dogs had overt congestive heart failure that resulted in death within 90 days, despite supportive therapy. Arrhythmias may occur at the time of treatment or within a variable period after treatment is complete. In humans with doxorubicin-induced cardiac diseases, significant dysrhythmias often occur in the absence of other physical or historical abnormalities.[5]

In animals with cardiomyopathy and fulminant congestive heart failure, clinical signs vary from anorexia, lethargy, and weakness to more common signs associated specifically with decreased cardiac output and ensuing congestive heart failure. Owners may complain that their pet has exercise intolerance; coughing spells late at night, which may develop into a persistent cough at all times of the day; abdominal distention; increased respiratory effort and rate; and generalized malaise.

The physical examination can reveal much useful information and may include identification of a jugular pulse; rapid heart and respiratory rates; ascites; cool extremities; blue mucous membranes; delayed capillary refill time; pitting edema of lower extremities; enlarged liver and spleen; and rapid, weak pulses. The chest may sound dull because of pleural effusion, or pulmonary edema may cause crackling lung sounds. Heart murmurs or an abnormal rhythm are frequently auscultated; heart sounds from dogs with atrial fibrillation may sound like "jungle drums" (i.e., irregularly irregular) on auscultation. Electrocardiography may suggest heart chamber enlargement or may be diagnostic for arrhythmias, which may be supraventricular or ventricular in origin.

Chest and abdominal radiographs are very valuable in identifying evidence of cardiac disease, including pericardial or pleural effusion, enlargement of the heart, liver, spleen, and pulmonary veins, and pulmonary edema, which usually is first noted around the hilar region. Echocardiography is extremely valuable for confirming pericardial effusion and for documenting chamber size, myocardial wall thickness, and parameters (e.g., ejection fraction, cardiac output, and contractility). Blood pressure measurements may assist in documentation of hypertension or hypotension. An elevated central venous pressure aids in making a diagnosis of cardiac insufficiency (Figure 3-6). Finally, there are more specific tests that can further clarify a diagnosis of drug- or radiation therapy-induced cardiac disease. These include fluid analysis of thoracic or abdominal effusion (usually a modified transudate with reactive mesothelial cells and macrophages) and contrast radiography. Unfortunately, no evaluation method can be performed routinely in veterinary practice to predict whether cardiotoxicity will occur in dogs that receive anthracycline agents or radiation therapy. This precludes withdrawal of therapy before overt signs of cardiac insufficiency occur. In humans, nuclear medicine imaging techniques may be able to predict the development of doxorubicin cardiomyopathy before it becomes clinically evident.

Therapy

The development of cardiomyopathy may be associated with a profound decrease in contractility without substantial alterations in quality

> **KEY POINT:**
>
> *Doxorubicin is the most common cause of chemotherapy-induced cardiomyopathy in dogs; the condition can occur after any dosage, but the risk increases significantly in animals with pre-existing cardiac disease and in those that have received more than 240 mg/m² total cumulative dose.*

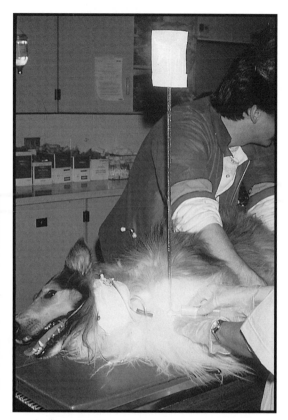

Figure 3-6: *Central venous pressure measurements can be used to ensure that a patient has increased venous pressure and to monitor therapy. With this procedure, values of less than approximately 5 mm of water are considered normal. Note that the base of the water column is at the level of the right atrium.*

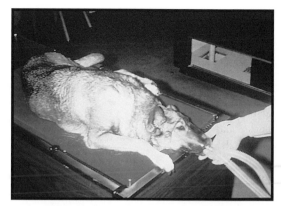

Figure 3-7: *Cancer patients with cardiac failure must be handled gently, and stress should be kept to a minimum. Oxygen often can be administered by a face mask to minimize the oxygen debt and reduce the risk of a fatal cardiac arrest during evaluation.*

of life. Other patients exhibit signs of heart failure. Once these alterations in cardiovascular performance are documented, doxorubicin administration should be discontinued indefinitely. The important lesson to be learned from these data is that the presence or absence of clinical signs should dictate whether chemotherapy or cardiac drugs should be initiated, rather than basing the decision on results of diagnostic tests.

Prevention

The hallmark of doxorubicin-induced heart disease is development of dilatative cardiomyopathy. Many methods to prevent the development of this condition have been explored. Vitamin E, thyroxine, and selenium treatments are ineffective for prevention of cardiomyopathy. In humans, weekly low-dose doxorubicin therapy reduces the prevalence of cardiomyopathy.[6] The compound ICRF-187 is more effective. This compound substantially reduces the occurrence of cardiomyopathy in dogs treated concurrently with doxorubicin.

Treatment

Treatment of cardiomyopathy begins with the indefinite discontinuation of the inciting cause (e.g., radiation therapy or doxorubicin). Diuretics, a low-salt diet, rest, oxygen therapy, positive inotropes, and vasodilators should be used as dictated by the clinical status of the patient. For example, furosemide may be used two to three times a day in a compensated animal, whereas the drug may be used every few hours, if necessary, in patients in respiratory distress from severe, fulminant pulmonary edema (Figure 3-7). Digoxin, a positive inotrope, can be given orally or parenterally in combination with a preload or afterload reducer. When given orally, therapeutic levels of digoxin generally are not achieved for a few days, which may be

TABLE 3-10
Potential therapeutic approach for dogs or cats with drug- or radiation-induced dilatative cardiomyopathy

General Principle	Specific Details, Drug Dosages, and Toxicities
Discontinue cardiotoxic agents	All cardiotoxic drugs should be discontinued indefinitely; additional radiation therapy to the heart should be avoided
Enforce complete rest	Avoidance of any stressful environment is essential; consider cage rest
Oxygenate	Acquire and maintain a patent airway
	Provide supplemental oxygen if needed; fifty percent oxygen should not be used for more than 24 hours to avoid pulmonary toxicity
	Perform thoracocentesis to reduce pleural effusion
	Initiate diuretic therapy for pulmonary edema (see below)
Reduce pulmonary edema	**Furosemide** (drug of choice; monitor for dehydration, hypokalemia, etc.) **Dogs:** 2–4 mg/kg IV or IM every 2–12 hours depending on the severity of edema; decrease to 1–4 mg/kg SID–TID PO for maintenance therapy **Cats:** 1–2 mg/kg IV or IM every 4–12 hours depending on the severity of edema; decrease to 1–2 mg/kg SID–TID PO for maintenance therapy
	Hydrochlorothiazide/spironolactone combination (use with furosemide or as maintenance therapy; monitor for dehydration and electrolyte abnormalities) **Dogs:** 2–4 mg/kg BID PO **Cats:** 1–2 mg/kg BID PO
Increase contractility	**Perform pericardiocentesis if pericardial effusion is present in significant amounts to reduce contractility**
	Digoxin (monitor blood levels to acquire and maintain therapeutic blood levels [1–2 ng/ml]; watch for anorexia, vomiting, diarrhea, and ECG abnormalities suggestive of digoxin toxicity) **Dogs:** Dogs <22 kg: 0.011 mg/kg BID PO; dogs >22 kg: 0.22 mg/m² BID PO **Cats:** Small cats <3 kg: ¼ of a 0.125-mg tablet QOD; medium to large cats 3–6 kg: ¼ of 0.125-mg tablet daily

TABLE 3-10 (continued)

General Principle	Specific Details, Drug Dosages, and Toxicities
	Dobutamine (monitor for tachycardia and arrhythmias) **Dogs and Cats:** 1–10 µg/kg/min constant rate infusion, usually in combination with a pre- or afterload reducer and furosemide in severe, fulminant congestive heart failure
	Milrinone (monitor for GI toxicity and hypotension) **Dogs and Cats:** 0.5–1.0 mg/kg BID PO
Redistribute blood volume	**Vasodilators** 2% nitroglycerin ointment; watch for hypotension **Dogs:** ¼ to ¾ inch on skin or in ear QID **Cats:** ⅛ to ¼ inch on skin or in ear QID
	Sodium nitroprusside 5–20 µg/kg/min constant rate infusion; watch for hypotension; prolonged use may result in cyanide toxicity
	Miscellaneous **Morphine** **Dogs only:** 0.05–0.5 mg/kg IV, IM, or SQ to reduce apprehension and to redistribute blood volume
Reduce afterload	**Enalapril** **Dogs and Cats:** 0.25–0.5 mg/kg SID or BID PO (do not use in conjunction with nitroprusside; monitor for hypotension)
	Hydralazine **Dogs:** 0.5–2.0 mg/kg BID PO (do not use in conjunction with nitroprusside; monitor for hypotension)
Control arrhythmias	See Table 3-11
Monitor response to therapy	Pulse, respiratory rate, ECG, body weight, central venous pressure, urine output, hydration, electrolytes, BUN, creatinine, blood gases, and quality of life; adjust therapy as indicated

adequate for animals that are relatively stable. Factors such as dehydration and electrolyte disturbances may promote development of digoxin toxicoses. Because digoxin toxicity is a serious problem that occurs frequently, intravenous loading dosages should not be used unless absolutely necessary. Regardless of the method of digitalization, periodic determination of serum digoxin concentration is essential for adjustment of drug dosage to maintain therapeutic levels.

In an acutely decompensated dying dog with car-

TABLE 3-11
Drugs used to treat supraventricular and ventricular bradyarrhythmias induced by anthracycline antibiotics or radiation therapy

Drug (Indications)	Specific Details and Drug Dosages
Atropine (sinus bradycardia, sinoatrial arrest, and AV block)	**Dogs and Cats:** 0.01–0.02 mg/kg IV; 0.02–0.04 mg/kg SQ; short acting (monitor for sinus tachycardia and paradoxic vagomimetic effects; redose to effect)
Glycopyrrolate (sinus bradycardia and sinoatrial arrest)	**Dogs and Cats:** 0.005–0.01 mg/kg IV; 0.01–0.02 mg/kg SQ (monitor for sinus tachycardia and paradoxic vagomimetic effects; redose to effect)
Isoproterenol (sinus bradycardia, sinoatrial arrest, and complete AV block)	**Dogs:** 1 mg in 250 ml 5% dextrose; administer IV at a rate of 0.01 µg/kg/min **Cats:** 0.5 mg in 250 ml 5% dextrose; administer IV to effect (monitor for CNS stimulation, arrhythmias, and emesis)

TABLE 3-12
Drugs used to treat supraventricular and ventricular tachyarrhythmias induced by anthracycline antibiotics or radiation therapy

Drug (Indications)	Specific Details and Drug Dosages
Digoxin (supraventricular premature complexes, supraventricular tachycardia, and atrial fibrillation)	**Dogs:** Dogs <22 kg: 0.011 mg/kg BID PO; dogs >22 kg: 0.22 mg/m^2 BID PO **Cats:** Small cats <3 kg: ¼ of 0.125-mg tablet QOD; medium to large cats 3–6 kg: ¼ of 0.125-mg tablet daily (monitor blood levels to acquire and maintain therapeutic blood levels [1–2 ng/ml]; watch for anorexia, vomiting, diarrhea, and ECG abnormalities suggestive of digoxin toxicity)
Lidocaine (premature ventricular contractions and ventricular tachycardia)	**Dogs:** 2–4 mg/kg IV slowly; can be repeated as a bolus (maximum 8 mg/kg) followed by 25–75 µg/kg/min constant rate infusion **Cats:** 0.25–1.0 mg/kg IV over 4–5 minutes, followed by 1–25 µg/kg/min (monitor for CNS excitation, seizures, vomiting, emesis, lethargy, and arrhythmias)
Tocainide (premature ventricular contractions and ventricular tachycardia)	**Dogs:** 5–20 mg/kg QID–TID PO (monitor for CNS signs or GI toxicity)

TABLE 3-12 (continued)

Drug (Indications)	Specific Details and Drug Dosages
Procainamide (premature ventricular contractions and ventricular tachycardia)	**Dogs:** 20–40 mg/kg QID PO, IM; 8–20 mg/kg IV; 25–50 µg/kg/min constant rate infusion
Propranolol (supraventricular premature complexes and tachyarrhythmias, atrial fibrillation, and ventricular premature complexes)	**Dogs and Cats:** 0.04–0.06 mg/kg IV slowly or 0.2–1.0 mg/kg BID–TID PO, often in combination with digoxin for supraventricular arrhythmias (monitor for decreased contractility and bronchoconstriction)
Diltiazem (supraventricular premature complexes and tachyarrhythmias and atrial fibrillation)	**Dogs:** 0.5–1.5 mg/kg TID PO **Cats:** 1.75–2.4 mg/kg BID–TID PO (monitor for bradyarrhythmias and hypotension)

diomyopathy, a constant rate infusion of dobutamine combined with intravenous furosemide and an intravenous (e.g., nitroprusside) or transdermal application (e.g., 2% nitroglycerin) of a preload or afterload reducer may be more logical than oral treatment. Dobutamine may increase cardiac output within minutes to hours, whereas improvement of cardiac output with oral digoxin therapy may take days. A more detailed treatment regimen for cardiomyopathy is outlined in Table 3-10.

Arrhythmias may occur during infusion of a chemotherapeutic agent (Tables 3-11 and 3-12). If arrhythmias persist, interfere with an animal's quality of life, or serve as a serious threat to the animal's survival, therapy should be instituted and the underlying cause identified and eliminated. In each case, the potential adverse effects of the antiarrhythmic agents must be evaluated and considered before therapy is initiated.

REFERENCES

1. Carter SK: Adriamycin: A review. *J Natl Canc Instit* 55:1265–1274, 1975.
2. Cotter SM, Kanki PJ, Simon M: Renal disease in five tumor-bearing cats treated with Adriamycin. *JAAHA* 21:405–411, 1985.
3. McChesney SL, Gillette EL, Powers BE: Radiation-induced cardiomyopathy in the dog. *Radiation Res* 113:120–132, 1988.
4. Maulin GE, Fox PR, Patnaik AK, et al: Doxorubicin-induced cardiotoxicosis: Clinical features of 32 dogs. *J Vet Intern Med* 6:82–88, 1992.
5. Jakacki RI, Larsen RL, Barber G, et al: Comparison of cardiac function tests after anthracycline therapy in childhood. *Cancer* 72:2739–2745, 1993.
6. Couto CG: Management of complications of cancer chemotherapy. *Vet Clin North Am Small Anim Pract* 4:1037–1053, 1990.

CLINICAL BRIEFING: CHEMOTHERAPY-INDUCED ANAPHYLAXIS AND HYPERSENSITIVITY

Anaphylaxis and Hypersensitivity

Diagnosis	*History:* Acute decompensation and collapse soon after the administration of a chemotherapeutic agent *Clinical Signs:* Pale or cyanotic mucous membranes, decreased capillary refill time, evidence of decreased cardiac output, alterations in heart rate, and cool extremities *Diagnostics:* Eliminate other causes with CBC, biochemical profile, urinalysis, and cardiac evaluation
Therapy	Eliminate the underlying cause Ensure a patent airway and adequate cardiac output Establish vascular access Initiate fluid therapy Treat with dexamethasone NaPO$_4$ or hydrocortisone, diphenhydramine, and epinephrine (if indicated)

CHEMOTHERAPY-INDUCED ANAPHYLAXIS AND HYPERSENSITIVITY

Although anaphylaxis or an anaphylaxis-like reaction can occur with any drug, these potentially life-threatening reactions usually happen soon after the administration of L-asparaginase. Hypersensitivity reactions can occur with any drug but most commonly occur with doxorubicin,[1] taxol,[2] and etoposide.[3]

L-asparaginase is well known for inducing anaphylaxis, hemorrhagic pancreatitis, diabetes mellitus, and coagulopathies in dogs and humans. Forty-eight percent of dogs given L-asparaginase intraperitoneally developed adverse effects[4]; 30% of these dogs exhibited signs of anaphylaxis.

KEY POINT:

The risk of L-asparaginase-induced anaphylaxis can be reduced substantially by giving the drug intramuscularly rather than intravenously or intraperitoneally.

These findings are similar to those in children that were given L-asparaginase intravenously.[5] The same study showed that administration of the drug intramuscularly completely eliminated signs associated with anaphylaxis but did not reduce remission rates (Figure 3-8).

L-asparaginase-induced anaphylaxis and hypersensitivity are common because of enzyme immunogenicity. Anaphylaxis usually is caused by IgE-mediated mast cell degranulation; however, certain substances (e.g., bacterial and fungal cell walls) can trigger anaphylaxis by activating the alternate complement pathway. During the activation of this alternate pathway, C3a and C5a are formed. These are known potent anaphylatoxins capable of degranu-

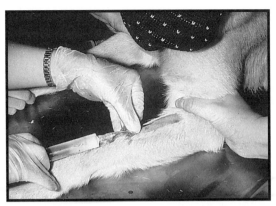

Figure 3-8: The rapid intravenous administration of chemotherapeutic agents, especially L-asparaginase, can result in anaphylaxis. Whenever possible, administer L-asparaginase intramuscularly.

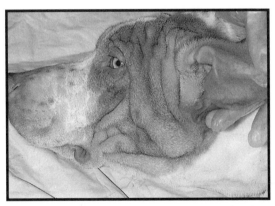

Figure 3-9: The carriers in such drugs as etoposide and taxol can induce a profound allergic reaction that can result in severe erythema, thickening of the skin, and pruritus, especially around the head and neck. This pointer was given etoposide, which resulted in an acute collapse and edema of the head and neck.

lating mast cells and basophils.[6] Although the exact mechanism of L-asparaginase-induced anaphylaxis in dogs is largely unexplored, induction of anaphylaxis in children with acute lymphoblastic leukemia is believed to result from complement activation induced by formation of immune complexes of L-asparaginase and specific antibodies.[7] Anaphylaxis

usually occurs within seconds to minutes after administration of L-asparaginase.

The hypersensitivity reaction secondary to doxorubicin therapy is believed to be related to mast cell degranulation. Cremophor EL and polysorbate 80, the carriers used in formulations of taxol and etoposide, respectively, are responsible for the hypersensitivity reaction induced by these drugs (Figure 3-9).

Predisposing Factors

One predisposing factor related to anaphylaxis secondary to L-asparaginase or other drug therapy is a history of prior exposure to the drug. Because L-asparaginase is a ubiquitous bacterial product in mammalian systems, anaphylaxis may occur after the first administration. In addition, anaphylactic and hypersensitivity reactions are worse in animals that have a prior condition such as atopy, which results in a buildup of mast cells and eosinophils prior to the drug treatment. As mentioned earlier, the route of administration of the drug may be a contributing factor to development of an anaphylactic or hypersensitivity reaction.

Diagnosis

The most common clinical signs associated with drug-induced anaphylaxis are acute collapse and cardiovascular failure, which lead to shock and death. The event usually occurs within minutes after a parenteral injection of the offending drug, although some anaphylactic reactions that occur hours to days after drug therapy have been reported. The patient generally is pale and weak and usually exhibits a bradycardia or tachycardia and a rapid, thready pulse. Mucous membranes generally are pale to cyanotic. Peripheral extremities are often cool to the touch, and blood pressure is low.

Hypersensitivity reactions may result in profound pruritus during or after administration of the drug. Pruritus may result in head shaking, and there may be swelling of the ears, lips, or paws or near the vein or area being treated. The erythematous reaction usually lasts for the duration of treatment. Occasionally, the edematous and erythematous reaction may last for hours after the treatment is finished.

TABLE 3-13
General approach to treatment of animals with drug-induced anaphylaxis

General Principle	Specific Details
Evaluate the patient	Initiate physical examination and ascertain temporal relationship to the drug treatment; discontinue drug infusion or injection indefinitely
Ensure a patent airway cardiac output	Initiate CPR if indicated: establish airway, breathe for the patient after endotracheal intubation, initiate cardiac compressions, and initiate drug therapy
Establish vascular access; initiate fluid and drug therapy	Establish indwelling intravenous catheter aseptically and initiate fluid therapy For shock: 70–90 ml/kg for the first hour followed by 10–12 ml/kg/hr; adjust as needed thereafter Concurrently, initiate drug therapy: Dexamethasone NaPO$_4$ (2 mg/kg IV) Diphenhydramine (2–4 mg/kg IM; watch for toxicoses, especially in cats) Epinephrine (0.1–0.3 ml of a 1:1000 solution IV or IM for severe reactions)

Therapy[6,8,9]
Prevention

Eighty-one dogs with histologically confirmed, measurable malignant tumors were used in a prospective study[8] to determine whether the prevalence of anaphylaxis associated with intramuscular administration of 232 doses of L-asparaginase (10,000 U/m^2). None of the dogs exhibited clinical signs associated with anaphylaxis. Therefore, to reduce the probability of anaphylaxis, L-asparaginase should be given IM rather than IV or intraperitoneally. In addition, because L-asparaginase is a potent inducer of anaphylaxis, administration of a test dose is advised.

Hypersensitivity reactions secondary to the administration of doxorubicin can be almost completely eliminated by diluting the drug into 150 to 500 ml of 0.9% NaCl and administering the drug over 20 to 40 minutes. Hundreds of doses of doxorubicin are administered each year at the Comparative Oncology Unit at Colorado State University, and less than 3% of patients show any signs of hypersensitivity reactions. Some advocate pretreatment with diphenhydramine and glucocorticoids prior to doxorubicin therapy to reduce the prevalence of hypersensitivity reactions.

The reactions secondary to the carriers in taxol and etoposide can be reduced by slowing the rate of infusion and by pretreating with dexamethasone (1–2 mg/kg IV), diphenhydramine (2–4 mg/kg IM), and cimetidine (2–4 mg/kg IV slowly) 1 hour before infusion of the chemotherapeutic agent. If a reaction is noted, the infusion can be discontinued temporarily until the animal is more comfortable.

Treatment

Anaphylaxis is a potentially fatal condition and should be treated immediately with supportive care, fluids, glucocorticoids, H$_1$ receptor antagonists, and epinephrine. The treatment outline is detailed in Table 3-13.

Hypersensitivity reactions can be treated by terminating drug therapy. Reactions usually subside within minutes. The patient can then be treated with H$_1$ receptor antagonists (see Table 3-13) prior to re-initiating drug treatment at a much slower rate.

REFERENCES

1. Ogilvie GK, Curtis C, Richardson RC, et al: Acute short term toxicity associated with the administration of doxorubicin to dogs with malignant tumors. *JAVMA* 195:1584–1587, 1989.
2. Ogilvie GK, Walters LM, Powers BE, et al: Organ toxicity of NBT taxol in the rat and dog: A preclinical study. *Proc 13th Ann Vet Canc Soc Conf:* 90–91, 1993.
3. Ogilvie GK, Cockburn CA, Tranquilli WJ, Reschke RW: Hypotension and cutaneous reactions associated with etoposide administration in the dog. *Am J Vet Res* 49:1367–1370, 1988.
4. Teske E, Rutteman GR, Heerde P van, Misdorp W: Polyethylene glycol-L-asparaginase versus native L-asparaginase in canine non-Hodgkin's lymphoma. *Eur J Cancer* 26:891–895, 1990.
5. Nesbit M, Chard R, Evans A, et al: Evaluation of intra-muscular versus intravenous administration of L-asparaginase in childhood leukemia. *Am J Pediatr Hematol Oncol* 1:9–13, 1979.
6. Degen MA: Acute hypersensitivity reactions, in Kirk RW (ed): *Current Veterinary Therapy X.* Philadelphia, WB Saunders, 1989, pp 537–542.
7. Fabry U, Korholz D, Jurgens H, et al: Anaphylaxis to L-asparaginase during treatment for acute lymphoblastic leukemia in children. Evidence of a complement-mediated mechanism. *Pediatr Res* 19:400–408, 1985.
8. Ogilvie GK, Atwater SW, Ciekot PA, et al: Prevalence of anaphylaxis associated with the intramuscular administration of L-asparaginase to 81 dogs with cancer: 1989–1991. *JAAHA* 3662–3665, 1994.
9. Couto CG: Management of complications of cancer chemotherapy. *Vet Clin North Am Small Anim Pract* 4:1037–1053, 1990.

CLINICAL BRIEFING: EXTRAVASATION OF CHEMOTHERAPEUTIC AGENTS

Diagnosis	*History:* Pain or discomfort during infusion and swelling at the injection site *Clinical Signs:* Initially, swelling and discomfort followed by severe tissue necrosis and a nonhealing lesion 1 to 4 weeks after infusion

Therapy	Stop the infusion, leave catheter in place, and aspirate as much fluid and drug as possible from the site
	Administer antidote
	    Doxorubicin antidote: Cold compresses and infuse with DHM3; possibly use topical DMSO or infiltrate area with intralesional hydrocortisone
	    Vinca alkaloid antidote: Warm compresses and instill hyaluronidase; possibly use topical DMSO or infiltrate area with intralesional hydrocortisone
	    Cisplatin antidote: Intralesional isotonic sodium thiosulfate for large amount of extravasation only

EXTRAVASATION OF CHEMOTHERAPEUTIC AGENTS

Many chemotherapeutic agents are known to induce significant tissue injury after extravasation. Some of these agents are severe irreversible vesicants; others induce irritation to tissue. The agents commonly used in veterinary medicine are listed in Table 3-14.

Management of extravasations in human and veterinary medicine is anecdotal and extremely controversial. Despite this controversy, guidelines (Table 3-15) have been established for clinical use.

Predisposing Factors

As expected, accurate and secure "first stick" catheter placement is absolutely essential when administering drugs that can cause tissue damage if extravasated perivascularly. Generally, only small-gauge (22- to 23-ga) indwelling intravenous catheters should be used when treatment volumes exceed 1 ml; 23- to 25-ga butterfly needles can be used for administering small volumes of drugs, such as vincristine. Everyone involved in patient care should note when and where blood samples are taken by venipuncture

TABLE 3-14
Drugs used in veterinary medicine that may be vesicants or irritants when administered extravascularly[1-4]

Actinomycin D	Mithramycin
Daunorubicin	Vinblastine
Doxorubicin	Vincristine
Epirubicin	Mitoxantrone
Etoposide	Cisplatin

and where catheters have been placed previously. This prevents administration of chemotherapeutic agents through veins that may leak because of previous procedures. Only catheters that have been very recently placed should be used for administration of chemotherapeutic agents. Extreme care should be taken when administering drugs to animals that have fragile veins (e.g., diabetics and some aged animals). The catheter should be checked for patency with a very large injection of saline (e.g., 12–15 ml) prior to

TABLE 3-15
General outline for immediate treatment of extravasation of drugs commonly used in veterinary medicine[1-4]

General Procedure/Specific Antidotes	Specific Details
Minimize amount of drug at site	Do *not* remove the catheter or needle
	With a syringe, immediately withdraw as much drug as possible from the tissue, tubing, and catheter
	Administer antidote (see below) or sterile saline to neutralize or dilute the drug
Doxorubicin, daunorubicin, epirubicin, idarubicin, and actinomycin D	Apply topical cooling with ice or cold compresses for 6–10 hours to inhibit vesicant cytotoxicity; *do not apply heat*
	Doxorubicin: inactivate by infiltrating site with bi(3,5-dimethyl-5-hydromethyl-2-oxomorpholin-3-yl) (also known as DHM3), if available
	Controversial: • Topical DMSO • Infiltrate area with 1 mg/kg hydrocortisone
	Surgical debridement or plastic surgery may be indicated in rare cases
Vincristine, vinblastine, and etoposide	Infiltrate area with 1 ml of hyaluronidase (150 units/ml) for every ml extravasated to enhance absorption and to disperse the drug
	Apply warm compresses to the site for several hours to enhance systemic absorption
	Controversial: • Topical DMSO • Infiltrate area with 1 mg/kg hydrocortisone
Cisplatin	Inject 1 ml of ⅙ molar isotonic sodium thiosulfate for each ml of cisplatin extravasated to inactivate the drug; treatment may be recommended for extravasation of large quantities of cisplatin

and after administration of the drug. In addition, it is mandatory that the catheter is checked for patency during infusion and that the injection site is checked during treatment.

Diagnosis

Usually, there is no doubt whether an extravasation has occurred. Some agents are very caustic if given perivascularly; animals may vocalize or physically

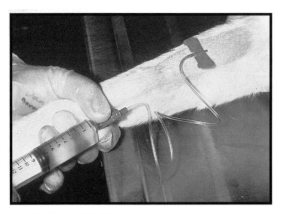

Figure 3-10: When an extravasation occurs, do not remove the catheter or needle. With a syringe, immediately withdraw as much drug as possible from the tissue, tubing, and catheter and administer an appropriate antidote to neutralize or dilute the drug.

react to pain at the injection site. Treatment for extravasation must begin immediately. Evidence of tissue necrosis generally does not appear for 1 to 10 days after injection and may progress for 3 to 4 weeks; these lesions may start as mild erythema and progress to open, draining wounds. These wounds will not heal without extensive debridement and plastic surgery weeks to months after the perivascular slough begins, when all damage is evident. The lesions occur early with vinca alkaloids and late with anthracycline antibiotics, such as doxorubicin.

Treatment[1–4]

Everyone involved with the administration of chemotherapeutic agents should be aware of procedures for treatment of extravasation (Figure 3-10). The procedures should be posted in a common area, and all materials needed to treat extravasations should be readily available and accessible. Because of their extensive use in veterinary practice, doxorubicin and the vinca alkaloids are the most common cause of perivascular sloughs. Unfortunately, no method effectively eliminates tissue necrosis. For example, sodium bicarbonate, corticosteroids, dimethyl sulfoxide (DMSO), α-tocopherol, N-acetylcysteine, glutathione, lidocaine, diphenhydramine, cimetidine, propranolol, and isoproterenol are not effective for the treatment of doxorubicin extravasations.[4]

Once tissue damage is identified, an Elizabethan collar and bandages with nonstick pads are essential to allow the area to heal without self-trauma. Bandages should be changed daily as long as the area is draining or has the potential for infection. If a bacterial infection is noted, culture and sensitivity testing and appropriate administration of antimicrobials are essential. Frequent cleansing and debridement may be necessary. In some cases, reconstructive surgical repair techniques are necessary.

REFERENCES

1. Couto CG: Management of complications of cancer chemotherapy. *Vet Clin North Am Small Anim Pract* 4:1037–1053, 1990.
2. Wittes RE, Hubbard SM: Chemotherapy: The properties and uses of single agents, in Wittes RE (ed): *Manual of Oncologic Therapeutics* 1991/1992. Philadelphia, JB Lippincott, 1991, pp 116–121.
3. Hubbard SM, Jenkins JF: Chemotherapy administration: Practical guidelines, in Chabner BA, Collins JM (eds): *Cancer Chemotherapy: Principals and Practice.* Philadelphia, JB Lippincott, 1990, pp 449–464.
4. Hubbard S, Duffy P, Seipp C: Administration of cancer treatments: Practical guide for physicians and nurses, in DeVita VT Jr, Hellman S, Rosenberg S (eds): *Cancer: Principles and Practice of Oncology,* ed 3. Philadelphia, JB Lippincott, 1989, pp 2369–2402.

CLINICAL BRIEFING: CHEMOTHERAPY-INDUCED ACUTE RENAL FAILURE

Acute Renal Failure

Diagnosis	*History:* Acute decompensation, anorexia, and vomiting *Clinical Signs:* Possible oliguria with increased body weight and central venous pressures with fluid therapy, uremic gastritis, and uremic breath *Diagnostics:* CBC, biochemical profile, urinalysis, central venous pressures, and urine output quantification
Therapy	Treat or eliminate the underlying cause Correct dehydration Administer fluids to meet daily needs and external losses and induce a mild to moderate diuresis Correct acid–base and electrolyte abnormalities Treat oliguria with dobutamine, furosemide, and dextrose (if indicated)

CHEMOTHERAPY-INDUCED ACUTE RENAL FAILURE

Cisplatin, doxorubicin, and methotrexate are commonly associated with renal failure in veterinary patients. In addition, renal failure is induced by a wide variety of malignant conditions, such as transitional cell carcinoma.

The most nephrotoxic chemotherapeutic agent is *cis*-diamminedichloroplatinum II (cisplatin), a heavy metal coordination compound that has antineoplastic activity when used to treat a variety of malignant tumors in dogs.[1-5] In dogs, 80% to 90% of the drug is eliminated in the urine within 48 hours. Nephrotoxicosis, characterized by reduced glomerular filtration rate and tubular injury, is the major dose-limiting toxicosis. Renal toxicosis may range from brief increases in serum urea nitrogen and creatinine concentrations to irreversible renal failure. However, renal damage generally is not a clinical problem if adequate hydration is maintained.[6,7] A variety of administration protocols have been suggested to limit or eliminate cisplatin nephrotoxicosis in the dog.[1-7] Each protocol includes the use of intravenous saline solution during the 1- to 24-hour diuresis period.

Doxorubicin also induces acute and chronic renal failure in dogs and cats. One study[9] suggests that the renal damage in cats is dose-dependent; however, this observation has not been repeated. Renal failure in dogs has been induced with variable cumulative doses of doxorubicin. Another unrelated drug, methotrexate, is eliminated primarily by the kidneys and has been associated with the development of nephrotoxicity.

Dogs with transitional cell carcinoma of the bladder, urethra, or prostate commonly have urethral obstruction that may lead to hydroureter, hydronephrosis, and renal dysfunction. The concurrent septic cystitis seen in most patients with bladder tumors may induce secondary pyelonephritis. This can result in acute and chronic renal failure.

Predisposing Factors

In veterinary medicine, the most common predisposing factors associated with the development of acute renal failure are cancer and nephrotoxic drugs, including chemotherapeutic agents. Therefore, when chemotherapeutic agents are used in veterinary patients, other nephrotoxic drugs, such as aminoglycosides, should be avoided. Other risk factors associated with the development of acute and chronic renal failure in dogs and cats are decreased cardiac output, urinary tract infection, sepsis, preexisting renal disease, advanced age, dehydration, fever, liver disease, hypokalemia, and hypercalcemia. Several studies have shown that pre-existing renal disease may be one of the most important predisposing factors for the development of cisplatin-induced acute renal failure.

Diagnosis

Acute and chronic renal failure are a result of decreased glomerular filtration rate, with or without tubular damage. Therefore, to diagnose these syndromes, the parameters used are related to damage of these structures. There may be significant renal disease for variable periods before clinical, hematologic, and biochemical abnormalities were identified, because at least two thirds of the kidney function must be abnormal before overt evidence of renal disease occurs.

Acute renal failure may occur with non-oliguria, oliguria, or anuria. Regardless of the amount of urine, it is usually isosthenuric or minimally concentrated with a high sodium content (>40 mEq/L). Glucose, protein, and renal epithelial cells may be noted in the urine. There is an acute rise in serum urea nitrogen, creatinine, and phosphorus concentrations. In oliguric or anuric renal failure, body weight, heart rate, and central venous pressure may increase if fluids are administered before urine flow is re-established.

Therapy

The best treatment for acute or chronic renal failure is prevention. Substantial data exist to show that cisplatin nephrotoxicity can be reduced and almost eliminated with adequate hydration. The incidence of doxorubicin- and methotrexate-induced renal failure can be reduced by not treating dogs with pre-existing renal disease and by increasing the duration of time the drug is administered. Because cisplatin is a profound nephrotoxin, a brief discussion on hydra-

tion schemes used to reduce kidney damage is followed by a review of acute renal failure treatment.

Prevention

Twenty-four-hour diuresis protocol. When cisplatin was first introduced to veterinary practice, care was taken to ensure that renal damage did not occur.[1] Saline diuresis for 24 hours at fluid rates of 66 to 132 ml/kg were reported effective for dogs.[1,2] The great expense and time involved led investigators to explore shorter diuresis protocols.

Six-hour diuresis protocol. A study completed using normal dogs suggested that one dose of cisplatin could be administered safely at 70 mg/m^2 of body surface using a 6-hour diuresis protocol.[7] In that study, cisplatin was administered IV to six healthy dogs over a 20-minute period after 0.9% NaCl solution was administered IV for 4 hours at a rate of 18.3 ml/kg/hr. After cisplatin injection, saline diuresis was continued at the same rate for 2 hours. All dogs vomited within 8 hours after the drug was administered. Clinical status, weight gain, and food consumption remained normal throughout the 27 days after the drug was administered. Nadirs in the daily neutrophil count were observed on days 6 and 15. There were no significant gross or histologic abnormalities referable to cisplatin administration when the dogs were necropsied at the conclusion of the study.

To ensure that the 6-hour diuresis protocol was safe and effective in older, tumor-bearing dogs, cisplatin (70 mg/m^2 body surface area IV every 21 days) was given to 61 dogs with malignant neoplasia for a total of 185 doses in one (n = 9 dogs), two (n = 26 dogs), three (n = 4 dogs), four (n = 9 dogs), five (n = 2 dogs), and six (n = 11 dogs) treatments. The cisplatin was given over a 20-minute period, after 0.9% NaCl solution (saline) was administered IV for 4 hours at a rate of 18.3 ml/kg/hr. After the cisplatin infusion, saline diuresis was continued at the same rate for 2 hours. Before each treatment with cisplatin, dogs were evaluated with at least a physical examination, CBC, serum urea nitrogen, and, in most cases, determination of serum creatinine and urine specific gravity. Four of the 61 dogs (6.6%) developed clinically evident renal disease after two (one dog), three (two dogs), and four (one dog) doses of cisplatin were administered. Three of the four dogs had pre-existing disease of the urinary tract prior to the beginning of therapy. Survival time in dogs that developed renal disease (median 145 days; range 15 to 150 days) was similar to all of the dogs in this study (median 154 days; range 30 to 500 days); 13 dogs were still alive at the conclusion of the study. Three of the four dogs that developed renal disease were euthanatized because of tumor-related causes and chronic renal failure; the fourth dog died as a direct result of the nephrotoxicity. Therefore, the 6-hour saline diuresis protocol used to administer cisplatin in this study seems to be effective in preventing nephrotoxicity in tumor-bearing dogs that did not have pre-existing urinary tract disease.

These studies suggest that the diuresis protocol used with the administration of cisplatin to normal and tumor-bearing dogs resulted in a clinically acceptable low incidence of nephrotoxicity. Because the procedure is extremely labor-intensive and expensive, interest was expressed in a shorter period of saline diuresis that would still protect dogs from nephrotoxicity induced by cisplatin.

Four-hour diuresis protocol. After the 6-hour diuresis protocol was determined to be safe and effective for administering cisplatin, a 4-hour diuresis protocol was designed.[10] In this study, cisplatin (70 mg/m^2 of body surface, IV, every 21 days) was given to 64 dogs that had malignant neoplasia for a total of 179 doses in one to four treatments. The cisplatin was given over a 20-minute period after 0.9% NaCl solution was administered IV for 3 hours at a rate of 25 mg/kg/hr. After cisplatin infusion, saline solution diuresis was continued at the same rate for 1 hour. Before each treatment with cisplatin, dogs were evaluated with at least a physical examination, CBC, and determination of serum phosphorus concentration and urine specific gravity. Exogenous creatinine clearance was evaluated in eight dogs. Five of the 64 dogs developed clinically evident renal disease after two and three doses of cisplatin were administered. Two of the five dogs had pre-existing disease of the urinary tract prior to the beginning of treatment. Median survival time in dogs that devel-

oped renal disease was 114 days; the range was from 5 to 586 days. Thirty dogs were still alive at the conclusion of the study. Three of the five dogs that developed renal disease were alive at the conclusion of the study, one died of the cancer, and the fifth dog died as a result of renal damage. The neutrophil counts decreased and the creatinine concentrations increased prior to the third and fourth treatments compared to pretreatment values. It was concluded from this study that up to four doses of cisplatin can be safely administered using the 4-hour diuresis protocol with minimal nephrotoxicity. Because the 4-hour diuresis protocol was relatively safe, an additional study was initiated to see if a 1-hour diuresis protocol was safe.

One-hour diuresis protocol. In this study,[11] four doses of cisplatin (70 mg/m^2 of body surface every 21 days) was administered IV to six healthy dogs over a 20-minute period after 0.9% NaCl solution (saline) was administered IV for 1 hour at a volume of 132 ml/kg$^{0.75}$. All dogs vomited at least once within 8 hours after each treatment. Clinical status, body weight, and food consumption were normal throughout the 12-week study for five of the six dogs. The sixth dog developed acute renal failure and became acutely blind and deaf within 3 days after the fourth dose of cisplatin. Electrolyte, creatinine, and serum urea nitrogen values remained within established normal limits in all dogs immediately prior to each treatment and in five of six dogs evaluated 3 weeks after the final treatment. The serum creatinine value (3.3 mg/dl) obtained from the dog euthanatized 2 weeks after the fourth treatment was above established normal values. Despite the normality of all but one of the creatinine values, the serum creatinine concentrations obtained 3 weeks after the final treatment with cisplatin were higher than pretreatment values. Important decreases in glomerular filtration rate as determined by exogenous and endogenous creatinine clearance tests were identified 3 weeks after the fourth treatment of cisplatin when compared to data from all other evaluation periods. Neutrophil counts decreased below pretreatment values at the third, fourth, and fifth evaluation period. Therefore, this protocol cannot be recommended.

TABLE 3-16
Example of fluid therapy needs for a 10-kg dog
that is 5% dehydrated and has diarrhea

Task	Calculation
Correct dehydration	5% (0.05) × 10 kg body weight = 0.5 kg of water needed to correct dehydration
	1000 ml/kg of water × 0.5 kg = 500 ml of water needed to correct dehydration
	75% (0.75) × 500 ml = 375 ml of fluid should be administered to replace 75% dehydration
Administer fluids to meet daily needs	66 ml/kg (daily requirements) × 10 kg body weight = 660 ml needed on a daily basis
	Increase this amount from 1.5–3 times to induce a mild to moderate diuresis in renal failure patients, ensuring urine output exceeds 2 ml/kg/hr
Replace ongoing losses	Estimated losses through diarrhea = 200 ml
Fluids needed (first 24 hrs)	375 ml + 660 ml + 200 ml = 1235 ml; increase fluid therapy judiciously to increase urine output, sustaining a mild to moderate diuresis

Treatment for Acute Renal Failure[12,13]

The initial goals for treating drug- and tumor-related acute renal failure in dogs and cats are to discontinue all drugs that may be nephrotoxic, document prerenal or postrenal abnormalities, and initiate fluid therapy (Table 3-16). The primary objectives for fluid therapy are to correct deficits (such as dehydration) and excesses (such as volume overload) seen in oliguric renal failure, supply maintenance needs, and supplement ongoing losses that occur with vomiting and diarrhea. Each patient must be assessed carefully, and a treatment plan must be tailored based on the hydration status, cardiovascular performance, and biochemical data. A general approach to patients in renal failure is shown in Table 3-17. Maintenance requirements vary from 44 to 110 ml/kg body weight; smaller animals require the larger amount. A simpler formula is to use 66 ml/kg/day plus an amount of fluid equal to external fluid losses, such as vomiting and diarrhea. This is the amount of fluid that is needed daily for maintenance. In patients with renal failure, 1.5 to 3 times this amount of fluid is administered daily to achieve a diuresis. The success of this diuresis can be monitored by documenting adequate urine output (>2 ml/kg/hr). Fluid therapy should meet daily needs, replace excessive losses, and correct dehydration. The percentage of dehydration should be determined; approximately 75% of the fluid needed to correct the dehydration should be administered during the first 24 hours. Fluid therapy should be altered to correct electrolyte and acid–base abnormalities. For animals in acute renal failure,

TABLE 3-17
General approach to dogs in renal failure

General Principle	Specific Details
Cease administration of nephrotoxins	For example, discontinue cisplatin, methotrexate, doxorubicin, and aminoglycosides; avoid anesthesia
Assess patient status	CBC, urinalysis, and biochemical profile Specifically, determine: 　Percentage of dehydration 　Amount of ongoing losses (e.g., vomiting, diarrhea, blood loss, etc.) 　Maintenance fluid requirements 　Electrolyte and biochemical abnormalities 　Cardiovascular performance 　Urine output
Select and administer specific fluids	Tailor therapy to needs of each patient: 　Isotonic polyionic fluid initially, preferably potassium-free (e.g., NaCl) 　Correct dehydration first over 6 to 8 hours to prevent further renal ischemia while watching carefully for pathologic oliguria and subsequent volume overload 　Meet maintenance requirements (approximately 66 ml/kg/day) 　Meet ongoing losses (e.g., vomiting and diarrhea) 　Induce a mild to moderate diuresis
Monitor urine output and ensure adequate output	Metabolism cage or indwelling catheter For inadequate output (<0.5–2.0 ml/kg/hr): 　Mannitol or dextrose 0.5–1.0 g/kg in a slow IV bolus 　Furosemide 2–4 mg/kg IV q 1–3 hours PRN 　Dopamine 1–3 µg/kg/min IV (50 mg dopamine in 500 ml of 5% dextrose = 100 µg/ml solution)
Correct acid–base and electrolyte abnormalities	Rule out hypercalcemia of malignancy; treat specifically for that, if identified
Provide mild to moderate diuresis	Urine output: 2–5 ml/kg/hr; monitor body weight, heart and respiratory rate, and central venous pressure for signs of overhydration
Consider peritoneal dialysis if not responsive	Temporary or chronic ambulatory peritoneal dialysis with specific dialysate solution may be helpful

TABLE 3-17 (continued)

General Principle	Specific Details
Initiate long-term plans	Continue diuresis until BUN and creatinine normalize or until these values stop improving despite aggressive therapy and a clinically stable patient, then gradually taper fluids
	Control hyperphosphatemia, if indicated (e.g., aluminum hydroxide, 500 mg at each feeding)
	Treat gastric hyperacidity, if indicated (cimetidine, 4 mg/kg every 6 hrs, IV or PO)

potassium-containing fluids generally are not good choices, because systemic hyperkalemia often occurs in these patients. Until more is known about the systemic effects of sepsis, lactate-containing fluids should be avoided, because sepsis and cancer are associated with hyperlactatemia, which worsens with the administration of lactate-containing fluids.

If oliguric renal failure is present, a diligent and aggressive approach should be made to increase urine output. This can be done by first increasing glomerular filtration rate and renal blood flow. Additionally, an osmotic diuresis can be used to increase urine flow. If urine output is less than 0.5 to 2.0 ml/kg/hr despite aggressive fluid therapy, furosemide should be administered every 1 to 3 hours. Furosemide will increase glomerular filtration rate and enhance diuresis in many patients. If furosemide is not effective, mannitol or 50% dextrose can be used as an osmotic diuretic to enhance urine production. The advantage of dextrose over mannitol is that dextrose can be detected on a urine glucose test strip. If the furosemide and osmotic diuretics are not effective, dopamine can be administered as a constant rate infusion. Dopamine enhances renal blood flow and increases urine output secondarily.

Treatment for acute renal failure should be continued until the patient improves substantially and until abnormal biochemical parameters have been corrected or are at least stabilized. The therapy should then be tapered off over several days, and a home treatment plan should be developed that includes avoiding nephrotoxic drugs; feeding a high-quality, low-quantity protein diet; maintaining a low-stress environment; and providing fresh, clean water ad libitum.

REFERENCES

1. Page R, Matus RE, Leifer CE, et al: Cisplatin, a new antineoplastic drug in veterinary medicine. *JAVMA* 186:288–290, 1985.
2. Mehlhaff CJ, Leifer CE, Patnaik AK, et al: Surgical treatment of pulmonary neoplasia in 15 dogs. *JAVMA* 20:799–803, 1984.
3. Himsel CA, Richardson RC, Craig JA: Cisplatin chemotherapy for metastatic squamous cell carcinoma in two dogs. *JAVMA* 89:1575–1578, 1986.
4. Shapiro W, Fossum TW, Kitchell BE, et al: Use of cisplatin for treatment of appendicular osteosarcoma in dogs. *JAVMA* 192:507–511, 1988.
5. LaRue SM, Withrow SJ, Powers BE, et al: Limb-sparing treatment for osteosarcoma in dogs. *JAVMA* 195:1734–1744, 1989.
6. Cvitkovic E, Spaulding J, Bethune V, et al: Improvement of cis-dichlorodiammineplatinum (NSC 119875): Therapeutic index in an animal model. *Cancer* 39:1357–1361, 1977.
7. Ogilvie GK, Krawiec DR, Gelberg HB, et al: Evaluation of a short-term saline diuresis protocol for the administration of cisplatin. *Am J Vet Res* 49:1076–1078, 1988.
8. Chiuten D, Vogel S, Kaplan B, et al: Is there cumulative or delayed toxicity for cis-platinum? *Cancer* 52:211–214, 1983.

9. Cotter SM, Kanki PJ, Simon M: Renal disease in five tumor-bearing cats treated with Adriamycin. *JAAHA* 21:405–412, 1985.

10. Ogilvie GK, Straw RC, Jameson VJ, et al: Prevalence of nephrotoxicosis associated with a four hour saline solution diuresis protocol for the administration of cisplatin to dogs with sarcomas: 64 cases (1989–1991). *JAVMA* 202:1845–1848, 1993.

11. Ogilvie GK, Fettman MJ, Jameson VJ, et al: Evaluation of a one hour saline diuresis protocol for the administration of cisplatin to dogs. *Am J Vet Res* 53:1666–1669, 1992.

12. Couto CG: Management of complications of cancer chemotherapy. *Vet Clin North Am Small Anim Pract* 21:1037–1053, 1990.

13. Kirby R: Acute renal failure as a complication of the critically ill animal. *Vet Clin North Am Small Anim Pract* 19:1189–1208, 1989.

CLINICAL BRIEFING: ENDOCRINE MANIFESTATIONS OF MALIGNANCY

Hypercalcemia

Diagnosis	*History:* Lethargy, anorexia, increased water consumption, increased urination, and vomiting due to hypercalcemic nephropathy *Clinical Signs:* Polyuria, polydipsia, vomition, constipation, bradycardia, skeletal muscle weakness, depression, stupor, coma, and seizures *Diagnostics:* Laboratory evidence of hypercalcemia and secondary renal damage. The underlying cause for this electrolyte abnormality may be identified with a CBC, biochemical profile, urinalysis, ionized calcium, bone-marrow aspirate, radiographs, ACTH stimulation, and, if indicated, parathyroid hormone or parathyroid hormone-related peptide concentrations
Treatment	Treat the underlying cause Therapy depends on the severity of clinical and laboratory signs. Consider saline diuresis and furosemide; give prednisone only after a diagnosis has been made In refractory cases, consider salmon calcitonin, biphosphonates, gallium nitrate, and mithramycin

Hypocalcemia

Diagnosis	*History:* Usually asymptomatic; occasional lethargy and anorexia *Clinical Signs:* Usually normal; occasional weakness, depression, and seizures *Diagnostics:* Electrolyte abnormality can be identified with a biochemical profile, urinalysis, ionized calcium, and (if indicated) parathyroid hormone concentration
Treatment	Treat the underlying cause In severe cases, administer 10% calcium gluconate IV; oral calcium supplementation, with or without vitamin D, may be effective

Hypoglycemia

Diagnosis	*History:* Weakness, confusion, seizures, and coma *Clinical Signs:* See history. Clinical signs are often paroxysmal and subtle in the earlier phases of the disease and are followed by seizures, coma, and death *Diagnostics:* CBC, biochemical profile, urinalysis, fasting blood glucose and insulin levels, radiographs, abdominal ultrasonography, exploratory surgery, and biopsy

Treatment	Treat the underlying cause Frequent feedings of a complex carbohydrate food Glucose infusion, prednisone, and diazoxide ± hydrochlorothiazide Propranolol may be of value in refractory cases

Syndrome of Inappropriate Secretion of Antidiuretic Hormone (SIADH)

Diagnosis	*History:* Anorexia, muscle stiffness, confusion or unresponsive state, and history of recent administration of drug that may cause hyponatremia or SIADH *Clinical Signs:* Anorexia, nausea, subtle neurologic symptoms, confusion, and coma *Diagnostics:* Biochemical profile to include serum sodium, urinalysis, fractional excretion of sodium, serum osmolality, and adrenal and thyroid function tests
Treatment	Treat the underlying cause Judicious water restriction Demeclocycline and furosemide Lithium carbonate, phenytoin, and hypertonic saline in refractory cases

Ectopic Cushing's Syndrome

Diagnosis	*History:* Most patients are asymptomatic; others exhibit polyuria, polydipsia, weakness, lethargy, and weight loss *Clinical Signs:* See history *Diagnostics:* Low-dose and high-dose dexamethasone suppression test, endogenous ACTH concentration, urine cortisol/creatinine ratio, CBC, biochemical profile, and urinalysis
Treatment	Treat the underlying cause Mitotane or ketoconazole

Cancer can induce clinical signs directly by altering the structure or function of the body through the physical presence of the tumor or indirectly by producing tumor-induced remote effects. These indirect effects are known as paraneoplastic syndromes. The most common paraneoplastic syndromes in veterinary medicine are caused by the production of polypeptide hormones. All paraneoplastic syndromes, especially those that result in endocrinologic changes secondary to a malignancy, are profoundly important to the practicing veterinarian because they can induce clinical signs that are more harmful to the animal than signs of the primary tumor. Detection of hormones or hormone-like substances that are elaborated directly or induced indirectly by the tumor can be used as a marker for the presence of the tumor. Clinical evidence of the endocrine-associated paraneoplastic syndrome also can be used as a tumor marker.

Therapy should be primarily directed at eliminating the underlying malignancy; however, modulation of tumor-induced hormones or hormone-like substances is an attractive alternative. In many cases, specific treatment of the paraneoplastic syndrome may be essential for the animal's survival.

When an endocrine manifestation of malignancy is suspected, several diagnostic differentials should be considered.[1] These include:

- a benign tumor responsible for the production of a hormone or hormone-like substance
- a hormone produced by a malignancy of endocrine origin
- an endocrine gland infiltrated by a tumor, resulting in the production of a hormone
- an endocrinopathy that develops secondary to administration of a therapeutic agent, such as a chemotherapeutic agent, or to the development of an infection
- a true paraneoplastic syndrome in which malignancy induces endocrinopathy as a remote effect unrelated to the tumor

The following is a brief description of hypercalcemia, hypocalcemia, hypoglycemia, ectopic arginine vasopressin production (syndrome of inappropriate secretion of antidiuretic hormone [SIADH]), and ectopic adrenocorticotrophic hormone (ACTH) syndrome.

ALTERED CALCIUM HOMEOSTASIS
Hypercalcemia of Malignancy
(also see Metabolic Emergencies chapter)

Cancer is the most common cause of hypercalcemia in dogs and cats.[1-4] The condition can result in an oncologic emergency and is covered in that context in the Metabolic Emergencies chapter in that section. The tumors most often associated with paraneoplastic syndrome are lymphoma, anal sac adenocarcinoma, multiple myeloma, and mammary gland adenocarcinoma, but any neoplastic process has the potential to elevate serum calcium. In 20% to 40% of dogs with lymphoma and hypercalcemia, the anterior mediastinum is involved. For dogs, therefore, chest radiographs are indicated whenever a persistent hypercalcemia is identified. Hypercalcemia as a paraneoplastic syndrome is

rare in cats but not in dogs. Parathyroid adenomas have been identified as malignancy-associated causes of hypercalcemia of malignancy in dogs and cats. It is not a true paraneoplastic syndrome, however.

The potential causes for hypercalcemia of malignancy include the following[1-6]:

- direct resorption of bone by tumor cells
- tumor-induced production of osteoclast-activating factors (OAFs), such as interleukins, tumor necrosis factor, lymphotoxin, colony-stimulating factors, and interferon-γ
- tumor-induced production of 1,25-dihydroxyvitamin D
- tumor-induced production of prostaglandins
- tumor-induced production of transforming growth factors
- tumor-induced production of parathyroid hormone-related peptide (PTHrP)

Tumors that probably are associated with local osteolytic hypercalcemia in veterinary medicine include multiple myeloma, lymphoma, and mammary neoplasia. Dogs with lymphoma and anal sac adenocarcinoma most commonly develop cancer-induced hypercalcemia from production of PTHrP.[5,6] The cDNA of PTHrP has been cloned and found to encode a 16,000-dalton protein in which 8 of 13 amino acids are identical to parathyroid hormone.

Clinical Presentation

Alterations in renal function cause the most common clinical manifestations of hypercalcemia of malignancy arising from malignant disease in the veterinary patient.[1,4] Polyuria and nocturia in the early phases of the disease are succeeded by anorexia, nausea, fatigue, dehydration, azotemia, and coma secondary to hypercalcemia-induced renal failure. Decreased sensitivity of the distal convoluted tubules and collecting ducts to antidiuretic hormone (ADH) causes polyuria and secondary polydipsia. Vasoconstrictive properties of calcium decrease renal blood flow and glomerular filtration rate, resulting in degenerative changes, necrosis, and calcification of the renal epithelium.[1-4] Other clinical signs (e.g., constipation, muscle weakness, seizures, etc.) may arise as a direct effect of the electrolyte abnormality.

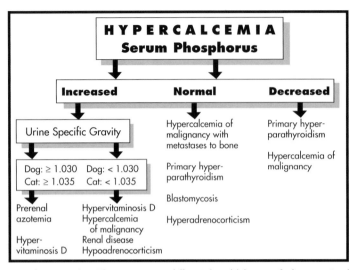

Figure 4-1: *The most common differentials and laboratory findings associated with hypercalcemia in dogs or cats.*

electrolyte is in the free, ionized fraction, which is increased by acidosis.

Ultimately, it may be difficult to identify malignancy as the cause of hypercalcemia. Laboratory abnormalities that may accompany true hypercalcemia include an elevated serum urea nitrogen, normophosphatemia or hypophosphatemia, hypercalciuria, hyperphosphaturia, hypernatriuria, and decreased glomerular filtration rate as determined by an exogenous or endogenous creatinine clearance study.

Treatment[1-4]

Eliminating the tumor is the first and most important therapy for hypercalcemia of malignancy. Clinical signs associated with hypercalcemia of malignancy can range from very mild to a full oncologic emergency. The approach to the treatment of this condition depends on the severity of the clinical signs.

Mild Hypercalcemia, Minimal Clinical Signs. This situation often can be controlled with adequate hydration. Monitoring of calcium, phosphorus, and creatinine levels is indicated until the underlying cause can be identified and eliminated or until the hypercalcemia and subsequent clinical signs progress to a point requiring additional therapy. Nephrotoxic drugs must be avoided at all costs. Whenever anesthesia is considered, concurrent intravenous hydration and careful postoperative monitoring are essential.

Moderate Hypercalcemia, Moderate Clinical Signs. More aggressive management is indicated in these patients, including administration of intravenous saline in volumes that exceed daily maintenance needs (>66 ml/kg/day or 1700 ml/m²/day) and result in urine output that exceeds 2 ml/kg/hour. Potassium chloride is often added to 0.9% NaCl to prevent

Diagnosis *(Figure 4-1)*

Clinical pathology must be combined with a good history and physical examination to rule in or rule out the following differentials: laboratory error; error in interpretation (e.g., in young, growing dogs); hyperproteinemia owing to dehydration; acute renal failure; vitamin D and calcium toxicosis; granulomatous disorders, such as blastomycosis and other fungal diseases; nonneoplastic disorders of bone; hypoadrenocorticism; and true hyperparathyroidism.[1-4] Calcium values must be interpreted in relation to serum albumin and blood pH. A correction formula that takes the albumin into account is as follows:

adjusted calcium (mg/dl) = (calcium [mg/dl] – albumin [g/dl]) + 3.5

Clinical signs associated with hypercalcemia are intensified when the

KEY POINT:

Premature and inappropriate administration of symptomatic therapy, especially any glucocorticoid in any dosage or route of administration, may interfere with the identification of the underlying cause of the electrolyte abnormality.

potassium depletion (20–30 mEq KCl/L of 0.9% NaCl). All electrolytes should be assessed and the therapy carefully tailored according to serum calcium and potassium levels. In addition, patients should be watched carefully for signs of overhydration and congestive heart failure. The administration of 0.9% NaCl intravenously is effective in expanding the extracellular fluid volume, increasing glomerular filtration rate, decreasing renal tubular calcium reabsorption, and enhancing calcium and sodium excretion.

In refractory cases, furosemide (2.2–8.8 mg/kg BID IV or PO) is often administered concurrently with NaCl to well-hydrated hypercalcemic patients to prevent calcium reabsorption in the kidneys. This drug is also effective for treating many cases of anuria or oliguria. Furosemide inhibits calcium resorption at the level of the ascending loop of Henle.

Prednisone (0.5–1.0 mg/kg BID PO) or any other glucocorticoid inhibits osteoclast-activating factor, prostaglandins, vitamin D, and the absorption of calcium across the intestinal tract; therefore, such drugs are effective for treating hypercalcemia of malignancy. Glucocorticoids are cytotoxic to lymphoma cells—the most common malignant cause of hypercalcemia in dogs—and therefore should not be used until a histologic diagnosis of suspect tissue is made. When administered, glucocorticoids may obscure the extent of the tumor and thus may delay diagnosis of lymphoma and prevent definitive therapy.

Severe Hypercalcemia, Severe Clinical Signs. This is considered an oncologic emergency; the reader is referred to the Metabolic Emergencies chapter for specific recommendations. Briefly, treatment is the same as for moderate hypercalcemia. In addition, the use of other agents, including calcitonin, mithramycin, prostaglandin-synthetase inhibitors, diphosphonate, gallium nitrate, and oral phosphate, can be considered to control the electrolyte abnormality.[2]

- Calcitonin: A dosage of 4 to 8 MRC units/kg SQ can cause a dramatic, rapid reduction in calcium levels, which may remain low for days.
- Mithramycin: This drug can be used at a dosage of 25 µg/kg IV, once or twice weekly. At higher dosages, it has anticancer properties.

- Diphosphonates: This class of agents is being explored for use in the therapy of hypercalcemia of malignancy. Didronal is the most commonly used member of this class in human medicine. Early work in human patients with severe hypercalcemia and severe clinical signs suggests that this class of drug is effective in long-term control of chronic hypercalcemia. Unlike phosphates, which bind calcium in the gastrointestinal tract, biphosphonates bind to hydroxyapatite in bone and inhibit the dissolution of crystals.[2]
- Gallium nitrate: This agent recently has been approved in human medicine for the treatment of hypercalcemia; it appears to inhibit bone resorption by binding to and reducing the solubility of hydroxyapatite crystals.[2]

Hypocalcemia

Hypocalcemia is an unusual complication in veterinary medicine. Hypocalcemia secondary to a malignancy or its treatment is much more common in human medicine.

Clinical Presentation

Hypocalcemia rarely causes clinical signs. In such cases, however, partial or generalized seizures are seen. In humans with bone metastases, hypocalcemia is more common than hypercalcemia.[3] In veterinary medicine, only a few possible causes have been documented. One potential cause of hypocalcemia is magnesium deficiency, which can occur from prolonged intestinal drainage procedures, parenteral hyperalimentation without magnesium supplementation, cisplatin therapy, and severe liver disease.[2,3] The hypomagnesemia seems to impair the effect of parathyroid hormone on its target organs, resulting in hypocalcemia. Tumor lysis syndrome may be associated with hypocalcemia secondary to elevated phosphate levels. This is an oncologic emergency and is discussed in that section.

Treatment[2,3,7]

The underlying cause of hypocalcemia should be identified and treated as soon as possible. If clinical signs are present, calcium should be administered intravenously slowly with ECG monitoring (10% calcium gluconate given over 10–20 minutes, 1.0–1.5 ml/kg; maintenance therapy of 2 ml/kg over 6–8 hours) followed by oral calcium supplements (i.e., calcium lactate, 400–600 mg/kg/day in 3–4 divided doses/day). Vitamin D supplementation may be indicated.

ALTERED GLUCOSE HOMEOSTASIS
Hypoglycemia
(also see Metabolic Emergencies chapter)

Hypoglycemia can cause a wide variety of clinical signs ranging from generalized weakness to seizures and death.[7-16] Insulinoma is the most common malignancy that is associated with hypoglycemia (blood glucose <70 mg/dl) in dogs,[8-11] but a wide variety of other non-islet cell tumors also have been shown to cause this condition in humans and dogs by inducing ectopic hormone production.[9-11] Non-islet cell tumors that cause hypoglycemia include hepatocellular carcinoma, hepatoma, plasmacytoid tumor, lymphoma, leiomyosarcoma, oral melanoma, hemangiosarcoma, and salivary gland adenocarcinoma.[9-11]

Insulinomas produce excessive quantities of insulin that cause very low blood glucose levels. In contrast, hypoglycemia of extrapancreatic tumors in dogs has been associated with low to low-normal insulin levels.[9-11] Extrapancreatic tumors cause hypoglycemia by secretion of an insulin-like substance, accelerating the utilization of glucose by the tumor, and by failure of gluconeogenesis and/or glycogenolysis by the liver.[9-11] The most common nonmalignant causes of hypoglycemia include hyperinsulinism, hepatic dysfunction, adrenocortical insufficiency, hypopituitarism, extrapancreatic tumors, starvation, sepsis, and laboratory error.

Clinical Signs
Neurologic signs including weak-ness, disorientation, behavioral changes, seizures, coma, and death predominate in animals with hypoglycemia secondary to a malignancy.[7-14] These clinical signs generally occur in dogs, cats, and ferrets when blood glucose falls below 45 mg/dl.

Catecholamines, growth hormone, glucocorticoids, and glucagon are released secondary to hypoglycemia and activate compensatory mechanisms to combat hypoglycemia by promoting glycogenolysis.

Diagnosis
Currently, it is not possible to identify the cause of hypoglycemia in many extrapancreatic tumors. Insulin-producing tumors, such as insulinomas, may be diagnosed by identifying elevated insulin levels in association with low blood glucose concentrations.[7,13,14] For accurate diagnosis, some patients require frequent evaluation of glucose and insulin concentrations during a 72-hour fast. Although controversial, the amended insulin:glucose ratio has been advocated as a method to help diagnose insulin-producing tumors in pets:

$$\frac{\text{serum insulin } (\mu U/ml) \times 100}{\text{serum glucose } (mg/dl) - 30} = \frac{\text{amended insulin:}}{\text{glucose ratio}}$$

Values above 30 are highly suggestive of a an insulinoma or other insulin-producing tumors.

KEY POINT:

Neurologic signs predominate in pets with hypoglycemia because carbohydrate reserve is limited in neural tissue and brain function depends on an adequate quantity of glucose.

Treatment
Surgery is the only method for eliminating the underlying cause of malignancy-associated hypoglycemia. Metastases are common in most malignant tumors associated with this condition. Therefore, surgery often is not curative. If an insulinoma is suspected, a partial pancreatectomy may be indicated. Complications include iatrogenic pancreatitis and diabetes mellitus. Medical management of the hypoglycemia is essential before, during, and after surgery because of the seri-

ous consequences of hypoglycemia and because of the high metastatic rate.[7–16] Animals with severe cases of hypoglycemia should be treated with intravenous administration of 2.5% to 5% dextrose in parenteral fluids, such as 0.9% NaCl or Ringer's solution. Animals that are convulsing should be given 0.5 g/kg dextrose intravenously slowly over 5 minutes. Prednisone (0.5–2.0 mg/kg divided BID PO) can induce hepatic gluconeogenesis and decrease peripheral utilization of glucose. Diazoxide (10–40 mg/kg divided BID PO), with or without hydrochlorothiazide (2–4 mg/kg daily PO), may be effective in elevating blood glucose levels by inhibiting pancreatic insulin secretion and glucose uptake by tissues, enhancing epinephrine-induced glycogenolysis, and increasing the rate of mobilization of free fatty acids.[15–17] Hydrochlorothiazide enhances the hyperglycemic effects of diazoxide. The β-adrenergic blocking agent, propranolol (0.2–1.0 mg/kg TID PO), may be effective in increasing blood glucose levels by blocking insulin release through the blockade of β-adrenergic receptors at the level of the pancreatic β cell, inhibiting insulin release by membrane stabilization, and altering peripheral insulin receptor affinity. Combined surgical and medical management of pancreatic tumors has been associated with remission periods of 1 year or more.[9,10]

ALTERED SODIUM HOMEOSTASIS
Syndrome of Inappropriate Secretion of Antidiuretic Hormone

Although the syndrome of inappropriate secretion of antidiuretic hormone (SIADH) is rarely identified in veterinary medicine, it is one of the best characterized and most frequently encountered ectopic hormone syndromes in human medicine.[2] It is likely that SIADH will be identified more frequently in animals as awareness of it grows.[7]

SIADH can be caused by in-

creased expression of ADH from the pituitary gland or as a true paraneoplastic syndrome secondary to the ectopic production of ADH. In addition, several drugs can indirectly cause SIADH by potentiating the release of ADH.[2]

Clinical Signs [2,7,17]

Most animals with SIADH are clinically normal. When sodium levels drop to 120 to 125 mEq/L, however, lethargy and mental dullness may be noted. When serum sodium levels drop below 115 mEq/L, more dramatic central nervous system (CNS) problems that may progress to convulsions and coma can develop. When this occurs, the animal must be treated for a medical emergency.

Diagnosis

The diagnosis of SIADH is based on the absence of hypovolemia and dehydration as well as on the following laboratory findings[2,7]:
- hypo-osmolality
- hyponatremia of extracellular fluids
- urine that is less than maximally dilute
- absence of volume depletion
- sustained renal excretion of sodium
- normal renal, pituitary, and adrenal function

Spurious or artifactual hyponatremia can occur in animals with marked increases in serum lipids or serum proteins. In addition, in animals with marked hyperglycemia, water can be drawn into the circulatory system, diluting electrolytes and causing hyponatremia.

Treatment

The treatment of choice for patients with SIADH is to eliminate the underlying cause. If clinical signs warrant treatment, the following measures may be helpful[2,7]:

Water Restriction. This is effective for mild cases in which the animal can be watched carefully for over- or underhydration. The objective is to

KEY POINT:

Drugs that can cause SIADH include chlorpropamide, vincristine, vinblastine, cyclophosphamide, opiates, histamine, thiazides, barbiturates, and isoproterenol.

raise the serum sodium level while restricting water intake to approximately 66 ml/kg/day.

Demeclocycline. This drug antagonizes the actions of ADH on the kidneys and thus causes reversible nephrogenic diabetes insipidus. In humans, nausea, vomiting, skin rashes, and hypersensitivity reactions are possible side effects. Demeclocycline is effective in treating patients with mild to moderate cases of SIADH. Other drugs such as lithium carbonate and phenytoin are not as effective as demeclocycline.

Hypertonic Sodium Chloride. This intravenous solution is generally reserved for patients that have significant clinical signs related to hyponatremia. A more detailed description of its use is described in the Oncologic Emergencies section.

ALTERED CORTICOSTEROID HOMEOSTASIS
Ectopic Cushing's Syndrome

The ectopic production of ACTH or related polypeptides has been described in dogs with primary lung tumors[18] as well as in a variety of human cancers, including small-cell lung cancer, bronchial carcinoids, islet cell tumors of the pancreas, medullary cancer, and pheochromocytoma.[2] The syndrome is caused by excessive steroid production from normal adrenal glands that are under the influence of the ectopic production of ACTH or ACTH-like substances.

Clinical Presentation

Most patients with this condition are asymptomatic. When clinical signs occur, however, they are similar to those of Cushing's disease.[2,7,18]

Diagnosis

Ectopic production of ACTH produces a syndrome identified by pronounced hypokalemia, metabolic alkalosis, glucose intolerance, and mild hypertension. In humans, plasma-cortisol concentrations are elevated and plasma ACTH levels generally are high. The tumors are rarely suppressible with dexamethasone.[2,7]

Treatment [2,7]

As in all paraneoplastic syndromes, elimination of the primary tumor is the treatment of choice. This is generally done while correcting any electrolyte or acid–base abnormalities. If sodium and water retention leads to clinical signs, thiazides or other diuretics may be indicated. If the underlying malignancy cannot be treated, the animal may need to be treated with mitotane (50 mg/kg/day PO for 5–10 days, then 25–50 mg/kg/week PO) or ketoconazole (dogs: 15 mg/kg BID PO; cats: 5–10 mg/kg TID–BID PO) using laboratory monitoring for Cushing's disease. In human cancer patients, aminoglutethimide, metyrapone, and RU 486 are viable alternative treatments.

REFERENCES

1. Meuten DJ: Hypercalcemia. *Vet Clin North Am Small Anim Pract* 14:891–910, 1984.
2. Griffin TW, Rosenthal PE, Costanza ME: Paraneoplastic and endocrine syndromes, in Cady B (ed): *Cancer Manual,* ed 7. Boston, American Cancer Society, 1986, pp 373–390.
3. Cryer PE, Kissane JM: Clinicopathologic conference: Malignant hypercalcemia. *Am J Med* 65:486–494, 1979.
4. Kruger JM, Osborne CA, Polzin DJ: Treatment of hypercalcemia, in Kirk RW (ed): *Current Veterinary Therapy. IX.* Philadelphia, WB Saunders, 1986, pp 75–90.
5. Weir EC, Nordin RW, Matus RE, et al: Humoral hypercalcemia of malignancy in canine lymphosarcoma. *Endocrinology* 122:602–612, 1988.
6. Weir EC, Burtis WJ, Morris CA, et al: Isolation of a 16,000-dalton parathyroid hormone-like protein from two animal tumors causing humoral hypercalcemia of malignancy. *Endocrinology* 123:2744–2752, 1988.
7. Ogilvie GK: Paraneoplastic syndromes, in Ettinger SJ, Feldman EC (eds): *Textbook of Veterinary Internal Medicine,* ed 4. Philadelphia, WB Saunders, 1994, in press.
8. Brennan MD: Hypoglycemia in association with non-islet cell tumors, in Service FJ (ed): *Hypoglycemic Disorders: Pathogenesis, Diagnosis, and Treatment.* Boston, GK Hall, 1983, pp 143–151.
9. Leifer CE, Peterson ME, Matus RE, Patnaik AK: Hypoglycemia associated with non-islet cell tumors in 13 dogs. *JAVMA* 186:53–55, 1985.
10. Strombeck DR, Krum S, Meyer D, et al: Hypoglycemia and hypoinsulinemia associated with hepatoma in the dog. *JAVMA* 169:811–812, 1976.
11. DiBartola SP, Reynolds HA: Hypoglycemia and polyclonal gammopathy in a dog with plasma cell dyscra-

sia. *JAVMA* 180:1345–1349, 1982.

12. deSchepper J, Vandestock J, deRick A: Hypercalcemia and hypoglycemia in a case of lymphatic leukemia in the dog. *Vet Rec* 94:602–603, 1974.

13. Allen TA: Canine hypoglycemia, in Kirk RW (ed): *Current Veterinary Therapy. VIII.* Philadelphia, WB Saunders, 1983, pp 845–850.

14. Feldman EC: Disease of the endocrine pancreas, in Ettinger SJ (ed): *Textbook of Veterinary Internal Medicine.* Philadelphia, WB Saunders, 1983, pp 1615– 1649.

15. Scandellari C, Zaccaria M, de Palo C, et al: The effect of propranolol on hypoglycemia: Observations in five insulinoma patients. *Diabetologia* 15:279–302, 1978.

16. Leifer CE, Peterson ME: Hypoglycemia. *Vet Clin North Am Small Anim Pract* 14:873–889, 1984.

17. Giger U, Gorman NT: Acute complications of cancer and cancer therapy, in Gorman NT (ed): *Oncology.* New York, Churchill Livingstone, 1986, pp 147–168.

18. Ogilvie GK, Weigel RM, Haschek WM, et al: Prognostic factors for tumor remission and survival in dogs after surgery for primary lung tumors: 76 cases (1975–1985). *JAVMA* 195:109–112, 1989.

CLINICAL BRIEFING: HEMATOLOGIC MANIFESTATIONS OF MALIGNANCY

Erythrocytosis

Diagnosis	*History:* Patient may be asymptomatic; lethargy, anorexia, polyuria, and polydipsia may be noted by the owner *Clinical Signs:* Polyuria, polydipsia, and red mucous membranes *Diagnostics:* Increased number of RBCs on CBC and hyperviscosity of the blood on visual inspection. Paraneoplastic syndrome: increased erythropoietin concentration, normal blood oxygenation, extramedullary hemapoiesis, and hyperplastic erythroid series on bone marrow examination. Nonparaneoplastic syndromes (including primary erythrocytosis): normal blood oxygenation and erythropoietin levels, malignant erythron on bone marrow examination. Secondary erythrocytosis caused by hypoxemia: elevated erythropoietin concentration, enlarged liver and spleen caused by extramedullary hematopoiesis and decreased arterial oxygen concentration. Secondary erythrocytosis caused by renal disease: evidence of renal disease on CBC, biochemical profile and urinalysis, normal arterial or venous oxygenation, and enlargement of spleen and liver caused by extramedullary hematopoiesis
Treatment	Treat the underlying cause and institute supportive care Phlebotomy Hydroxyurea in selected cases

Anemia

Diagnosis	*History:* Lethargy, weakness, and exercise intolerance *Clinical Signs:* Pale mucous membranes, lethargy, and weakness *Diagnostics:* CBC, biochemical profile, bone-marrow aspirate and biopsy, serum iron, total iron-binding capacity, slide agglutination test, antinuclear antibody, and Coomb's test (if indicated)
Treatment	Treat the underlying cause Consider iron supplementation, erythropoietin, and immune modulation after specific diagnosis is identified Transfusion after cross-match

Thrombocytopenia

Diagnosis	*History:* Bleeding from any site and into any body cavity without an obvious cause

	Clinical Signs: Petechiation, ecchymotic hemorrhages, bleeding from any site without cause (especially epistaxis), pale mucous membranes, weakness, and shock *Diagnostics:* CBC; biochemical profile; bone-marrow aspirate; and coagulation profile, including ACT, OSPT, APTT, fibrinogen, antithrombin III, platelet factor III, and FDPs
Treatment	Treat the underlying cause Correct acid–base abnormalities, volume contraction, and dehydration Fresh whole blood or platelet-rich plasma

Leukocytosis

Diagnosis	*History:* Patient usually asymptomatic; otherwise, lethargy and anorexia *Clinical Signs:* Bone marrow packing can result in shifting leg lameness due to bone pain; lethargy; and possibly splenomegaly, if the reticuloendothelial system is actively clearing abnormal cells *Diagnostics:* CBC, bone marrow aspirate and biopsy, and special stains for abnormal cells; look for other cause with chest and abdominal radiographs, biochemical profile, and urinalysis
Treatment	Treat the underlying cause Beware of and treat any underlying infection

ERYTHROCYTOSIS

An increase in the number of red blood cells (RBCs) (erythrocytosis) is common in veterinary patients, but only a fraction of the cases can be classified as true paraneoplastic syndromes and are an indirect result of malignancy.[1–7] Erythrocytosis also can be caused by dehydration and secondary volume contraction, pulmonary and cardiac disorders, venoarterial shunts, Cushing's disease, chronic corticosteroid administration, and polycythemia vera. Erythrocytosis can produce significant clinical signs and a diagnostic dilemma.

An elevated RBC mass secondary to malignancy occurs either directly by tumor production of erythropoietin or secondary due to hypoxia produced by the physical presence of a tumor that induces production of erythropoietin. Erythropoietin is normally produced by the kidney in dogs and cats; thus, it is not surprising that kidney tumors are associated with erythrocytosis.[1–4] In addition to renal tumors, hepatic tumors and lymphoma have been associated with erythrocytosis.[1–7] When erythrocytosis is secondary to elevated erythropoietin concentrations, four possible mechanisms may be responsible[1–7]:

- erythropoietin produced directly by the tumor
- erythropoietin produced either in response to tumor-initiated hypoxia or vascular obstruction
- erythropoietin produced by the kidney in response to a tumor-induced factor
- tumor-induced change in metabolism of erythropoietin

Clinical Presentation

Many animals with erythrocytosis are asymptomatic.[1–9] Others exhibit lethargy, anorexia, polydipsia, and polyuria. If the erythrocytosis is caused by gener-

TABLE 4-1

Results of common diagnostic tests and various classifications of erythrocytosis

Classification	Erythropoietin Levels	Blood Oxygen	Bone Marrow	Renal Status	Extramedullary Hematopoiesis
(1°) Polycythemia vera	OK to Low	OK	Malignant	OK	No
(2°) Paraneoplastic syndrome	Increased	OK	Hyperplastic	OK	Yes
(2°) Tissue hypoxia	Increased	Low	Hyperplastic	OK	Yes
(2°) Renal disease	Increased	OK	Hyperplastic	Abnormal	Yes

alized hypoxia, clinical signs referable to decreased oxygenation (which, in rare cases, may include cardiovascular decompensation, exercise intolerance, ascites, dyspnea, and cyanosis) may predominate.

Diagnosis

The diagnosis of erythrocytosis is based on the results of a hemogram, biochemical profile, blood gas analysis, erythropoietin levels, chest and abdominal radiographs, cardiovascular examination, renal imaging, and a splenic aspirate (Table 4-1).[1,2,5–9] Animals with erythrocytosis of paraneoplastic origin have normal renal structure and function but show signs of extramedullary hematopoiesis and a hyperplastic erythroid series in the bone marrow; animals with secondary polycythemia have decreased arterial oxygen saturation or renal disease.[1,2,5–7] Polycythemia vera is a myeloproliferative disorder that results from clonal proliferation of RBC precursors. The diagnosis generally is made using histology and cytology of a bone marrow core biopsy specimen and aspirate after ruling out the presence of local or systemic hypoxia and elevated erythropoietin concentrations.

Treatment

Patients with erythrocytosis usually require no treatment. Specific therapy for the underlying cause of the tissue hypoxia should be instituted in appropriate cases.[1,2,5–9] Phlebotomies may assist temporarily to reduce the RBC load. This procedure is performed by withdrawing approximately 20 to 40 ml/kg of blood through a large-bore needle (e.g., 14-ga) while simultaneously replacing the volume being removed with crystalloid fluids. With polycythemia vera, the chemotherapeutic agent hydroxyurea (30 mg/kg/day PO for 7 days, then 15 mg/kg/day) can be used to induce reversible bone marrow suppression and reduce RBC production[1,2,7] (see Bone Marrow Neoplasia chapter).

ANEMIA

Anemia occurs frequently in veterinary cancer patients and may result from increased blood loss, decreased RBC production (e.g., abnormal bone marrow function), or increased RBC destruction (e.g., immune-mediated diseases).[1,2,4–6] More specific causes of malignancy-associated anemia include anemia of chronic disease, bone marrow invasion by tumor cells, marrow suppression by chemotherapy, hypersplenism, immune-mediated disease, megaloblastic anemia, vitamin and iron deficiency, microangiopathic hemolytic anemia, and pure red cell aplasia.[1,2,5] Anemia of any cause arising as an indirect effect of the tumor is indeed a paraneoplastic syndrome. In

KEY POINT:

The treatment of choice for the erythropoietin-producing tumor or the tumor that induces regional or systemic hypoxia is surgical removal. Phlebotomies and hydroxyurea can be used if needed.

most patients, a clear cause of the anemia is not found and the diagnosis of "anemia of chronic disease" is made.

Blood loss anemia is seen in many types of cancer. It can occur as a direct effect of the cancer or indirectly as a result of coagulopathies linked with hemangiosarcomas, thyroid carcinomas, and inflammatory mammary carcinomas. Histamine released from mast cell tumors may activate parietal cells in the stomach, increasing production of hydrochloric acid and inducing gastric or duodenal ulceration and consequent blood loss. If anemia is secondary to blood loss, the cause may be obvious (as with bleeding superficial tumors) or inconspicuous (as with bladder or GI tumors).

Microangiopathic hemolytic anemia is commonly seen in dogs with splenic hemangiosarcoma and occurs secondary to hemolysis because of damage to arteriolar endothelium or fibrin deposition within the artery.[1–3,5] Disseminated intravascular coagulation (DIC) is an important cause of this type of anemia. Although hemangiosarcoma is the most common cause of DIC, a variety of other neoplastic diseases, such as thyroid carcinoma and inflammatory mammary adenocarcinoma, may result in anemia because of DIC.

In animals, immune-mediated hemolytic anemia is sometimes triggered by tumors. The result is premature destruction of RBCs by immune mechanisms.[1,2,5] Antibodies can be directed against the RBC or against a hapten (e.g., virus or drug) that is associated with the RBC.

Chemotherapy-induced nonregenerative anemia is common in animals. The condition frequently is associated with chronic drug therapy. Although chemotherapeutic agents often decrease the number of white blood cells (WBCs) and platelets, anemia associated with administration of chemotherapeutic agents generally is mild and is not associated with clinical signs.

Less common causes of cancer-induced anemia include leukoerythroblastic anemia, hematopoietic

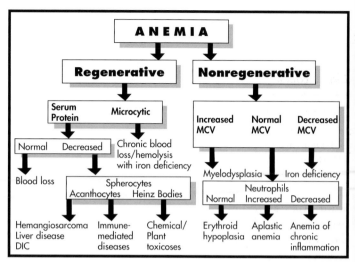

Figure 4-2: Diagnostic differentials and laboratory findings associated with anemia.

dysplasia, hypersplenism, erythrophagocytosis, megaloblastic anemia, and red cell aplasia.[1,2]

Clinical Presentation

Many of the mechanisms previously described work alone or in concert to decrease the population of RBCs.[1–3,5,6] Although clinical signs relating to the anemia may be overshadowed by aspects of the underlying neoplastic condition, the anemia can nevertheless impair the quality of life of the cancer-bearing animal. The majority of patients remain asymptomatic if anemia develops gradually or if the number of RBCs are only slightly decreased. As the anemia progresses, lethargy and exercise intolerance may arise. Mucous membranes may be pale.

Diagnosis (Figure 4-2)

The anemia must first be classified as regenerative or nonregenerative. If the anemia is regenerative (i.e., >1% corrected reticulocytosis in dogs, 0.04 corrected aggregate count in cats, or polychromasia) and if serum proteins are decreased, blood loss may be considered.[1,2,5] If serum proteins are increased, differentials of RBC destruction by immune-mediated diseases (e.g., immune-mediated hemolytic anemia), physical trauma (e.g., DIC or parasites), or toxins (e.g., methylene blue) must be considered. If the anemia is nonregenerative, a bone marrow aspiration or biopsy should be performed to evaluate erythroid hypoplasia (causes such as anemia of chronic disease, endocrine deficiencies, renal disease, or lead toxicity), aplastic anemia (causes such as estrogen toxicity, feline leukemia virus, or phenylbutazone), myeloproliferative disorders, and iron deficiency.

Anemia of chronic disease in cancer patients is associated with a shortened erythrocyte life span, depressed bone marrow response, and disordered iron metabolism and storage.[1,2,5,6] Clinically, anemia of chronic disease is recognized as normocytic and normochromic, with normal bone marrow cellularity and reticuloendothelial iron sequestration. Blood loss anemia is recognized clinically when the RBCs are microcytic and hypochromic because of decreased hemoglobin synthesis.[1,2,5,6] Poikilocytosis, microleptocytosis, inadequate reticulocytosis, increased total iron-binding capacity, decreased serum-iron concentrations, and elevated platelet counts may also be seen with blood loss. Hemolysis and schistocytosis are the hallmarks of microangiopathic hemolytic anemia. The diagnosis of immune-mediated hemolytic anemia is based on finding antibody or complement on the surface of the patient's RBCs by a Coomb's test or slide agglutination test and, in dogs only, spherocytosis, paired with nonregenerative anemia. Histologically, chemotherapy-induced changes include bone marrow hypoplasia of the erythroid or other cell lines that subsequently cause inadequate reticulocytes and decreased red cell mass with normal erythrocytic indices.[1,2,5,6]

Treatment

As with all paraneoplastic syndromes, the best treatment is eliminating the underlying cause.[1,2,5,6] Symptomatic treatment is usually needed only if the anemia produces clinical signs or if the animal is to undergo surgery. If acute correction of the condition is warranted, it is common to administer RBCs after a cross match. The following general guidelines for transfusion should be followed. A more detailed description can be found in the chapter on Transfusion Support.

General Rule: Amount to Transfuse

$$\text{ml donor} = [(2.2 \times \text{wt}_{kg}) \times (40_{dog} \text{ or } 30_{cat})] \times \frac{(\text{PCV}_{desired} - \text{PCV}_{recipient})}{\text{PCV}_{donor}}$$

Note: 2.2 ml of whole blood/kg or 1 ml/kg of packed red blood cells raises PCV 1% (transfused whole blood has a PCV of 40%).

General Rule: Rate of Transfusion

Dogs: 0.25 ml/kg/30 minutes or faster (22 ml/kg/day) with close patient monitoring

Cats: 40 ml/30 minutes with close patient monitoring

Human recombinant erythropoietin (75–100 U/kg/day SQ three times a week; decrease to once or twice weekly when the desired hematocrit level is reached) is being used more commonly for a variety of anemias.[2] Because recombinant erythropoietin is somewhat species-specific, patients may develop antibodies to the recombinant protein, which may cross with the patient's own erythropoietin. Recombinant erythropoietin is most effective when endogenous erythropoietin levels are low and when adequate erythrocyte precursors are present in the bone marrow and other structures. If anemia is attributable to blood loss, the source of bleeding should be identified and eliminated. Medical management of immune-mediated hemolytic anemia can include prednisone (2 mg/kg daily PO); in addition, azathioprine (2 mg/kg daily for 4 days, then 0.5–1.0 mg/kg every other day PO) may be indicated if resolution of the underlying neoplastic condition is delayed.[1–3] Cyclosporine (5 mg/kg BID; dose adjusted by monitoring blood levels) is sometimes effective. Contrary to some reports, cyclophosphamide may be of limited value in treating immune-mediated hemolytic anemia and associated conditions in the dog.[1,2]

THROMBOCYTOPENIA

Mechanisms associated with diminished platelet numbers in dogs with cancer include reduced platelet production from bone marrow, sequestration of platelets in capillaries, increased platelet consumption as in DIC, increased platelet destruction, and reduction of hematopoietic growth factors. Consumption of platelets is considered the primary hemostatic abnormality in tumor-bearing dogs.[1,2]

Diminished platelet numbers and elevated plasma-fibrinogen concentrations are common in animals with extensive tumors involving spleen or marrow.[1,2,10,11] DIC, a common cause of platelet consumption, occurs in 39% of dogs with tumors that involve these structures.[11] In these dogs, eliminating the neoplastic condition and administering intravenous fluids and heparin may be of therapeutic value. Immune-mediated thrombocytopenia also significantly decreases platelet numbers in some dogs with cancer.[1,2,10,11]

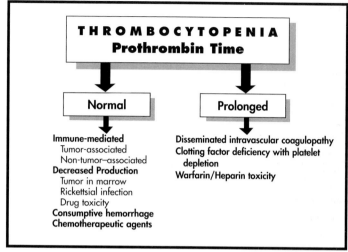

Figure 4-3: *Diagnostic differentials and laboratory findings associated with thrombocytopenia.*

Clinical Presentation

Animals with thrombocytopenia may be clinically normal, or they may bleed for no reason into any part of the body. For example, these animals may bleed excessively from a simple venipuncture and may have petechial or ecchymotic hemorrhages on physical examination.

Diagnosis (Figure 4-3)

Complete blood count (CBC), platelet count, clotting profile, and bone marrow evaluation are essential to diagnose and evaluate the cause of thrombocytopenia in dogs or cats.[1,2] Combined with a complete history and physical examination, this information helps to determine whether thrombocytopenia results from decreased production (e.g., tumor-induced myelophthisis or chemotherapy-induced marrow suppression), increased consumption (e.g., DICs secondary to any malignancy, including hemangiosarcoma), or increased loss. If DIC is suspected, prolongation of clotting times (activated clotting time [ACT], one-step prothrombin time [OSPT], activated partial thromboplastin time [APTT]) and elevated fibrinogen levels may be identified. Thrombocytopenia attributable to an immune mechanism is diagnosed when antibodies against bone-marrow megakaryocytes are detected. In addition, thrombocytopenia can be a true paraneoplastic syndrome, which is diagnosed by eliminating all other causes and by determining whether the animal responds to removal of an apparently unrelated tumor.

Treatment

Obviously, animals with thrombocytopenia should be kept quiet. The primary treatment for the paraneoplastic syndrome is removal of the

> **KEY POINT:**
>
> *Vincristine and platelet transfusions should be administered only when the thrombocytopenia is transient and the animal is stable, as in instances of transient thrombocytopenia that follow chemotherapy.*

tumor.[1,2,10,11] Malignancy-associated, immune-mediated thrombocytopenia has been resolved successfully in dogs by treatment with immunosuppressive drugs, such as prednisone (2 mg/kg daily) and azathioprine (2 mg/kg daily for 4 days followed by 0.5–1.0 mg/kg every other day).[1–4] Cyclosporine may be helpful in refractory cases. In any case of thrombocytopenia secondary to a malignancy, vincristine (0.5–0.75 mg/m^2) can be used to increase the number of platelets temporarily; response is directly proportional to the number of megakaryocytes and the rate of platelet removal from the body. Platelet counts increase 4 days after vincristine is given. In academic or large private-practice settings, platelet transfusions can be administered to specific cases that are, or have a high likelihood of, bleeding uncontrollably. The amount of random donor platelet transfusion generally is about 3 U/m^2 body surface area or 0.1 U/kg body weight. Each unit should be administered with 30 to 60 ml of plasma/U of platelets. When acute bleeding is not responsive to other treatments or procedures, epsilon aminocaproic acid (Amicar®) can be given intravenously or orally (250 mg/m^2 QID).

LEUKOCYTOSIS

An increased WBC count attributable to either increased production, decreased loss, or decreased destruction is common in veterinary cancer patients.[1,2,12–14] Any cell line can be involved. When leukocytosis is a remote effect of underlying malignancy, the laboratory finding may be classified as a paraneoplastic syndrome. Paraneoplastic leukocytosis in animals arises from a variety of malignancies, including lymphoma and hemangiosarcoma.[1,2,4,5,12–14] Although some cases of leukocytosis are caused by malignant clonal prolifera-

tion of a specific WBC line, they are not considered paraneoplastic syndromes.

Clinical Presentation

Animals with paraneoplastic leukocytosis are often clinically normal. Human patients occasionally describe bone pain due to the high proliferative rate in the bone marrow.

Diagnosis

The diagnosis is based on a CBC and bone marrow examination. Occasionally, special stains may be performed by the clinical pathology laboratory to determine whether the increased number of leukocytes are from a neoplastic clone.

Treatment

The condition is not generally of clinical significance and requires no therapy.

REFERENCES

1. Ogilvie GK: Paraneoplastic syndromes, in Withrow SJ, MacEwen EG (eds): *Clinical Oncology.* Philadelphia, JB Lippincott, 1989, pp 29–40.
2. Ogilvie GK: Paraneoplastic syndromes, in Ettinger SJ, Feldman EC (eds): *Textbook of Veterinary Internal Medicine,* ed 4. Philadelphia, WB Saunders, 1994, in press.
3. Griffin TW, Rosenthal PE, Costanza ME: Paraneoplastic and endocrine syndromes, in Cady B (ed): *Cancer Manual,* ed 7. Boston, American Cancer Society, 1986, pp 373–390.
4. Giger U, Gorman NT: Acute complications of cancer and cancer therapy, in Gorman NT (ed): *Oncology.* New York, Churchill Livingstone, 1986, pp 147–168.
5. Madewell BR, Feldman BF: Characterization of anemias associated with neoplasia in small animals. *JAVMA* 176:419–425, 1980.
6. Comer KM: Anemia as a feature of primary gastrointestinal neoplasia.

> **KEY POINT:**
>
> *The mechanism of the malignancy-associated leukocytosis is not known but may involve the direct or indirect production of hematopoietic growth factors, such as granulocyte colony-stimulating factor, granulocyte-macrophage colony-stimulating factor, or interleukin-3 or may occur as a result of tissue necrosis and granulocyte breakdown with positive feedback that increases neutrophil production.[1,2]*

Compend Contin Educ Pract Vet 12(1):13–22, 1990.

7. Couto CG, Boudrieau RJ, Zanjani ED: Tumor associated erythrocytosis in a dog with nasal fibrosarcoma. *J Vet Intern Med* 3:183–185, 1989.

8. Peterson ME, Randolph JF: Diagnosis and treatment of polycythemia vera, in Kirk RW (ed): *Current Veterinary Therapy VIII*. Philadelphia, WB Saunders, 1983, pp 406–408.

9. Hammond D, Winnick S: Paraneoplastic erythrocytosis and ectopic erythropoietin. *Ann N Y Acad Sci* 230:219–226, 1974.

10. Helfand SC, Couto CG, Madewell BR: Immune-mediated thrombocytopenia associated with solid tumors in dogs. *JAAHA* 21:787–794, 1985.

11. Hargis AM, Feldman BE: Evaluation of hemostatic defects secondary to vascular tumors in dogs: 11 cases (1983–1988). *JAVMA* 198:891–894, 1991.

12. Chinn DR, Myers RK, Matthews HA: Neutrophilic leukocytosis associated with metastatic fibrosarcoma in the dog. *JAVMA* 186: 806–809, 1985.

13. Couto CG: Tumor-associated eosinophilia in the dog. *JAVMA* 184:837– 838, 1984.

14. Center SA, Randolph JF, Erb HN, Reiter S: Eosinophilia in the cat: A retrospective study of 312 cases (1985–1986). *JAAHA* 26:349–358, 1990.

CLINICAL BRIEFING: HYPERGAMMAGLOBULINEMIA

Diagnosis	*History:* Anorexia, lethargy, polyuria, polydipsia, and spontaneous bleeding *Clinical Signs:* Bleeding from any site, petechial and ecchymotic hemorrhages, evidence of volume expansion, cardiovascular problems, blindness due to retinal hemorrhages, and bone pain *Diagnostics:* CBC, biochemical profile, urinalysis, immunoelectrophoresis demonstrating monoclonal gammopathy in blood and urine, increased blood pressure, and chest and abdominal radiographs and/or ultrasonography and bone marrow aspirate to help rule in or out neoplastic etiology
Therapy	Eliminate underlying cause: surgery, chemotherapy (e.g., melphalan and prednisone), and radiation therapy Restore tissue perfusion with fluids; stabilize cardiovascular system; and reduce viscosity (if needed) with fluids, plasmapheresis, or plasma harvests from patient

HYPERGAMMAGLOBULINEMIA

Hypergammaglobulinemia, also known as M-component disorder or hyperviscosity syndrome, is common in animals with a variety of malignancies, particularly multiple myeloma.[1-8] These diseases result from excessive secretion of immunoglobulin by a monoclonal line of immunoglobulin-producing cells. These globulins include IgG, IgA, IgM, and light-chain protein classes. Light chains, also known as Bence-Jones proteins, may be present in the urine. Tumors of plasma cells, termed *plasma cell* or *multiple myeloma*, exhibit M-component disorders about 75% of the time. Other tumors or disorders associated with the production of large quantities of immunoglobulins include lymphoma, lymphocytic leukemia, a variety of solid tumors, and primary macroglobulinemia.[1,2,5,8] Paraneoplastic syndromes occur only in tumors that increase globulin concentration as an indirect, distant effect of the malignancy.

Clinical Presentation

Clinical signs associated with M-component disorders arise from increased viscosity associated with elevated globulins and from the tumor's direct effect on surrounding structures. Excessive bleeding from any site results from elevated proteins that interfere with normal platelet function.[1,2,5,8] Hyperviscosity syndrome, which decreases blood fluidity, causes polydipsia, CNS signs, retinopathies, visual disturbances, secondary renal problems, and congestive heart failure. Renal decompensation often succeeds renal amyloidosis or Bence-Jones proteinuria; increased serum viscosity decreases renal perfusion, and concentrating ability is impaired. Neurologic signs arise when altered blood flow and diminished delivery of oxygen to neural tissue produce hypoxia in the CNS. Increased blood volume and viscosity place greater demands on the heart. This can produce decompensation of stable pre-existing cardiac conditions or development of a hypertrophic cardiomyopathy-like state.

Diagnosis

Each case of hypergammaglobulinemia must be assessed to determine the underlying cause by performing the following baseline tests[1-3,5,6,8]:
- CBC, biochemical profile, and urinalysis
- immunoelectrophoresis of serum and urine (± Bence-Jones protein test of urine)

- bone marrow aspiration and cytology
- chest and abdominal radiographs
- survey skeletal radiographs (± nuclear scintigraphy of skeletal system)
- retinal examination
- coagulogram (APTT, OSPT, ACT, platelet count, fibrin degradation products (FDPs), and antithrombin III)
- *Ehrlichia* titer

Initial screening tests are performed primarily to detect evidence of bone marrow involvement by tumor or *Ehrlichia*, monoclonal gammopathy, renal failure secondary to hyperglobulinemia, coagulopathy distinct from increased globulins, lytic bone lesions suggestive of multiple myeloma, myelophthisis, or hypertension and bleeding. Because it determines not only whether monoclonal gammopathy is present but also which class of immunoglobulins is involved, immunoelectrophoresis generally is preferred to general electrophoresis. Multiple myeloma, which does not engender paraneoplastic syndrome, is covered in a later chapter; it is diagnosed by the prescence of monoclonal gammopathy, Bence-Jones proteinuria or monoclonal proteinuria, "punched out" bone lesions that may appear with a nuclear bone scan, and by more than 20% to 30% plasma cells in bone marrow. Resolution of clinical signs occurs when malignancy is controlled. If increased globulin concentrations are in response to *Ehrlichia* infection, titers should disclose the organism.

Treatment

The treatment of choice for multiple myeloma is melphalan (0.1 mg/kg daily for 10 days, then 0.5 mg/kg every other day PO) and prednisone (0.5 mg/kg daily for 21 days, then every other day thereafter

PO); this combination produces a median survival time of 18 months.[1–6,8] An alternative protocol is found in the Chemotherapy chapter on page 81. Radiation therapy for areas of bone involvement may be palliative. Lymphoma can be treated with doxorubicin as a single agent or with combinations of such drugs as cyclophosphamide, vincristine, prednisone, and doxorubicin.[7] Plasmapheresis rapidly reduces protein levels and is useful in cases where hyperviscosity requires symptomatic treatment.[1,2,8]

Other supportive care involves fluid therapy for dehydration. Because myeloma cells are believed to secrete a substance that suppresses macrophage and lymphocyte function, antibiotics may be indicated.

KEY POINT:

Because plasmapheresis requires specialized equipment, blood from animals with clinically significant hypergammaglobulinemia can be harvested into plastic collection bags; the plasma can then be siphoned off and the RBCs resuspended in an equal volume of 0.9% NaCl for immediate reintroduction into the patient.

REFERENCES

1. Ogilvie GK: Paraneoplastic syndromes, in Withrow SJ, MacEwen EG (eds): *Clinical Veterinary Oncology.* Philadelphia, JB Lippincott, 1989, pp 29–40.
2. Ogilvie GK: Paraneoplastic syndromes, in Ettinger SJ, Feldman EC (eds): *Textbook of Veterinary Internal Medicine,* ed 4. Philadelphia, WB Saunders, 1994, in press.
3. Griffin TW, Rosenthal PE, Costanza ME: Paraneoplastic and endocrine syndromes, in Cady B (ed): *Cancer Manual,* ed 7. Boston, American Cancer Society, 1986, pp 373–390.
4. Giger U, Gorman NT: Acute complications of cancer and cancer therapy, in Gorman NT (ed): *Oncology.* New York, Churchill Livingstone, 1986, pp 147–168.
5. MacEwen EG, Hurvitz AI: Diagnosis and management of monoclonal gammopathies. *Vet Clin North Am Small Anim Pract* 7:119–132, 1977.
6. Dewhirst MW, Stump GL, Hurvitz AI: Idiopathic monoclonal (IgA) gammopathy in a dog. *JAVMA* 170: 1313–1316, 1977.
7. Cotter SM, Goldstein MA: Comparison of two protocols for maintenance of remission in dogs with lymphoma. *JAAHA* 23:495–499, 1987.
8. Matus RE, Leifer CE: Immunoglobulin-producing tumors. *Vet Clin North Am Small Anim Pract* 15:741–753, 1985.

CLINICAL BRIEFING: CANCER CACHEXIA AS A MANIFESTATION OF MALIGNANCY

Diagnosis	*History:* Weight loss in the face of adequate nutritional intake *Clinical Signs:* Weight loss despite adequate energy intake; increased toxicoses in response to radiation therapy, surgery, and chemotherapy; decreased response to therapy *Diagnostics:* Elevated serum lactate and insulin concentrations; abnormal amino acid and lipid profiles
Therapy	Eliminate underlying cause: surgery, chemotherapy, and radiation therapy Feed complex carbohydrates and high-quality proteins; moderate amounts of fats, possibly enriched with n-3 eicosanoids Encourage oral feeding (when possible); use nasogastric, gastrostomy, or jejunostomy feeding (when necessary) Parenteral support should be employed, if enteral feeding fails

CANCER CACHEXIA

Cancer cachexia produces involuntary weight loss even when caloric intake is adequate.[1–4] As with all other paraneoplastic syndromes, this condition is a remote effect of cancer. Cancer cachexia arises from dramatic alterations in carbohydrate, lipid, and protein metabolism that occur before clinical evidence of cachexia is detectable.[1–16] This paraneoplastic syndrome is encountered by every practitioner who treats animals with cancer. The actual cause of cancer cachexia is not known, but its metabolic effects are wide ranging and thus impair quality of life, response to therapy, and overall survival. A detailed description of this paraneoplastic syndrome and its treatment are found in the chapter on Nutritional Support.

Recent research demonstrates that elevated serum insulin and lactate concentrations in dogs with lymphoma and other malignancies rise higher still, compared with those in control dogs, in response to glucose-tolerance tests.[7]

Increased lactate and insulin levels in dogs with cancer do not normalize even after a complete remission is obtained after doxorubicin chemotherapy or surgery.[5] Dogs with lymphoma have even higher lactate and insulin levels on re-evaluation after relapse and show signs of cachexia.[5] Additional studies suggest that dogs with lymphoma may have a postreceptor defect, further indicating that dietary therapy may be effective in combating the problem. Hyperlactatemia becomes more pronounced on administration of lactate-containing parenteral fluids (e.g., lactated Ringer's solution) to dogs with lymphoma as compared with control animals.[6] Dogs with cancer show alterations in protein and lipid metabolism that remain after chemotherapy or surgery effects remission.[4] Dogs with lymphoma

> **KEY POINT:**
>
> *Dramatic alterations in carbohydrate, lipid, and protein metabolism are documented in cancer patients even before clinical evidence of cachexia is noted; these alterations fail to resolve following remission achieved with either surgery or chemotherapy.*

have significant reductions in threonine, glutamine, glycine, valine, cystine, and arginine. In contrast, their isoleucine and phenylalanine levels are significantly increased.[1] Dogs with untreated lymphoma have significantly higher free fatty acid, total triglycerides, and very low-density lipoprotein and triglyceride serum concentrations compared to untreated control animals. High-density lipoprotein cholesterol (HDL-CH) levels in dogs with lymphoma are significantly lower than in control dogs. After doxorubicin treatment, dogs with lymphoma develop significantly elevated total cholesterol levels, as noted in humans with cancer.

Indirect calorimetry has been used in clinical cancer patients to quantify nutritional and water requirements.[9–11] It demonstrates that energy expenditure and caloric needs in dogs with lymphoma and other malignancies are equal to or less than in normal dogs.[9,10] Furthermore, it demonstrates that major or minor surgery fails to increase significantly the energy expenditure of normal or cancer-bearing dogs.

These discoveries are important to the practitioner because they suggest that alterations in metabolism affect a diverse population of dogs with a wide variety of cancers and that therapy to improve these alterations must begin early and continue even after surgery or other treatment eliminates the malignancy. Because carbohydrates exacerbate hyperlactatemic and non-insulin-dependent diabetic states, a study of dogs with lymphoma recently compared a few dogs fed high-carbohydrate diets with those fed diets high in fat. Dogs fed diets high in fat were much more likely to go into remission. This research was continued and also demonstrated that a diet high in arginine and the eicosanoid n-3 series caused significant improvements in many alterations in metabolism. This demonstrates for the first time in biomedical science that dietary therapy can be an important adjunctive treatment for cancer in dogs.

Clinical Presentation

Animals with cancer cachexia show no clinical signs of the paraneoplastic syndrome in the early

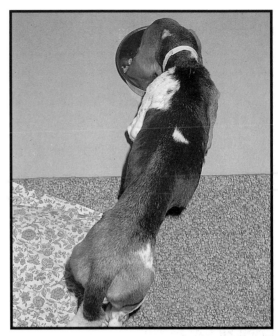

Figure 4-4: Dog with lymphoma that has dramatic weight loss despite adequate nutritional intake, the hallmark for the paraneoplastic syndrome, cancer cachexia. The metabolic alterations associated with this condition occur even before clinical signs are noted and continue after the animal is rendered free of the malignancy.

stages. As the syndrome progresses, weight loss is noted despite a good appetite (Figure 4-4). Later, weight loss, anorexia, lethargy, and depression predominate.

Diagnosis

As discussed earlier, alterations occur early in the course of malignant disease. Dogs in the preclinical or silent phase of cancer cachexia may only show exercise intolerance, lethargy, and anorexia. Later in the course of the disease, there is overt wasting and loss of body condition despite adequate nutritional intake. This is followed by death due to failure of one or more organ systems.

Treatment

Detailed therapeutic strategies are found elsewhere. A review of some general principles follows:

- Ensure that the patient consumes an adequate quantity of highly bioavailable nutrients presented in a palatable form.

- A diet composed of modest amounts of complex carbohydrates, minimal quantities of rapidly absorbed simple carbohydrates, high-quality but relatively modest amounts of bioavailable proteins, and a modest amount of fat may be ideal for supporting cancer patients without enhancing tumor growth.

- Animals should be fed enterally whenever possible. If appropriate, methods such as warming the food, increasing palatability, and using pharmacologic agents (e.g., megestrol acetate, benzodiazepine derivatives, or cyproheptadine) to enhance appetite and stimulate oral feeding should be employed before considering nasogastric, gastrostomy tube, or jejunostomy tube feeding.

- When enteral feeding is not feasible, parenteral feeding should be employed by using minimal simple carbohydrates.

- Avoid diets with simple carbohydrates as the principle source of calories because they may enhance hyperlactatemia and hyperinsulinemia.

- When possible, avoid lactate- and glucose-containing fluids, as they may produce lactate and insulin. A clear exception is in cases of septic shock or during an insulin overdose, when glucose-containing fluids may be required specifically to treat hypoglycemia.

- Adequate calories should be provided; however, it may not be necessary to provide more nutrients than needed by disease-free animals. The following formula is a general approximation of the amount of metabolizable food to feed (Kcal/day): $2(30 \times \text{body weight [kg]}) + 70$.

REFERENCES

1. Ogilvie GK, Vail DM: Nutrition and cancer: Recent developments. *Vet Clin North Am Small Anim Pract* 20:1–15, 1990.
2. Ogilvie GK: Paraneoplastic syndromes, in Withrow SJ, MacEwen EG (eds): *Clinical Veterinary Oncology.* Philadelphia, JB Lippincott, 1989, pp 29–40.
3. Vail DM, Ogilvie GK, Wheeler SL: Metabolic alterations in patients with cancer cachexia. *Compend Contin Educ Pract Vet* 12:381–387, 1990.
4. Ogilvie GK: Alterations in metabolism and nutritional support for veterinary cancer patients: Recent advances. *Compend Contin Educ Pract Vet* 15:925–937, 1993.
5. Ogilvie GK, Vail DM, Wheeler SL, et al: Effects of chemotherapy and remission on carbohydrate metabolism in dogs with lymphoma. *Cancer* 69:233–238, 1992.
6. Vail DM, Ogilvie GK, Fettman MJ, et al: Exacerbation of hyperlactatemic by infusion of LRS in dogs with lymphoma. *J Vet Intern Med* 4:228, 1990.
7. Vail DM, Ogilvie GK, Wheeler SL, et al: Alterations in carbohydrate metabolism in canine lymphoma. *J Vet Intern Med* 4:8–11, 1990.
8. Ogilvie, GK, Ford RD, Vail DM, et al: Alterations in lipoprotein profiles in dogs with lymphoma. *J Vet Intern Med* 8:62–66, 1994.
9. Ogilvie GK, Walters LM, Fettman MJ, et al: Energy expenditure in dogs with lymphoma fed two specialized diets. *Cancer* 71:3146–3152, 1993.
10. Walters LM, Ogilvie GK, Fettman MJ, et al: Repeatability of energy expenditure measurements in normal dogs by calorimetry. *Am J Vet Res* 54:1881–1885, 1993.
11. Ogilvie GK, Vail DM: Unique metabolic alterations associated with cancer cachexia in the dog, in Kirk RW (ed): *Current Veterinary Therapy. XI.* Philadelphia, WB Saunders, 1992, pp 433–438.
12. Ogilvie GK: Paraneoplastic syndromes, in Withrow SJ, MacEwen EG (eds): *Clinical Veterinary Oncology.* Philadelphia, JB Lippincott, 1989, pp 29–40.
13. Krishnaswamy K: Effects of malnutrition on drug metabolism and toxicity in humans. *Nutritional Toxicology* 2:105, 1987.
15. Fields ALA, Cheema-Dhadli S, et al: Theoretical aspects of weight loss in patients with cancer. *Cancer* 50:2183, 1982.
16. Chlebowski RT, Heber D: Metabolic abnormalities in cancer patients: Carbohydrate metabolism. *Surg Clin North Am* 66:957, 1986.

CLINICAL BRIEFING: MISCELLANEOUS CONDITIONS—FEVER, NEUROLOGIC SYNDROMES, AND HYPERTROPHIC OSTEOPATHY

Fever

Diagnosis	*History:* Lethargy and anorexia *Clinical Signs:* Lethargy, anorexia, increased body temperature, and weight loss (if condition is prolonged) *Diagnostics:* Confirm that elevated body temperature persists in a quiet patient. Rule out infections and inflammatory or immune-mediated causes with a CBC; biochemical profile; urinalysis; echocardiogram; antinuclear antibody test; and cultures of blood, urine, and lung. Rule in or out disease of the hypothalamus with history, physical examination, brain-imaging studies, and a CSF tap (if indicated)
Treatment	Eliminate the underlying cause Therapy depends on the severity of clinical and laboratory parameters; consider fluids and steroidal and nonsteroidal anti-inflammatory agents

Neurologic Syndromes

Diagnosis	*History:* Abnormalities referable to the brain, spinal cord, peripheral nerves, and muscle and neuromuscular junctions *Clinical Signs:* See history. Clinical signs are often subtle in the earlier phases but can include behavioral abnormalities and CNS upper motor neuron as well as central and peripheral nervous system lower motor neuron dysfunction *Diagnostics:* CBC, biochemical profile, and evaluation of thyroid and adrenal function; specific disease of nervous system diagnosed by imaging (CT, MRI, myelogram, etc.), CSF tap (if indicated), electrodiagnostics, biopsy of nervous tissue, and response tests (e.g., with tensilon)
Treatment	Treat the underlying cause Treat symptomatically for specific disease with glucocorticoids, mannitol, or surgical decompression as indicated

Hypertrophic Osteopathy

Diagnosis	*History:* Shifting leg lameness *Clinical Signs:* Swollen, warm extremities; may also involve ribs and pelvis

	Diagnostics: Radiographs of affected bones to demonstrate unique periosteal reaction. Search for underlying malignancy with chest radiograph, followed by abdominal radiography or ultrasonography, CBC, biochemical profile, and urinalysis
Treatment	Treat the underlying cause Anti-inflammatory agents

FEVER

Fever is a common complication of cancer.[1-3] In many cases, pyrexia is caused by infection. Although other noninfectious causes, such as drug toxicity and adrenal insufficiency, have been associated with fever, elevated body temperature can be a sign of neoplastic disease.[2] Tumor-associated fever is usually defined as unexplained elevated body temperature that coincides with growth or elimination of a tumor. Tumor-induced fevers may result from release of pyrogens from tumor cells as well as from normal leukocytes or other normal cells. These tumor-elaborated pyrogens may act on the hypothalamus to reset temperature regulation of the body. Although the incidence of cancer-associated fever is unknown in animals, in humans, up to 40% of fevers of unknown origin are found to be caused by cancer.[3]

Clinical Signs

Clinical signs are directly related to the underlying malignant disease, elevated body temperature, and associated increase in energy expenditure. These can result in depression, anorexia, lethargy, and weight loss.

Diagnosis

The diagnosis of this paraneoplastic syndrome is essentially a diagnosis of exclusion and is supported by determining whether eliminating the underlying tumor resolves the elevated body temperature. All nontumor-related causes of increased body temperature are eliminated with the following procedures: CBC, biochemical profile, urinalysis, blood and urine cultures, chest radiographs, echocardiography (look-ing for bacterial endocarditis), and (if indicated) an antinuclear antibody test, a brain-imaging study (CT and MRI), myelogram, and a cerebrospinal fluid (CSF) tap to evaluate for hypothalamic dysfunction (because the hypothalamus governs thermoregulation).

Treatment

This paraneoplastic syndrome can be used as a tumor marker to document response to therapy.[1-3] Excessive fever that induces clinical signs and is directly related to malignant disease can be treated symptomatically with antipyretics or nonsteroidal anti-inflammatory agents. Resolution of the underlying malignant condition usually eliminates the fever.

NEUROLOGIC SYNDROMES

In both human and veterinary patients, the remote effects of cancer on the nervous system induce a wide variety of clinical signs[1-9] of unknown causes. Cancer-induced neuropathies in dogs include cases of peripheral neuropathy, trigeminal nerve paralysis, and Horner's syndrome.[4-9] Animals also exhibit neurologic signs secondary to endocrine, fluid, and electrolyte disturbances attributable to neoplasia. Examples of these include hypercalcemia, hyperviscosity syndrome, and hepatoencephalopathy. The neurologic syndromes of myasthenia gravis (e.g., megaesophagus and acetyl cholinesterase-responsive neuropathy) secondary to thymoma are well described in the literature.[1-9]

Clinical Signs

Manifestations of neurologic paraneoplastic syndrome comprise virtually any change in normal ner-

TABLE 4-2
Paraneoplastic syndromes of the nervous system and resulting neurologic syndromes[1-9]

Site Involved	Syndrome
Brain	Cerebellar degeneration
	Optic neuritis
	Progressive multifocal leukoencephalopathy
Spinal cord	Subacute necrotic myelopathy
	Subacute motor neuropathy
Peripheral nerves	Sensory neuropathy
	Peripheral neuropathy
	Autonomic GI neuropathy
Muscle and neuromuscular junction	Dermatomyositis and polymyositis
	Myasthenic syndrome (Eaton-Lambert syndrome)
	Myasthenia gravis

vous system function. These abnormalities include behavioral changes; peripheral and spinal cord neuropathies; and alterations in the function of the cerebrum, cerebellum, medulla, and neuromuscular junction in both humans and animals. Some of these aberrations are noted in Table 4-2.

Diagnosis

The diagnosis of this paraneoplastic syndrome includes eliminating nonneoplastic causes using CBC, biochemical profile, urinalysis, tests of the thyroid and adrenal axes, brain or spinal cord imaging (CT, MRI, and contrast radiography), biopsy of the affected nerves, CSF tap, and (if indicated) electrodiagnostics.

Treatment

Elimination of the neoplastic condition may result in resolution of neurologic syndromes. Immune-mediated conditions of the CNS or peripheral nervous system may require the use of immunosuppressive therapy, including glucocorticoids.

HYPERTROPHIC OSTEOPATHY

Hypertrophic osteopathy is a relatively common disease that primarily occurs in the bones of the extremities. The disease primarily affects dogs and is rare in cats. This paraneoplastic syndrome is often associated with primary and metastatic lung tumors.[2] Other neoplastic and nonneoplastic conditions have been associated with this disorder. These include esophageal sarcoma, rhabdomyosarcoma of the urinary bladder, pneumonia, heartworm disease, congenital and acquired heart disease, and focal lung atelectasis.[2] Other factors include hyperestrogenism, deficient oxygenation, and increased blood flow.[2]

Clinical Signs

The disease produces an increase in peripheral blood flow and a periosteal proliferation along the shafts of long bones, often beginning with the digits and extending as far proximally as the femur and humerus. Initially, there is soft tissue proliferation. This is succeeded by osteophytes, which tend to radiate from the cortices at a 90-degree angle. The cause of this unique syndrome is unknown; however, successful treatment by vagotomy suggests a neurovascular mechanism that may involve a reflex emanating from the tumor and nearby pleura that is transmitted through afferent vagal fibers.[2]

Diagnosis (Figure 4-5)

Radiographs of affected limbs and the contralateral extremity often show an increased soft tissue density and a unique osteophyte reaction that radiates outward at a 90-degree angle from the cortex of the bone. When hypertrophic osteopathy is identified, radiographs of the chest (and of the abdomen, when indicated) should be done to identify the underlying cause. Although a biopsy is definitive, the classic history, physical examination, and radiographic changes often are enough to permit a definitive diagnosis of hypertrophic osteopathy.

Treatment

Prednisone offers temporary improvement in clinical signs and may reduce swelling.[1,2] Removal of the tumor can effect almost immediate resolution of clinical signs; regression of bony and soft tissue changes may take months or years. Other treatments, such as the use of analgesics, unilateral vagotomy on the side of the lung lesion, incision through the parietal pleura, subperiosteal rib resection, or bilateral cervical vagotomy have been suggested.

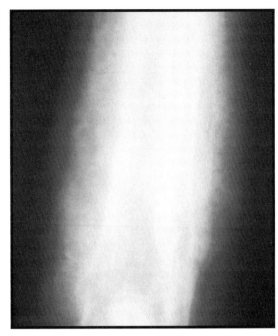

Figure 4-5: *Radiograph of a limb affected with hypertrophic osteopathy showing an increased soft tissue density and a unique osteophyte reaction that radiates outward at a 90-degree angle from the cortex of the bone.*

REFERENCES

1. Ogilvie GK: Paraneoplastic syndromes, in Withrow SJ, MacEwen EG (eds): *Clinical Veterinary Oncology.* Philadelphia, JB Lippincott, 1989 pp 29–40.
2. Ogilvie GK: Paraneoplastic syndromes, in Ettinger SJ, Feldman EC (eds): *Textbook of Veterinary Internal Medicine,* ed 4. Philadelphia, WB Saunders, 1994, in press.
3. Griffin TW, Rosenthal PE, Costanza ME: Paraneoplastic and endocrine syndromes, in Cady B (ed): *Cancer Manual,* ed 7. Boston, American Cancer Society, 1986, pp 373–390.
4. Shahar R, Rosseau C, Steiss J: Peripheral polyneuropathy in a dog with functional islet B-cell tumor and widespread metastases. *JAVMA* 187:175, 1985.
5. Bergman PJ, Bruyette DS, Coyne BE, et al: Canine clinical peripheral neuropathy associated with pancreatic cell carcinoma. *Prog Vet Neurol* 5:57–62, 1994.
6. Duncan ID: Peripheral neuropathy in the dog and cat. *Prog Vet Neurol* 2:111–121, 1990.
7. Manana KR, Luttgen PJ: Endocrine-associated neuropathies in dogs and cats. *Compend Contin Educ Pract Vet,* 1994, in press.
8. Braund KG, McGuire JA, Henderson RA: Peripheral neuropathy associated with malignant neoplasms in dogs. *Vet Pathol* 24:16–24, 1987.
9. Braund KG: Remote effects of cancer on the nervous system. *Semin Vet Med Surg [Small Anim]* 5:262–273, 1990.

CLINICAL BRIEFING: THEORY AND PRACTICE

This introductory chapter on Theory and Practice provides an overview of how Section V is organized and how best to utilize the chapter format in the management of the veterinary cancer patient.

At the beginning of each chapter in Section V, a Clinical Briefing box is provided. The Clinical Briefing is a synopsis and is not meant to replace the text in that chapter. It does, however, provide the busy practitioner with an outline of the clinical presentation, biological behavior, and treatment options for each relevant tumor type. Following the Clinical Briefing box, each chapter provides a textual discussion of different tumor types found in cats and dogs. This discussion is divided into the following headings:

Incidence, Signalment, and Etiology

• Clinical Presentation and History • Staging and Diagnosis

• Prognostic Factors • Treatment

Please read this introductory chapter carefully. Although each chapter in Section V stands alone, it is important to understand some common theory in order to derive maximum benefit from the information provided in the text.

INCIDENCE, SIGNALMENT, AND ETIOLOGY

Much of the data on incidence and signalment for tumors in cats and dogs is derived from studies that emphasize pathologic descriptions and rarely involve animals that were presented for treatment. Often, data are limited to small numbers of case series; nonetheless, we have attempted to provide the reader with some basic background information as to age and gender of the affected population. Most animals with cancer are old, and true gender predisposition is difficult to assess, as some reports are conflicting, and other studies are based on limited numbers of animals. Owners often ask the question, "What caused my pet's cancer?" but the etiology of most neoplasms in dogs and cats remains obscure. We list causative agents when there is clear epidemiologic evidence to support their inclusion. Also provided in this subsection are data on the most common tumor types and the sites at which they occur.

CLINICAL PRESENTATION AND HISTORY

Cancer affects an old population of animals. Regardless of the tissue of origin, cancer causes metabolic disturbances that lead to common clinical signs and owner observations. Such nonspecific signs as lethargy, inappetence, depression, and weight loss are common to most tumor types, and each of the following chapters provides details on only those signs that may assist the veterinarian in making a specific diagnosis.

Physical examination is extremely important in evaluating any animal with cancer, and old animals may have other diseases or even other cancers that could otherwise escape detection. Specific physical findings for each tumor type are provided.

STAGING AND DIAGNOSIS

When evaluating an animal for treatment of cancer, it is important not only to obtain a definitive diagnosis but also to assess the general health of the patient by clinical examination and ancillary diagnostics. This involves determining the extent of organ involvement with the tumor as well as identifying unrelated or secondary conditions that need to be treated or controlled before instituting appropriate therapy.

Staging is a clinical process that enables the veterinarian to quantitate the extent of cancer involvement in the patient. Staging often carries prognostic significance and enables the veterinarian and client to make informed and rational decisions regarding the type of therapy best suited to the patient. Most staging systems are based on assessment of three major components of the malignant process:

- The size of the primary tumor (T)
- Lymph node metastasis (N)
- Distant metastasis (M)

These components are further modified by the use of subscript numbers to indicate increase in tumor size (T_0, T_1, T_2, and T_3), progressive involvement of regional lymph nodes (N_0, N_1, and N_2), and the presence or absence of distant metastasis (M_0 and M_1). To obtain this information, ancillary diagnostics are very important and sophisticated imaging techniques are often used (Figure 5-1).

Physical Examination

A complete physical examination is essential to the staging process. All lymph nodes, especially those that provide lymphatic drainage from the site of the primary tumor (so-called regional lymph nodes), should be palpated. The primary tumor and involved lymph nodes should be measured, and those measurements should be recorded to assist the veterinarian in assessing response to therapy or in planning surgery and adjunctive therapy.

Clinical Pathology

The results of a complete blood count, serum chemistry profile, or urinalysis rarely provide definitive information regarding the type of cancer or whether it has metastasized. Such information is discussed in the Staging and Diagnosis section for each tumor type

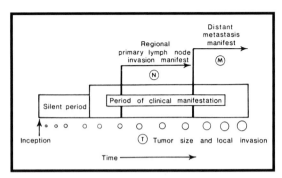

Figure 5-1: *Schematic diagram showing progression of a tumor from inception to metastasis. Subscript numerical values assigned to each of T, N, and M assist the clinician in evaluating the patient for appropriate therapy. (From Beahrs OH, Henson DE, Hutter RVP, et al: Manual for Staging of Cancer, ed 3. Philadelphia, JB Lippincott, 1988; with permission.)*

only if specific prognostic information can be obtained. It is assumed, however, that routine blood work and an urinalysis will be performed as part of a general health screen for every animal with cancer.

Anemia in animals with cancer is common, but it is usually low grade and characterized as normocytic, normochromic, which is compatible with anemia of chronic disease. Moderate to severe anemia may be present in animals experiencing blood loss from gastrointestinal involvement with the tumor, coagulopathies, or, occasionally, from paraneoplastic immune-mediated destruction. White cell counts and differentials rarely assist the clinician in staging a dog or cat with cancer. Neutrophilia may result from inflammation, tumor necrosis, or stress and does not automatically imply infection, but it should prompt further investigation for an underlying cause. Similarly, abnormalities in other cell lines may not be specific for the animal's tumor but should be investigated by thoracic radiographs, ultrasonography, or, possibly, bone marrow aspiration. Some tumors cause changes in the hemogram or serum chemistry profile as a paraneoplastic syndrome, and these changes are noted in the relevant chapters.

Serum chemistry profiles are essential to establish the health of an animal with cancer. When complicated surgical procedures or multiple radiation therapies that require repeated or prolonged anesthesia are

MANAGEMENT OF SPECIFIC DISEASES

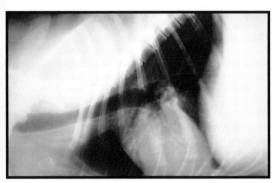

Figure 5-2: Thoracic radiograph of a 6-year-old, female Bernese mountain dog in right lateral recumbency. This dog has malignant histiocytosis. Note the lack of evidence for pulmonary metastatic disease (see Figure 5-3).

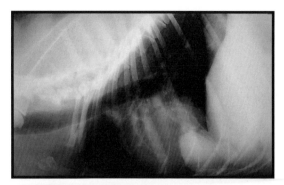

Figure 5-3: Left lateral thoracic radiograph of the same dog as in Figure 5-2. A pulmonary nodule is clearly visualized but was not evident on the right lateral view. Two lateral views of the thorax should always be performed.

planned, acceptable renal and hepatic functions are vital. In addition, some chemotherapeutic agents that are metabolized or excreted by the liver or kidneys may require reduction in dosage if these organs are functionally compromised (see the chapter on Chemotherapeutic Agents). Paraneoplastic conditions, such as hypercalcemia or hypoglycemia, may be observed that would direct the clinician to search for an otherwise unsuspected neoplasm.

Urinalysis may disclose evidence of infection that can occur as a consequence of tumor-related immunosuppression or general debility. Initiation of appropriate antibiotic therapy is recommended, particularly when myelosuppressive chemotherapy is anticipated as a treatment modality.

Radiography and Ultrasonography

Radiographs of the thorax and abdomen are valuable in determining the clinical stage of disease. Thoracic radiographs may permit identification of lymphadenopathy of sternal or tracheobronchial nodes. In addition, a mediastinal mass, pulmonary metastasis, or pleural effusion may be present. Proper radiographic assessment of the lungs requires both a right and left lateral view as well as a dorsoventral view (Figures 5-2 and 5-3). Radiographs of the abdomen are used to identify a mass, organomegaly, or lymphadenopathy, particularly of the sublumbar nodes. Some tumors are

calcified and are easily visualized on radiographs.

If biopsy of a mass located in one of the body cavities is considered (particularly if effusion is present), ultrasonography provides an accurate and relatively safe guide for obtaining a tissue or fluid sample. In addition, when involvement of abdominal viscera is suspected, ultrasonography allows evaluation of organ homogeneity and architecture and can be used to detect the presence of enlarged lymph nodes as well as gastrointestinal involvement. Ultrasonography has the advantage of providing no risk of exposure to radiation and does not require an anesthetized patient.

Computed Tomography

Computed tomography (CT) is becoming more widely available for veterinary use, particularly at teaching institutions and large specialty practices. The major advantage of CT over conventional radiography is its ability to discriminate between tissues that have only minor differences in radiodensity that would not be appreciated on plain radiographs (Figure 5-4). For example, CT can discriminate hepatic metastases from normal liver. Objects that are close together, however, may be difficult to depict separately. Computed tomography has advantages over ultrasonography in imaging lesions that are shielded by bone or gas (e.g., lung or intracranial tumors); however, unlike ultrasonography, CT requires general anesthesia.

MANAGEMENT OF SPECIFIC DISEASES

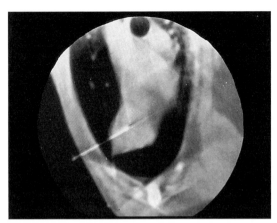

Figure 5-4: Microcore biopsy tract shown on this CT image of a small thymoma located in the anterior mediastinum. The accuracy of this method allows a definitive diagnosis to be reached prior to an exploratory surgery. (Courtesy of A.S. Tidwell)

Imaging Tumors of Specific Sites

For diagnostic purposes, conventional radiography, preferably with high-detail film, is effective in imaging nasal and oral tumors, whereas ultrasonography is often useful for retrobulbar lesions. Computed tomography is probably the modality of choice for imaging tumors of the brain as well as nasal, oral, and retrobulbar tumors. Computed tomography is particularly useful when the veterinarian is trying to determine tumor margins in these sites prior to surgery or radiation therapy. Lesions of the brain stem may be difficult to image accurately with CT.

Ultrasonography is the imaging modality of choice for tumors of the heart. For most other thoracic lesions, conventional radiography provides a more global view. Computed tomography is best for assessing tumor margins and the tissue of origin (e.g., mediastinum versus lung). Computed tomography imaging may also detect pulmonary metastases that are too small to be seen or are equivocal lesions on conventional radiographs.

Ultrasonography is considered by some to be the first choice for imaging the abdomen, although conventional radiography will provide a global aspect.

Computed tomography may be useful if organs are obscured by gas. In addition, CT is very useful in assessing margins of large soft tissue tumors anywhere in the body. An even newer modality, magnetic resonance imaging (MRI), is sometimes available to veterinarians through large human hospitals. This modality provides excellent resolution and is particularly useful for imaging tumors of the brain or spine.

PROGNOSTIC FACTORS

When possible, we describe factors relating to the patient, tumor, staging of the tumor, and treatment regimen that have been found to influence tumor response to therapy and patient survival. Much of the information regarding prognosis is contradictory or controversial, usually because of the small number of animals in each study. When two conflicting results are available, both have been provided. Graphic representations in the form of survival curves are provided to compare two or more different prognostic factors.

This subsection has not been included for many tumor types because no prognostic variables have been identified. Future studies may identify new prognostic factors or confirm existing ones; the reader is encouraged to keep up to date with the veterinary literature for such information.

TREATMENT

For each tumor type, the relevant veterinary literature has been reviewed and treatments that have been found to be effective for cats and dogs have been provided. Although information regarding treatment of the same tumor types in humans is often available, there are considerable differences in biological behavior and tumor response between species. We have therefore chosen to use only the veterinary literature for this section. When information is not published but a treatment has been observed to be effective, it is reported here as anecdotal and the source (usually a personal communication) is provided.

Therapies that deal with the primary tumor are still the mainstay of veterinary oncology, and surgery is the primary modality used in private practice. The

MANAGEMENT OF SPECIFIC DISEASES

TABLE 5-1
Definitions of objective tumor remissions and
responses following anticancer therapy

Tumor Response	Tumor Size
Complete (CR)*	Disappearance of all evidence of cancer in all sites for a defined period of time (e.g., one intertreatment interval of 3 weeks).
Partial (PR)*	Decrease in size of all tumors by 50% or greater as measured by the sum of the products of two diameters for each tumor. These diameters should be the largest tumor diameter and the diameter perpendicular to it. There should be sustained decrease in tumor size, as defined for CR, and no new tumors should arise.
Stable disease (SD)	Decrease of <50% or an increase of <25% in the sum of the products of the diameters as measured for PR.
Progressive disease (PD)	Increase of 25% or more in the sum of the products of tumor diameters or the appearance of a new tumor.

*CR + PR = Objective response rate.

results of surgical treatment are provided, but detailed discussion of specific surgical techniques is beyond the scope of this text. The reader is referred to the primary references for such information.

The results of radiation therapy for treatment of various tumor types has been largely based on early studies using low cumulative doses and coarse fractionation. Recent advances in radiation oncology have led to daily fractionation and to smaller treatment fractions, which allow higher cumulative radiation doses to be delivered to cats and dogs with tumors. With these advances, many of the tumors that were previously reported as nonresponsive actually may prove to be well controlled by radiation therapy. This is a rapidly changing field, and the most current results available have been provided in the relevant chapters.

Chemotherapy for cats and dogs is also a changing field, and with more careful evaluation of available drugs as to their efficacy as single agents, we can expect combination chemotherapy protocols to become available for a number of different cancers. Only those protocols and drugs for which published

data existed have been provided in this book. Many complicated chemotherapy protocols have been adapted from human oncology, but their relevance and efficacy for the treatment of tumors in cats and dogs have been largely untested. The reader is encouraged to keep up to date with the literature, as this is a rapidly advancing field.

Results of other treatment modalities, such as biological response modifiers, photodynamic therapy, and hyperthermia are provided for individual tumors in which responses have been noted.

The effects of different treatment modalities influence two major factors: the response of the tumor and the survival of the patient. Tumor responses are reported in this book as complete response (or remission), partial response, stable disease, or progressive disease. The definitions of these terms are found in Table 5-1. Ultimately, however, it is the survival of the patient that is important, although tumor response may be an important component in improving quality of life. When known, the survival times and remission durations for animals with different tumors are provided.

CLINICAL BRIEFING: LYMPHOMA

Lymphoma in Dogs

Common Clinical Presentation	Generalized peripheral lymphadenopathy (clinical stage III)
Common Histologic Types	Diffuse large cell, immunoblastic, and small lymphocytic
Epidemiology and Biological Behavior	All breeds, middle-aged; systemic disease
Prognostic Factors	*Clinical Stage:* Stages IV and V worse than I–III; dogs with clinical signs worse than if asymptomatic *Hypercalcemia:* Worse when associated with an anterior mediastinal mass *Sex:* Female dogs better than male dogs *Body Size:* Small dogs better than large dogs *Pretreatment Corticosteroids:* Worse *High Grade:* Higher response rate and longer duration of remission

Treatment
Single Agent
  Prednisone, cyclophosphamide, and vincristine
  Doxorubicin
 	
Combinations
  Cyclophosphamide, vincristine, and prednisone (COP)
  COP plus L-asparaginase and methotrexate
  COP plus doxorubicin
  COP plus doxorubicin and L-asparaginase
	
	50% in CR for median 1–6 months
	
	60%–75% in CR for median 6–8 months
	
	70% in CR for median 5 months
	
	80% in CR for median 5 months
	
	80% in CR for median 7 months
	80% in CR for median 9 months

Lymphoma in Cats

Common Clinical Presentation	Anterior mediastinal or alimentary involvement
Common Histologic Type	Not known

MANAGEMENT OF SPECIFIC DISEASES

Epidemiology and Biological Behavior	Often FeLV positive but dependent on anatomic location of lymphoma; occurs in all breeds with a bimodal age peak
Prognostic Factors	*Clinical Stage:* Stage I better than all other stages *FeLV Positive:* Worse survival rate; no effect on response to therapy

Treatment
  Combinations
    Cyclophosphamide, vincristine, and prednisone, (COP)
	50% to 80% in CR for median 5 months

Vincristine, cyclophosphamide, and methotrexate (VCM)	50% in CR for median 4 months
VCM plus L-asparaginase	60% in CR for median <7 months
CR = complete remission.	

The terms *lymphoma* and *lymphosarcoma* are interchangeable in veterinary medicine. Lymphoma is the most common hematopoietic tumor of both dogs and cats. The natural history and progression of lymphoma is well described in both species, and chemotherapy has been shown to be very effective in altering that progression and prolonging quality of life in most animals.

The following sections briefly review lymphoma and its incidence in both dogs and cats. The most common presenting signs and clinical history and ancillary testing needed to diagnose the disease definitely and to assess the patient for prognostic factors found to influence remission and survival as well as common treatment for this disease are discussed.

LYMPHOMA IN DOGS
Incidence, Signalment, and Etiology

Lymphoma is the most common malignancy that involves cells of the hematopoietic system, and it is the most responsive to chemotherapy.

Lymphoma accounts for approximately 90% of canine hematopoietic tumors.

Lymphoma is uncommon in young dogs; affected dogs are typically middle-aged. Neither gender nor neutering is a predisposing factor for developing lymphoma.

In two studies of canine tumor epidemiology, boxers had a significantly greater number of lymphoma cases than expected. Their risk of developing lymphoma was approximately 10 times greater than for all dogs combined.[1,2] In a group of 59 bullmastiffs, nine dogs developed lymphoma over a 3-year course and cases seemed to follow a familial distribution.[3] Other reports documented that German shepherds and poodles were more often affected, and recent anecdotal evidence suggests a high incidence in golden retrievers.

Evidence suggests that high exposure to some herbicides, notably 2,4 dichlorophenoxyacetic acid (2,4D), is associated with an increased risk of non-Hodgkin's lymphoma in humans. A case-controlled study found that dogs with lymphoma were exposed

> **KEY POINT:**
>
> *Exposure to the herbicide 2,4D has been associated with an increased risk of a dog developing lymphoma by as much as two-fold.*

MANAGEMENT OF SPECIFIC DISEASES

to 2,4D more frequently than were control dogs. In addition, the risk of a dog developing lymphoma increased two-fold if the owner applied 2,4D to the lawn four or more times per year.[4]

Virus particles resembling a C-type retrovirus have been observed in cases of canine lymphoma and leukemia as well as in tissue cultures of canine lymphoma cells.[3,5] The purported retrovirus also has been found in normal dogs, however, and no etiologic involvement has been confirmed. In view of the lack of an early age–incidence peak for dogs with lymphoma and the lack of reports of "clustering" of cases, it seems unlikely that a viral etiology of the type seen for feline lymphoma is present in the dog.

Clinical Presentation and History

The most common physical finding in dogs with lymphoma is peripheral lymphadenopathy, which is usually generalized but may be localized to a single lymph node or a region of the body. Involvement of other organs, such as spleen, liver, or bone marrow are indications of advanced disease. Involvement of other (extranodal) sites is rare in dogs.

Most canine patients with lymphoma present with generalized lymphadenopathy, often because their owners have noticed mandibular lymphadenopathy when patting or grooming the pet (Figure 5-5). Most commonly, there are few, if any, clinical signs of illness, although owners may report reduced exercise tolerance, fatigability, and mild inappetence. This is in contrast with most systemic infections (e.g., fungal, bacterial, rickettsial, viral, and protozoal) that cause obvious signs of illness, as do immune-mediated diseases causing lymphadenopathy. Lymphoma should always be suspected in a middle-aged, apparently healthy dog with lymphadenopathy.

If the disease is advanced and involves other organs, dogs may show weakness, depression, anorexia, vomiting, or diarrhea. Terminally ill dogs may be cachectic, dyspneic due to respiratory tract obstruction by lymph nodes, pyrexic (dogs with lymphoma are immunocompromised and therefore are at high risk of developing severe infections, such as pneumonia), and have episodes of collapse.

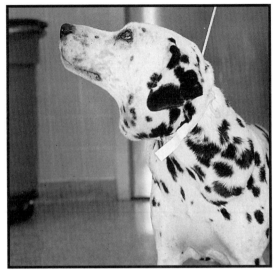

Figure 5-5: This 6-year-old Dalmatian has extremely large peripheral lymph nodes. The dog had no organomegaly or evidence of bone marrow involvement and was clinically well. The lymphoma was therefore classified as clinical stage IIIa. Complete remission was achieved with combination chemotherapy.

Untreated lymphoma progresses rapidly (1–2 months) from presentation to terminal stages. With chemotherapy, however, considerable improvement in the duration and quality of the patient's life can be expected.

Staging and Diagnosis

When evaluating an animal for treatment of lymphoma, it is important not only to obtain a definitive diagnosis but also to assess the general health of the patient by clinical examination and ancillary diagnostics. Lymphoma is a systemic disease; therefore, it is important to determine the extent of organ involvement with lymphoma and to identify unrelated or secondary conditions that need to be treated or controlled before instituting appropriate therapy.

Staging is a clinical process that enables the veterinarian to quantitate the extent of lymphoma involvement in the patient. Staging carries prognostic significance and enables the veterinarian and client to make

MANAGEMENT OF SPECIFIC DISEASES

TABLE 5-2
Clinical stages of canine lymphosarcoma (WHO)[6]

Clinical Stage*	Criteria
Stage I	Involvement limited to single node or lymphoid tissue in single organ (excluding the bone marrow)
Stage II	Regional involvement of many lymph nodes, with or without involvement of the tonsils
Stage III	Generalized lymph node involvement
Stage IV	Involvement of liver and/or spleen, with or without generalized lymph node involvement
Stage V	Involvement of blood, bone marrow, and/or other organs

*Stages are further classified to clinical substage a (no clinical signs) or b (with clinical signs). For example, Stage IIIa describes a dog with generalized lymphadenopathy and no clinical signs..

informed and rational decisions as to the type of therapy best suited for the patient. In dogs, the most widely used scheme is the one developed by the World Health Organization (Table 5-2). Each dog is clinically staged based on the results of physical examination, clinical laboratory testing (i.e., CBC, biochemical profile, urinalysis, and bone marrow cytology), and imaging procedures (i.e., radiography and ultrasonography). In each case, a biopsy of the affected lymphoid tissue is necessary to confirm the diagnosis and determine the cell type (histologic grading).

The clinical stage of a dog with lymphoma is often determined on physical examination. All lymph nodes should be palpated; accurate measurements should be recorded to help the clinician assess response to therapy. The eyes should be assessed for lymphoid infiltrate and/or anterior uveitis. Abdominal palpation may reveal organomegaly, and lymphomatous infiltration of the spleen or liver can be confirmed with ancillary tests, such as fine-needle aspiration or biopsy.

Radiographs of the thorax and abdomen are valuable in determining the clinical stage of disease. In one report, 75 of 100 dogs with lymphoma had abnormalities detected radiographically.[7] Thoracic radiographs may allow appreciation of lymphadenopathy of sternal or tracheobronchial nodes. In addition, a mediastinal mass, pulmonary infiltration, or pleural effusion may be seen (Figure 5-6). Radiographs of the abdomen principally are used to identify hepatosplenomegaly or lymphadenopathy of the sublumbar nodes.

If biopsy of a mediastinal mass is being considered, particularly if pleural effusion is present, ultrasonography provides an accurate guide and a relatively safe means of obtaining a tissue or fluid sample (Figure 5-7). In addition, when involvement of abdominal viscera is suspected, ultrasonography allows evaluation of spleen and liver homogeneity and renal architecture and can be used to detect the presence of enlarged lymph nodes as well as gastrointestinal (GI) involvement.

KEY POINT:

Accurate measurements of all affected lymph nodes or extranodal sites will assist the veterinarian in assessing response to chemotherapy.

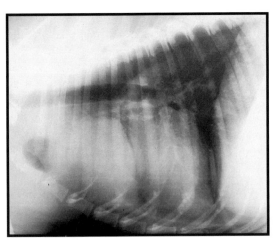

Figure 5-6: A dog with anterior mediastinal lymphoma. This disease may be associated with pleural effusion and dyspnea or may cause dyspnea due to space-occupying pressure on the trachea. This anatomic form of lymphoma also may be associated with paraneoplastic hypercalcemia. The concurrent findings of hypercalcemic and anterior mediastinal lymphoma warrant a poor prognosis. (Courtesy D.G. Penninck)

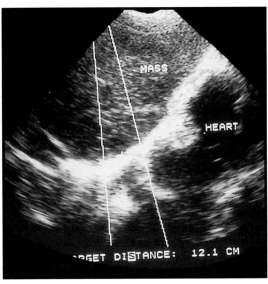

Figure 5-7: Ultrasound image of the same dog as in Figure 5-6. Ultrasound-guided biopsy is a relatively noninvasive method of confirming a diagnosis of anterior mediastinal lymphoma. The technique is safe and effective. (Courtesy D.G. Penninck)

Anemia is common in animals with lymphoma, but it is usually low grade and characterized as normocytic, normochromic, which is compatible with anemia of chronic disease. Moderate to severe anemia may be present in animals that are experiencing blood loss from GI involvement and occasionally may result from immune-mediated destruction. Anemia is rarely a consequence of bone marrow infiltration, particularly if granulocyte and platelet counts are normal. This is because of the relatively long life span of mature erythrocytes (120 days) compared to that of platelets (5–6 days) or neutrophils (6 hours).[8]

Thrombocytopenia, particularly in association with neutropenia, may indicate bone marrow infiltration by lymphoma, and bone marrow aspiration should be performed. Immune-mediated thrombocytopenia may occur in dogs with lymphoma. In addition, thrombocytopenia may be a sign of disseminated intravascular coagulopathy (DIC), which is a life-threatening complication that can occur in dogs with lymphoma. Evaluation of both intrinsic and extrinsic clotting pathways should be performed

and appropriate therapy begun (see Oncologic Emergencies section).

Lymphopenia (due to stress of disease) or normal lymphocyte counts may be found on the hemogram of animals with lymphoma. Lymphocytosis should prompt critical evaluation of lymphocyte morphology, as circulating lymphoblasts imply bone marrow involvement and a higher clinical stage (stage V) and a correspondingly worse prognosis for remission. In this situation, bone marrow aspiration should be performed. If the lymphocyte count is elevated and there is bone marrow infiltration but no other clinical findings, the disease is designated as a lymphoid leukemia (see chapter on Bone Marrow Neoplasia) and evaluation of lymphocyte morphology is critical for an accurate prognosis.

When cytopenias other than anemia occur in an animal with lymphoma, neoplastic infiltration of the bone marrow must be suspected and should be confirmed by aspiration or biopsy (see Biopsy section). For animals with neoplastic infiltration, myelosuppressive chemotherapeutic agents should not be used until the segmented neutrophil and platelet counts are in a noncritical range (>3000 segmented neutrophils/µl; >50,000 platelets/µl).

An animal with lymphoma is often immunosuppressed and therefore susceptible to urinary tract infections, which may be subclinical. Bacterial cultures should be performed if abnormalities in the urinalysis suggest infection; in this situation, antibiotics should be administered concurrently with chemotherapy. Animals with urinary tract infections are at high risk for sepsis when myelosuppressive chemotherapy drugs are used.

Serum chemistry profiles are useful in staging animals with lymphoma. Elevated hepatic enzyme levels, particularly in the presence of cranial abdominal organomegaly, imply infiltration of the liver with lymphoma. If severe disturbances in liver function occur, the use of some chemotherapeutic agents should be re-evaluated. Cyclophosphamide is metabolized to an active form in the liver, and it may therefore be ineffective if liver function is impaired. Doxorubicin is metabolized in the liver, so liver function impairment may lead to higher than expected serum concentrations and greater toxicity. Doxorubicin dosages should be reduced in dogs with poor liver function. Elevated blood urea nitrogen (BUN) or serum creatinine levels may be associated with hypercalcemia in dogs. Primary renal involvement with lymphoma is rare in this species.

Hypercalcemia in association with lymphoma occurs in 10% to 15% of affected dogs. It is most commonly associated with mediastinal involvement. With high serum calcium levels (>14 mg/gl), polyuria, polydipsia, weakness, and anorexia may develop. If serum calcium levels remain elevated, calcium nephropathy and resultant renal failure may ensue. A complete discussion of the treatment of hypercalcemia can be found in the Oncologic Emergencies section. Briefly, calcium levels may be reduced with saline diuresis (0.9% NaCl) or furosemide diuretic treatment. In addition, prednisone may be used to increase renal losses, decrease GI calcium absorption, and reduce osteoclast activity. A confirmed histologic diagnosis should be obtained before commencing prednisone therapy, as complete clinical remission of lymphoma may occur, leaving the clinician uncertain as to the true cause of the hypercalcemia. The clinician should not delay obtaining a diagnosis while trying to reduce the calcium levels. It is important to obtain a diagnosis and begin chemotherapy quickly, as this will result in rapid normalization of serum calcium.

Another paraneoplastic syndrome rarely seen in dogs with lymphoma is a monoclonal gammopathy, which may be detected by serum electrophoresis. Most malignancy-associated monoclonal gammopathies in dogs are associated with multiple myeloma.

The diagnosis of lymphoma can be confirmed by cytologic or histologic demonstration of malignant lymphoid infiltration in organs that do not ordinarily contain such cells.

Cytologic examination of lymph nodes may be suggestive of, or compatible with, a diagnosis of lymphoma but rarely provides a definitive diagnosis. In the presence of lymphadenopathy, a definitive diagnosis of lymphoma is based on histologic examination of a surgically resected lymph node. This is preferable to a needle or wedge biopsy because an entire lymph node can be examined for key histopathologic evidence of malignancy, such as dis-

---

KEY POINTS:

If a dog with lymphoma is neutropenic, nonmyelosuppressive chemotherapeutic agents should be used, such as prednisone, vincristine, and L-asparaginase.

For hypercalcemic dogs, it is important to obtain a diagnosis and begin chemotherapy quickly rather than to delay while attempting to reduce serum calcium by other means.

MANAGEMENT OF SPECIFIC DISEASES

ruption of architecture and invasion of the capsule. Examination of nodal architecture enables the pathologist to assign a grade, which is important for prognosis. The most accessible, most easily removed lymph node is the popliteal lymph node, which is the preferred site of biopsy if the node is enlarged.

Prognostic Factors

General statistics for survival of canine lymphoma patients can be derived from reports of the efficacy of different chemotherapy protocols, but there is little information available to help form a prognosis for the individual patient. As more information becomes available, it is becoming clear that good clinical staging and ancillary laboratory testing provide important prognostic information.

In the future, histopathologic "subtyping" of lymphoma using specific antibodies and cell markers may provide prognostic information for individual patients. At present, however, the features known to be important in predicting outcome for dogs with lymphoma patients are described below:

Stage of Disease

Various studies have shown the prognostic importance of clinical staging; however, the details remain controversial. Some studies have suggested that dogs with less extensive diseases (i.e., stage I to III lymphoma) are more likely to achieve complete remission (CR) than are dogs in clinical stages IV and V.[9] In other studies, however, the percentage of dogs achieving remission was not correlated with stage of disease, but the duration of remission and survival were significantly higher in dogs with stage I to III lymphoma (Figure 5-8).[10–12] In some studies, the stage of disease was not of prognostic significance,[13] but the presence or absence of clinical illness (substage b or a, respectively) did predict remission duration and survival; dogs in substage b had shorter remission and survival times (Figure 5-9).[13–15]

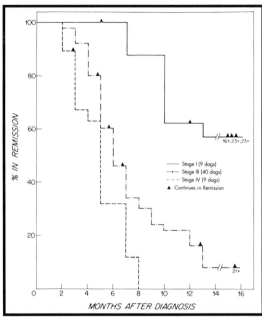

Figure 5-8: *Populations of dogs treated for lymphoma using combination chemotherapy (COP) separated according to clinical stage. Dogs with localized disease at diagnosis (stages I and II) have longer remissions than dogs with more advanced disease. (From Cotter S: Treatment of lymphoma and leukemia with cyclophosphamide, vincristine and prednisone: I. Treatment of dogs. JAAHA 19:159–165, 1983; with permission.)*

Hypercalcemia

Hypercalcemia is often associated with anterior mediastinal lymphoma; therefore, thoracic radiographs should always be considered in dogs with confirmed hypercalcemia. A dog with lymphoma and hypercalcemia is, by convention, considered to be in clinical substage b. Early studies found that the presence of hypercalcemia in dogs with lymphoma did not affect response to therapy or remission duration when these data were compared to historical controls. Mean survival time for hypercalcemic dogs, however, was shorter than for nonhypercalcemic dogs (118 and 198 days, respectively).[16]

> **KEY POINT:**
>
> *Dogs with advanced lymphoma, particularly if they are clinically ill, have a poor prognosis compared to healthy dogs with limited disease.*

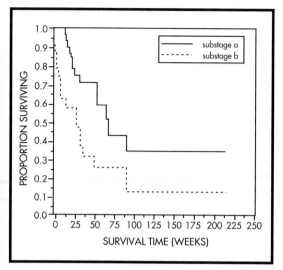

Figure 5-9: Survival curves for dogs with lymphoma, treated with the Madison-Wisconsin protocol, separated according to clinical substage (with or without clinical signs of illness). Substage a (no clinical signs) is associated with longer survival than substage b (clinical signs of illness present). (From Keller E, MacEwen E, Rosenthal R, et al: Evaluation of prognostic factors and sequential combination chemotherapy for canine lymphoma. J Vet Intern Med, 7:289–295, 1993; with permission.)

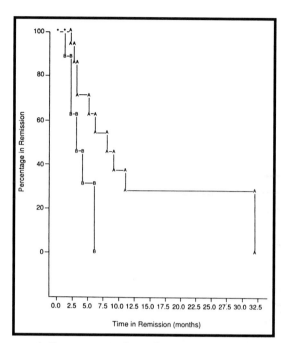

Figure 5-10: Correlation of remission duration and absence (A) or presence (B) of an anterior mediastinal mass in dogs with lymphoma and hypercalcemia treated with AMC-2 protocol. (From Rosenburg M, Matus R, Patnaik A: Prognostic factors in dogs with lymphoma and associated hypercalcemia. J Vet Intern Med 5:268–271, 1991; with permission.)

In a more recent study, 37 dogs with lymphoma and hypercalcemia were staged according to WHO criteria. An anterior mediastinal mass was found in 16 of 37 dogs (43%), and 15 of 37 (41%) had cytologic evidence of bone marrow involvement. For 26 dogs treated with chemotherapy, the median remission was 180 days. Of multiple factors studied, only the presence of an anterior mediastinal mass (AMM) was prognostic; dogs that did not have a mass had longer remission and survival times (280 days versus 90 days with AMM). Clinical stage, calcium concentration, and presence of azotemia were unrelated to prognosis.[17] Twenty-five percent of the dogs were alive at one year. Hypercalcemia, particularly in association with AMM, should be considered a poor prognostic sign (Figure 5-10).

> **KEY POINT:**
>
> *Dogs with lymphoma that have hypercalcemia and an anterior mediastinal mass have a poor prognosis.*

Sex

Some studies have found that female dogs, both sexually intact and spayed, had significantly longer remission and survival times than male dogs.[13,18]

Regardless of disease, female dogs have a longer age-adjusted, overall survival than do their male counterparts.[19] This is particularly important in evaluating the reported prognostic value of sex on response to chemotherapy for dogs with lymphoma.

Body Weight

Dogs that weighed less than or equal to 15 kg had longer survival times than larger dogs.[11] Drug dosages in this study were based on a mg/kg basis, which may tend to

MANAGEMENT OF SPECIFIC DISEASES

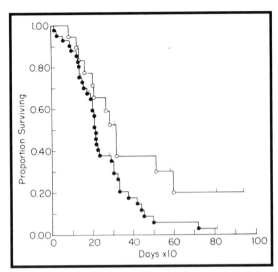

Figure 5-11: Correlation of survival with body weight for dogs with lymphoma that weigh less than or equal to 15 kg (open circles) or more than 15 kg (full circles) following chemotherapy using AMC-1 protocol. (From MacEwen E, Hayes A, Matus R, Kurzman I: Cyclic combination chemotherapy of canine lymphosarcoma. JAVMA 178:1178–1181, 1981; with permission.)

deliver relatively higher doses to smaller animals compared to dosages based on a m^2 body surface area (Figure 5-11). Other studies in which chemotherapeutics are dosed on both a mg/lb or mg/m^2 basis have not confirmed this association between body weight and survival.[13,20]

Response to Therapy

Survival times of patients with canine lymphoma are often biased because of persistence in treatment by the veterinarian and the owner, and most dogs are euthanatized at the owner's request rather than dying of natural causes. Response to therapy and quality of life are, therefore, important criteria in prolonging survival. If a dog shows only a partial remission (PR), its survival time is significantly shorter than if it achieved a complete remission (CR).[9,13]

Histologic Type

A variety of histologic grading schemes, including the Rappaport system, have not shown any correlation between histologic classification and prognosis. *Histiocytic lymphoma* is a little-used term in current pathologic description, and despite anecdotal reports of poor prognosis associated with this type of lymphoma, there is no statistical evidence for such an association.

Although the Rappaport system was not found to be of prognostic use, a system of histologic classification for canine lymphoma based on the *NCI Working Formulation* for classification of non-Hodgkin's lymphomas has shown some prognostic significance.[12] Canine lymphoma is morphologically heterogeneous, almost always diffuse (versus nodular), and usually high grade. Most canine lymphomas seem to fit into three morphologic groups: diffuse large cell, immunoblastic, and small lymphocytic (high grade).

Curiously, dogs with high-grade lymphomas are more likely to achieve complete clinical remission than dogs with intermediate-grade lymphoma, possibly due to a higher proportion of "cycling" cells in the tumor.[12] In addition, remission and survival times are usually longer in dogs with high-grade lymphomas.[21] In two studies, dogs with an immunoblastic cell type had higher CR rates and longer remission duration and survival times.[14,20] In some studies, however, no differences in remission duration or survival have been noted. Low-grade lymphoma is rare in dogs. In the few reported cases of low-grade lymphoma, response rates have been lower than for high- or intermediate-grade lymphoma, but survival times are often long, owing to a more indolent clinical course. Further studies that address the issue of histologic grades are needed to elucidate the prognostic significance of these data.

Pretreatment Steroid Therapy

It has been postulated that administration of glucocorticoids prior to

KEY POINT:

Dogs with immunoblastic-type lymphoma have a higher remission rate and longer survival than do dogs with other cell types.

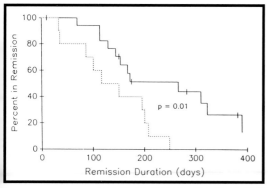

Figure 5-12: Remission duration for dogs with lymphoma treated with combination chemotherapy. Dogs that received corticosteroids prior to receiving chemotherapy had shorter remission (broken line) than dogs that did not receive corticosteroids prior to chemotherapy (solid line). (From Price G, Page R, Fischer B, et al: Efficacy and toxicity of doxorubicin/cyclophosphamide maintenance therapy in dogs with multicentric lymphosarcoma. J Vet Intern Med 5:259–262, 1991; with permission.)

other chemotherapeutic agents may change the staging of dogs by causing incomplete remission, thereby masking more advanced disease, which is known to be a poor prognostic sign. It is also possible that glucocorticoid therapy may induce multiple drug resistance in the malignant cells, as has been observed in human patients.[22]

In one study, 11 of 28 dogs with lymphoma received glucocorticoids before initiation of combination chemotherapy. They had significantly shorter remissions than dogs that did not receive glucocorticoids before treatment (134 versus 267 days). Duration of glucocorticoid treatment (more than 2 weeks compared to less than 2 weeks) did not influence this finding (Figure 5-12).[23]

Hypoalbuminemia

Hypoalbuminemia (albumin <2.8 g/dl) that was present before initiation of chemotherapy was a poor prognostic sign in one study; hypoalbuminemic dogs had a mean remission time of 108.5 days compared with 208 days for dogs with normal serum albumin. The cause of the low serum albumin was not investigated, although no dogs had proteinuria.[23]

Treatment
Discussion With the Owner

Once a definitive diagnosis has been obtained and after the patient has been staged accurately, the veterinarian should schedule a discussion with the owner regarding prognosis and treatment. This consultation should allow enough time to discuss the chances and the length of remission and survival balanced against costs and side effects. One of the most important distinctions to make for the client is between remission and cure. Remission is the absence of clinical evidence of lymphoma, whereas cure really only becomes a reality when remissions have been sustained for more than two years. When toxicities are discussed, the owner should be given criteria by which to distinguish mild side effects from those that can be life-threatening. A copy of the protocol to be administered, with scheduled treatments, rechecks, and blood counts, will assist owners in remembering much of the information they receive at this time. Well-informed owners whose pets are receiving chemotherapy are reliable, cooperative, and appreciative of a veterinarian's efforts to treat lymphoma.

First-Line Therapy

In this section, therapy for canine lymphoma is discussed under the subheadings "First-Line Therapy," which pertains to drugs and protocols used to induce remission in animals that have received no prior therapy, and "Rescue Therapy," which details drugs and protocols used to re-induce remission when lymphoma relapses on treatment with chemotherapy. Dogs with lymphoma in relapse are generally more difficult to induce into a subsequent remission. A graphic comparison of different chemotherapeutic protocols is seen in Figure 5-13.

> **KEY POINT:**
>
> *Glucocorticoids should not be given to dogs with lymphoma if future combination chemotherapy is planned.*

MANAGEMENT OF SPECIFIC DISEASES

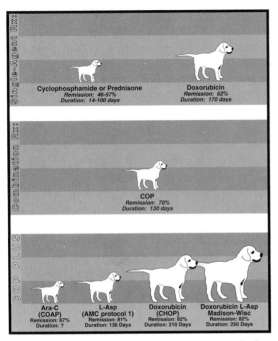

Figure 5-13: A graphic representation comparing the clinical responses and remission lengths for dogs with lymphoma when treated with chemotherapy.

Single-Agent Chemotherapy

Vincristine, cyclophosphamide, and prednisone provide the basis for most combination protocols to treat canine lymphoma, but surprisingly little information exists as to their efficacy as single agents. The results of studies using these and other drugs as single agents are summarized in Table 5-3.

Prednisone: Approximately 50% of dogs treated with prednisone have a partial or CR to treatment,[24–26] and that response usually lasts between 14 and 240 days[10,24,25] with an average of 53 days.[10]

Cyclophosphamide: Cyclophosphamide is probably more effective than prednisone as a single agent. More CRs occur for a median of 165 days.[25] The response rate apparently is dose-related. In one early study, successful treatment with cyclophosphamide was hindered by high-dosage regimens (240 mg/m² PO for 5 consecutive days) that resulted in mortality due to bone marrow aplasia.[27] Lower doses given in

combination with prednisone produced a response rate similar to that of prednisone alone.[10]

Vincristine: Vincristine was found to be more efficacious and less toxic than vinblastine (which is myelosuppressive) in treating canine lymphoma; however, no studies comparing vincristine with other single chemotherapeutic agents have been reported in detail.[28]

Chlorambucil: This alkylating agent was not as successful as cyclophosphamide in causing remission, even when used in conjunction with prednisone.[25] The major clinical use of chlorambucil is to substitute it for cyclophosphamide if animals develop hemorrhagic cystitis.

L-asparaginase: This agent has been used widely for the treatment of canine lymphoma because of its low rate of toxicity. Although the CR rate is low when used as a single agent, most dogs show a PR to L-asparaginase; therefore, it is a useful addition to combination protocols.[29,30] L-asparaginase and vincristine cause severe myelosuppression if given at the same time; this is presumably due to decreased hepatic clearance of the vincristine. If both drugs are to be used, it is best to separate their administration by at least 24 hours.[13,31]

The most common toxicity to L-asparaginase is hypersensitivity (anaphylaxis) to circulating antibodies. The covalent attachment of polyethylene glycol (PEG) conjugates to L-asparaginase produces a compound that is active, stable, without significant immune response, and has a greatly extended plasma half-life. Trials comparing "native" L-asparaginase with PEG-conjugated L-asparaginase in dogs demonstrated no differences in response rate, time to relapse, or overall survival between the two groups.[29,30] Adverse (allergic) reactions were uncommon in both groups; this was attributed to the intramuscular route of administration (compared with the intraperitoneal route, which produces a 20% to 47% adverse reaction rate).[11,30,32,33] L-asparaginase should be given intramuscularly to dogs.

Doxorubicin: Doxorubicin is considered the most active single agent in the treatment of canine lymphoma. It was reported to be successful as a "rescue"

MANAGEMENT OF SPECIFIC DISEASES

TABLE 5-3
Canine lymphoma treatment with single agents

Drug	Number of Dogs in CR	Total Dogs Treated	Percentage in CR (%)	Remission Range (Days)	Reference
Prednisone	26	57	46	14–210	10, 25
Cyclophosphamide	17	30	57	62–111	25, 59
Chlorambucil	2	9	22	?–615	25
Vincristine	—	—	—	<60	15
Vinblastine	5	8	63	30–180	43
Methotrexate	1	3	33	—	43
L-asparaginase	26	134	20	—	29, 30
Mitoxantrone	10	40	25	49–440	38
Ara-C	0	10	0	—	40
Epirubicin	26	37	70	—	41

agent (to reinduce clinical remission when the tumor was resistant to chemotherapy).[34] The response rates and durations for studies using doxorubicin as a single induction agent are found in Table 5-4. Overall, doxorubicin causes CR in about 70% of dogs treated, for a median of 165 days.

Toxicities are relatively common in dogs treated with doxorubicin at a dose of 30 mg/m², but they are usually mild and well tolerated by dogs and their owners. Of 37 dogs with lymphoma treated with doxorubicin in one study, toxicities occurred in 21 dogs (5 anaphylaxis, 3 cardiomyopathy, 9 GI, and 4 hematologic) and were mild in most dogs. Large dogs apparently were at greater risk of developing cardiomyopathy, whereas smaller dogs were more likely to develop other toxicities.[35]

The standard dose for doxorubicin in dogs is 30 mg/m² every 3 weeks, but there is evidence that weekly administration of a lower dose decreases the prevalence of cardiotoxicity in humans.[36] Nine dogs with lymphoma were treated with 15 weekly treatments of doxorubicin at a dose of 10 mg/m². This protocol was found to be safe in the dogs treated but was generally ineffective in achieving remission rates comparable to those provided by the standard protocol. Of 9 dogs, two had a CR (for 14 and 231 days) and five had a PR. Median remission duration was 14 days. Mild toxicosis was seen in three dogs.[37]

Mitoxantrone: When this drug was given as a single agent at a dose of 5 mg/m² IV to 40 dogs with untreated lymphoma, it induced a CR rate of 25% (10 dogs) with a median remission duration of 94 days (range 49 to 440 days).[38]

Mitoxantrone was delivered as a 1-hour intravenous infusion at a dose of 5 mg/m² every 3 weeks to 10 dogs with lymphoma that had achieved CR with L-asparaginase and prednisone. The median remission time was 119 days (range 28 to 483+ days) with five dogs in remission. Toxicities were similar to those described for mitoxantrone given as a bolus injection.[39]

Recent evidence suggests that 6.0

KEY POINT:

Doxorubicin is considered the most active single agent in the treatment of canine lymphoma.

TABLE 5-4
Canine lymphoma treatment with doxorubicin

Number of Dogs in CR	Total Dogs Treated	Percentage in CR (%)	Remission (Days)			Reference
			Mean	Median	Range	
28	38	74	—	180	—	42
7	11	64	—	124	21–218	55
22	37	59	—	151	44–734	35
16	21	76	190	206	—	12
18	38	47	—	38	—	20

TABLE 5-5
Canine lymphoma treatment with cyclophosphamide, vincristine, and prednisone (COP)

Number of Dogs in CR	Total Dogs Treated	Percentage in CR (%)	Remission (Days)			Reference
			Mean	Median	Range	
15	19	79	184	—	30–282	10
13	20	65	106	80	40–640	60
58	77	75	—	180	—	9
20	30	67	—	—	—	28
14	20	70	100	129	—	12
36	67	54	—	45	—	20

mg/m² may be a more appropriate dosage in dogs as toxicities below that dosage are uncommon and mild in nature.

Cytosine Arabinoside (ara-C): At various doses and schedules, cytosine arabinoside was not found to be a useful induction agent in one early study.[28] This was supported by a more recent trial in which 15 dogs with lymphoma received cytosine arabinoside (300 mg/m² for 2 consecutive days given as a continuous IV infusion) as an induction agent.[40] No dog responded to this treatment, and although the use of cytosine arabinoside has been recommended in combination protocols, its efficacy must be ques-

tioned. There was evidence of myelosuppression (principally thrombocytopenia) in this study (10 of 15 dogs). Although ara-C may be more effective in combination with alkylating agents, such as cyclophosphamide, care should be used in such combination protocols.[40]

Epirubicin: This derivative of doxorubicin has equivalent antitumor activity to doxorubicin in the treatment of human cancer but puts patients at considerably less risk of cardiotoxicity. Epirubicin was compared with doxorubicin for efficacy in the treatment of canine lymphoma. Dogs were given six treatments of either doxorubicin or epirubicin (both at a dose of 30 mg/m^2 IV) at 3-week intervals. For doxorubicin, 74% of 38 dogs achieved CR, whereas 70% of 37 dogs treated with epirubicin achieved CR. The median durations of remission were 180 and 143 days for doxorubicin and epirubicin, respectively. This drug is not currently available for the treatment of canine lymphoma.[41,42]

Actinomycin D: At a weekly dose of 0.75 mg/m^2 IV, actinomycin D caused remission in three of four dogs with lymphoma.[43] In a more recent study, actinomycin D (0.5 to 0.9 mg/m^2 IV every 3 weeks) was used to treat 12 dogs with lymphoma. Complete responses were seen in 5 of 12 dogs for a median duration of 63 days (range 21 to 105 days). Three of these dogs had not received prior treatment and had either a CR (84, 63 days) or a PR (42 days).[44] The efficacy of actinomycin D as a single induction agent is still uncertain.

Vinblastine: Vinblastine given at a weekly dose of 1.5 mg/m^2 IV resulted in objective responses in five of eight dogs. Remissions lasted one to six months.[43]

Methotrexate: At a weekly dose of 30 mg/m^2, methotrexate resulted in an objective response in one of three dogs.[43] Gastrointestinal toxicity is commonly encountered during treatment with methotrexate.

6-mercaptopurine: This drug was not found to be a useful induction agent for the treatment of canine lymphoma.[28]

Combination Protocols

COP Protocol: Much of the information regarding efficacy of treatment for canine lymphoma has come from studies using combinations of cyclophosphamide, vincristine, and prednisone. This combination has become known colloquially as COP (Cytoxan®, Oncovin®, prednisone) and forms the foundation for most currently used chemotherapy protocols (see COP PROTOCOL 1 and COP PROTOCOL 2).

The efficacy of COP protocol has been evaluated in seven published reports. There were minor variations in dosage and schedule. COP is a relatively nontoxic protocol and is relatively inexpensive. A brief summary of these studies is included in Table 5-5, and the two most commonly used COP protocols are schematically represented in the boxes. The two protocols illustrated appear equal in efficacy, and the choice between them is solely one of familiarity and comfort. Overall, COP chemotherapy causes complete remission in about 70% of dogs with lymphoma for a median of 130 days.

COP, L-asparaginase, and Methotrexate: Methotrexate is not widely used as a single agent for treating canine lymphoma; however, it does have some role in combination with other drugs for maintenance of remission. One hundred forty-seven dogs with lymphoma were treated with vincristine, L-asparaginase, cyclophosphamide, and methotrexate according to the protocol in the box (see AMC PROTOCOL 1). Complete response was achieved in 77% of the dogs, and PRs were seen in 17.7%. For dogs showing a CR, the median remission duration was 140 days and the median survival was 290 days.[13]

COP PROTOCOL 1[9]

Vincristine is administered at 0.75 mg/m^2 IV. Cyclophosphamide* is given at 300 mg/m^2 (*250 mg/m^2* may be a safer dosage in dogs) PO. The dose for prednisone is 1 mg/kg daily for 7 days, then QOD PO.

Week	Vincristine	Cyclophosphamide*	Prednisone
1	•	•	
2	•		
3	•		
4	•	•	
5			
6			
7	•	•	
10	•	•	
	⇓	⇓	↓

every three weeks

*If hemorrhagic cystitis occurs, chlorambucil is substituted on the same schedule at 15 mg/m^2 PO daily for 4 consecutive days (or 6 to 8 mg/m^2 PO daily continuously).

MANAGEMENT OF SPECIFIC DISEASES

COP PROTOCOL 2[60]

Vincristine is administered at 0.5 mg/m² IV. Cyclophosphamide* is given at 50 mg/m² daily for 4 consecutive days PO. The dose for prednisone is 10 mg/m² BID for 7 days, then 10 mg/m² daily.

Week	Vincristine	Cyclophosphamide*	Prednisone
1	•	•	
2	•	•	
3	•	•	
4	•	•	
5	•	•	
6	•	•	
7	•	•	
8	•	•	
	⇓	⇓	

The cycle is repeated to week 8, then repeated every 2 weeks to week 24, then every 3 weeks to week 48, and finally every 4 weeks.
*Chlorambucil 2 mg/m² PO is substituted on the same schedule from week 8.

A similar protocol in which L-asparaginase was given on days 7 and 14 did not improve either remission duration or survival, although a higher proportion of dogs appeared to enter CR.[11]

COP and Cytosine Arabinoside (COAP): Cytosine arabinoside recently has been shown to be ineffective as a single induction agent[40]; however, reported synergy with alkylating agents has been the basis for including it with COP. This synergy has not been marked in reported studies in which cytosine arabinoside at a dose of 100 mg/m² IV for the first 4 days of the first week was added to the protocol (COP PROTOCOL 2). CRs occurred in 67% of dogs, which was essentially the same response rate seen for the protocol without cytosine arabinoside.[15] Duration of the response was not evaluated.

Vincristine, Cyclophosphamide, Prednisone, and Doxorubicin (COPA): The exceptional efficacy of doxorubicin as an induction agent led to two studies using doxorubicin in combination with vincristine, cyclophosphamide, and prednisone. In one study, doxorubicin was used for the maintenance of remission induced by COP.[45] Surprisingly, overall remission durations and survival did not differ greatly from COP protocol; however, it is possible that the scheduling of doxorubicin in only the maintenance phase of the protocol may have influenced the outcome.

In a randomized study comparing COP and COP plus doxorubicin, more dogs achieved remission and that remission lasted longer if doxorubicin was administered.[46] Overall survival times did not differ, however.

Vincristine, Cyclophosphamide, Prednisone, Doxorubicin, and L-asparaginase Combination Protocols: A maintenance schedule identical to that just described (COP and doxorubicin[45]) was given to 41 dogs that were induced into remission using weekly doses of a combination of vincristine, L-asparaginase, and prednisone. Thirty one (76%) attained a CR for a median of 330 days, and 48% were still in remission at one year.[31] This group of dogs had longer remission times both overall and for dogs in clinical stage III than did dogs receiving COPA.[45] The protocol is summarized as ACOPA-1 in the box. Toxicity of this protocol was most marked during the induction phase; five dogs (12%) died during this period.[31] Myelosuppression was marked during induction and was somewhat unexpected, as the three induction drugs are not considered potent myelosuppressive agents. L-asparaginase, however, decreases hepatic clearance of vincristine, leading to more pronounced myelosuppression. It is inadvisable to administer L-asparaginase and vincristine on the same day.

A similar protocol (see ACOPA-2 PROTOCOL) used doxorubicin and prednisone for induction of remission and had a similar maintenance phase to the protocol just described. ACOPA-2 was found to induce fewer dogs into remission than ACOPA-1 (44 dogs, 65%), and the dogs that achieved remission had a shorter median remission time (228 days; 34% still in remission at 1 year). ACOPA-2 protocol was found to have a lower rate of induction toxicity than ACOPA-1.[47] These data imply that an aggressive induction is important for long-term remission.

AMC PROTOCOL 1[13]

Vincristine is administered at 0.7 mg/m² IV. Cyclophosphamide is given at 200 to 250 mg/m² IV. The dose for L-asparaginase is 400 IU/kg IP *(IM is a better route of administration)*. Methotrexate is given at 0.6 to 0.8 mg/kg PO.

Week	Vincristine	L-asparaginase	Cyclophosphamide	Methotrexate
1	●	●		
2			●	
3	●			
4				●
5	●			
6			●	
7	●			
8				●
	⇓		⇓	⇓
	every 2 weeks		every 4 weeks	every 4 weeks

ACOPA-1 PROTOCOL[31]

Vincristine is administered at 0.75 mg/m² IV. Cyclophosphamide* is given at 250 mg/m² PO. The dose for L-asparaginase is 10,000 IU/m² IM *(may be safer to give the day after each vincristine)* (maximum total dose per treatment = 10,000 IU). Doxorubicin is administered at 30 mg/m² IV. Prednisone is given at 40 mg/m² PO daily for 7 days, then QOD.

Week	Vincristine	L-asparaginase	Cyclophosphamide*	Doxorubicin	Prednisone
1	●	●			
2	●	●			
3	●	●			
4	●	●			
5					
6					
7	●		●		
10	●			●	
13	●		●		
16	●		●		

Repeat weeks 10 to 16 every 9 weeks until week 75 then cease.
*If hemorrhagic cystitis occurs, chlorambucil is substituted on the same schedule at 15 mg/m² PO daily for 4 consecutive days.

MANAGEMENT OF SPECIFIC DISEASES

ACOPA-2 PROTOCOL[47]

Vincristine is administered at 0.75 mg/m^2 IV. Cyclophosphamide* is given at 250 mg/m^2 PO. The dose for L-asparaginase is 10,000 IU/m^2 IM (maximum total dose 10,000 IU). Doxorubicin is administered at 30 mg/m^2 IV. Prednisone is given at 40 mg/m^2 PO daily for 7 days, then QOD.

Week	Doxorubicin	Vincristine	Cyclophosphamide*	L-asparaginase	Prednisone
1	•				
2					
3					
4		•	•		
5					
6					
7			•	•	
8				•	
10	•	•			
13		•	•		
16		•	•		
19	•	•			
22		•	•		
25				•	
26				•	
29					

From week 29 repeat weeks 10 to 16 every 9 weeks until week 75, then stop.
*If hemorrhagic cystitis occurs, chlorambucil is substituted on the same schedule at 15 mg/m^2 PO daily for 4 consecutive days.

Fifty-five dogs were treated with a sequential chemotherapy protocol that used vincristine and cyclophosphamide in combination with L-asparaginase, doxorubicin, and prednisone for induction of remission, and in combination with methotrexate for maintenance of remission (MADISON-WISCONSON PROTOCOL). Complete remission was achieved in 46 dogs (84%) for a median of 252 days. Fifty-two percent of the dogs were still alive one year after starting chemotherapy. Toxicities that required dose reduction occurred in 40% of the dogs.[18]

Fifty-five dogs with high- and intermediate-grade lymphoma that did not have hypercalcemia were treated with a combination chemotherapy protocol (AMC PROTOCOL 2). These dogs may have a slightly better prognosis than hypercalcemic dogs with lymphoma. Complete remission was achieved in 49 dogs (89%) for a median of 255 days. Approximately 50% of the dogs were still alive one year after starting chemotherapy.[21]

Current Recommendations

It is important that the client be given all the options and that the best option be used first. As a general rule, combination chemotherapy is superior to single-agent therapy. Each time an effective drug is

MANAGEMENT OF SPECIFIC DISEASES

added to the COP protocol, the remission time improves. Although the remission time increases with the addition of a drug, so does the cost and the potential for toxicity. It is also important that clients realize that a second or third remission is possible with appropriate therapy. These subsequent remissions are more difficult to attain and their duration is generally half the duration of the previous remission.

For clients who cannot afford or will not accept a combination chemotherapy protocol due to the risks of toxicity, a protocol using prednisone alone (40 mg/m² daily PO for 7 days then QOD) or in combi-

> **KEY POINT:**
>
> *Combination chemotherapy using vincristine, cyclophosphamide, prednisone, doxorubicin, and L-asparaginase provides long remission times with good quality of life for dogs with lymphoma.*

nation with chlorambucil (6 to 8 mg/m² QOD PO) may provide palliation with few risks of side effects. A complete blood count (CBC) should be collected every 2 to 3 weeks to make sure that myelosuppression is not occurring.

The COP protocol (either version) is a relatively inexpensive chemotherapy protocol with a low risk of toxicity. Dogs tolerate the treatments, and veterinarians find the protocol very manageable. Complete blood counts should be taken one week after each dose of cyclophosphamide to ensure that myelosuppression (if it occurs) is not severe and that doses do not need to be adjusted.

MADISON-WISCONSIN PROTOCOL[18]

Vincristine is administered at 0.5 to 0.7 mg/m² IV. L-asparaginase is given at 400 IU/kg IM. The dose for cyclophosphamide* is 200 mg/m² IV. Doxorubicin is administered at 30 mg/m² IV. Methotrexate is given at 0.5 to 0.8 mg/kg IV. The dose for prednisone is 2.0 mg/kg PO, week 1; 1.5 mg/kg PO, week 2; 1.0 mg/kg PO, week 3; and 0.5 mg/kg PO, week 4.

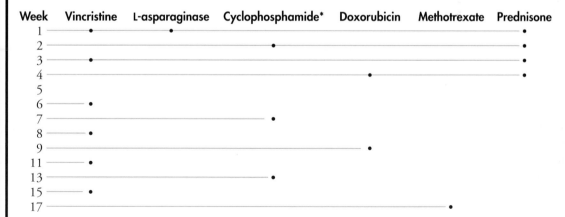

From week 17, repeat weeks 11 to 17 every two weeks. After week 25, treatments given every 3 weeks. After week 49, treatments given every 4 weeks.
*Replace with chlorambucil 1.4 mg/kg PO from week 11 if dog is in CR.

AMC PROTOCOL 2

Doxorubicin is administered at 30 mg/m^2 IV. Total cumulative dose of doxorubicin is 180 mg/m^2. Doses are the same as in the AMC PROTOCOL 1.

Week	Vincristine	L-asparaginase	Cyclophosphamide	Doxorubicin	Prednisone
1	•	•			•
2			•		•
3				•	•
4	•				
5			•		
6				•	

Repeat weeks 4–6 at 14-day intervals for 2 cycles, then repeat weeks 4–6 at 21-day intervals for 2 cycles.

Doxorubicin administered every 3 weeks for 5–8 treatments at a dosage of 30 mg/m^2 (1 mg/kg for small dogs) is the most effective single chemotherapeutic agent. This treatment regimen results in a relatively high remission rate with relatively few serious life-threatening toxicities (<5%). With the advent of generic doxorubicin, the cost is reasonable for most clients. Because the drug is given every three weeks, this treatment approach is less time intensive than most chemotherapeutic protocols. It appears that the second remissions are more likely if a dog is treated with doxorubicin and then COP to attain a second remission than if COP is used first.[12] Remission times for the two-protocol treatment approach is similar to the COPA protocol.[45]

By far, the most effective chemotherapy protocols to date use a five-drug combination of L-asparaginase, vincristine, cyclophosphamide, doxorubicin, and prednisone. Similar remission rates and survival times have been obtained for the protocols detailed as ACOPA-1, VELCAP (see box), AMC-2, and MADISON-WISCONSIN. The protocol ACOPA-2 is not recommended. Although these protocols require more intense client–veterinarian communication and monitoring for toxicity; the overall level of satisfaction for owners, pets, and veterinarians is high.

Other Treatment Modalities for Canine Lymphoma

Chemoimmunotherapy: The potential use of chemoimmunotherapy appears promising, and as further information is obtained using antibodies with different chemotherapeutic protocols, it may prove to be an efficacious and well-tolerated treatment modality.

Based on the premise that immunotherapy is presumably more effective after reduction of tumor burden, some dogs with lymphoma that achieved CR with chemotherapy have been treated with immunotherapy.

Early studies used an autochthonous tumor vaccine, which is made from tumor cells that have been extracted and acetoacetylated. This vaccine is administered intramuscularly to dogs in CR with Freunds complete adjuvant at 2, 3, 4, 6, and 8 weeks after finishing chemotherapy. Results of early studies did not show any benefit to this therapeutic approach.[48]

Antibody 231: Monoclonal antibodies were obtained from mice immunized with cultured canine lymphoma cells. One of these antibodies (CL/MAb 231, Synbiotics Corporation, San Diego, CA) bound to the cells of 73% of 15 lymphomas tested.[49] In vitro studies showed enhanced antibody-dependent

VELCAP PROTOCOL

Vincristine is administered at 0.75 mg/m² IV. Cyclosphosphamide* is given at 250 mg/m² PO. The dose for L-asparaginase is 10,000 IU/m² IM (maximum treatment dose = 10,000 IU). Doxorubicin† is administered at 25 mg/m² IV. Prednisone is given at 40 mg/m² SID PO for 7 days, then QOD.

Week	Vincristine	Cyclophosphamide*	L-asparaginase	Doxorubicin†
1	•			
2	•			•
3	•			
4				•
5				
6				
7	•	•	•	
8			•	
9			•	
12	•	•		
15	•	•		
18	•			•
21	•	•		
24		•	•	
25			•	
27	•			•

From week 28, repeat weeks 12 to 18 every 9 weeks until week 75, then stop.
*If hemorrhagic cystitis occurs, chlorambucil is substituted on the same schedule at 15 mg/m² PO daily for 4 consecutive days (or 6 to 8 mg/m² PO daily continuously).
†Echocardiograms are performed prior to each doxorubicin administration starting at sixth treatment.

cell-mediated cytotoxicity against canine lymphoma cells when canine mononuclear cells were combined with these antibodies.[50] A weekly cyclic chemotherapy protocol (L-asparaginase 400 IU/kg IP or SQ, week 1; vincristine 0.75 mg/m² IV, week 2; cyclophosphamide 75 mg/m² PO daily for 4 days, week 3; and doxorubicin 30 mg/m² IV, week 4) was repeated, with a 2-week interval between cycles. After a 3-week interval, CL/MAb 231 was administered daily for 5 days to dogs in CR.

Fifty-eight (75%) of 77 dogs achieved CR, and 42 of these dogs received monoclonal antibody (CL/MAb 231). Preliminary results showed a medi-an survival time of 591 days, with 17 dogs still alive. Median first remission duration was 128.5 days. The median number of chemotherapy cycles (4 weeks) received in the first year was three, and the median number of CL/MAb 231 cycles was one.[51] For a further 65 dogs treated with the same protocol, median survival was 633 days (range = 111–848 days). It is important to remember that CL/MAb 231 should only be administered to dogs in CR. This antibody is currently undergoing further evaluation.

Rescue Therapy

Durable first remissions in dogs with lymphoma

are achievable with available schedules and protocols, and most efforts are directed toward reducing toxicity and cost of therapy. In contrast, success in achieving durable second remissions is rare. Most "rescue" protocols result in remission rates of 30% or less, and the duration of these second remissions is generally short. More work is needed to develop efficacious "rescue" protocols.

> **KEY POINT:**
>
> *For most dogs with lymphoma, second remissions are difficult to obtain and are of short duration.*

Single-Agent Chemotherapy

Mitoxantrone: Mitoxantrone was given as a single agent at a dose of 5 mg/m² IV to 34 dogs that had failed to respond or relapsed from other chemotherapy. Twenty-six percent of the dogs (n = 9) had a CR for a median of 126 days (range = 42–792 days).[38] Although the response rate is low, it is interesting to note that it is similar to that for mitoxantrone used for induction of remission in previously untreated dogs (see page 239).

Actinomycin D: In one study, this drug was given to dogs that had failed previous chemotherapy, and a high response rate was seen.[44] In another study, however, 30 dogs that had relapsed on combination chemotherapy protocols were treated with actinomycin D at a dose of 0.5 to 0.9 mg/m² IV every 3 weeks.[52] None of the dogs in this group responded despite a higher average dose rate than the previous study. The efficacy of actinomycin D as a rescue agent for dogs that have received doxorubicin appears poor, possibly as a result of tumor-cell cross-resistance to these two agents.

Etoposide (VP-16): A dosage of 100 mg/m² IV or 25 mg/m² IV for 4 days of etoposide was given to 13 dogs that had failed to respond to, or had relapsed on, combination chemotherapy. Only one dog responded completely for 30 days (and partially for another 90 days). Eleven of 13 dogs showed cutaneous reactions; these reactions were severe in three dogs and were not alleviated by diphenhydramine or corticosteroids. Six dogs were sedated using ketamine and diazepam to minimize discomfort.[53] These toxic reactions are believed to result from canine sensitivity to polysorbate 80, a drug-delivery vehicle used in etoposide.[54] Intravenously administered etoposide is *not* recommended for routine use in dogs, and oral etoposide has not been well evaluated for the treatment of lymphoma in dogs.

Combination Chemotherapy

Dacarbazine (DTIC) and Doxorubicin: Dacarbazine has not been evaluated for single-agent activity in the treatment of canine lymphoma. Owing to observed synergy with doxorubicin in the treatment of human lymphoma patients, DTIC was given in combination with doxorubicin to nine dogs with lymphoma. Six dogs had failed to respond to doxorubicin; five of these six dogs achieved CR with the combination for a median of 87 days (range = 32–281 days). Another three previously untreated dogs that were treated with the combination achieved CR for 30, 89, and 106 days, respectively. The DTIC dosage was 133 to 167 mg/m² IV as a 5-day course every 3 weeks. The doxorubicin dose ranged from 36.5 to 40.0 mg/m² every 3 weeks.[55]

Doxorubicin and DTIC were given to 15 dogs with lymphoma resistant to a combination chemotherapy protocol that had included doxorubicin. Doxorubicin dosage was 30 mg/m² every 3 weeks, and dacarbazine was given at 200 mg/m² IV for 5 days every 3 weeks. Complete remission was achieved in 5 of 15 dogs.[56]

MOPP: The combination of mechlorethamine, vincristine, procarbazine, and prednisone (MOPP) has been relatively effective in the treatment of Hodgkin's disease in humans. As a rescue protocol, MOPP was given on a 28-day cycle to 17 dogs with relapsed lymphoma. Mechlorethamine (6 mg/m² IV) and vincristine (0.7 mg/m² IV) were given on day 1, and procarbazine (100 mg/m² PO) and prednisone (30 mg/m² PO) were given daily from day 1 through 14. Severe myelosuppression necessitated reductions in dose to 3 mg/m² mechlorethamine and 50 mg/m² procarbazine. Complete remission was seen in 35%

of dogs (53% showing a PR) for a median remission duration of 28 days (mean = 50 days). This protocol was severely myelosuppressive; two thirds of the dogs became leukopenic, and six died from this toxicity.[57]

At the lower dosages described, MOPP was used to treat another 12 dogs with resistant lymphoma. Median remission duration was still 28 days (range = 0–224 days), and toxicities were considerably less common.[57] Anecdotal information suggests improved second remission duration as more dogs are treated.

Cisplatin and Cytosine Arabinoside: Ten dogs with resistant lymphomas were treated with cisplatin (50 mg/m^2 IV every 3 weeks) and cytosine arabinoside (100 mg/m^2 every 7 days; IV on day 0 and SQ on day 7 and 14). Although this protocol had little associated toxicity, only one dog had a CR, which lasted 56 days, and two dogs had PRs for 30 and 108 days.[58]

LYMPHOMA IN CATS
Incidence, Signalment, and Etiology

Lymphoma accounts for approximately 90% of the hematopoietic tumors in both dogs and cats, and cats have a higher incidence of lymphoma than do dogs or humans.

The average age of occurrence for feline lymphoma is 3 years for feline leukemia virus (FeLV)-positive cats and 7 years for FeLV-negative cats. The majority of cats with lymphoma are FeLV-positive (70%); however, both FeLV-positive and FeLV-negative lymphoma cells can have tumor-specific feline oncornavirus-associated cell membrane antigen (FOCMA) on their membranes, indicating that FeLV may cause both types of feline lymphoma.[62]

Neutering reduces the incidence of lymphoma by 40% to 50% in female cats, and age at neutering apparently is important in this effect.[19] Intact male and female cats were at high risk of developing lymphoma, which is consistent with the epidemiology of FeLV-associated diseases.

No breed predilection has been noted for cats. Manx and Burmese breeds, however, were found to be at increased risk in one study.[63]

As previously stated, the majority of reported feline lymphomas occur in FeLV-positive cats. In addition, the anatomic distribution of lymphoma in cats varies with the concurrence of FeLV. For example, although approximately 80% of cats with multicentric or mediastinal lymphoma test positive for FeLV, fewer than 25% of cats with alimentary lymphoma test positive.[64]

Clinical Presentation and History

In contrast to dogs, most cats present with visceral involvement rather than generalized lymphadenopathy. The most common sites of occurrence for feline lymphoma are the alimentary tract, anterior mediastinum, liver, spleen, and kidneys. Less common sites include the skin, eyes, and central nervous system.

These lymphoma types have been grouped according to anatomic distribution by a number of investigators. The most commonly used classification recognizes alimentary, mediastinal, multicentric, and miscellaneous categories for feline lymphoma. Some investigators have designated renal lymphoma as a distinct entity, and extranodal lymphomas are often classified as miscellaneous lymphoma. The term *multicentric* is confusing, as some investigators include liver and spleen involvement as well as renal lymphoma in this category. We recommend using the staging system found on page 251 in conjunction with the above anatomic distribution to describe the lymphoma accurately.

In one study, multicentric feline lymphoma was the most commonly observed form; it occurred in 43.6% of 454 cats. Mediastinal (38.3%) and alimentary (15.2%) were the next most common sites of lymphoma.[64] In another study of 150 cats with lymphoma, the alimentary form was more common (46.7% of the cases) than were the mediastinal

> **KEY POINT:**
>
> *Most cats with mediastinal lymphoma are FeLV antigenemic; alimentary lymphoma, however, is rarely associated with FeLV antigenemia.*

MANAGEMENT OF SPECIFIC DISEASES

(25.4%) or multicentric (18.6%) forms.[65] The definition of the multicentric type of lymphoma, however, varied between the two studies. At Tufts University, alimentary lymphoma is the most common type of lymphoma diagnosed, accounting for more than 30% of the cases.

Alimentary lymphoma is defined as involving the GI tract itself or the mesenteric lymph nodes. It is rarely associated with FeLV antigenemia and affects old cats. The clinical presentation for 29 cats with alimentary lymphoma was recently reviewed at Tufts University. FeLV antigenemia was present in four of these cats, which represented an older population with no gender predilection. Presenting signs included vomiting (15 cats) and diarrhea (5 cats), but interestingly, 13 cats showed only anorexia or weight loss as an indication of GI disease. Most of the 29 cats had a palpable abdominal mass, and GI or mesenteric lymph node involvement was confirmed by ultrasonography, endoscopy, and/or exploratory surgery (Figure 5-14).[66]

Cats with renal lymphoma present with signs of acute renal failure and on physical examination have very large, occasionally painful, kidneys. Cats with renal lymphoma have been reported to have a high rate of relapse in the central nervous system compared to lymphoma of other primary sites.[67]

Spinal lymphoma is the most common cause of posterior paresis in cats. Cats with spinal lymphoma often are FeLV-positive, and most have bone marrow that contains lymphoblasts.[68] This is important in deciding whether to perform a laminectomy to obtain a definitive diagnosis of lymphoma, as confirmation may be best made by bone marrow aspiration (see also the chapter on Tumors of the Nervous System).

Generalized peripheral lymphadenopathy, as seen in dogs, is rarely associated with lymphoma in cats. Feline lymphoid hyperplasia is the most common cause of lymphadenopathy. Hyperplasia may occur due to a number of causes, including bacterial infection, der-

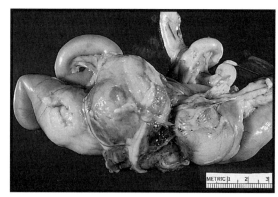

Figure 5-14: Intestinal lymphoma from a 4-year-old cat, showing transmural infiltration with secondary rupture and localized peritonitis. Intestinal lymphoma is usually diffuse and often is associated with abdominal adhesions, making surgical intervention difficult.

matitis, or other antigenic stimulus. Many cats, however, have lymphadenopathy with no identifiable cause. In one report, 82 of 132 cats with lymphadenopathy were classified as having idiopathic hyperplasia.[69] In two other studies, affected cats were young (most younger than 1 year of age) and nodes were two to three times normal size.[70,71] The lymphadenopathy regressed without therapy within four months in all cats.

In cats with generalized lymphadenopathy, dermatologic or systemic disease should be considered. Both FeLV and feline immunodeficiency virus (FIV) have been associated with lymphadenopathy, and tests for these viruses should be performed. Nodes should be measured, their size monitored, and the cat observed for other signs of illness. Lymph node aspirates are unlikely to provide a diagnosis unless organisms are found (e.g., cryptococcus) or metastatic neoplasia is discovered. Occasionally, a misdiagnosis of lymphoma may be made from cytologic specimens and an excisional biopsy is mandatory to distinguish lymphoma from hyperplasia. Use of corticosteroids to treat benign lymphoid hyperplasia is contraindicated, as immunosuppression

KEY POINT:

Spinal lymphoma is the most common cause of posterior paresis in cats.

MANAGEMENT OF SPECIFIC DISEASES

TABLE 5-6
Clinical stages of feline lymphosarcoma[67]

Clinical Stage	Criteria
Stage I	A single tumor (extranodal) or single anatomic area (nodal), including anterior mediastinum
Stage II	A single tumor (extranodal) with regional lymph node involvement Two or more nodal areas or extranodal tumors on the same side of the diaphragm A resectable primary GI tract tumor, with or without involvement of associated lymph nodes
Stage III	Two or more nodal areas or extranodal tumors above and below the diaphragm All unresectable intra-abdominal disease All paraspinal or epidural tumors
Stage IV	Stages I–III with involvement of the liver and/or spleen
Stage V	Stages I–IV with involvement of the CNS, bone marrow, or both

may allow an undetected agent to escape immuno-logic control.

Staging and Diagnosis

When evaluating an animal for treatment of lymphoma, it is important not only to obtain a definitive diagnosis but also to assess the general health of the patient by clinical examination and ancillary diagnostics. These include blood work, urinalysis and viral serology, thoracic and abdominal radiographs, bone marrow aspiration, and biopsy of lymphomatous tissue. This will also allow accurate evaluation of the extent of involvement of all the patient's organs and systems with lymphoma and will enable other unrelated or secondary conditions to be treated or controlled before instituting therapy.

A staging system similar to that used in dogs has been devised for cats; however, the high rate of visceral involvement in cats makes the staging process more difficult. The staging system (Table 5-6) provides some prognostic information, but cats should also be evaluated as to the anatomic location of their lymphoma. The procedures for staging are similar to those in dogs, and this section focuses on the specific differences in procedures for clinically staging cats.

The clinical stage of a cat affected with lymphoma is often determined by physical examination. Abdominal palpation may reveal organomegaly, and lymphomatous infiltration of the spleen or liver can be confirmed with further ancillary testing, such as fine-needle aspiration or biopsy. Abdominal masses are usually composed of adhesions between lymphomatous intestinal tract and associated lymphadenopathy. The thorax should be carefully auscultated and palpated, as some cats with anterior mediastinal lymphoma may have an incompressible thorax.

On thoracic radiographs, it may be possible to appreciate a mediastinal mass or pleural effusion. If biopsy of a mediastinal mass is being considered, particularly if pleural effusion is present, ultrasonography provides an accurate guide and a relatively safe means of obtaining a tissue or fluid sample. In addition, when involvement of abdominal viscera is suspected, ultrasonography allows evaluation of spleen and liver homogeneity as well as renal architecture and can be used to detect enlarged lymph nodes or

MANAGEMENT OF SPECIFIC DISEASES

GI involvement. Ultrasound-guided biopsy, particularly in cats with GI tract involvement, has proven to be efficacious in obtaining diagnostic samples.[72]

Anemia in cats with lymphoma is common, but it is usually low grade and characterized as normocytic, normochromic, which is compatible with anemia of chronic disease. Moderate to severe anemia may be present in animals experiencing blood loss from GI involvement or is occasionally due to immune-mediated destruction. Anemia is rarely a consequence of bone marrow infiltration, particularly if granulocyte and platelet counts are normal, because of the relatively long life span of the mature erythrocyte (73 days) compared to platelets (5 to 6 days) or neutrophils (10 hours).[8] Anemia in cats with lymphoma may also occur secondary to FeLV infection. A bone marrow aspirate may demonstrate red cell aplasia or myelofibrosis.

Lymphocytosis should prompt critical evaluation of lymphocyte morphology, because circulating lymphoblasts imply bone marrow involvement and a worse prognosis for remission. In this situation, bone marrow aspiration should be performed. If there is bone marrow infiltration without other clinical findings, the disease is designated as a lymphoblastic leukemia (see the chapter on Bone Marrow Neoplasia).

Serum chemistry profiles may be used to stage cats with lymphoma. Elevated hepatic enzyme levels, particularly in the presence of cranial abdominal organomegaly, may imply infiltration of the liver with lymphoma. Elevated BUN or serum creatinine levels are rarely associated with hypercalcemia in cats, which differs from dogs with lymphoma. Azotemic cats may have renal lymphoma. Another paraneoplastic syndrome that may occur in cats with lymphoma is monoclonal gammopathy, which may be detected by serum electrophoresis. This syndrome may be associated with hyperviscosity (see the chapter on Plasma Cell Tumors).

KEY POINT:

The majority of cats with spinal lymphoma have lymphoblastic infiltration of bone marrow. Bone marrow aspiration may be a less invasive, more rapid method of diagnosis than laminectomy.

Endoscopy can be used to obtain diagnostic samples from the stomach, duodenum, and colon. The advantages of endoscopy are that it is minimally invasive and does not cause the morbidity associated with laparotomy. In many cases, deep biopsies are required to make a histologic diagnosis. Although endoscopic biopsy is effective for obtaining superficial biopsy specimens, surgical biopsies may be needed to obtain submucosal samples.

All cats with lymphoma should be tested for FeLV antigenemia and presence of antibodies to FIV. Both viruses are associated with feline lymphoma, and the presence of FeLV has prognostic significance for survival.

In cats with lymphadenopathy, a definitive diagnosis of lymphoma is based on histologic examination of a surgically resected lymph node. This is preferable to a needle or a wedge biopsy, because an entire lymph node can be examined for key histopathologic evidence of malignancy, such as disruption of architecture and invasion of the capsule. In cats with generalized lymphadenopathy, cytologic evaluation does not help differentiate lymphoma from lymphoid hyperplasia; therefore, a biopsy is mandatory.

The diagnosis of lymphoma also may be confirmed by cytologic demonstration of malignant lymphoid cellular infiltration in organs or organ systems (e.g., GI tract or anterior mediastinum) that do not ordinarily contain lymphoid cells.

Prognostic Factors

General statistics for survival of feline lymphoma patients can be derived from reports of the efficacy of different chemotherapy protocols, but there is little information available to help form a prognosis for an individual cat. As more information becomes available, it is becoming clear that good clinical staging and ancillary laboratory testing provide important prognostic information.

MANAGEMENT OF SPECIFIC DISEASES

Stage of Disease

The stage of disease was significantly related to response to therapy in one study. Complete response rates were as follows: stage I (93%), stage II (48%), stage IV (42%), and stage V (58%). The stage of disease also was related to survival; cats with less advanced disease (stages I and II) had median survival times of 7.6 months, compared with 3.2 months for cats in stages III and IV, and 2.6 months for those in stage V (Figure 5-15).[73]

Stage of disease was important for prognosis in cats with lymphoma primarily involving the kidneys. Interestingly, the presence of azotemia was not a prognostic indicator in these cats[67] and often resolved with treatment of the lymphoma.

Anatomic Site

Mediastinal lymphoma had the highest rate of CR in one study (89%); median remission duration was 24 weeks.[74] By contrast, in another study, only 45% of 31 cats with mediastinal lymphoma attained complete remission for a median remission of 8 weeks.[75] Peripheral lymphadenopathy without other system involvement carried a good prognosis in both studies; most cats achieved CR for a median of over 2 years. To confuse the issue, it is possible that some of these cats may have had "atypical" feline lymphoid hyperplasia rather than lymphoma, thereby accounting for the high response rate.

Response to Therapy

Cats that achieve a CR after chemotherapy have longer survival than do cats that obtain a PR.[73, 74] In addition, cats that were induced into remission with chemotherapy, but not given further chemotherapy, relapsed more rapidly than did those that received continued treatment, indicating the importance of maintenance chemotherapy beyond the induction phase.[76]

FeLV Status

FeLV test status has been shown in some studies to have some prognostic significance for survival of cats with lymphoma. Cats positive for FeLV antigen have

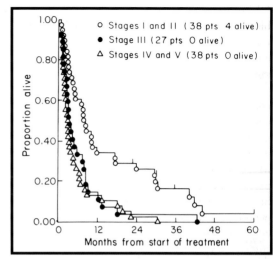

Figure 5-15: *Correlation of survival time and stage of lymphoma for cats treated with VCM plus L-asparaginase. Cats with less advanced disease (stages I and II) lived significantly longer than cats with more advanced disease (stages III, IV, and V). Pts = patients. (From Mooney S, Hayes A, MacEwen E, et al: Treatment and prognostic factors in lymphoma in cats: 103 cases (1977–1981). JAVMA 194:696–699, 1989; with permission.)*

shorter survival times[73]; however, FeLV status does not influence response to therapy.[73,74] Therefore, survival data may actually be influenced by other concurrent FeLV-related diseases, such as anemia and immunosuppression, rather than by the cancer itself.

Stage and FeLV

There was no difference in survival times for cats in stages III, IV, and V regardless of FeLV status; however, cats in stage I and II with a positive FeLV test result had a median survival of 4 months compared to 17.5 months for FeLV-negative cats with stage I or II lymphoma (Figure 5-16).[73] Similarly, for 28 cats with renal lymphoma, prognosis was best for FeLV-negative cats with stage II disease.[67]

Treatment

Cats have a higher incidence of lymphoma than do dogs or humans; however, although major advances have been made in the treatment of canine lym-

phoma with agents such as doxorubicin and L-asparaginase and the cre-
ation of multidrug chemotherapy
protocols, the treatment of feline
lymphoma has received scant attention. As newer drugs and protocols
are evaluated, improved remission
and survival times for cats with lymphoma can be expected.

median remission duration for these
18 cats was 183 days (range =
30–825 days) with two cats still alive
and off treatment at 351 and 825
days. One cat died in remission at
220 days of unknown causes.[79] The
dose-limiting toxicities are leukopenia and anorexia, as reported with
other anthracycline derivatives, such
as doxorubicin. The ease and nonin-
vasive nature of administration makes idarubicin an
attractive option for the client, and the remissions
seen imply that other anthracyclines (e.g., doxorubicin) may be useful in the treatment of feline lymphoma. Unfortunately, there is little reported information as to the efficacy of doxorubicin in this
disease. Preliminary results of a study using doxorubicin in combination with other chemotherapeutics
are detailed below.

Mitoxantrone: This agent (6.5 mg/m² IV every 3
weeks) did not seem to treat feline lymphoma effectively; only 1 of 11 cats had an objective response to
treatment.[80]

First-Line Therapy
Single-Agent Chemotherapy

Prednisone/Cyclophosphamide/Chlorambucil: Six
cats with lymphoma were treated with prednisone
(n = 2), cyclophosphamide (n = 1), chlorambucil
(n = 2) and chlorambucil plus prednisone (n = 1).
Responses were seen in all three cats treated with
prednisone, either alone or with chlorambucil. The
cat treated with cyclophosphamide had a CR for 14
months. The two cats treated with chlorambucil
alone did not respond.[25] Other responses to cyclophosphamide and to cyclophosphamide and prednisone were reported in early studies; however, the
duration of these responses was rarely provided.

Vincristine: Cats that were resistant to the above
combination achieved remission when treated with
vincristine, and this agent resulted in long-term
remissions and even cures when used as a single
agent.[28,77]

L-asparaginase: The use of this agent resulted in an
unmaintained remission of 2 months in one of four
cats.[78] Two cats achieved CR in stage III and V disease.[78]

Idarubicin: This agent is an anthracycline derivative that is more active in vitro than its parent compound, daunorubicin, but it is less cardiotoxic in vitro. In addition, the drug is active by both parenteral
and oral routes of administration.

Idarubicin (2 mg/day PO for 3 consecutive days,
every 21 days) treatment resulted in CRs in two cats
with lymphoma. In a study of the utility of idarubicin for treatment of feline lymphoma, 18 cats that
achieved remission following vincristine, cyclophosphamide, and prednisone (COP) therapy were treated from week 4 with idarubicin as a single agent. The

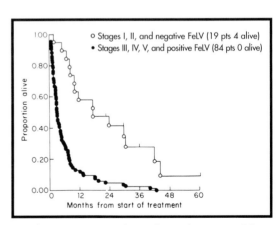

Figure 5-16: *Correlation of survival time, stage of disease,
and FeLV status in 103 cats with lymphoma treated with
VCM plus L-asparaginase. FeLV-negative cats with less
advanced disease have considerably longer survival times.
FeLV does not influence whether a cat achieves remission;
however, it does influence overall survival. Pts = patients.
(From Mooney S, Hayes A, MacEwen E, et al: Treatment and
prognostic factors in lymphoma in cats: 103 cases (1977–
1981). JAVMA 194:696–699, 1989; with permission.)*

MANAGEMENT OF SPECIFIC DISEASES

Combination Chemotherapy

As with dogs treated for lymphoma, a combination protocol using the three most effective single chemotherapeutic agents has been used to treat a number of cats. Vincristine, cyclophosphamide, and prednisone (COP protocol) still provide the basis of most chemotherapy protocols for feline lymphoma.

Vincristine, Cyclophosphamide, and Prednisone (COP): Thirty-eight cats with lymphoma were treated with vincristine (0.75 mg/m² IV weekly for 4 weeks, then every 3 weeks), cyclophosphamide (300 mg/m² PO every 3 weeks), and prednisone (2 mg/kg/day).[74] Complete remission was attained in 79% of cats. Remission durations ranged from 42 days to more than 42 months (median = 150 days). Remission rates varied with anatomic site; highest rates were for mediastinal (92% CR; 2–29 months, median = 6 months) or peripheral lymphadenopathy. Cats had a lower CR rate than did dogs treated with the same chemotherapy protocol and were more likely to relapse early in therapy than dogs; however, when compared to dogs, a higher percentage of cats remained in CR after 12 months.

In a series of 21 cats with spinal lymphoma, nine cats were treated with COP chemotherapy and one cat with surgical decompression and chemotherapy. Of six cats receiving vincristine, cyclophosphamide, and prednisone, three attained a CR, with a median duration of 14 weeks (range = 5–28 weeks). Three cats attained a PR (median = 6 weeks; range = 4–10 weeks). Three cats were given prednisone alone. Of those cats, one cat had no response and two had a PR for 4 and 10 weeks, respectively. The cat treated with surgery and chemotherapy had a CR for 62 weeks. On relapse, treatment with doxorubicin (30 mg/m² IV) resulted in a further CR.[68]

Twenty-eight cats with alimentary lymphoma were treated with COP chemotherapy. Eleven cats received other drugs, including doxorubicin, L-asparaginase, chlorambucil, idarubicin, and mitoxantrone after failing to achieve or maintain remission with COP. Response to therapy was determined by improvement in clinical signs, reduction in the size of a palpable mass, or by ultrasonography. The lymphoma primarily involved the intestinal tract (rather than stomach) in approximately 70% of the cats. Median survival with chemotherapy was 50 days; however, the mean was 239 days (range = 2–2120 days). Nine cats had a CR for a median of 213 days (mean = 545 days). Although most cats responded poorly to chemotherapy, a subpopulation of cats had long survival times and four cats survived more than one year.[66] Survival times did not seem to be influenced by the extent of the lymphoma within the GI tract, nor by the anatomic location or clinical stage. Response to therapy may be the most reliable indicator for prognosis of cats with GI lymphoma.

Nutritional support is extremely important in cats with alimentary lymphomas, as anorexia and vomiting are two of the major clinical signs associated with this form of the disease. It may be necessary to place a feeding tube to maintain alimentation (and hence body weight) in a cat undergoing treatment for GI lymphoma. If vomiting occurs in association with the lymphoma, a jejunostomy tube may be required. If the cat is not vomiting, a nasogastric, pharyngostomy, or gastrotomy tube can be used.

Vincristine, Cyclophosphamide, and Methotrexate (VCM): In another protocol, lymphoma was treated in 75 cats with vincristine (0.025 mg/kg IV, weeks 1 and 3), cyclophosphamide (10 mg/kg IV, week 2), and methotrexate (0.8 mg/kg PO [IV if GI lymphoma], week 4).[75] This 4-week cycle was continued. Of 62 cats that had follow-up examinations, 32 (52%) attained CR for a median of 16 weeks. Forty-four cats also received prednisone, and 36 also received L-asparaginase. Cats with mediastinal lymphoma did not fare as well in this study, with only 45% of cats achieving CR for a median of 8 weeks.

VCM plus L-asparaginase: The same protocol just described (with the addition of L-asparaginase at 400 IU/kg IP on week 1 of cycle 1) was given to 103 cats with lymphoma.[73] Responses were classified as CR if there was a 75% or greater reduction in tumor volume. Sixty-four cats (62%) had a CR, with median survival of 7 months (response durations not given). Thirty percent of cats showing CR were alive at one year. Stage of disease was related to response and sur-

MANAGEMENT OF SPECIFIC DISEASES

vival, whereas FeLV status adversely affected survival but not response to therapy.

VCM plus L-asparaginase and Cytosine Arabinoside (Renal Lymphoma): A series of 28 cats with renal lymphoma was treated with the same protocol just described, with the addition of cytosine arabinoside (ara-C) (600 mg/m² SQ) in 10 cats. Response criteria were the same as for the earlier series. Seventeen cats (61%) had a CR with median remission duration of 127 days (range = 20–2542+ days). Forty percent of the cats not treated with ara-C developed CNS lymphoma, and none of the cats treated with ara-C developed CNS relapse.[67] This association has not been reported by other investigators.

COP plus Doxorubicin: Thirty-six cats with lymphoma were treated with COP chemotherapy. Eighteen cats that achieved CR of their lymphoma were randomized at week 7 of therapy to receive maintenance chemotherapy that was either COP or single-agent doxorubicin for a total duration of six months. Median remission in 11 cats that continued to receive COP was 83 days. The median remission for seven cats that received doxorubicin was 259 days[81] (A.S. Moore, unpublished data).

Current Recommendations

The COP protocol[74] remains a moderately effective, relatively nontoxic and inexpensive method of treating feline lymphoma. The most commonly observed toxicities that occur during the first four weeks of vincristine therapy are anorexia and vomiting, which result in weight loss. If severe, these signs warrant a short delay before administering the next therapy (7 days or less) and a reduction in dose (from 0.75 to 0.65 mg/m² is usually sufficient). Supportive measures, such as subcutaneous fluid administration and appetite stimulants (e.g., cyproheptadine 2–4 mg BID–TID PO), assist in rapid recovery. Hemorrhagic cystitis following cyclophosphamide

administration is rare in cats; however, myelosuppression often occurs seven days after administration. A CBC should be performed one week after each cyclophosphamide dose, and the dosage for all subsequent treatments should be reduced by 25% if the segmented neutrophil count is below 1000 cells/μl.

If the lymphoma proves resistant to COP, doxorubicin at a dose of 25 mg/m² IV every 3 weeks may be used as a "rescue" agent. Anorexia seems to be the most common doxorubicin-induced toxicity in cats, and myelosuppression results in a neutrophil nadir at 7 to 10 days. Supportive therapy should be provided as for vincristine toxicity, and a dose reduction to 20 mg/m² in the case of neutropenia (as noted earlier) is usually sufficient to prevent recurrence of doxorubicin toxicity. Doxorubicin-induced cardiomyopathy is less common in cats than in dogs; however, some investigators believe that doxorubicin produces a cumulative renal toxicity. It is probably prudent to monitor renal function in cats receiving long-term doxorubicin therapy until this toxicity is further evaluated.

The success of COP plus doxorubicin implies that changing the chemotherapeutic maintenance protocol may result in longer remission times.[81] Doxorubicin should also be evaluated for the induction of remission in cats with lymphoma.

Other chemotherapeutic agents, such as L-asparaginase and chlorambucil, are rarely effective in treating feline lymphoma; however, toxicities are uncommon with these two drugs, and their use may be warranted in refractory cases. L-asparaginase (10,000 IU/m² IM) and chlorambucil (2 mg/cat QOD PO) appear to be safe dosages in the cat.

Radiation Therapy

Ten cats with localized (stage I) lymphoma that involved the nasal cavity (n = 3), retrobulbar area (n = 3), mediastinum, subcutaneous tissue, maxilla, and mandible (n = 1 each) were treated with radiation therapy. Four cats also received

> **KEY POINT:**
>
> *Combination chemotherapy using doxorubicin, vincristine, cyclophosphamide, and prednisone provides long remission times with good quality of life for cats with lymphoma.*

chemotherapy. Overall, median remission time for the eight cats that achieved CR was 114 weeks (range = 4–227 weeks). Total radiation dose varied from 6 Gy to 40 Gy and did not seem to predict duration of response. Three cats had recurrence of lymphoma at sites other than the irradiated area, indicating that a combination of radiation and chemotherapy is necessary to delay or prevent progression of localized lymphoma.[82]

Radiation therapy causes a rapid reduction in tumor burden, and may also be considered for cats that have life-threatening obstructive or space-occupying lymphoma (e.g., large mediastinal masses or pharyngeal/laryngeal disease). Owing to the relatively low doses needed to achieve a response, toxicities due to radiation therapy are unlikely. The contribution to remission duration is uncertain, however, and studies defining the role of palliative adjunctive radiation therapy have yet to be published.

REFERENCES

1. Dorn C, Taylor D, Schneider R: The epidemiology of canine leukemia and lymphoma. *Bibl Haemat* 36:403–415, 1970.
2. Priester W: Canine lymphoma: Relative risk in the boxer breed. *J Natl Cancer Inst* 39:843–845, 1967.
3. Onions D: RNA-dependent DNA polymerase activity in canine lymphosarcoma. *Europ J Cancer* 16:345–350, 1980.
4. Hayes HM, Tarone RE, Cantor KP, et al: Case-control study of canine malignant lymphoma: Positive association with dog owners use of 2,4-dichlorophenoxyacetic acid herbicides. *J Natl Cancer Inst* 83:1226–1231, 1991.
5. Tomley F, Armstrong S, deSouza P, et al: Retrovirus particles associated with canine lymphosarcoma and leukemia. *Br J Cancer* 45:644, 1982.
6. Owen L: *TNM Classification of Tumors in Domestic Animals.* Geneva, World Health Organization, 1980, pp 46–47.
7. Ackerman N, Madewell BR: Thoracic and abdominal radiographic abnormalities in the multicentric form in lymphosarcoma. *JAVMA* 176:36–40, 1980.
8. Jain NC: The neutrophils, in Jain NC (ed): *Schalm's Veterinary Hematology,* ed 4. Philadelphia, Lea & Febiger, 1986, pp 676–730.
9. Cotter S: Treatment of lymphoma and leukemia with cyclophosphamide, vincristine, and prednisone: I. Treatment of dogs. *JAAHA* 19:159–165, 1983.
10. Squire R, Bush M, Melby E, et al: Clinical and pathologic study of canine lymphoma: Clinical staging, cell classification and therapy. *J Natl Cancer Inst* 51:565–574, 1973.
11. MacEwen E, Hayes A, Matus R, Kurzman I: Cyclic combination chemotherapy of canine lymphosarcoma. *JAVMA* 178:1178–1181, 1981.
12. Carter R, Harris C, Withrow S, et al: Chemotherapy of canine lymphoma with histopathological correlation: Doxorubicin alone compared to COP as first treatment regimen. *JAAHA* 23:587–596, 1987.
13. MacEwen E, Hayes A, Matus R, Kurzman I: Evaluation of some prognostic factors for advanced multicentric lymphosarcoma in the dog: 147 cases (1978–1981). *JAVMA* 190:564–568, 1987.
14. Greenlee P, Filippa D, Quimby F, et al: Lymphomas in dogs: A morphologic, immunologic and clinical study. *Cancer* 66:480–490, 1990.
15. Theilen G, Worley M, Benjamini E: Chemoimmunotherapy for canine lymphosarcoma. *JAVMA* 170:607–610, 1977.
16. Weller R, Theilen G, Madewell B: Chemotherapeutic responses in dogs with lymphosarcoma. *JAVMA* 181:891–893, 1982.
17. Rosenburg M, Matus R, Patnaik A: Prognostic factors in dogs with lymphoma and associated hypercalcemia. *J Vet Intern Med* 5:268–271, 1991.
18. Keller E, MacEwen E, Rosenthal R, et al: Evaluation of prognostic factors and sequential combination chemotherapy for canine lymphoma. *J Vet Intern Med* 7:289–295, 1993.
19. Schneider R: Comparison of age- and sex-specific incidence rate patterns of the leukemia complex in the cat and the dog. *J Natl Cancer Inst* 70:971–977, 1983.
20. Hahn K, Richardson R, Teclaw R, et al: Is maintenance chemotherapy appropriate for the management of canine malignant lymphoma? *J Vet Intern Med* 6:3–10, 1992.
21. Meleo K, Matus R, Patnaik A, Greenlee P: Prognostic factors and response to therapy in 55 dogs with high and intermediate grade, multicentric lymphoma [Abstr]. *Proc Vet Cancer Soc 10th Annu Conf:*63, 1990.
22. Thompson E, Harmon J: Glucocorticoid receptors and glucocorticoid resistance in human leukemia in vivo and in vitro. *Adv Exp Med Biol* 196:111–127, 1986.
23. Price G, Page R, Fischer B, et al: Efficacy and toxicity of doxorubicin/cyclophosphamide maintenance therapy in dogs with multicentric lymphosarcoma. *J Vet Intern Med* 5:259–262, 1991.
24. Moldovanu G, Friedman M, Miller D: Experience with the management of malignant lymphoma in dogs. *Sangre* 9:253–262, 1964.

MANAGEMENT OF SPECIFIC DISEASES

25. Brick J, Roenigk W, Wilson G: Chemotherapy of malignant lymphoma in dogs and cats. *JAVMA* 153:47–52, 1968.
26. Bell R, Cotter S, Lillquist A, et al: Characterization of glucocorticoid receptors in animal lymphoblastic disease: Correlation with response to single-agent glucocorticoid treatment. *Blood Vol* 63:380–383, 1984.
27. Moldovanu G, Friedman M, Miller D: Treatment of canine malignant lymphoma with surgery and chemotherapy. *JAVMA* 148:153–156, 1966.
28. Squire R, Bush M: The therapy of canine and feline lymphosarcoma. *Bibl Haemat* 39:189–197, 1973.
29. MacEwen E, Rosenthal R, Fox L, et al: Evaluation of L-asparaginase: Polyethylene glycol conjugate versus native L-asparaginase combined with chemotherapy. A randomized double-blind study in canine lymphoma. *J Vet Intern Med* 6:230–234, 1992.
30. Teske E, Rutteman C, Heerde V, et al: Polyethylene glycol-L-asparaginase versus native L-asparaginase in canine non-Hodgkin's lymphoma. *Eur J Cancer* 26:891–895, 1990.
31. Stone M, Goldstein M, Cotter S: Comparison of two protocols for induction of remission in dogs with lymphoma. *JAAHA* 27:315–321, 1991.
32. Bowles C, Lucus D, Norton L, Graw R: Immunologic studies of canine lymphosarcoma: Mixed leukocyte reactivity following chemotherapy. *Clin Immunol Immunopathol* 9:211–217, 1978.
33. Ogilvie G, Atwater S, Ciekot P, et al: Prevalence of anaphylaxis associated with the intramuscular administration of L-asparaginase to 81 dogs with cancer: 1989–1991. *JAAHA* 30:62–64, 1994.
34. Calvert C, Leifer C: Doxorubicin for treatment of canine lymphosarcoma after development of resistance to combination chemotherapy. *JAVMA* 179:1011–1012, 1981.
35. Postorino N, Susaneck S, Withrow S, et al: Single-agent therapy with adriamycin for canine lymphosarcoma. *JAAHA* 25:221–225, 1989.
36. Chlebowski R, Paroly W, Pugh R, et al: Adriamycin given once on a weekly schedule without loading course: Clinically effective with reduced incidence of cardiotoxicity. *Cancer Treat Rep* 64:47–51, 1980.
37. Ogilvie G, Vail D, Klein M, et al: Weekly administration of low-dose doxorubicin for treatment of malignant lymphoma in dogs. *JAVMA* 198:1762, 1991.
38. Moore A, Ogilvie G, Ruslander D, et al: Mitoxantrone for the therapy of canine lymphoma. *JAVMA* 204:1903–1905, 1994.
39. Hauck M, Movotney C, McEntee M, et al: Toxicity, pharmacokinetics and efficacy of mitoxantrone administered as a 1-hour infusion in dogs with lymphoma [Abstr]. *Proc 11th Ann Conf Vet Cancer Soc*:45–46, 1991.
40. Ruslander D, Moore A, Gliatto J, Cotter S: Cytosine arabinoside as a single agent for the induction of remission in canine lymphoma. *J Vet Intern Med*, 1993, in press.
41. Hahn K, Hahn E: Epirubicin (4′-epi-doxorubicin) chemotherapy, in Kirk RW, Bonagura JD (eds): *Current Veterinary Therapy XI.* Philadelphia, WB Saunders, 1992, pp 393–395.
42. Vonderhaar M, Morrison W, DeNicola D, et al: Comparison of duration of first remission using doxorubicin versus epirubicin as single agent therapy for canine multicentric malignant lymphoma [Abstr]. *Proc 11th Ann Conf Vet Cancer Soc*:87–88, 1991.
43. Engstrom D, Shumway J, Jonas A, Bertino J: Dog lymphosarcoma as a model system for experimental chemotherapy. *Clin Res* 13:337, 1965.
44. Hammer A, Couto C, Ayl R, Shauk K: Treatment of tumor-bearing dogs and cats with actinomycin D. *J Vet Intern Med* 8:236–239, 1994.
45. Cotter S, Goldstein M: Comparison of two protocols for maintenance of remission in dogs with lymphoma. *JAAHA* 23:495–499, 1987.
46. Crow S, Carter R: Chemotherapy of canine lymphoma: CHOP vs. COP [Abstr]. *Proc 10th Ann Conf Vet Cancer Soc*:11–12, 1990.
47. Myers N, Moore A, Cotter S: Comparison of two protocols for the induction and maintenance of remission in dogs with lymphoma. *JAVMA*, 1994, submitted for publication.
48. Weller R, Theilen G, Madewell B, et al: Chemoimmunotherapy for canine lymphosarcoma: A prospective evaluation of specific and nonspecific immunomodulation. *Am J Vet Res* 41:516–521, 1980.
49. Steplewski Z, Jeglum K, Rosales C, Weintraun N: Canine lymphoma-associated antigens defined by murine monoclonal antibodies. *Cancer Immunol Immunother* 24:197–201, 1987.
50. Rosales C, Jeglum K, Obrocka M, Steplewski Z: Cytolytic activity of murine anti-dog lymphoma monoclonal antibodies with canine effector cells and complement. *Cellular Immunol* 115:420–428, 1988.
51. Jeglum K, Sorenmo K, Steplewski Z, Shofer F: Adjuvant immunotherapy of canine lymphoma with monoclonal antibody 231. *Synbiotics Corporation, San Diego, CA.*
52. Moore A, Ogilvie G, Vail D: Actinomycin-D as a rescue agent for canine lymphoma. *J Vet Intern Med,* 8:343–344, 1994.
53. Hohenhaus A, Matus R: Etoposide (VP-16): Retrospective analysis of treatment in 13 dogs with lymphoma. *J Vet Intern Med* 4:239–241, 1990.
54. Ogilvie G, Cockburn C, Tranquilli W, et al: Hypoten-

sion and cutaneous reactions associated with intravenous administration of etoposide (VP-16-213) in the dog. *Am J Vet Res* 49:1367–1370, 1988.

55. Gray K, Raulston G, Gleiser C, Jardine J: Histologic classification as an indicator of therapeutic response in malignant lymphoma in dogs. *JAVMA* 184:814–817, 1984.

56. VanVechten M, Helfand S, Jeglum K: Treatment of relapsed canine lymphoma with doxorubicin and dacarbazine. *J Vet Intern Med* 4:187–191, 1990.

57. Rosenberg M, Matus R: The use of MOPP as rescue treatment for dogs with lymphoma [Abstr]. *Proc 11th Ann Conf Vet Cancer Soc*:56, 1991.

58. Ruslander D, Moore AS, Cotter SM: Cisplatin and ara-C as rescue treatment for dogs with lymphoma [Abstr]. *Proc 11th Ann Conf Vet Cancer Soc*:61, 1991.

59. McClelland R: Cyclophosphamide therapy in lymphoma of the dog. *Cornell Vet* 53:319–322, 1963.

60. Madewell B: Chemotherapy for canine lymphosarcoma. *Am J Vet Res* 36:1525–1528, 1975.

61. Bowles C, Lucas D: Clinical and immunological response of lymphoma in dogs following chemotherapy and irradiation. *Comp Immun Microbiol Infect Dis* 3:317–326, 1980.

62. Francis D, Cotter S, Hardy W Jr, Essex M: Comparison of virus positive and virus negative cases of feline leukemia and lymphoma. *Cancer Res* 39:3866–3870, 1979.

63. Priester WA, McKay FW: *The Occurrence of Tumors in Domestic Animals*. Washington DC, National Institutes of Health, Monograph 54, November, 1980.

64. Hardy W Jr: Epidemiology of primary neoplasms of lymphoid tissues in animals. In: The immunopathology of lymphoreticular neoplasms. *Plenus Publ Corp*:129–180, 1978.

65. Meincke J, Hobbie W Jr, Hardy W Jr: Lymphoreticular malignancies in the cat: Clinical findings. *JAVMA* 160:1093–1099, 1972.

66. Mahony O, Moore A, Cotter S: Allimentary lymphoma in cats: 28 cases (1988–1993). *JAVMA*, 1994, in press.

67. Mooney S, Hayes A, Matus R, MacEwen E: Renal lymphoma in cats: 28 cases (1977–1984). *JAVMA* 191:1473–1477, 1987.

68. Spodnick G, Berg J, Moore F, Cotter S: Spinal lymphoma in cats: 21 cases (1976–1989). *JAVMA* 200:373–376, 1992.

69. Moore F, Emerson W, Cotter S, Delellis R: Distinctive peripheral lymph node hyperplasia of young cats. *Vet Pathol* 23:386–391, 1986.

70. Lucke V, Davies J, Wood C, Whitbread T: Plexiform vascularization of lymph nodes: An unusual but distinctive lymphadenopathy in the cat. *J Comp Pathol* 97: 109–119, 1987.

71. Mooney SC, Patnaik AK, Hayes AA, MacEwen EG: Generalized lymphadenopathy resembling lymphoma in cats: Six cases (1972–1976). *JAVMA* 190:897–900, 1987.

72. Penninck D, Moore A, Tidwell A, et al: Ultrasonography of alimentary lymphosarcoma in the cat. *Vet Radiol*, 1994, in press.

73. Mooney S, Hayes A, MacEwen E, et al: Treatment and prognostic factors in lymphoma in cats: 103 cases (1977–1981). *JAVMA* 194:696–699, 1989.

74. Cotter S: Treatment of lymphoma and leukemia with cyclophosphamide, vincristine and prednisone: II. Treatment of cats. *JAAHA* 19:166–172, 1983.

75. Jeglum K, Whereat A, Young K: Chemotherapy of lymphoma in 75 cats. *JAVMA* 190:174–178, 1987.

76. Cotter S, Essex M, McLane M, et al: Chemotherapy and passive immunotherapy in naturally occurring feline mediastinal lymphoma. *Elsevier North Holland Inc*:219–225, 1980.

77. McClelland R: Chemotherapy in reticulum-cell sarcoma in five dogs and a cat and in mast cell leukemia in a cat. *Cornell Vet* 61:477–481, 1971.

78. Carpenter J, Holzworth J: Treatment of leukemia in the cat. *JAVMA* 158:1130–1131, 1971.

79. Moore A, Ruslander D, Rand W, et al: Toxicity and efficacy of oral idarubicin administration to cats with neoplasia. *JAVMA*, 1995, in press.

80. Ogilvie G, Moore A, Obradovich J, et al: Toxicoses and efficacy associated with the administration of mitoxantrone to cats with malignant tumors. *JAVMA* 202:1839–1844, 1993.

81. Moore AS, Frimberger AE, L'Heureux DA, Cotter SM: Doxorubicin vs. COP for the maintenance of remission in feline lymphoma. *Proc 14th Ann Conf Cancer Vet Soc*, 1994.

82. Elmslie R, Ogilvie G, Gillette E, McChesney-Gillette S: Radiotherapy with and without chemotherapy for localized lymphoma in 10 cats. *Vet Radiol* 32:277–280, 1991.

CLINICAL BRIEFING: BONE MARROW NEOPLASIA (MYELOPROLIFERATIVE DISEASE)

Myelodysplasia in Dogs and Cats

Common Clinical Presentation	Reflects cytopenias (e.g., fever and neutropenia or petechiation and thrombocytopenia)
Common Histologic Type	Differentiated from leukemias by <30% blasts in a dysplastic bone marrow
Epidemiology and Biological Behavior	No age, gender, or breed predilection; usually progresses to an acute leukemia in cats (most are FeLV antigenemic)
Prognostic Factors	None identified

Treatment
    Supportive Treatment
    Differentiating Agents
	Antibiotics and transfusions of blood and blood products
	Cytosine arabinoside (ara-C) and retinoids are under investigation

Acute Nonlymphoid Leukemia in Dogs

Common Clinical Presentation	Nonspecific, lethargy and weight loss; clinical signs also result from cytopenias
Common Histologic Types	Not clinically relevant to distinguish because of poor prognosis, but terminology includes acute myeloid (granulocytic), myelocytic, promyelocytic, monocytic, monoblastic, myelomonocytic, megakaryocytic, and erythroleukemic; myelomonocytic is most common
Epidemiology and Biological Behavior	Females, large breeds, all ages; median age is 6 years; rapidly progressive; pancytopenia due to myelophthisis
Prognostic Factors	None identified

Treatment
    Supportive Treatment
    Chemotherapy
	Antibiotics and transfusions of blood and blood products
	No real efficacy in this disease; aggressive chemotherapy often causes marrow ablation and death

MANAGEMENT OF SPECIFIC DISEASES

Acute Lymphoblastic Leukemia in Dogs

Common Clinical Presentation	Acute onset lethargy and anorexia; splenomegaly common; mild lymphadenopathy
Common Histologic Type	Lymphoblasts; differentiate from stage V lymphoma
Epidemiology and Biological Behavior	No age or gender predilection; large-breed dogs; rapidly progressive; pancytopenia due to myelophthisis
Prognostic Factors	None identified

Treatment
   Supportive Treatment
   Chemotherapy
	Antibiotics and transfusions of blood and blood products
	Use nonmyelosuppressive agents, at least initially (e.g., prednisone, vincristine, and L-asparaginase) until normal neutrophil counts are obtained, then use standard lymphoma protocols; median survival is 120 days, with a 40% response rate to vincristine and prednisone

Chronic Lymphocytic Leukemia in Dogs

Common Clinical Presentation	Nonspecific; often asymptomatic
Common Histologic Type	Mature lymphocytosis; differentiate from reactive lymphocytosis and well-differentiated lymphoma
Epidemiology and Biological Behavior	Old dogs; often slow to progress
Prognostic Factors	None identified

Treatment
   Observation
 	
   Chemotherapy
	Repeated monitoring by blood counts may be all that is required for asymptomatic animals
	Prednisone and chlorambucil provide long-term remissions in symptomatic dogs

Primary Erythrocytosis in Dogs

Common Clinical Presentation	Polyuria, polydipsia, bleeding, seizures, and hyperemic mucous membranes

MANAGEMENT OF SPECIFIC DISEASES

Common Histologic Type	Mature erythrocytosis; rule out relative and secondary polycythemia
Epidemiology and Biological Behavior	Middle-aged dogs; no breed predilection; bleeding and seizures due to hyperviscosity; elevated red cell mass without increase in erythropoietin
Prognostic Factors	None identified
Treatment Phlebotomy Chemotherapy	 Periodic removal eventually induces iron deficiency and microcytic cells that may assist in palliation Hydroxyurea gives long-term control

Acute Nonlymphoid Leukemia in Cats

Common Clinical Presentation	Rapid onset of inappetence and lethargy; clinical signs reflect cytopenias; hepatosplenomegaly
Common Histologic Type	Not clinically relevant to distinguish due to poor prognosis; see acute nonlymphoid leukemia in dogs (above)
Epidemiology and Biological Behavior	Young cats (median age is 4 years); possible male predilection; FeLV antigenemia in 90% or more of cats; rapidly progressive; organ infiltration common
Prognostic Factors	None identified
Treatment Supportive Treatment Chemotherapy	 Antibiotics and transfusions of blood and blood products Not efficacious

Acute Lymphoblastic Leukemia in Cats

Common Clinical Presentation	Rapid onset of anorexia and weight loss; lymphadenopathy is common
Common Histologic Type	Lymphoblasts; differentiate from lymphoma
Epidemiology and Biological Behavior	Young cats (median age is 5 years); no breed or gender predilection; most cats are FeLV antigenemic
Prognostic Factors	None identified

MANAGEMENT OF SPECIFIC DISEASES

Treatment
  Supportive Treatment
  Chemotherapy
	Antibiotics and transfusions of blood and blood products
	COP protocol gives 65% remission rate for median
	remission of 7 months

Hypereosinophilic Disease in Cats

Common Clinical Presentation	Gastrointestinal signs due to eosinophilic infiltration; often, chronic history
Common Histologic Type	Mature eosinophilia; rule out allergic diseases and eosinophilic granuloma complex
Epidemiology and Biological Behavior	Adult cats (median age is 8 years); females may be predisposed; cats may have widespread organ infiltration
Prognostic Factors	None identified
Treatment Chemotherapy	Prednisone and hydroxyurea may be palliative, but this is still under investigation

Primary Erythrocytosis in Cats

Common Clinical Presentation	Neurologic disturbances (e.g., seizures and ataxia) due to hyperviscosity; dark mucous membranes
Common Histologic Type	Mature erythrocytosis; rule out relative and secondary polycythemia
Epidemiology and Biological Behavior	Median age is 6 years; male predominance; hyperviscosity causes signs (above)
Prognostic Factors	None identified

Treatment
  Phlebotomy
  Chemotherapy
	Periodic removal of blood is palliative
	Hydroxyurea gives long-term control

Other Myeloproliferative Disorders Reviewed

Chronic myeloid leukemia in dogs and chronic lymphocytic leukemia in cats

MANAGEMENT OF SPECIFIC DISEASES

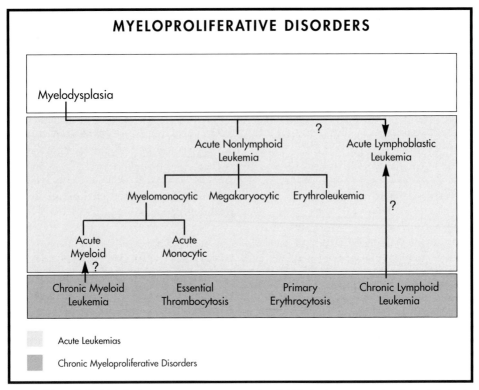

MYELOPROLIFERATIVE DISORDERS

Figure 5-17: Myelodysplasia may progress to acute nonlymphoid leukemia or to acute lymphoblastic leukemia. Chronic myeloproliferative disorders, such as chronic lymphocytic leukemia and chronic myeloid leukemia, occasionally progress to an acute leukemia, but this is rare in animals.

It is more realistic to think of neoplastic disorders of the bone marrow elements as presenting a continuum of disease rather than as a number of discrete pathophysiologic entities. The earliest stages in myeloproliferative disease reflect decreased or inappropriate bone marrow production; signs may reflect functional problems without overt evidence of neoplasia. When cytopenias and morphologic abnormalities are detected, these conditions are termed *myelodysplasia* or *preleukemia*. Myelodysplasia may progress to a true neoplastic process or leukemia, which may be "aleukemic" when it involves only bone marrow, not peripheral blood. Leukemias may affect any of the cell lines in the marrow, and the nomenclature of leukemia reflects the type of cell from which it is derived (Figure 5-17). Clinically, it is important to distinguish chronic leukemias and myeloproliferative diseases from acute leukemias and to distinguish acute lymphoblastic leukemia (ALL) from acute nonlymphoid leukemia (ANLL).

MYELODYSPLASIA (PRELEUKEMIA) IN DOGS

Incidence, Signalment, and Etiology

In dogs, myelodysplasia (MDS) is rarely recognized, but the true prevalence of this disease may be underestimated because it is difficult to diagnose. Theoretically, defects in stem cells impair hematopoiesis, which produces a wide variety of abnormalities, including disordered granulopoiesis accompanied by abnormal cellular morphology or maturation arrest. There are no apparent breed, gender, or age predilections toward canine myelodysplasia. Most affected dogs range from 4 to 11 years of age.[1] Because the disease may initially be unrecognized in animals, it is often described retrospectively after development of acute leukemia. Myelodysplasia is usually defined as peripheral cytopenia with hypercellular bone marrow that manifests abnormalities in nuclear and cytoplasmic maturation but is composed of less than 30% blast cells in the marrow. In contrast, more than 30% of nucleated bone marrow cells are blast cells in leukemia.[2]

Clinical Presentation and History

Peripheral cytopenias may produce a number of clinical signs and physical findings. Fever is common and may reflect production of pyrogens in response to the disease or, more often, may arise from infections that the neutropenic animal is unable to overcome.[1,3,4] Anemia and thrombocytopenia may cause petechiation, pallor, and lethargy. Inappetence and other nonspecific signs of illness can be seen. On clinical examination, hepatomegaly and splenomegaly may be detected, which possibly arise from extramedullary hematopoiesis or from increased sequestration and destruction of abnormal cells.

Staging and Diagnosis

Staging for animals with myelodysplasia includes a CBC, biochemical profile, urinalysis, bone marrow cytology, and special stains of abnormal cells. The hemogram of MDS usually reveals cytopenias involving any or all of the hematopoietic cell lines. Dogs with MDS have been reported to have pancytopenia with marked normoblastemia.[1] Nucleated red blood cells are often present in numbers disproportionate to reticulocytosis, and large or bizarre platelets may be seen. Granulocytes may be immature or show abnormal morphology.

The bone marrow of animals with MDS is usually cellular and often contains an increased number of plasma cells and macrophages.[1] Megakaryocytes may be numerous but are often dysplastic, with small nuclei or cytoplasmic vacuolization. There may be an abnormal progression in the granulocyte maturation series with an increased percentage of progranulocytes as well as cells with abnormal nuclear to cytoplasmic maturation, skipped mitoses, giant granulocytes, or megaloblastic cells. Blast cells may be absent; if present, they may account for up to 30% of the marrow without fulfilling the criteria for leukemia. Progression to acute leukemia is often rapid and has been reported to occur in dogs within 5 to 10 weeks.[1,4]

Treatment

In human medicine, treatment for MDS is controversial. Some authors recommend no therapy until development of acute leukemia. Treatment with so-called differentiating agents, such as low-dose cytosine arabinoside (5 to 10 mg/m^2/day SQ) has been of benefit for some human patients, but its use has rarely been reported in dogs. Other differentiating agents being explored include etretinate and *cis*-retinoic acid. Transfusions are considered supportive for anemic patients but must be given at frequent intervals to maintain a reasonable quality of life for the dog.[1,4]

Supportive treatment with transfusions and broad-spectrum antibiotics for neutropenic animals should be considered for dogs with myelodysplasia. Aggressive chemotherapy is not warranted; however, differentiating agents may be worth considering on an investigational basis.

ACUTE LEUKEMIAS IN DOGS
Acute Nonlymphoid (Myeloid) Leukemia

Although the cell of derivation for an acute leukemia can often be suspected on the basis of conventionally stained blood or bone marrow cytologic preparations, it is usually necessary to use special cytochemical

---

KEY POINT:

Myelodysplasia is characterized by a bone marrow that contains abnormalities in cellular maturation but with less than 30% blast cells.

MANAGEMENT OF SPECIFIC DISEASES

stains to confirm the lineage of a particular leukemia. For the veterinary clinician, the primary application of these stains is to distinguish ALL from ANLL. The prognosis for ANLL is poor, and further delineation of the specific leukemia cell type is often clinically unnecessary but can be of academic interest.

Acute nonlymphoid leukemia is probably a better term for this condition than acute myeloid leukemia (AML), which also has been used to describe granulocytic leukemia and may exclude leukemias that are erythroid in derivation.

Incidence, Signalment, and Etiology

There are some reports that ANLL is more common than ALL in dogs, and it accounts for approximately 70% of leukemias described in three studies.[5-7] The most common subclassification is acute myelomonocytic leukemia.[5,6,8] Acute nonlymphoid leukemia is more likely to affect female dogs than males.[6,8-11] There seems to be no breed predisposition, although large-breed dogs may be overrepresented.[8-10] The ages of affected dogs range widely from 1 to 12 years, with a median age of 6 years.[6,8]

Clinical Presentation and History

Nonspecific clinical signs, such as lethargy, anorexia, and sudden weight loss are most commonly noticed by owners.[6,9-11] In one study, more than one third of dogs had a shifting limb lameness that was attributed to subperiosteal infiltration by malignant cells or bone infarcts.[6] The duration of signs is rarely longer than one month and is often less than two weeks.[9]

On physical examination, the most frequent findings are splenomegaly, lymphadenopathy, and hepatomegaly.[6,8,10,11] Dogs frequently have pale mucous membranes, sometimes with petechiation.[6,10] Ocular changes are more frequently described in association with ANLL than with ALL. Ocular changes include hyphema; glaucoma; retinal detachment, often with hemorrhage; chorioretinitis; chemosis; and conjunctivitis. These changes occur in approximately 30% of dogs with ANLL.[6,8]

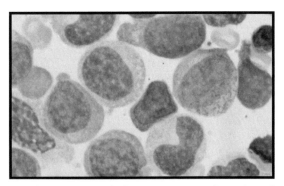

Figure 5-18: *This bone marrow aspirate from a dog with acute nonlymphoid leukemia shows a predominant population of blast cells. It is necessary to perform special cytochemical stains to determine whether nonlymphoid or lymphoblastic leukemia is present. (Courtesy S.M. Cotter)*

Staging and Diagnosis

Staging should be performed as described in the previous section. Dogs with acute leukemia have a predominance of blast cells in their blood and bone marrow, which makes this disease difficult to diagnose accurately using only morphologic criteria (Figure 5-18). Cytochemical stains are required to determine the cell of origin. Some authors believe that bone marrow blast cells stain with greater intensity than do cells in the peripheral circulation,[12] whereas others believe that cells in a buffy coat preparation provide better morphology.[5] To improve specificity, dogs with leukemia should have cytochemical stains performed on samples of bone marrow as well as peripheral blood. Cytochemical staining provided the basis for changing the diagnosis from ALL to ANLL or vice versa in 7 of 22 cases of leukemia in one study[12] and in 8 of 17 cases in another.[5] Techniques such as electron microscopy and cytogenetics are not readily available nor reliable for distinguishing leukemic cells from normal cells.[7,13]

Most dogs with ANLL are truly leukemic (i.e., abnormal cells circulate rather than appear only in bone marrow), and mean or median leucocyte counts are between 85,000 and 95,000 cells/µl,[6,9] with a range of 1500 ("aleukemic") to 191,000.[9] Affected dogs are often pancytopenic, although anemia and thrombocytopenia are more common than other hematologic abnormalities in dogs with ANLL.[8] A leukoerythroblastic reaction may be seen (increases in nucleated red blood cells and immature granulocytes) due to crowding of the bone marrow and disruption to the marrow–blood barrier.[6] Some dogs with ANLL have circulating micromegakaryocytes.[14]

Treatment

Chemotherapy for ANLL in dogs has been uniformly disappointing; death commonly occurs either from progressive disease or from marrow ablation by overzealous treatment. In one series of 10 dogs with ANLL, treatment with vinblastine, prednisone, cyclophosphamide, and cytosine arabinoside produced an average survival of 3 weeks, with a range of 1 day to 6 weeks.[5, 9] Similarly, in two other studies, treated dogs survived from 4 to 12 weeks,[6] and 1 to 42 days (median = 10 days).[7] Death occurred as a result of sepsis or from hemorrhage due to thrombocytopenia. Cytosine arabinoside (100 mg/m^2 IV every 12 hours for 4 days), 6-thioguanine (40 mg/m^2 BID PO for 4 days), and prednisone (20 mg/m^2 BID PO reduced to 10 mg/m^2 BID QOD) were used to treat a dog with ANLL and central nervous system (CNS) infiltration. The dog responded but relapsed 120 days later. Re-induction of remission was successful for an additional 120 days, at which time the dog was euthanatized.[8] Two other dogs treated with the same regimen were euthanatized 10 days after starting treatment.

In human patients with ANLL, doxorubicin is a useful agent, as is another anthracycline, daunorubicin. In two veterinary reports that used doxorubicin (30 mg/m^2 IV) in combination with prednisone and cyclophosphamide[10] or with vincristine, 6-thioguanine, and prednisone,[11] death occurred within 7 and 30 days, respectively. The dog treated with the latter regimen had less than 5% blasts in the bone marrow after treatment; however, normal marrow elements also were ablated. Six other dogs treated with doxorubicin and prednisone did not respond and had short survival (S.M. Cotter, personal communication, 1994). The use of related chemotherapeutic agents, such as daunorubicin and idarubicin, has not been evaluated in dogs with ANLL.

The prognosis for dogs with ANLL is poor due to lack of proven efficacy for chemotherapeutic agents at currently used dosages and lack of adequate support by specialized transfusions (e.g., granulocytes) and antimicrobial coverage. The use of colony-stimulating factors to support normal marrow elements is controversial, as these factors may also stimulate the growth of malignant cells. Stimulated growth may make tumor cells more susceptible to chemotherapy, however.

Acute Lymphoblastic Leukemia
Incidence, Signalment, and Etiology

Acute lymphoblastic leukemia (ALL) is a term used to describe a lymphoid malignancy that primarily involves bone marrow, which is hypercellular and usually replaced by blasts.

ALL affects dogs of all ages.[6,9,15] German shepherds and other large-breed dogs may be overrepresented.[9,15] There seems to be no strong gender predilection for ALL.[6,9,15]

Clinical Presentation and History

Clinical signs are usually acute with ALL and occur for 1 to 12 weeks prior to diagnosis; the median duration is two weeks.[15] Nonspecific signs such as lethargy and anorexia are common; vomiting, diarrhea, abdominal pain, polyuria, polydipsia, and shifting lameness occasionally are seen.[6, 9, 15]

Affected dogs are usually thin. Between 50% and 60% have lymphadenopathy, which is often mild compared to the dramatic lymphadenopathy seen in dogs with lymphoma. Splenomegaly, hepatomegaly, and pale mucous membranes are the most common abnormalities

KEY POINT:

Chemotherapy for ANLL in both dogs and cats has not met with any success. The prognosis for these animals is very poor.

MANAGEMENT OF SPECIFIC DISEASES

detected on physical examination and occur in up to 70% of dogs. Infiltration of the CNS with lymphoblasts may occur, and dogs may be presented for incoordination and depression or acute paresis.[6]

This condition should be distinguished from stage V lymphoma, in which the disease primarily involves marked lymphadenopathy and may also cause splenomegaly and hepatomegaly. Dogs with lymphoma are frequently in good clinical condition. The prognosis for stage V lymphoma is guarded, whereas the prognosis for ALL is poor (see also the chapter on Lymphoma).

Staging and Diagnosis

Staging for dogs with ALL is as described in previous sections. As with ANLL, dogs with ALL often have a predominance of primitive undifferentiated cells that are difficult to identify definitively. Cytochemical staining is important to distinguish ALL from ANLL. Both diseases are difficult to treat but may differ somewhat in their prognoses.

White blood cell counts are frequently high in ALL. Counts of greater than 100,000 cells/μl were reported in one study,[15] and counts were greater than 600,000/μl in another study.[6] Some dogs may be "aleukemic" or pancytopenic because of myelophthisis.[15] Thrombocytopenia and anemia are frequent in dogs with ALL.[6,15] It should be noted that white cell counts may rapidly normalize after treatment with corticosteroids,[6] so these drugs should be avoided until samples needed to reach a definitive diagnosis have been obtained.

Treatment

If thrombocytopenia and anemia are present, particularly if the dog is slow to respond to chemotherapy, supportive therapy with blood products, such as fresh whole blood and platelet-rich plasma, should be initiated. As mentioned earlier, hematopoietic

---

KEY POINT:

Dogs with ALL may be pancytopenic because of myelophthisis. Nonmyelosuppressive drugs, such as vincristine, L-asparaginase, and prednisone should be used in these dogs.

---

growth factors may be useful to increase the number of neutrophils, but there may be some risk that these factors may enhance the growth of the tumor cells.

In one study, nine dogs that received either no treatment (n = 3) or single-agent treatment with prednisone (n = 3) or cyclophosphamide (n = 3) did not achieve remissions.[15] All nine dogs died within 60 days. Median survival was 12 days. Another 21 dogs received vincristine (0.025 mg/kg/week IV) and prednisone (2.2 mg/kg SID PO). Four dogs (20%) achieved a complete remission (CR) and four dogs achieved a partial remission (PR). The median survival for these 8 dogs was 120 days and ranged from 8 to 241 days. The median time to achieve a measurable response was 14 days, and the dogs that responded earlier lived longer.[15]

Dogs with ALL are often pancytopenic because of bone marrow crowding by tumor cells, and this pancytopenia may be exacerbated by aggressive chemotherapy. Neither vincristine nor prednisone is strongly myelosuppressive, which is important in allowing normal marrow elements to repopulate while the dog enters remission. In addition, prednisone is one of the few drugs that crosses the blood–brain barrier, which is important in view of the risk of CNS involvement with ALL.[6] L-asparaginase is another nonmyelosuppressive chemotherapeutic agent that has indirect action across the blood–brain barrier by reducing asparagine levels. Care should be taken when administering L-asparaginase at the same time as vincristine, as the combination is extremely myelosuppressive (see the chapter on Lymphoma).

Prednisone (40 mg/m² SID PO for 3 weeks, then every other day) and vincristine (0.75 mg/m² IV every 7 days) followed 1 day later by L-asparaginase (10,000 IU/m² IM every 7 days) should be used until the neutrophil count is above 3000 cells/μl. This

MANAGEMENT OF SPECIFIC DISEASES

induction chemotherapy reduces the tumor-cell burden while maintaining normal marrow elements. Then, more aggressive use of myelosuppressive agents, such as cyclophosphamide and doxorubicin, may be used to "consolidate" the remission when normal myeloid elements are restored. Even with this approach, prognosis is guarded for dogs with ALL, as dogs frequently relapse when the intensity of the chemotherapeutic regimen is eased into a maintenance phase.

MYELODYSPLASIA (PRELEUKEMIA) IN CATS

Incidence, Signalment, and Etiology

Myelodysplasia is considerably more common in cats than in dogs, largely because of the role of feline leukemia virus (FeLV) in this disease. Experimental infection of cats with FeLV leads to the development of myeloid and erythroid leukemias, and it is possible that certain strains of the virus may determine the pathologic outcome. Subgroup C FeLV has been associated with pure red cell aplasia, whereas defective FeLV may cause MDS.[16]

Myelodysplasia is distinguished from the acute leukemias by the presence of less than 30% abnormal blast cells in bone marrow on aspiration. The distinction may be clinically irrelevant, however, as affected cats are frequently very ill, and survival beyond one week from diagnosis is rare.[17] Cats with MDS are usually FeLV-positive[18-20] and are often young, although affected cats without detectable FeLV[18,21] have been described. In one study, 15 of 21 cats with MDS were FeLV antigenemic.[17] The ages ranged from 6 months to 15 years with a median of 3 years. Most cats were domestic shorthair or domestic longhair, and 75% were male. In one cat, MDS progressed to ANLL 90 days after peripheral blood changes of macrocytic red blood cells and large platelets were seen.[22]

Clinical Presentation and History

As with dogs, cats with MDS are usually anorexic and lethargic.[3,18,21] Weight loss and fever are occasionally noted. Despite pancytopenia, some cats are initially asymptomatic but they usually progress to show signs similar to those just listed.[18] Clinical examination may reveal pallor, weight loss, and, often, hepatosplenomegaly. Retinal hemorrhages have been described in cats with MDS.[17] Clinical signs are rarely present more than three weeks prior to presentation and may be of shorter duration.[17]

Staging and Diagnosis

A bone marrow aspirate is warranted in any cat with nonregenerative anemia or other unexplained cytopenias. Although clinical signs usually relate to anemia, pancytopenia is the most common finding on the hemogram.[18,19,21] In one study, all but one of 21 cats with MDS were anemic. Large platelets are often seen in circulation. Bone marrow cytology usually reveals hypercellular marrow that often shows a preponderance of early granulocyte precursors with the same morphologic abnormalities that occur in dogs. In one study of 16 cats with MDS, nine (56%) had evidence of myelofibrosis.[23] Progression to acute leukemia (ALL or ANLL) may be rapid or may occur after many months of persistent cytopenias.[18,19,22]

Treatment

Supportive therapy, such as transfusions, antibiotics (if the cat is febrile or severely neutropenic), corticosteroids, and anabolic steroids have been used in cats with MDS. Some authors recommend monitoring asymptomatic cats with serial blood counts and providing supportive care only to animals that develop life-threatening cytopenias. The use of differentiating agents, such as low-dose cytosine arabinoside (ara-C), has not been reported for cats. In one study, 3 of 21 cats lived for 6 weeks (after two blood transfusions), 5 months, and 9 months, respectively. The two cats that survived longer had no cytopenias at diagnosis.[17] One cat treated supportively developed ANLL within 15 weeks of treatment. Another untreated cat devel-

> **KEY POINT:**
>
> *Most cats with myelodysplasia are FeLV antigenemic.*

MANAGEMENT OF SPECIFIC DISEASES

oped ANLL after 11 months of persistent neutropenia. Chemotherapy is not warranted for MDS, and the prognosis is very poor.

ACUTE LEUKEMIAS IN CATS
Acute Nonlymphoid Leukemia
Incidence, Signalment, and Etiology

Both ANLL and ALL are more common in cats than in dogs. Most cats present with ANLL, but progression from MDS to ANLL has been described.[22] In one study, ANLL was more frequently described than MDS and occurred in 39 of 60 cats with nonlymphoid hematopoietic neoplasms.[17]

The age of cats with ANLL varies from 7 months to 16 years; the median age of affected cats is 4 years.[17,24] No obvious gender predilection was found in one study of 39 cats,[17] although a review of 110 cases found that 78 cats were male and 32 were female. Most affected cats are domestic shorthair or domestic longhair.[17]

Feline leukemia virus is associated with ANLL, and FeLV antigen has been detected in 88% to 97% of cats with ANLL.[16,17,25,26] In one study, the only cats not infected may have had hypereosinophilic disease, not ANLL.[25]

Clinical Presentation and History

Cats with ANLL have a rapid onset of clinical signs that are often seen between 2 and 11 days before presentation.[24] Many affected cats have shown signs for less than one week.[17]

Clinical signs are nonspecific and are related to cytopenias as well as circulating leukemic cells. Inappetence, lethargy, weakness, and weight loss are most commonly described. Physical findings are similar to those in dogs with ANLL. One third of cats with ANLL have an enlarged spleen or liver or both.[17,24] Fever (presumably due to concurrent neutropenia and sepsis) may be present, and some cats are dyspneic, possibly due to profound anemia.[17,24] Retinal hemorrhages may occur in cats with ANLL.[17]

Staging and Diagnosis

Absolute classification of the cell of origin for any feline acute leukemia is difficult on the basis of mor-

phologic criteria alone. As with dogs, it is clinically important to distinguish ANLL from ALL using cytochemical stains.

Anemia is common in cats with ANLL and occurs in nearly all affected cats.[17,24] Median packed cell volume (PCV) is 14%.[24] An inappropriate number of nucleated red blood cells were seen in 62 of 110 cats with ANLL, and the average count in these cats was 83/100 leukocytes.[24] Other cytopenias, such as neutropenia, may be seen.[24] Cytopenias may be due simply to overcrowding and growth inhibition of the marrow by malignant cells. One study, however, found that more than 60% of cats with ANLL had myelofibrosis.[23] Possibly, FeLV may play a role in bone marrow suppression.[25]

Not all cats have circulating blast cells, which causes white cell counts to vary widely from 1300/µl to 369,000/µl.[17] Bone marrow aspiration may be necessary to confirm a diagnosis. A bone marrow aspirate that contains more than 30% abnormal blast cells is diagnostic for either ALL or ANLL; less than 30% blasts with abnormal maturation is consistent with MDS. Cats with either ANLL or ALL are likely to have malignant cellular infiltrates in organs other than bone marrow. In one study, such infiltrates were found in spleen, liver, kidney, and lymph nodes, whereas cats with MDS had no other organ infiltration.[17]

Treatment

Most cats with ANLL are euthanatized at diagnosis,[17] but occasionally supportive treatment, including transfusions, is used. Three cats treated supportively in this way lived 14, 19, and 72 days.[17] In another study, three cats treated with transfusions lived for a median of 14 days.[24] Two of these cats were also treated with plasmapheresis or with cytosine arabinoside and L-asparaginase.[24] Chemotherapy is rarely reported. When a daunorubicin derivative, idarubicin, was used to treat five cats with ANLL, no cat responded to treatment.[27]

Acute Lymphoid Leukemia
Incidence, Signalment, and Etiology

Acute lymphoid leukemia is less common than

lymphoma in cats, accounting for 15 of 53 cats (28%) in one study of lymphoid malignancies.[28]

Cats with ALL have a similar signalment to cats with ANLL. The average age of affected cats is younger than 5 years; in a review of 57 cases, ages ranged from 6 months to 14 years.[24] There is no obvious gender or breed predilection. Feline leukemia virus infection is frequently associated with ALL, although this association is less common than that between FeLV and ANLL.[17,25,26]

Clinical Presentation and History

As with ANLL, clinical signs of ALL are nonspecific; anorexia, lethargy, weight loss, and fever are most commonly reported. Lymphadenopathy is common in cats with ALL.[24]

Staging and Diagnosis

The staging scheme for cats with ALL is as described in previous sections. Blast cells found in the circulation or in bone marrow aspirates are difficult to identify definitively on morphologic criteria alone; therefore, cytochemical staining, as discussed previously, is warranted for all cases of acute leukemia.

Most cats with ALL are anemic; the average PCV is 16%.[24] Leukopenia may be present.[24] Blast cells may account for up to 83% of circulating cells, with an average of 18%. Some cats with ALL have cytopenia without circulating blasts; therefore, bone marrow aspiration is warranted in any cat with nonregenerative anemia or other unexplained cytopenias.

Treatment

In a report of 15 cats treated with COP protocol (vincristine [0.75 mg/m² IV], cyclophosphamide [300 mg/m² PO every 3 weeks], and prednisone [40 mg/m² SID PO]) (see the chapter on Lymphoma), four cats achieved CR and six cats had PRs.[28] Remission lasted between 1 and 24 months with a median of 7 months. The

prognosis for cats with ALL is considerably better than for cats with ANLL.

CHRONIC LEUKEMIAS AND MYELOPROLIFERATIVE DISORDERS
Chronic Lymphocytic Leukemia in Dogs
Incidence, Signalment, and Etiology

Chronic lymphocytic leukemia (CLL) is an uncommon myeloproliferative disease characterized by an increased number of circulating lymphocytes with normal morphology; the bone marrow often is infiltrated with similar cells. Affected dogs are usually old (median age = 10.5 years).[29-34] There is no obvious sex or breed predisposition.

Clinical Presentation and History

Dogs may be asymptomatic, in which case the diagnosis may be made only when a hemogram is evaluated for some other reason.[29,33] The most common owner complaint is lethargy (>50% of affected dogs); inappetence, sporadic vomiting, polyuria, polydipsia, and lymphadenopathy each occur in about 20% of the cases. Other signs include lameness and diarrhea, both of which may be intermittent, and weight loss. Infiltration by abnormal lymphocytes produces such signs as buccal ulceration[32] and pruritic dermatitis.[34] On clinical examination, mild lymphadenopathy is noted in up to 80% of affected dogs.[29] Splenomegaly and hepatomegaly, attributable to cellular infiltration or to extramedullary hematopoiesis,[30] are often found.[29,32] The duration of these signs is often long, and some dogs have been known to have an elevated lymphocyte count for up to 2.5 years prior to definitive treatment.[30,34]

Staging and Diagnosis

Unlike acute leukemias, definitive diagnosis of chronic leukemias is rarely problematic. Hematologic evaluation reveals a lymphocytosis composed of well-differentiated cells (Figure 5-19). Occasionally, "reactive" forms are noted. Lymphocyto-

KEY POINT:

FeLV infection is frequently associated with both ANLL and ALL in cats.

MANAGEMENT OF SPECIFIC DISEASES

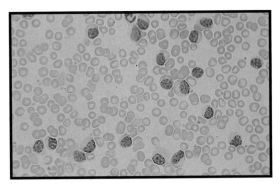

Figure 5-19: Chronic lymphocytic leukemia is characterized by a very high number of circulating lymphocytes that are morphologically normal. Lymphocyte counts in excess of 100,000/μl can occur with this disease; however, the prognosis with treatment is very good. (Courtesy S.M. Cotter)

sis varies widely with counts from 6000 to over 100,000 in one study.[29] Dogs with unexplained or persistent lymphocytosis should have a bone marrow aspirate evaluated cytologically as confirmation is by bone marrow cytology, which discloses infiltration by small lymphocytes. Infiltration explains other hematologic abnormalities, such as nonregenerative anemia and thrombocytopenia,[29,30] which are usually mild with a hematocrit level above 20% and a platelet count above 100,000/μl.[29] Unlike in acute leukemias, severe cytopenias are rare, as marrow is rarely replaced. CLL apparently occurs in three distinct stages: an asymptomatic period, which may last for months despite a high number of circulating lymphocytes; a symptomatic stage when therapy is required; and a third stage, malignant transformation (blast crisis), which is rarely recognized in dogs.[29] Three dogs with CLL developed lymphoma after achieving stable remission between 460 and 730 days.[29] This may represent a transformation of an otherwise well-differentiated disease to a more malignant stage.

Neoplastic cells are usually B lymphocytes, which may produce abnormal paraproteins. Globulin levels may be normal, but nearly 70% of 22 dogs in one study had monoclonal gammopathy.[29] In order of prevalence, the abnormal proteins were IgM (9 dogs),

IgA (4 dogs), and IgG (2 dogs). Hyperviscosity is uncommon despite the high incidence of paraproteinemia; signs due to hyperviscosity are rare but include retinal hemorrhage.[29,31] Light-chain (Bence-Jones) proteinuria was confirmed in nearly half the dogs with a monoclonal gammopathy.

Protein electrophoresis and immunoelectrophoresis should be performed, particularly if the globulin concentration is increased. Abnormal immunoglobulins may interfere with normal immune function as well as with coagulation and circulation (see the chapter on Plasma Cell Tumors).

Treatment

Patients with chronic lymphocytic leukemia are very responsive to treatment. For asymptomatic dogs, however, the clinician should consider a trial period of observation during which serial hematologic evaluations are performed every three months. One dog observed in this manner showed no clinical deterioration for 23 months.[33]

The presence or development of clinical signs should lead to prompt chemotherapy. Chlorambucil and prednisone are the most active agents in dogs as well as in humans. In a study of 20 dogs treated for 1 to 3 weeks with vincristine (0.75 mg/m² IV every 7 days), followed by chlorambucil (6 mg/m² PO daily for 1 week, then 3 mg/m² PO daily) and prednisone (30 mg/m² PO daily decreasing over 3 weeks), 14 achieved long-term remission for an average survival of 452 days (median = 348 days; range = 30–1000 days). Three dogs died or were lost to follow-up, and three dogs failed to respond. Some dogs took up to three months to achieve a remission.[29,31] Similar results, however, have been achieved with chlorambucil and prednisone alone; in other studies, chlorambucil and prednisone, even on intermittent schedules, have caused remissions of 10 months to 3 years.[30,31,34] Vincristine, cyclophosphamide, and cytosine arabinoside have been reported to assist in control of the disease; however, the excellent results with chlorambucil and prednisone make it unnecessary to use these agents.[31,34]

MANAGEMENT OF SPECIFIC DISEASES

Chronic Lymphocytic Leukemia in Cats
Incidence, Signalment, and Etiology

This disease is very rare in cats. Three cases were reported in old castrated male cats.[35] An 11-year-old female cat was diagnosed with CLL.[36] Three other cases occurred in castrated males of 12 and 5 years of age and in a spayed female that was 12 years of age (A.S. Moore, unpublished observations). White cell counts were above 55,000/µl in five cats, and the white cell count was 13,500/µl in one. Three cats were FeLV- and FIV-negative on serology.

Clinical Presentation and History

Anemia may be a feature of this disease in cats as in dogs; however, three of six cats had normal hematocrit levels. Although appetite may be normal, weight loss, as well as mild diarrhea and lethargy, may occur.

Staging and Diagnosis

Circulating mature lymphocytosis in a cat should prompt the clinician to evaluate bone marrow cytology. Infiltration of the bone marrow with more than 15% mature lymphocytes confirms the diagnosis of CLL in cats. Unlike dogs, normal cats may have lymphocytes as part of their bone marrow.

Treatment

Observation of asymptomatic cats with CLL may be justified. One cat with splenomegaly, thrombocytopenia, and presumed hypersplenism secondary to CLL that remained neutropenic and anemic after chlorambucil administration was treated with splenectomy, and all medications were discontinued. The cat remained asymptomatic with a stable lymphocytosis five years later. Two cats treated with prednisone achieved remissions of several months[35,36]; another cat failed to respond to vincristine and prednisone.[36] Chlorambucil and prednisone resulted in a long remission in one cat.[35] Two cats remained in remission for one and three years on the combination of chlorambucil (2 mg/cat, QOD) and prednisone (40 mg/m² QOD) (A.S. Moore, personal observations). The prognosis for cats with CLL seems to be similar to that of dogs with CLL, and the combination of chlorambucil and prednisone is the treatment of choice for symptomatic cats.

Chronic Myeloid Leukemia in Dogs
Incidence, Signalment, and Etiology

Chronic myeloid leukemia (CML) is extremely rare in dogs, and lack of defined diagnostic criteria makes it difficult to diagnose except by elimination of other diseases, such as systemic infections, immune-mediated disease, and other inflammatory diseases. The finding of granulocyte series overproduction in the absence of other causes is the best diagnostic criterion. Chromosomal abnormalities that are seen in human chronic granulocyte leukemia and used to confirm the diagnosis of CML have not been identified in dogs.

The median age of affected dogs is 7 to 8 years.[37-40] There are no obvious gender or breed predilections.

Clinical Presentation and History

Affected dogs have nonspecific signs, such as lethargy, weight loss, and inappetence for months prior to diagnosis of CML.[39,40] Some dogs may be asymptomatic.[37] Enhanced neutrophil activity, including phagocytosis, superoxide generation, and secretion of elastase and lysozyme, may cause degranulation in the circulation and thus contribute to clinical signs such as intermittent fever.[39] Although neutrophil function may increase, some dogs show signs of immune compromise.[38] Hepatosplenomegaly is common[37,40] and is due to organ infiltration by abnormal cells or to extramedullary hematopoiesis.

> **KEY POINT:**
>
> *Clinical improvement is usually evident soon after treatment for CLL is started, but lymphocyte counts may not drop appreciably until the dog has been treated for up to three months.*

MANAGEMENT OF SPECIFIC DISEASES

Staging and Diagnosis

Leukocyte counts with CML range from 16,000 cells/µl[38] to 169,000 cells/µl[37]; the median in one study was 98,000 cells/µl.[37] Anemia and thrombocytopenia are common, and nucleated red blood cells are a consistent finding.[38]

On bone marrow aspiration cytology, the myeloid:erythroid (M:E) ratio ranges from 3:1 to 24:1.[37] Clearly, a bone marrow aspirate is difficult to interpret accurately as is the circulating leukocyte pattern. Therefore, the definitive diagnosis is one of exclusion. The primary differential diagnosis for chronic myeloid leukemia is leukemoid reaction to another tumor; however, in leukemoid responses, anemia and thrombocytopenia are not characteristic findings.[39]

Treatment

Hydroxyurea was used to treat six dogs with CML at a dose of 50 mg/kg PO daily for 14 days. If the dog was in remission, the treatment interval was lengthened to two days and then to three days. All six dogs attained CR within one month.[37,38] Acute leukemia (blast crisis) occurred terminally in three of these six dogs,[37,38] and in another two dogs that were untreated. Survival in treated dogs ranged from 41 to more than 690 days. The two untreated dogs died 80 and 703 days after diagnosis. One dog required transfusions every two months to treat persistent anemia. This dog developed multisystemic and meningeal neoplastic infiltrates 660 days after treatment was initiated.[38] Busulfan (Myleran®, Burroughs Wellcome, NC) at a dose of 2 to 8 mg/dog/day has been recommended for treatment of patients with CML, although details and response rates were not provided.[3] Busulfan 0.1 mg/kg PO daily was used to treat a dog with chronic basophilic leukemia—with no response—and hydroxyurea (50 mg/kg BID PO) was substituted. The dog subsequently achieved CR within 5 weeks and was still in remission 62 weeks after diagnosis,

despite receiving no treatment for 32 weeks.[41] Therefore, hydroxyurea at the described dosage is the treatment of choice for dogs with CML.

Hypereosinophilic Disease in Cats
Incidence, Signalment, and Etiology

This is a rare condition that is diagnosed by exclusion rather than by other defined criteria. Causes of mature eosinophilia in cats include flea-allergy dermatitis and eosinophilic granuloma complex,[42] although the eosinophil count in these conditions does not usually reach the levels seen with hypereosinophilic disease. In a review of 13 cases, all but one occurred in adult cats, with a median age of 8 years.[43] Affected cats ranged from 10 months to 10 years of age. Nine of 13 cats reviewed were female.

Eosinophilic leukemia is a term used when eosinophilia is not ordered and immature blast forms are seen in increased numbers, either in the circulation or in the bone marrow.[44] Hypereosinophilia is usually an ordered progression, similar to CML, although metamyelocyte forms may be seen in the circulation.

Clinical Presentation and History

Hypereosinophilia in cats and dogs is usually associated with gastrointestinal signs, presumably arising from gastrointestinal infiltration by eosinophils. Affected cats often have diarrhea, weight loss, vomiting, and anorexia.[44] On physical examination, bowel loops may be thickened, lymphadenopathy is palpable, and splenomegaly and hepatomegaly may be detected. Fever, and pruritus from cutaneous involvement are less commonly noted.[44] Clinical signs have often been present for a long time.[44]

Staging and Diagnosis

Diagnosis is usually made on the basis of mature hypereosinophilia without other causes. Eosinophil counts in one study ranged from 3200 to 130,000 cells/µl with a mean of 42,000 cells/µl.[44] No other

> **KEY POINT:**
>
> *Hypereosinophilia is usually associated with gastrointestinal signs due to eosinophilic bowel and lymph node infiltration.*

cell lines were affected. Cats may be mildly anemic. Bone marrow may be heavily infiltrated with eosinophil precursors. Numerous other organs, most commonly the small intestine, spleen, mesenteric lymph nodes, and liver, may be involved.[43]

Cats with eosinophilia should be carefully evaluated for causative diseases. When these diseases have been excluded, bone marrow aspiration should be performed. The finding of an increased number of eosinophil precursors without a preponderance of blast forms leads to a diagnosis of hypereosinophilic disease.

Treatment

Treatment is not very efficacious for this disease. Prednisone was used to treat six cats, but despite decreasing the eosinophil count in some cats and improving the attitude in others, five died due to their disease within four months. In one cat, hypereosinophilia resolved with prednisone (2 mg/kg BID PO), and the cat became normal for eight months.[46] On relapse, increasing prednisone doses and adding hydroxyurea (15 mg/kg/day) had no effect on the disease. Hydroxyurea was ineffective in treating another cat.[47] Treatment using hydroxyurea in combination with prednisone may be warranted, but this use is still considered investigational.

Polycythemia in Dogs and Cats

Polycythemia is characterized by an increase in the PCV, hemoglobin concentration, and red blood cell count. This increase may follow changes in plasma volume, such as occur with dehydration, and is termed *relative* polycythemia. Absolute polycythemia may be *primary* (polycythemia vera, primary erythrocytosis) or *secondary* to an increase in serum erythropoietin. Conditions that cause secondary polycythemia include systemic hypoxia arising from cardiopulmonary disease, hemoglobinopathies, or high altitude. Some breeds of dogs, such as greyhounds, have a higher normal range of PCV. Erythropoietin may also be secreted by tumors, particularly renal tumors, leading to secondary polycythemia. In dogs, renal carcinomas and renal lymphoma have

been reported to result in increased serum erythropoietin levels.

Polycythemia vera results from a clonal proliferation of the erythroid series and does not require erythropoietin for continued stimulus. In humans, this disorder usually includes thrombocytosis and hepatosplenomegaly and progresses to myelofibrosis or acute leukemia. In dogs and cats, these manifestations are not reported; therefore, *primary erythrocytosis* may be a more appropriate term.

Primary Erythrocytosis in Dogs
Incidence, Signalment, and Etiology

Primary erythrocytosis is rarely reported in dogs. When it occurs, this disease affects middle-aged dogs.[48-51] There is no apparent gender or breed predilection.

Clinical Presentation and History

Affected dogs are reported to have hyperemic (brick-red) mucous membranes.[48-51] They may also have polyuria and polydipsia, lethargy, inappetence, or restlessness. Other clinical signs include bleeding, which has been reported as hematochezia; hematemesis and hematuria[48,51]; and such neurologic disturbances as seizures,[48,51] posterior weakness, ataxia, and blindness.[48] Increased blood viscosity leading to dilation and weakening of peripheral vessels may cause bleeding. Dogs with primary erythrocytosis have dilated retinal vessels.[50] Seizures and other neurologic manifestations are presumably due to the same cause. Signs have been reported to occur from 1 week to 12 months prior to diagnosis, with an average of 6 weeks.[50] Mild splenomegaly is occasionally noted.[48,51]

Staging and Diagnosis

The PCV of dogs reported to have primary erythrocytosis ranges from 65% to 82%; the median in one study was 78%.[48] Once absolute polycythemia is confirmed, possible causes of secondary polycythemia must be ruled out. Thoracic radiographs may detect changes consistent with chronic pulmonary disease or cardiac changes, and echocardiography can detect

MANAGEMENT OF SPECIFIC DISEASES

underlying cardiac disease. Arterial blood gas measurement is the best method to rule out systemic hypoxia, although it is usually not available in general practice. Renal architecture may be examined by intravenous pyelography; however, abdominal ultrasonography is a simple and reliable alternative.

The diagnosis of primary erythrocytosis after ruling out causes of secondary polycythemia may be confirmed by serum erythropoietin assay. Erythropoietin levels should be low or normal in a dog with primary erythrocytosis. Serum erythropoietin measurements have been undetectable in affected dogs.[49,50]

Treatment

Phlebotomy may be used successfully to manage dogs with primary erythrocytosis and should be performed as the initial therapy in all dogs. The procedure usually followed is to remove 20 ml/kg body weight of blood, which reduces the PCV by approximately 15%. This volume is replaced with crystalloid solutions.

Repeated phlebotomy will maintain the PCV in the high-normal range. Iron supplementation is not required, as iron deficiency will produce erythrocyte microcytosis and assist in controlling the red cell mass. The PCV should be checked every 3 to 4 weeks, and phlebotomy should be performed when appropriate. Phlebotomy every 2 to 4 weeks successfully maintained a high normal PCV in one dog.[51] The disadvantage of phlebotomy is that repeated procedures may decrease patient tolerance, but it is safe.

Other treatments have been attempted in dogs with primary erythrocytosis. Radiophosphorus (^{31}P) accumulates in bone and results in bone marrow irradiation and myelosuppression. It is difficult to assess the response of dogs to this therapy, as doses have varied from 1.5 mCi (total dose)[48] to 3.25 mCi/m^2 and were sometimes combined with phlebotomy and busulfan (2 mg PO daily).[48] Of four dogs treated with ^{31}P alone, one achieved a CR for two years, and

> ### KEY POINT:
>
> *Phlebotomy to remove 20 ml/kg body weight of blood will reduce the animal's PCV by approximately 15%.*

another dog had a PR for a number of months. In the dogs that failed or relapsed, repeated phlebotomy or chemotherapy with hydroxyurea controlled the disease.[50] Radiophosphorus treatment is not widely available and probably has an adjunctive role in the treatment of canine primary erythrocytosis, but it is difficult to draw conclusions on the basis of the available literature.

Chemotherapy with hydroxyurea is probably the treatment of choice for dogs with primary erythrocytosis.[50,51] Initial phlebotomy to reduce the PCV was followed by a "loading" dose of 30 mg/kg/day PO for 7 days, then 15 mg/kg/day PO for maintenance. Three dogs treated in this way achieved a normal PCV in 2 to 6 weeks.[51] Two dogs relapsed on treatment at 2 years and at 8 months following initial treatment, and both were successfully reinduced with a 7-day loading dose. It is important to monitor the PCV of dogs receiving hydroxyurea every one to three months, and doses should be individualized. Anecdotally, less frequent administration of 500-mg capsules to smaller dogs results in a similar long-term control while protecting the handler from the risk of exposure when splitting capsules for daily dosage (A.S. Moore, personal observations).

Primary Erythrocytosis in Cats
Incidence, Signalment, and Etiology

Polycythemia vera is defined as an increase in the red cell mass accompanied by thrombocytosis and organomegaly. Because it does not progress to myelofibrosis or leukemia, *primary erythrocytosis* is probably a better term for the disease in cats, which are rarely affected. It is characterized by an increase in the number of erythrocytes in the presence of normal or low serum erythropoietin levels.

In a review of 11 reported cases of primary erythrocytosis,[52] affected cats ranged from 3 to 15 years of age (median = 6 years). Male cats were predominantly affected (8 of 10 cats). There was no obvious breed predisposition.

MANAGEMENT OF SPECIFIC DISEASES

Clinical Presentation and History

Neurologic disturbances, such as seizures, are common in cats with erythrocytosis and occurred in 7 of 11 reported cases.[52] Blindness, ataxia, or abnormal behavior may occur. Less common signs include depression, lethargy, anorexia, polyuria, and polydipsia. Dark mucous membranes may be noted. Splenomegaly is rare, and hepatomegaly has not been recorded.

Staging and Diagnosis

To confirm a diagnosis of primary erythrocytosis in a normally hydrated cat, secondary erythrocytosis should be ruled out. Causes of secondary erythrocytosis include cardiopulmonary diseases, other causes of hypoxia, and abnormal production of erythropoietin due to renal neoplasia. Thoracic radiographs should be obtained to evaluate cardiopulmonary structures; if cardiac disease is suspected, echocardiography should be performed. Hypoxemia can be ruled out by performing blood gas analysis. Renal structure may be assessed by ultrasonography, and any suspicious lesions should be biopsied. Serum erythropoietin levels can confirm the diagnosis, although this test is still in the process of validation for use in cats. In 11 reported cases of primary erythrocytosis, initial PCV was 63% to 82%.[52] Increases in white cell counts were seen in three cats, and the platelet count was increased in one cat. Serum erythropoietin level was low or normal in all eight cats for which a sample was obtained.[52]

Treatment

Survival times in two cats that did not receive treatment were 6 weeks[53] and more than 20 weeks.[54] Phlebotomy alone every 2 to 3 months was used to manage one cat for longer than 20 months.[55]

Hydroxyurea either alone or in combination with phlebotomy was used to treat eight cats, and all survived more than one year. Two cats survived more than six years. The dose of hydroxyurea to induce

> ### KEY POINT:
>
> *Care should be taken when administering large, single doses of hydroxyurea to cats, as methemoglobinemia may occur.*

and maintain remission is variable. Doses of less than 500 mg require capsules to be split, which introduces inaccuracy and risk of drug exposure to the handler. A cat treated with a single hydroxyurea dose of 500 mg developed severe methemoglobinemia and hemolytic anemia with Heinz bodies (A.S. Moore, unpublished observations); therefore, although some cats tolerate 500 mg orally every 5 to 7 days, it may be prudent to start treatment at 125 mg/cat every 2 days for 2 weeks, followed by 250 mg/cat twice weekly for 2 weeks, then 500 mg weekly, or as often as is necessary to maintain a normal hematocrit level. The cat should be hospitalized for 24 hours following treatment to check for methemoglobinemia each time the dose is increased; it may be prudent to store blood collected from the cat prior to treatment for autotransfusion if necessary. Signs of methemoglobinemia include dyspnea and dark-brown mucous membranes.

REFERENCES

1. Weiss DJ, Raskin R, Zerbe C: Myelodysplastic syndrome in two dogs. *JAVMA* 187:1038–1040, 1985.
2. Jain NC, Blue JT, Grindem CB, et al: Proposed criteria for classification of acute myeloid leukemia in dogs and cats. *Vet Clin Pathol* 20:63–82, 1991.
3. Gorman NT, Evans RJ: Myeloproliferative disease in the dog and cat: Clinical presentations, diagnosis and treatment. *Vet Rec* 121:490–496, 1987.
4. Couto CG, Kallet AJ: Preleukemic syndrome in a dog. *JAVMA* 184:1389–1392, 1984.
5. Grindem CB, Stevens JB, Perman V: Cytochemical reactions in cells from leukemic dogs. *Vet Pathol* 23:103–109, 1986.
6. Couto CG: Clinicopathologic aspects of acute leukemias in the dog. *JAVMA* 186:681–685, 1985.
7. Grindem CB: Cytogenetic analysis of leukemic cells in the dog: A report of 10 cases and a review of the literature. *J Comp Pathol* 96:623–635, 1986.
8. Jain NC, Madewell BR, Weller RE, Geisster MC: Clinical-pathological findings and cytochemical characterization of myelomonocytic leukaemia in 5 dogs. *J Comp Pathol* 91:17–31, 1981.
9. Grindem CB, Stevens JB, Perman V: Morphological classification and clinical and pathological characteris-

MANAGEMENT OF SPECIFIC DISEASES

tics of spontaneous leukemia in 17 dogs. *JAAHA* 21: 219–226, 1985.

10. Hamlin RH, Duncan RC: Acute nonlymphocytic leukemia in a dog. *JAVMA* 196:110–112, 1990.

11. Rohrig KE: Acute myelomonocytic leukemia in a dog. *JAVMA* 182:137–141, 1983.

12. Facklam NR, Kociba GJ: Cytochemical characterization of leukemic cells from 20 dogs. *Vet Pathol* 22:363–369, 1985.

13. Grindem CB: Ultrastructural morphology of leukemic cells from 14 dogs. *Vet Pathol* 22:456–462, 1985.

14. Canfield PJ, Watson ADJ, Begg AP, Dill-Macky E: Myeloproliferative disorder in four dogs involving derangements of erythropoiesis, myelopoiesis and megakaryopoiesis. *J Small Anim Pract* 27:7–16, 1986.

15. Matus RE, Leifer CE, MacEwen EG: Acute lymphoblastic leukemia in the dog: A review of 30 cases. *JAVMA* 183:859–862, 1983.

16. Tzavaras T, Stewart M, McDougall A, et al: Molecular cloning and characterization of a defective recombinant feline leukaemia virus associated with myeloid leukaemia. *J Gen Virol* 71:343–354, 1990.

17. Blue JT, French TW, Kranz JS: Non-lymphoid hematopoietic neoplasia in cats: A retrospective study of 60 cases. *Cornell Vet* 78:21–42, 1988.

18. Madewell BR, Jain NC, Weller RE: Hematologic abnormalities preceding myeloid leukemia in three cats. *Vet Pathol* 16:510–519, 1979.

19. Maggio L, Hoffman R, Cotter SM, et al: Feline preleukemia: An animal model of human disease. *Yale J Biol Med* 51:469–476, 1978.

20. Evans RJ, Gorman NT: Myeloproliferative disease in the dog and cat: Definition, aetiology and classification. *Vet Rec* 121:437–443, 1987.

21. Harvey JW, Shields RP, Gaskin JM: Feline myeloproliferative disease: Changing manifestations in the peripheral blood. *Vet Pathol* 15:437–448, 1978.

22. Raskins RE, Krehbiel JD: Myelodysplastic changes in a cat with myelomonocytic leukemia. *JAVMA* 187:171–174, 1985.

23. Blue JT: Myelofibrosis in cats with myelodysplastic syndrome and acute myelogenous leukemia. *Vet Pathol* 25:154–160, 1988.

24. Grindem CB, Perman V, Stevens JB: Morphological classification and clinical and pathological characteristics of spontaneous leukemia in 10 cats. *JAAHA* 21:227–236, 1985.

25. Hardy WD Jr: Hematopoietic tumors of cats. *JAAHA* 17:921–940, 1981.

26. Cotter SM, Hardy WD Jr, Essex M: Association of feline leukemia virus with lymphosarcoma and other disorders in the cat. *JAVMA* 166:449–454, 1975.

27. Moore AS, Ruslander D, Cotter SM, et al: Toxicity

and efficacy of oral idarubicin administration to cats with neoplasia. *JAVMA*, 1994, in press.

28. Cotter SM: Treatment of lymphoma and leukemia with cyclophosphamide, vincristine, and prednisone: II. Treatment of cats. *JAAHA* 19:166–172, 1983.

29. Leifer CE, Matus RE: Chronic lymphocytic leukemia in the dog: 22 cases (1978–1984). *JAVMA* 189:214–217, 1986.

30. Hodgkins EM, Zinkl JG, Madewell BR: Chronic lymphocytic leukemia in the dog. *JAVMA* 177:704–707, 1980.

31. Kristensen AT, Klausner JS, Weiss DJ, et al: Spurious hyperphosphatemia in a dog with chronic lymphocytic leukemia and an IgM monoclonal gammopathy. *Vet Clin Pathol* 20:45–48, 1991.

32. Olivry T, Atlee BA: Leucemie lymphoide chronique avec ulcerations buccales chez un chien. *Pract Med Chir Anim Compag* 27:177–181, 1992.

33. Harvey JW, Terrell TG, Hyde DM, Jackson RI: Well-differentiated lymphocytic leukemia in a dog: Long-term survival without therapy. *Vet Pathol* 18:37–47, 1981.

34. Couto GC, Sousa C: Chronic lymphocytic leukemia with cutaneous involvement in a dog. *JAAHA* 22:374–379, 1986.

35. Cotter SM, Holzworth J: Disorders of the hematopoietic system, in Holzworth J (ed): *Diseases of the Cat. Medicine and Surgery.* Philadelphia, WB Saunders, 1987, pp 755–807.

36. Thrall MA: Lymphoproliferative disorders: Lymphocytic leukemia and plasma cell myeloma. *Vet Clin North Am Small Anim Pract* 11:321–347, 1981.

37. Leifer CE, Matus RE, Patnaik AK, MacEwen EG: Chronic myelogenous leukemia in the dog. *JAVMA* 183:686–689, 1983.

38. Grindem CB, Steven JB, Brost DR, Johnson DD: Chronic myelogenous leukaemia with meningeal infiltration in a dog. *Compar Haematol Int* 2:170–174, 1992.

39. Thomsen MK, Jensen AL, Skak-Nielsen T, Kristensen F: Enhanced granulocyte function in a case of chronic granulocytic leukemia in a dog. *Vet Immunol Immunopathol* 28:143–156, 1991.

40. Ndikuwere J, Smith DA, Obwolo MJ, Masvingwe C: Chronic granulocytic leukaemia/eosinophilic leukemia in a dog? *J Small Anim Pract* 33:553–557, 1992.

41. MacEwen EG, Drazner FH, McClelland AJ, Wilkins RJ: Treatment of basophilic leukemia in a dog. *JAVMA* 166:376–380, 1975.

42. Center SA, Randolph JF, Erb NH, Reiter S: Eosinophilia in the cat: A retrospective study of 312 cases (1975–1986). *JAAHA* 26:349–358, 1990.

43. Neer TM: Hypereosinophilic syndrome in cats. *Comp*

Contin Educ Pract Vet 13:549–555, 1991.

44. Simon N, Holzworth J: Eosinophilic leukemia in a cat. *Cornell Vet* 57:579–597, 1967.

45. Muller VD: Dietl Fallbericht uber die eosinophilen-leukamie bei einer katze. *Mh Vet Med* 45:98–100, 1990.

46. Harvery RG: Feline hypereosinophilia with cutaneous lesions. *J Small Anim Pract* 31:453–456, 1990.

47. Scott DW, Randolph JF, Walsh KM: Hypereosinophilic syndrome in a cat. *Feline Pract* 15:22–30, 1985.

48. McGrath CJ. Polycythemia vera in dogs. *JAVMA* 164:1117–1122, 1974.

49. Quesnel AD, Kruth SA: Polycythemia vera and glomerulonephritis in a dog. *Can Vet J* 33:671–672, 1992.

50. Smith M, Turrell JM: Radiophosphorus (^{32}P) treatment of bone marrow disorders in dogs: 11 cases (1970–1987). *JAVMA* 194:98–102, 1989.

51. Peterson ME, Randolph JF: Diagnosis of canine primary polycythemia and management with hydroxyurea. *JAVMA* 180:415–418, 1982.

52. Watson ADJ, Moore AS, Helfand SC: Primary erythrocytosis in the cat. Treatment with hydroxyurea. *J Small Anim Pract* 35:320–325, 1994.

53. Reed C, Ling GV, Gould D, Kaneko JJ: Polycythemia vera in a cat. *JAVMA* 157:85–91, 1970.

54. Duff BC, Allan GS, Howlett CR: A presumptive case of polycythemia vera in a cat. *Austr Vet Pract* 3:78–79, 1973.

55. Foster ES, Lothrop CD Jr: Polycythemia vera in a cat with cardiac hypertrophy. *JAVMA* 192:1736–1738, 1988.

CLINICAL BRIEFING: PLASMA CELL TUMORS

Multiple Myeloma in Dogs

Common Clinical Presentation	Anemia and secondary infections due to myelophthisis; lameness and pain from bone lytic lesions; polyuria and polydipsia from hypercalcemia, renal disease, and paraproteinuria; hemorrhage due to hyperviscosity
Epidemiology and Biological Behavior	Median age is 8 to 9 years; most cases occur in purebred dogs; systemic disease
Prognostic Factors	Dogs with hypercalcemia, extensive bone lysis, or light-chain (Bence-Jones) proteinuria have a worse prognosis
Treatment Prednisone Melphalan and Prednisone Other Agents Radiation Therapy	 Palliative only; median survival is 220 days Complete remission in 40% and partial remission in 50% of dogs for median survival of 540 days Cyclophosphamide or chlorambucil may be effective Palliative for localized bone lesions

Multiple Myeloma in Cats

Common Clinical Presentation	Nonspecific clinical signs; most cats are anemic; lytic bone lesions are rare
Epidemiology and Biological Behavior	Old cats; mostly domestic shorthair; no association with FeLV
Prognostic Factors	None identified
Treatment Melphalan and Prednisone	 Remission in 40% of cases for median survival of 170 days

Cutaneous and Extramedullary Plasmacytomas in Dogs

Common Clinical Presentation	Solitary cutaneous mass in trunk or limbs; may affect oral cavity, ears, and head; less commonly, may occur in multiple or other sites, such as diffuse GI tumors

MANAGEMENT OF SPECIFIC DISEASES

Epidemiology and Biological Behavior	Old dogs; cutaneous tumors are usually benign; plasmacytomas of other sites (e.g., GI) may metastasize
Prognostic Factors	None identified

Treatment
   Surgery
 	
   Radiation Therapy
   Chemotherapy
	
	Surgery with wide surgical margins is curative in most cases of cutaneous plasmacytomas
	Radiation-sensitive tumor
	Melphalan, prednisone, and doxorubicin have all caused tumor responses, often for a long duration in dogs with extramedullary plasmacytomas

In small animals, most plasma cell neoplasms involve the bone marrow and are accompanied by other clinical features, which are distinct from the physical presence of the tumor, that may lead to a diagnosis of multiple myeloma. Although the term *extramedullary plasmacytoma* indicates a lack of bone marrow involvement and hence includes all plasmacytomas other than myeloma, we have made a distinction between plasmacytomas of skin and those of other sites based on an apparent difference in biological behavior.

MULTIPLE MYELOMA IN DOGS

The diagnosis of multiple myeloma may be made in a dog or a cat when two or more of the following criteria are detected:

- Monoclonal gammopathy
- Lytic bone lesions
- Bence-Jones (light-chain) proteinuria
- Neoplastic plasma cells or bone marrow plasmacytosis

By strict definition, *multiple myeloma* is the term used when monoclonal IgG, IgA, or light chains are produced, whereas *Waldenstrom's macroglobulinemia* is associated with IgM overproduction. Monoclonal gammopathies may be seen with other neoplasms (such as lymphoma) or with infectious diseases (such as ehrlichiosis), in which plasmacytosis may also be found on bone marrow aspiration.

Incidence, Signalment, and Etiology

Most published data regarding multiple myeloma in dogs are case reports. There are, however, two large reviews: one series of 60 dogs[1] and one retrospective study of 20 dogs.[2] The median age for dogs with multiple myeloma is between 8 and 9 years; ages range from 18 months[3] to 16 years.[2] There is no apparent gender predilection. German shepherds were found to be at higher risk in one study,[1] accounting for more than 20% of affected dogs. Most reported cases have occurred in purebred dogs.

Clinical Presentation and History

The pathophysiology of multiple myeloma is complex and affects multiple systems. Clinical signs vary and are usually noticed by owners for a month or more before the dog is presented to the veterinarian.[1] Tumor proliferation in the bone marrow causes myelophthisis when plasmacytosis becomes severe. Peripheral blood counts may reflect this occurrence, and affected dogs are often anemic and thrombocytopenic; some are neutropenic. In one group of dogs, nearly 70% were anemic, 25% were leukopenic, and 30% were thrombocytopenic.[1] Neutropenic patients are at increased risk for developing infections, partic-

MANAGEMENT OF SPECIFIC DISEASES

ularly if normal immunoglobulin levels are also suppressed. Dogs may present with signs referable to secondary infections, such as cystitis.[4,5]

Bone involvement may manifest as multiple lytic lesions that primarily affect the axial skeleton, or affected dogs may appear diffusely osteoporotic. These changes result from osteoclast activation, which may also cause hypercalcemia. Pathologic fractures, if severe, may cause lameness; if the axial skeleton is involved, there may be paresis. Dogs may also have pain from fractured ribs or may become acutely paralyzed from vertebral body collapse. Weakness was a presenting sign in more than 60% of 60 dogs.[1] Nearly half of these dogs were lame from paresis or pain. Lameness, paresis, and pain were the reasons for presentation in 17 of 41 other reported cases.[2,4,6–11]

Most reported cases of canine multiple myeloma involve overproduction of IgA or IgG. In one survey, IgA and IgG were each found in 30 of 60 dogs.[1] Of other reported cases, IgA was found in 11 dogs[5,9–15] and IgG in 5 dogs[4,5,11] with multiple myeloma.

Normal immunoglobulin production is often suppressed; thus, it is possible for a dog with multiple myeloma and an abnormal monoclonal immunoglobulin level to still have a normal total globulin level. Serum protein electrophoresis or immunoelectrophoresis is necessary to confirm a diagnosis in these dogs. Abnormal immunoglobulin may be produced as incomplete fragments, which are usually "light chains" of myeloma protein. Occasionally, they may be heavy chains.[14] These abnormal proteins are excreted in the urine (Bence-Jones proteins), but they are undetectable on routine urinalysis.

Abnormal immunoglobulin, particularly IgM or IgA (which, as dimers, may form high molecular weight polymers in circulation), may produce hyperviscosity of the blood when high protein levels are reached. Hyperviscosity is recognized clinically as bleeding due to paraprotein coating of platelets and as "sludging" of blood in vessels. Bleeding is often

> ## KEY POINT:
>
> *Normal immunoglobulin levels are often suppressed; therefore, a dog with multiple myeloma may still have a normal total globulin level.*

compounded by interference with normal coagulation and absolute thrombocytopenia due to bone marrow infiltration by plasma cells. Hyperviscosity may cause such central nervous system (CNS) signs as dementia, confusion, and seizures as well as funduscopic changes and retinal detachment. In one study, 19 of 60 dogs had evidence of hyperviscosity; 14 of these dogs had an elevation in IgA, and five had IgG paraproteinemia.[1] There were signs of bleeding in 37% of 60 dogs,[1] and bleeding was a presenting sign (i.e., petechiation, epistaxis, and hematuria) in another 7 of 21 case reports.[2,4,11,12,15,16] Signs referable to the CNS were less common and were seen in 12% of 60 dogs.[1]

Paraprotein light chains (Bence-Jones proteins) and hypercalcemia may contribute to renal dysfunction; these changes may be exacerbated by renal infiltration with neoplastic plasma cells. Light-chain nephropathy, renal tubular damage from hypercalcemia, and glomerulosclerosis may all contribute to irreversible azotemia; however, azotemia may be prerenal in dogs with hypercalcemia and thus is often reversible when chemotherapy succeeds. Polydipsia and polyuria may be noticed by owners and was a reason for presentation in 15 of 60 dogs.[1] In the same study, azotemia was documented in 20 dogs and hypercalcemia was noted in 10 dogs. Bence-Jones proteinuria was found in 24 of 60 dogs with multiple myeloma in the same study and in 11 of 19 other dogs reported.[2,4,9–13,15,16]

Staging and Diagnosis

Complete staging of a dog with suspected multiple myeloma involves collection of a complete blood count (CBC), serum profile, whole body radiographs, electrophoresis and immunoelectrophoresis of serum and urine, and bone marrow aspiration.

A CBC should be obtained to identify patients at increased risk for infection arising from neutropenia or bleeding from thrombocytopenia. A serum chemistry profile may identify an increase in total protein levels that is primarily serum globulins. In addition, dogs with azotemia should be evaluated for both renal dysfunction and hypercalcemia. Urinalysis can provide information about the patient's renal function, particularly if azotemia is present; however, although proteinuria may be an indication of glomerular damage, it is not an indication of Bence-Jones proteinuria. Urine-protein detection strips detect albumin, and as mentioned earlier, special heat-precipitation methods are needed to detect Bence-Jones proteinuria. Urine immunoelectrophoresis may be a more sensitive method than heat precipitation to document Bence-Jones protein[15] and detect heavy chains in the urine.[14]

Serum protein electrophoresis should be performed even in dogs with a normal globulin level. Suppression of normal circulating immunoglobulin levels may cause overall normal serum globulin in a dog that actually has a monoclonal immunoglobulin spike. A monoclonal spike may be further evidenced by immunoelectrophoresis, which differentiates IgA, IgG, or IgM among an increase in monoclonal antibodies. Immunoelectrophoresis of the urine may also detect abnormal light- or heavy-chain paraproteins.

Bone lesions from multiple myeloma are almost purely lytic, with very little new bone production; therefore, radionuclide bone scans may not be effective for imaging myeloma-induced bone lesions.[6] Plain radiograph skeletal surveys are the most sensitive method for detecting such abnormalities.

Bone marrow aspiration should be performed from any of the routinely used sites (see Biopsy section). Some investigators consider plasma cells that comprise more than 30% of nucleated bone marrow cells diagnostic for multiple myeloma, but most believe that between 5% and 20% of affected cells support such a diagnosis.[1] For dogs with large lytic bone lesions, samples may be obtained for histopathology by fluoroscopically guided biopsy; aspiration can secure samples for cytology.

In dogs that are not treated or that fail to respond to treatment, neoplastic plasma cells are frequently found as discrete masses (which may be quite large) in several organs.[2,12] Sites of involvement include lymph nodes, pharynx, esophagus, gastrointestinal (GI) tract, liver, pancreas, skin, muscle, and lung.

In a series[1] of 38 dogs with multiple myeloma that died from their disease, six dogs with spinal cord paralysis were euthanatized at the time of diagnosis. Pancytopenia was the reason that three dogs were euthanatized later, and 11 others died from hemorrhage or infection. Progressive renal failure was the cause of death in 13 dogs; another five dogs failed to respond to chemotherapy.

Prognostic Factors

There has only been one study of sufficient magnitude to identify prognostic factors in dogs with multiple myeloma.[1] In this study of 60 patients, dogs that were hypercalcemic, had extensive bone lysis, or had evidence of myeloma light chains in the urine (Bence-Jones proteinuria) all had significantly shortened survival times (Figure 5-20).

Gender, class of immunoglobulin (IgA or IgG), presence of hyperviscosity, and azotemia did not affect survival (Figure 5-21). Of the 49 dogs that were treated, chemotherapy with a combination of alkylating agents and prednisone enabled significantly longer survival than treatment with prednisone alone[1] (see below).

Treatment

As mentioned previously, dogs with multiple myeloma are at high

> **KEY POINTS:**
>
> *Dogs with multiple myeloma that are hypercalcemic, have extensive bony lysis, or have light-chain proteinuria do not survive as long as dogs without these findings.*
>
> ---
>
> *Combination chemotherapy using melphalan and prednisone often results in long survival for dogs with multiple myeloma.*

MANAGEMENT OF SPECIFIC DISEASES

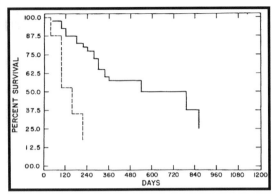

Figure 5-20: *Survival data for dogs with multiple myeloma that were treated with melphalan and prednisone. The solid line indicates 31 dogs with a normal serum calcium (<11.5 g/dl) and the broken line indicates 6 dogs that were hypercalcemic. The difference is significant. (From Matus RE, Leifer CE, MacEwen EG, Hurvitz AI: Prognostic factors for multiple myeloma in the dog. JAVMA 188:1288–1292, 1986; with permission.)*

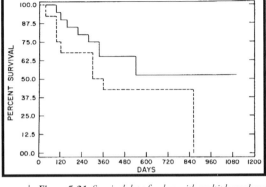

Figure 5-21: *Survival data for dogs with multiple myeloma that were treated with melphalan and prednisone. The solid line indicates 24 dogs that were not azotemic, and the broken line indicates 13 dogs that were azotemic. The difference is not significant. (From Matus RE, Leifer CE, MacEwen EG, Hurvitz AI: Prognostic factors for multiple myeloma in the dog. JAVMA 188:1288–1292, 1986; with permission.)*

risk for infection due to effects on the bone marrow and on humoral immunity. Dogs with fever or other evidence of infection require immediate antibiotic therapy.

Dogs with renal dysfunction, particularly those with hypercalcemia, should be supported with aggressive fluid therapy to maintain hydration and to enhance renal perfusion. Dogs with hypercalcemia also should be treated with furosemide while receiving 0.9% sodium chloride diuresis. Chemotherapy should be started in these patients as soon as diagnosis is confirmed. Care should be taken when administering melphalan to dogs with renal dysfunction. Melphalan-induced myelosuppression is more severe in dogs with renal dysfunction when delivered intravenously, probably because of decreased clearance of the drug and resultant longer half-life.[17] Absorption is more varied with oral administration; therefore, careful monitoring of blood counts when melphalan is administered, rather than an empiric dose reduction, is recommended. Exercise should be restricted for dogs with

severe bone lysis, particularly of the vertebrae. If the lesions in these dogs are large and localized, radiation therapy may resolve these lytic lesions.[6] A pathologic fracture of the femur was treated with 36 Gy of teletherapy and internal fixation; it healed progressively over six months.[6] For hyperviscous dogs, chemotherapy will usually cause improvement within weeks of initiation. In critical situations, plasmapheresis can reduce plasma protein levels.[18]

Most reported dogs are treated with chemotherapy or euthanatized at diagnosis. Three dogs that received no treatment for their disease[2,4,11] and one dog that failed to respond to treatment[3] all died within 40 days of initial presentation.

Chemotherapy is the treatment of choice for canine multiple myeloma. In a series of 12 dogs treated with prednisone (0.5 mg/kg SID PO) for palliation, median survival was 220 days.[1] In the same study,[1] another 37 dogs received melphalan (0.1 mg/kg SID PO for 10 days, then 0.05 mg/kg SID PO) and prednisone (0.5 mg/kg SID PO for 10 days, then 0.5 mg/kg QOD PO).

KEY POINT:

Lytic bone lesions seem to be rare in cats with multiple myeloma.

MANAGEMENT OF SPECIFIC DISEASES

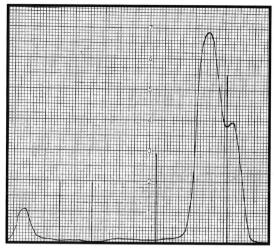

Figure 5-22: *Electrophoretogram of a 6-year-old dog showing a monoclonal globulin spike. Total serum protein for this dog was 12.0 mg/dl. The dog was hypoalbuminemic at presentation.*

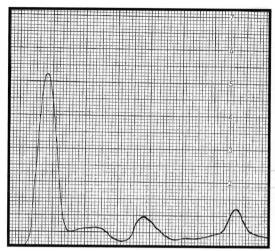

Figure 5-23: *Electrophoretogram of the same dog as Figure 5-22 three months after starting treatment with melphalan and prednisone. Note the decrease in the globulin spike. The total serum protein is now 6.2 mg/dl, and the albumin is normal.*

Twenty-one of these 37 dogs also received a single initial dose of cyclophosphamide (7 mg/kg IV). Of these 37 dogs, only three (8%) failed to respond to treatment. Complete remission was attained in 16 dogs (43%), and partial remission (PR) occurred in 18 (49%). Median survival for these 37 dogs was 540 days, which was significantly longer than for dogs treated with prednisone alone. Interestingly, the addition of cyclophosphamide did not influence survival times. Complete response to therapy was associated with longer survival, however.[1]

Other dogs have been treated with combinations of melphalan and prednisone, with or without cyclophosphamide[6,10,16] or vincristine.[6,16] Survival times of 9, 14, 18, and 22 months were reported in four dogs[6,9,10]; these times do not differ greatly from survival times of dogs treated with melphalan and prednisone alone.

Once resistance to melphalan and prednisone arises, most dogs are euthanatized. In one report, a second PR was obtained with cyclophosphamide administered for two months in a dog resistant to the former combination.[6] There is a report of a dog that relapsed

after a five-month remission, which had been achieved with prednisone and melphalan, and then responded for another seven months to chlorambucil (4 mg/m² for 5 days every three weeks PO).[5] A dog obtained a second remission of 18 months with cyclophosphamide (50 mg/m² QOD PO) and chlorambucil (6 mg/m² QOD PO) chemotherapy when it became resistant to melphalan and prednisone after 26 months of treatment (Figures 5-22 and 5-23) (A.S. Moore, personal observation). Thus, second remissions may be possible with appropriate therapy. Chlorambucil has also been recommended for treatment of macroglobulinemia.[19]

MULTIPLE MYELOMA IN CATS
Incidence, Signalment, and Etiology

Reports of multiple myeloma in cats are infrequent, and no series describes more than six cats.[19] Of 21 reported cases,[19–26] all were domestic cats with the exception of one Burmese.[20] Sixteen affected cats were male and five were female. The average age was 10.5 years. All of the cats tested negative for the presence of FeLV antigen.

MANAGEMENT OF SPECIFIC DISEASES

Clinical Presentation and History

Most cats present with nonspecific signs of lethargy, anorexia, and weight loss, which is often severe. One cat had a 16-month history of intermittent vomiting and anorexia.[24] Polydipsia and polyuria and secondary infections affecting the upper respiratory tract or skin[20] or pleural cavity[24] are sometimes reported. Two cats presented with peritoneal or pleural effusion caused by bacterial infection and plasma cell infiltrate.[24,25] Neurologic signs, including seizures[23] or circling,[22] have been associated with hyperviscosity of the serum. Hyperviscosity is also associated with retinal hemorrhage and detachment in some cats.[22–24] There is a report of one cat that had cutaneous lesions as well as systemic involvement. Another cat had diffuse intestinal involvement and constipation, and a third cat had tetraplegia due to extradural plasmacytomas.[26] Most affected cats are anemic.

Staging and Diagnosis

The staging and diagnosis of cats with multiple myeloma are similar to that of dogs. Of cats in which serum immunoelectrophoresis was performed, 13 had an IgG paraprotein,[19,20,22,23,25] two had IgA,[20,24] and one had IgM.[19] Bence-Jones proteins were detected in the urine of 10 of 17 cats. Skeletal lesions, which are relatively common in dogs, were reported in only one cat with multiple myeloma.[19]

Hyperviscosity was reported in four of 11 cats[19,22–24] and was associated with retinal hemorrhage and/or neurologic signs. Three cats with hyperviscosity had an abnormal IgG,[22,23] and one cat had an abnormal IgA.[22]

As feline skeletal lesions are rare, diagnosis of multiple myeloma is based on detecting two of three possible signs: monoclonal gammopathy, Bence-Jones proteinuria, or neoplastic plasma cells in bone marrow or elsewhere.

Treatment

As for dogs, supportive treatment for cats with multiple myeloma is important and consists of maintaining adequate renal function and, when infection occurs, initiating aggressive antimicrobial therapy. Many cats with multiple myeloma die from infection[20,23,24] or renal disease[20] either before receiving chemotherapy or during treatment.

Definitive antineoplastic therapy with melphalan and prednisone was documented in 10 cats[19,20,23]; six failed to respond to treatment. Plasmapheresis was attempted in one cat seven weeks after treatment began. Cyclophosphamide was used in place of melphalan, but the cat died five weeks later.[23] The four cats that responded improved clinically and had reduced serum protein levels and Bence-Jones proteinuria as well as improved hematologic parameters. Survival times in these cats was for 10,[23] 24, 28, and 63 weeks.[20] The cats died from infections (i.e., pyoderma and *Sporothrix* pyoderma), nephrotic syndrome, or anemia. When cyclophosphamide and prednisone were used to treat one cat,[21] initial clinical improvement was seen but treatment was discontinued because of mild leukopenia in the third week; the cat worsened and died 10 weeks after treatment began.

Response to chemotherapy for cats with multiple myeloma seems considerably poorer than that reported for dogs. Overall, cats had a 40% response rate and a median survival of 170 days, compared to a 92% response rate for a median of 540 days in dogs.

MONOCLONAL GAMMOPATHY FROM LYMPHOMA IN CATS

Monoclonal gammopathies have been reported in association with lymphoma in six cats,[19,25,27,28] of which five were 2 years of age or younger. Four cats were males. One of the three cats tested for FeLV antigenemia had a positive result.[27]

IgG was abnormal in five cats, and IgM was abnormal in the other cat.[27] Hyperviscosity was present in two of four cats tested.[27,28] Bence-Jones proteinuria was not present in

> **KEY POINT:**
>
> *Response to chemotherapy is considerably poorer in cats with multiple myeloma when compared to dogs with the disease.*

four cats tested. Clinical signs were similar to those reported with multiple myeloma; most cats were lethargic and anorexic. Retinal hemorrhages occurred in both cats with hyperviscosity. Two cats had cutaneous lymphoma.[27,28] Treatment was not reported in any of these cats.

PLASMA CELL TUMORS OF EXTRAMEDULLARY SITES

Extramedullary is a term given to neoplasms of plasma cells that occur in sites outside the marrow. These tumors rarely produce abnormal paraproteins and are not classified as multiple myeloma. There seems to be a clear difference in biological behavior between cutaneous plasmacytomas and plasmacytomas of other sites that we have called "extramedullary."

PLASMA CELL TUMORS OF SKIN AND ORAL MUCOSA IN DOGS
Incidence, Signalment, and Etiology

The most common sites for canine extramedullary plasmacytomas are skin and oral cavity. Comparatively, this is a recently diagnosed tumor, and there are no published reports prior to 1987. Five reports since that time have documented tumors in 282 dogs.[29-34] Plasma cell tumors of the skin and oral mucosa occur with approximately equal prevalence in males and females, with no obvious breed predilection, although mixed-breed dogs accounted for more than 25% of 206 dogs.[30,31] The mean age of affected dogs is between 9 and 10 years; affected dogs range in age from 2 to 22 years.

Clinical Presentation and History

Few clinical signs are associated with cutaneous or mucosal plasma cell tumors. Most tumors appear as smooth, pink-to-red raised nodules[29,31] that are occasionally polypoid (particularly in the ear canal)[32] and sometimes ulcerated (especially on the digits).[32] Tumors range in diameter from 0.2 to 10.0 cm, but most measure between 1 and 2 cm. Tumors occur most frequently on the trunk and limbs (131 of 273

> **KEY POINT:**
>
> *Cutaneous plasmacytomas are benign tumors and are rarely associated with other signs of multiple myeloma.*

or 48%),[29-33] on the head (83 of 273 or 30%), and in the oral cavity (59 of 273 or 22%). Forty-one of the 83 tumors on the head occurred in the ear canal or on the pinna.

Most cutaneous plasmacytomas are solitary, but multiple tumors were seen in 13 of 269 dogs. One dog with nearly 200 cutaneous tumors had evidence of systemic plasma cell tumors and may have had multiple myeloma.[34] Owners often report that tumors grow rapidly. Clinical signs are rare; however, dogs with aural tumors often have signs of otitis.

Staging and Diagnosis

Plasmacytomas of the skin and oral mucosa are rarely associated with systemic disease. In one study, 2 of 131 dogs had elevated serum protein levels (although most dogs did not have protein levels measured), and neither dog had serum protein electrophoresis performed.[30] One of these two dogs also had a rectal tumor and bled excessively after surgery, which may have indicated that this dog had multiple myeloma. The dog was euthanatized two months later.

In another study, two dogs with a solitary cutaneous plasmacytoma also had multiple myeloma with lytic vertebral lesions.[31] Amyloid deposits were found in six tumors; such tumors have been infrequently reported.[33] Although presence of amyloid implies immunologic activity, no behavioral difference in the cutaneous tumors containing amyloid has been detected. Only one canine cutaneous plasmacytoma was documented to have metastasized to regional lymph nodes.[35]

Most cutaneous plasmacytomas are benign. If the clinician wishes to be complete, however, patients should still be evaluated with immunoelectrophoresis, radiographs, hemogram, biochemistry profile, and urinalysis.

Treatment

For dogs with solitary plasmacytomas, surgical

excision is nearly always curative. In one study, surgical excision completely controlled the tumors in 194 of 213 dogs treated.[29–33] Local recurrences occurred in 11 dogs,[30,32,33] and one dog had both distant and local recurrences.[33] One study found that eight of nine local recurrences were predictable because of incomplete surgical excision; four of these dogs had oral lesions that were difficult to excise completely.[30]

Based on responses seen in multiple myeloma, this tumor is probably sensitive to radiation. To date, however, radiation therapy has been reported in only two dogs with plasmacytoma. One dog received radiation treatment with ^{137}Cs after four surgical excisions failed to control the tumor; the dog was free of disease three months later.[30] Another dog with a recurrent oral tumor was treated with ^{60}Co teletherapy, and there was no recurrence by six months after treatment.[36]

Chemotherapy has been reported in only a few dogs with multiple cutaneous or mucosal plasmacytomas, and responses are difficult to assess because of apparent intermittent spontaneous regressions. One dog was treated with melphalan and prednisone and had a 7-month remission.[29] On relapse, the dog was treated homeopathically and the tumors again regressed. Another dog had tumor regression after treatment with cyclophosphamide and prednisone, but new tumors appeared despite continued treatment.[33] Two dogs had tumor regression and were disease free 16 months after treatment with melphalan and prednisone.[32] Intermittent spontaneous regression was seen in a dog with multiple cutaneous plasmacytomas that received no treatment (S.M. Cotter, personal communication, 1994).

EXTRAMEDULLARY PLASMACYTOMAS IN DOGS
Incidence, Signalment, and Etiology

Most extramedullary plasmacytomas in dogs occur in the GI tract, particularly the rectal mucosa[31,37,38]; other sites are rare. Plasmacytomas also have been found in the esophagus[39] and gastric mucosa.[34,38,40] One extramedullary plasmacytoma was found in the lung,[34] and another was found in the spleen.[34] Plas-

macytomas have been reported in the kidneys and the vertebral canal.[41] Reported cases occur in old dogs (range = 3 to 10 years). There are no obvious breed or gender predilections.

Clinical Presentation and History

Clinical signs depend on the area of the GI tract involved. Vomiting was a presenting sign in four dogs with gastric[34,38,40] or esophageal[39] tumors. Rectal prolapse with tenesmus and hematochezia occurs in most dogs with rectal plasmacytoma.[31,37,38] Tumors can be multiple or can diffusely infiltrate the GI wall, making excision difficult.

Staging and Diagnosis

Extramedullary plasmacytomas are more aggressive than their cutaneous counterparts. Regional lymph node metastasis was documented in two dogs with rectal plasmacytoma[37,41] and in one dog with gastric plasmacytoma.[40] In addition, widespread visceral metastasis was described in a dog with a rectal tumor[37]; this dog also had an IgG paraprotein detected on serum immunoelectrophoresis.[37] Another canine rectal tumor progressed into multiple myeloma.[42] Dogs with GI plasmacytomas should be examined carefully for evidence of metastasis using thoracic radiography and abdominal ultrasonography. These dogs should also be investigated for signs consistent with multiple myeloma in the manner previously described.

Treatment

Complete excision for nonmetastatic extramedullary plasmacytomas may have a good prognosis.[30,31] Excision can be difficult, however, due to multiple tumors or diffuse infiltration. Plasma cells are very sensitive to the cytotoxic effects of radiation therapy, but there are no reports of this modality for treatment of extramedullary plasmacytomas. Solitary tumors that cannot be excised may be best treated with radiation therapy, as are some cutaneous plasmacytomas.[30,36]

Chemotherapy, usually with alkylating agents and prednisone, has been reported. Two dogs with respective gastric and rectal plasmacytomas that were not excised completely received melphalan (0.1 mg/kg SID PO) and prednisone (0.5 mg/kg SID PO); one dog also received cyclophosphamide (7 mg/kg IV once).[38] These dogs were free of disease at 33 and 22 months, respectively. Another dog with metastatic rectal plasmacytoma also responded to treatment with melphalan and prednisone and was free of disease nine months after starting therapy.[37] One dog with gastric plasmacytoma metastatic to the regional lymph node was free of disease 30 months after receiving two doses of doxorubicin (25 mg/m^2 IV).[40]

CUTANEOUS PLASMACYTOMA IN CATS

Two case reports of cutaneous extramedullary plasmacytoma indicate that these tumors can have a similar benign course to cutaneous tumors in the dog,[29,34] although one cat had regional lymph node metastasis and a monoclonal gammaglobulin spike.[43] This cat responded to treatment with melphalan and prednisone for six weeks and then died from widespread metastatic disease.

REFERENCES

1. Matus RE, Leifer CE, MacEwen EG, Hurvitz AI: Prognostic factors for multiple myeloma in the dog. *JAVMA* 188:1288–1292, 1986.
2. Osborne CA, Perman V, Sautler JH, et al: Multiple myeloma in the dog. *JAVMA* 153:1300–1319, 1968.
3. Stone RW: The unexpected diagnosis of multiple myeloma in a Shiba Inu incidental to warfarin intoxication. *Canine Pract* 18:26–28, 1993.
4. Orr CM, Higginson J, Baker JR, Jones DRE: Plasma cell myeloma with IgG paraproteinaemia in a bitch. *J Small Anim Pract* 22:31–37, 1981.
5. Pechereau D, Lanore D, Martel PH: Le Myelome multiple: Mise au point a partir de neuf cas. *Pract Med Chir Anim Compag* 26:369–378, 1991.
6. MacEwen EG, Patnaik AK, Hurvitz AI, Bradley R: Non-secretory multiple myeloma in two dogs. *JAVMA* 184:1283–1286, 1984.
7. Oduye OO, Lasos GJ: Multiple myeloma in a dog. *J Small Anim Pract* 13:257–263, 1972.
8. Brener W, Colbatzky F, Platz S, Hermanns W: Immunoglobulin-producing tumours in dogs and cats. *J Comp Pathol* 109:203–216, 1993.
9. Maeda H, Ozaki K, Abe T, et al: Bone lesions of multiple myeloma in three dogs. *JAVMA* 40:384–392, 1993.
10. Cayzer J, Jones BR: IgA multiple myeloma in a dog. *N Z Vet J* 39:139–144, 1991.
11. Finnie JW, Wilks CR: Two cases of multiple myeloma in the dog. *J Small Anim Pract* 23:19–27, 1982.
12. Day MJ, Penhale WJ, McKenna RP, et al: Two cases of IgA multiple myeloma in the dog. *J Small Anim Pract* 28:147–156, 1987.
13. Zinkl JG, LeCouteur RA, Davis DC, Saunders GK: "Flaming" plasma cells in a dog with IgA multiple myeloma. *Vet Clin Pathol* 12:15–19, 1983.
14. Hoenig M: Multiple myeloma associated with the heavy chains of immunoglobulin A in a dog. *JAVMA* 190:1191–1192, 1987.
15. Kirschner SE, Niyo Y, Hill BL, Betts DM: Blindness in a dog with IgA forming myeloma. *JAVMA* 193:349–350, 1988.
16. Jacobs RM, Couto CG, Wellmann ML: Biclonal gammopathy in a dog with myeloma and cutaneous lymphoma. *Vet Pathol* 23:211–213, 1986.
17. Alberts DS, Chen H-SG, Benz D, Mason NL: Effect of renal dysfunction in dogs on the disposition and marrow toxicity of melphalan. *Br J Cancer* 43:330–334, 1981.
18. Matus RE, Leifer CE, Gordon BR: Plasma plasmapheresis and chemotherapy of hyperviscosity syndrome associated with monoclonal gammopathy in the dog. *JAVMA* 183:215–218, 1983.
19. MacEwen EG, Hurvitz AI: Diagnosis and management of monoclonal gammopathies. *Vet Clin North Am Small Anim Pract* 7:119–132, 1977.
20. Drazner FH: Multiple myeloma in the cat. *Compend Contin Educ Pract Vet* 4:206, 1982.
21. Farrow BRH, Penny R: Multiple myeloma in a cat. *JAVMA* 158:606–611, 1971.
22. Hribernik TN, Barta O, Gaunt SD, Boudreaux MK: Serum hyperviscosity syndrome associated with IgG myeloma in a cat. *JAVMA* 181:169–170, 1982.
23. Forrester SD, Greco DS, Relford RL: Serum hyperviscosity syndrome associated with multiple myeloma in two cats. *JAVMA* 200:79–82, 1992.
24. Hawkins EC, Feldman BF, Blanchard PC: Immunoglobulin A myeloma in a cat with pleural effusion and serum hyperviscosity. *JAVMA* 188:876–878, 1986.
25. Kehoe JM, Hurvitz AI, Capra JD: Characterization of three feline paraproteins. *J Immunol* 109:511–516, 1972.
26. Carpenter JL, Andrews LK, Holzworth J: Tumors and tumor-like lesions, in Holzworth J (ed): *Diseases of the Cat. Medicine and Surgery.* Philadelphia, WB Saunders, 1987, pp 406–596.
27. Williams DA, Goldschmidt MH: Hyperviscosity syn-

drome with IgM monoclonal gammopathy and hepatic plasmacytoid lymphosarcoma in a cat. *J Small Animal Pract* 23:311–323, 1982.

28. Dust A, Norris AM, Vail VEO: Cutaneous lymphosarcoma with IgG monoclonal gammopathy serum hyperviscosity and hypercalcemia in a cat. *Can Vet J* 23:235–239, 1982.

29. Lucke VM: Primary cutaneous plasmacytomas in the dog and cat. *J Small Anim Pract* 28:49–55, 1987.

30. Clark GN, Berg J, Engler SJ, Bronson RT: Extramedullary plasmacytomas in dogs: Results of surgical excision in 131 cases. *JAAHA* 28:105–111, 1992.

31. Rakich PM, Latimer KS, Weiss R, Steffans WL: Mucocutaneous plasmacytomas in dogs: 75 cases (1980–1987). *JAVMA* 194:803–810, 1989.

32. Baer KE, Patnaik AE, Gilbertson SR, Hurvitz AI: Cutaneous plasmacytomas in dogs: A morphologic and immunohistochemical study. *Vet Pathol* 26:216–221, 1989.

33. Rowland PH, Valentine BA, Stebbons KE, Smith CA: Cutaneous plasmacytomas with amyloid in six dogs. *Vet Pathol* 28:125–130, 1991.

34. Walton GS, Gopinath C: Multiple myeloma in a dog with some unusual features. *J Small Anim Pract* 13:703–708, 1972.

35. Trigo FJ, Hargis AM: Canine cutaneous plasmacytoma with regional lymph node metastasis. *Vet Med Small Anim Clin* 78:1749–1751, 1983.

36. Morton LD, Barton CL, Elissalde GS, Wilson SR: Oral extramedullary plasmacytoma in two dogs. *Vet Pathol* 26:637–639, 1986.

37. Trevor PB, Saunders GK, Waldrom DR, Leib MS: Metastatic extramedullary plasmacytoma of the colon and rectum in a dog. *JAVMA* 203:406–409, 1993.

38. MacEwen EG, Patnaik AK, Johnson GF, Hurvitz AI: Extramedullary plasmacytoma of the gastrointestinal tract in two dogs. *JAVMA* 184:1396–1398, 1984.

39. Carpenter JL: Esophageal plasmacytoma in the dog. *JAVMA* 204:1210–1211, 1994.

40. Brunnert SR, Dee LA, Herron AJ, Altman NH: Gastric extramedullary plasmacytoma in a dog. *JAVMA* 200:1501–1502, 1992.

41. Kyriazidou A, Brown PJ, Lucke VM: An immunohistochemical study of canine extramedullary plasma cell tumors. *J Comp Pathol* 100:256–266, 1989.

42. Lester SJ, Mesfin GM: A solitary plasmacytoma in a dog with progression to a disseminated myeloma. *Can Vet J* 21:284–286, 1980.

43. Carothers MA, Johnson GC, DiBartola SP, et al: Extramedullary plasmacytoma of the gastrointestinal tract and immunoglobulin-associated amyloidosis in a cat. *JAVMA* 195:1593–1597, 1989.

CLINICAL BRIEFING: TUMORS OF THE NERVOUS SYSTEM

Tumors of the Canine Brain

Common Clinical Presentation	Seizures and temperament changes
Common Histologic Type	Meningioma
Epidemiology and Biological Behavior	Mixed breeds and boxers; old dogs (10 years of age and older); slight male predilection; locally invasive, rare metastases
Prognostic Factors	Worse prognosis with severe neurologic dysfunction, abnormal cerebrospinal fluid, or multiple tumors

Treatment
  Palliation
  Surgery
  Radiation Therapy
 	
  Chemotherapy
	
	Corticosteroids and anticonvulsants
	May be beneficial for meningiomas
	Treatment of choice for gliomas; useful alone or as an adjunct to surgery for meningiomas
	Hindered by blood–brain barrier; possible role for carmustine and lomustine

Tumors of the Feline Brain

Common Clinical Presentation	Sudden-onset visual deficits, seizures, and neurologic dysfunction
Common Histologic Type	Meningioma
Epidemiology and Biological Behavior	Old cats (75% >9 years of age); locally invasive, rare metastases
Prognostic Factors	None identified

Treatment
  Surgery
  Radiation Therapy
	
	Treatment of choice due to slow regrowth of meningioma
	May be useful adjunct to incomplete excision

MANAGEMENT OF SPECIFIC DISEASES

Tumors of the Canine Spine

Common Clinical Presentation	Pain; slow onset of ataxia and paresis
Common Histologic Types	Extradural tumors; vertebral body
Epidemiology and Biological Behavior	Large-breed dogs, young to middle-aged; locally invasive
Prognostic Factors	None identified
Treatment 　Surgery 　Radiation Therapy	Treatment of choice for extradural and intradural-extramedullary tumors; intramedullary tumors are not amenable to surgical excision May be a useful adjunct to incomplete surgery

Tumors of the Feline Spine

Common Clinical Presentation	Acute paresis
Common Histologic Type	Lymphoma
Epidemiology and Biological Behavior	70% of cats are FeLV positive and 85% have bone marrow that contains lymphoma; most tumors are extradural
Prognostic Factors	None identified
Treatment 　Surgery 　Radiation Therapy 　Chemotherapy	Rarely indicated because of systemic disease May give local palliation Drugs described in the Lymphoma chapter may give complete remission

Tumors of the Peripheral Nerves

Common Clinical Presentation	Slowly progressive lameness
Common Histologic Type	*Dogs:* Neurofibrosarcoma *Cats:* Lymphoma

MANAGEMENT OF SPECIFIC DISEASES

Epidemiology and Biological Behavior	*Dogs:* Large-breed dogs; middle-aged dogs (average age is 7 years); local disease, rare metastasis *Cats:* Systemic disease
Prognostic Factors	None identified
Treatment **Surgery**	 Surgical resection of tumor for small masses; amputation and resection for large masses or if severe neurologic deficits are present
Radiation Therapy	Used for incompletely excised tumors
Chemotherapy	Most effective for lymphoma

Tumors of the nervous system are rare in dogs and cats. Brain tumors are more common than spinal cord tumors. Tumors of the nervous system rarely metastasize; their effects occur as a result of slow expansion and displacement or destruction of surrounding nervous tissue. Therefore, signs may be mild and overlooked by owners until the advent of more serious neurologic disturbances, such as seizures or paresis.

TUMORS OF THE CANINE BRAIN
Incidence, Signalment, and Etiology

Although most canine brain tumors are meningiomas, tumors of neuroectodermal origin (e.g., astrocytomas, gliomas, ependymomas, and choroid-plexus papillomas) have been described (Table 5-7). In dogs, brain tumors most commonly occur in the cerebrum rather than in the brain stem or cerebellum. The cerebrum is the most accessible area for surgery. Most studies of canine brain tumors do not separate data by histologic type, so much of the information refers to a conglomerate of tumor types. Overall, affected dogs are old (mean age = 9 to 10 years; range = 1 to 17 years).[1,2] There is a slightly higher incidence in males than females (1.5:1).[1,2] In two recent studies, mixed-breed dogs were the most commonly affected. Boxers were the purebreds most often affected.[1-3]

Clinical Presentation and History

An early study found that temperament changes and locomotor deficiencies were the most common clinical signs associated with cerebral tumors.[3] A more recent study, however, reported that seizures were the most common sign, occurring in 22 of 43 dogs.[2] Interestingly, 31 of 43 dogs had a normal neurologic examination on presentation despite a history of seizures, but 25 of these 31 dogs later developed persistent deficits, usually within three months. Lack of persistent neurologic deficits at presentation was ascribed to involvement of the rostral cerebrum, which contains neither motor nor sensory areas. Progression of the tumor to involve other structures could produce more permanent deficits later.[2]

Visual deficits are recognized as an uncommon presenting sign in dogs with cerebral neoplasia[3] and may signal neoplasia with involvement of the optic chiasm.[4] This manifestation, however, is rare even for pituitary macroadenomas and adenocarcinomas.[4,5] Blindness may occur without other neurologic signs and may persist even after tumor excision. Meningiomas are associated with slow progression of clinical signs.[1]

Nasal tumors are occasionally the cause of neurologic signs such as seizures because of extension through the cribriform plate. It should be noted that these tumors may occur with no sign of nasal disease.[2,6]

MANAGEMENT OF SPECIFIC DISEASES

TABLE 5-7
Primary tumors involving the cerebrum in dogs

Tumor	Number of 56 Dogs[1]* (%)	Number of 39 Dogs[2] (%)
Meningioma	27 (48)	13 (33)
Astrocytoma	7 (12)	7 (18)
Neuroblastoma	Not reported	5 (13)
Ependymoma	Not reported	1 (3)
Nasal tumor (by extension)	4 (7)	13 (33)
Choroid plexus	6 (11)	Not reported

*Only 44 of 56 reported tumors are included in this table.

Staging and Diagnosis

If a brain tumor is suspected, metabolic causes of signs should be eliminated by routine blood work and urinalysis. In addition, thoracic radiographs and computed tomography (CT) or magnetic resonance imaging (MRI) of the brain should be performed.

In private practice, it can be difficult to confirm the presence of a brain tumor. Radiographs of the cranium rarely reveal changes, although meningiomas occasionally may be associated with hyperostosis or skull lysis. Cerebrospinal fluid (CSF) is rarely abnormal in dogs with brain tumors; when abnormalities occur, they often indicate only nonspecific inflammation or necrosis.[1,2] Computed tomography (CT scanning) reconstructs an image of a cross section of the body. CT scans can be used to localize tumors and delineate tissue margins within structures. The scans locate the tumor precisely, which increases the accuracy of surgery and radiation therapy and thereby reduces injury to surrounding normal tissue. CT scans can sometimes indicate probable tumor type. Delineation between tumor and normal tissue during CT scanning is enhanced with an intravenous contrast material that pools within the imperfect microvasculature of the tumor. Although much of this information is extrapolated from human studies, uniformly contrast-enhanced, well-marginated, broad-based lesions that are located peripherally are commonly meningiomas (Figure 5-24). Tumors associated with hemorrhage are more likely to be high-grade astrocytomas or glioblastomas[7] (Figure 5-25). Many veterinary schools and a growing number of private practices have access to CT scanners. Although CT necessitates the use of general anesthesia, there is little other risk to the patient. Magnetic resonance imaging is becoming more common in veterinary practice and provides better resolution for intracranial structures than CT scanning.

Biopsy of brain lesions prior to surgery is rarely performed in veterinary medicine, partly because of difficulties in positioning the biopsy needle accurately. Therefore, definitive diagnosis is usually made at the time of surgery or at necropsy.

Rarely a primary brain tumor will metastasize outside the cranial vault. Pulmonary metastases of meningiomas were described in four dogs.[8,9] For this reason, complete staging should include thoracic radiographs.

Prognostic Factors

Dogs with mild or moderate neurologic impairment at presentation

> **KEY POINT:**
>
> *Computed tomography is usually required to localize brain tumors and to delineate the extent of tissue involvement.*

MANAGEMENT OF SPECIFIC DISEASES

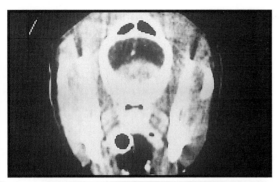

Figure 5-24: CT scans usually reveal meningiomas as peripherally located, broad-based lesions. A CT scan assists in planning surgery radiation therapy. (Courtesy A.S. Tidwell)

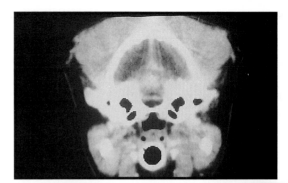

Figure 5-25: An astrocytoma of the cerebellum is demonstrated by CT scan. A CT scan allows accurate planning for megavoltage radiation therapy. (Courtesy A.S. Tidwell)

have a more favorable prognosis than dogs with severe initial neurologic signs.[1] Dogs with multiple tumors or intracranial metastasis have a shorter survival than dogs with a solitary tumor, and dogs with normal CSF fluid analysis have longer survival times.[1] Dogs with meningiomas live longer than dogs with other types of brain tumors.[1]

In one retrospective study, dogs receiving ^{60}Co teletherapy, with or without other treatment modalities, lived longer than dogs undergoing surgery or supportive care only.[1]

Treatment

Many neurologic signs and impairments seen in dogs with brain tumors arise from peritumoral edema that pressures normal tissue. Neurologic status, and, therefore, quality of life can be improved with corticosteroids (e.g., prednisone, 1 mg/kg SID or QOD PO) and anticonvulsants, such as phenobarbital. Supportive measures do not improve survival times.[1]

Definitive therapy consists of surgery, which is usually reserved for superficial tumors (e.g., meningiomas), or radiation therapy, which is used for more deep-seated tumors.

Surgery is at least moderately successful for treatment of meningiomas; however, incomplete excisions are common because these tumors have poorly defined borders. Regrowth of meningiomas is usual-

ly slow; therefore, survival is prolonged. Perioperative mortality from bleeding and edema may be a problem following excision of large tumors. Careful selection of anesthesia during surgery can help prevent increases in intracranial pressure that could cause brain herniation and death. Administering mannitol and corticosteroids, elevating the animal's head, and hyperventilating the patient help to control intracranial pressure.

Radiation therapy, used alone or as an adjunct to surgery, is important in treating brain tumors and prolonging survival in dogs.[1] Because of the depth of these tumors and protection by overlying bony structures, megavoltage (rather than orthovoltage) teletherapy is recommended. Megavoltage radiation also allows "splitting" of doses, thereby reducing damage to normal surrounding brain tissues. Median survival for 16 dogs with meningiomas treated with radiation alone was 233 days. For 10 dogs with gliomas treated solely by radiation, median survival was 176 days.[10] In another study, five dogs that received megavoltage (linear-accelerator) radiation therapy alone had a median survival of 360 days.[11] Another study found that regardless of tumor type, dogs receiving radiation had a median survival of approximately 150 days, whereas dogs with meningiomas that were irradiated had a median survival that approached 270 days.[1] Dogs treated with radiation for meningiomas seem to have longer survival

MANAGEMENT OF SPECIFIC DISEASES

times than dogs treated with radiation for other types of brain tumors. For example, median survival of 18 dogs with meningioma receiving 45 Gy of radiation alone was 150 days; five dogs survived 10 months or longer after treatment.[12]

Despite apparent disadvantages of orthovoltage radiation in treating deep-seated tumors, 14 dogs treated with orthovoltage alone for brain tumors had a median survival of 412 days; dogs receiving a higher dose (45 Gy rather than 39 Gy) survived even longer.[13]

Laser therapy caused localized tumor reduction and resolution of clinical signs for seven months in a boxer with an invasive meningioma.[14]

Chemotherapy is largely inconsequential in treatment of brain tumors because of poor penetration of most drugs across the blood–brain barrier. Carmustine and lomustine are nitrosourea compounds unique because of their lipid solubility. Both agents enter the CSF in animals to achieve concentrations of 15% to 30% of concurrent plasma levels. Lomustine is completely absorbed orally and is well tolerated by this route. Carmustine is administered intravenously. Both compounds have been evaluated clinically for treatment of brain tumors in dogs.

Lomustine was administered orally to eight dogs with brain tumors.[15] The dose used was 60 to 80 mg/m² every 6 to 8 weeks, and the major toxic side effect was myelosuppression, with a leukocyte nadir at 1 to 4 weeks after treatment. Occasional vomiting was reported. Clinical response is difficult to assess, as five of eight dogs received lomustine after surgery to remove the tumor. For these five dogs, median survival was 90 days (range = 28 to 630 days), with two dogs still alive at last report. Of the three dogs with measurable disease, one had complete remission, one had stable disease, and one had progression of the disease. Histopathology was not available for these three dogs.

Carmustine was administered intravenously to 15 dogs with brain tumors at a dose of 50 mg/m² every 6 weeks.[16] Neutropenia occurred at a nadir of 7 to 9

KEY POINT:

Radiation therapy is an effective modality in the treatment of brain tumors.

days after treatment and remained low for 15 days. One dog developed histologic evidence of pulmonary fibrosis without clinical signs after eight treatments with carmustine. Six of these dogs and one other dog[17] all had gliomas; all had partial remissions. The median survival of dogs with glioma was 218 days; responders had a median survival of 288 days,[16] which is comparable to radiation therapy. Both carmustine and lomustine should be further evaluated for treatment of canine gliomas.

PITUITARY MACROADENOMAS AND ADENOCARCINOMAS
Incidence, Signalment, and Etiology

Although most pituitary ACTH-secreting tumors are microadenomas, macroadenomas (diameter >1 cm) occasionally are reported. In 320 dogs with pituitary-dependent hyperadrenocorticism, 40 (12.5%) had a large tumor of the pituitary, and all showed neurologic dysfunction. Tumors may occur in any area of the pituitary gland, and carcinomas may invade thalamus and hypothalamus, causing hemorrhage and death.[18] Any dog with hyperadrenocorticism that develops neurologic signs should be evaluated for presence of a pituitary mass. These tumors affect old dogs (10 to 12 years of age on average). There is no sex predilection.[18] Small-breed dogs commonly develop pituitary-dependent hyperadrenocorticism.[5] Large pituitary tumors are rare in cats.[5]

Clinical Presentation and History

Clinical signs of hyperadrenocorticism include polydipsia and polyuria, truncal alopecia, and abdominal enlargement (i.e., pot-bellied appearance). The most common neurologic signs in dogs with pituitary macroadenoma are stupor, nystagmus, and behavior changes; pacing, circling, lethargy, and seizures also may occur.[18,19] Symmetric tetraparesis was common in one group of dogs.[18] Despite the proximity of these tumors to the optic chiasm, blindness is uncommon.[5,20] The absolute size of a pituitary tumor may be less important than other relative fac-

MANAGEMENT OF SPECIFIC DISEASES

tors, such as calvarium size and tumor location and growth rate. Hence, small dogs may show neurologic signs with quite small (<1 cm) tumors.[5]

Dogs that develop neurologic signs while being treated with mitotane (o,p'-DDD) for pituitary-dependent hyperadrenocorticism should be evaluated for a large pituitary tumor. Mitotane is cytotoxic for the adrenal cortex but will not affect growth of a pituitary tumor.[18,19] Inadequate serum cortisol suppression during a high-dose dexamethasone-suppression test may indicate an adrenal tumor. In an animal with pituitary-dependent hyperadrenocorticism, inadequate suppression may indicate the potential for subsequent development of a large or invasive pituitary tumor.[18] Large pituitary tumors are capable of producing very high levels of ACTH and are not easily suppressed by exogenous corticosteroid administration. In one study, dogs that had large pituitary tumors and eventually developed neurologic signs had higher average plasma ACTH levels at presentation than dogs with small tumors.[5]

Staging and Diagnosis

In any dog suspected of having a pituitary tumor, staging should include endogenous ACTH levels, low and high dose dexamethasone suppression tests, thoracic radiographs, and CT or MRI imaging of the brain. A presumptive diagnosis of pituitary macroadenoma or adenocarcinoma may be made by CT scan on detection of a mass in the sella turcica. Evidence of compression of surrounding structures as well as displacement and dilation of the third and lateral ventricles are common. CSF analysis is not useful to diagnose this type of tumor. Definitive diagnosis by biopsy is rare unless surgical resection is performed. Occasionally, pituitary adenocarcinoma may metastasize intracerebrally.[21]

Treatment

When hypophysectomy was used to treat a dog with a pituitary macroadenoma, the dog was still alive eight months after surgery.[19] This surgery is technically difficult, particularly if the tumor is large.

Radiation therapy is the preferred treatment for large pituitary tumors. For dogs with confirmed macroadenoma of the pituitary, 40 to 45 Gy of megavoltage radiation to the tumor and 1 cm of adjacent normal tissue resolved neurologic signs within six months of therapy in all reported cases[22]; tumor shrinkage often continued for more than one year.[23] Resolution of signs of hyperadrenocorticism was more variable. ACTH levels decreased to normal over a period of months in some dogs, but other dogs required concurrent mitotane therapy. Hypopituitarism was not noted in any dog treated with radiation therapy. In six dogs with large pituitary tumors treated with radiation, median survival was 740 days (range = 157 to 1298 days).[23] Some reports suggest that prophylactic megavoltage (^{60}Co) irradiation of dogs with small pituitary tumors may prevent the onset of neurologic signs.[5] The cost of this treatment should be weighed against the apparently low likelihood of most dogs with hyperadrenocorticism developing neurologic signs. For dogs that do develop neurologic signs from an expanding pituitary tumor, radiation teletherapy is an effective treatment.

TUMORS OF THE FELINE BRAIN
Incidence, Signalment, and Etiology

Meningioma is the most common intracranial tumor in cats. More than 75% of cats with meningiomas are older than 9 years of age[24]; these tumors are rare in cats less than 5 years of age.[24,25] There seems to be no breed predilection. Meningiomas may occur more frequently in male cats.[24] Pituitary tumors[4] and ependymomas[24] have been described in cats but are far less common than meningiomas. Ependymomas and neuroblastomas may arise in the olfactory epithelium and erode the cribriform plate to extend caudally.[24] Tumors in this location have been associated with FeLV infection.[26]

> **KEY POINT:**
>
> *Dogs that develop neurologic signs while being treated for hyperadrenocorticism should be evaluated by CT scan for a large pituitary tumor.*

MANAGEMENT OF SPECIFIC DISEASES

Clinical Presentation and History

Signs referable to a meningioma are usually obvious to owners only briefly (5 weeks in one study)[27] before the animal is presented to the veterinarian. The most common clinical signs are impaired vision (>90% in one study),[27] paresis, seizures, and behavioral or demeanor changes (e.g., pacing, dullness, or lethargy). Less common signs include ataxia, circling, or head tilting.[28]

Staging and Diagnosis

As for dogs, absence of metabolic causes for clinical signs should be confirmed by routine blood work and urinalysis. Thoracic radiographs and CT and MRI of the brain should also be performed.

Nearly half of the cats with meningioma have evidence of hyperostotic bone adjacent to the tumor on CT scan, although this may be difficult to see on skull radiographs. Most cats have solitary meningioma. Multiple tumors may be seen in approximately 15% of cats with meningioma,[27] but distant metastasis is rare. Thoracic radiographs are therefore rarely necessary other than as a screen for other diseases.

On CT scan, the tumor appears as a peripherally located mass with a broad base and distinct tumor margins that are enhanced uniformly by contrast injection. This appearance may be sufficient to at least make a tentative diagnosis of meningioma,[7] and meningiomas should be strongly considered in any old cat with a recent history of neurologic impairment.

Ependymomas are uncommon in cats; when they occur, they may metastasize.[24]

Prognostic Factors

No prognostic factors for feline meningiomas have been identified. Factors that did not affect prognosis for survival in one study included age of the cat, loca-

KEY POINTS:

Most meningiomas in cats are solitary; however, they may be multiple in approximately 15% of cats.

Two thirds of the cats that have a meningioma removed are alive 1 year after surgery, and half are alive 2 years after surgery.

tion of the tumor, and whether tumors were multiple or single.[27]

Treatment

Feline meningiomas tend to be more discrete than their canine counterparts and hence are more amenable to surgical excision. Surgery is the preferred treatment for feline meningioma. Two series of cats (17 cats[28] and 42 cats[27]) were treated by surgical excision. The most common complications were problems in completely excising deep or adherent meningiomas, and occurrence of postoperative hemorrhage and anemia. Perioperative mortality approached 20% in both studies and was mainly attributed to cerebral edema, brain herniation, or both. In the cats that recovered from surgery, improvement in demeanor and in most neurologic dysfunction occurred within 48 hours to 1 week. Visual impairment was least likely to resolve.

Overall survival after surgery was 66% at one year and 50% at two years.[27] There was local recurrence, either confirmed or presumed on the basis of recurrent neurologic deficits, in 20% to 25% of these cats. Recurrence often occurred 2 to 4 years after the original surgery, indicating that regrowth may be slow. Particularly in old cats, this fact should be remembered when considering adjunctive therapy after surgery.

In humans and dogs with meningiomas, radiation is a useful adjunct to surgical excision. In cats, the local recurrence rate for surgically excised meningiomas is low and usually takes a long time to occur. For this reason, radiation therapy probably is applicable only in treatment of meningiomas that are incompletely excised or that recur after surgery. There is little published data regarding the usefulness of radiation therapy for feline meningioma.[29]

Palliative Therapy

Anecdotally, cats with recurrent meningioma and

MANAGEMENT OF SPECIFIC DISEASES

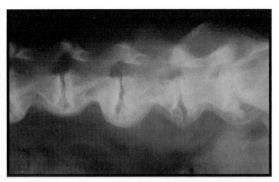

Figure 5-26: An osteosarcoma of the sixth lumbar vertebra causing extradural compression of the associated spinal cord. Surgical decompression may relieve symptoms, but definitive surgery requires vertebral removal and is unlikely to achieve complete resection (Courtesy J. Berg)

neurologic deficits have "done well" on corticosteroid and anticonvulsant medication. There are no controlled studies, however, to determine whether this treatment improves survival times, because similar palliation treatment does not seem to improve the length of survival of dogs.

TUMORS OF THE CANINE SPINE
Incidence, Signalment, and Etiology

Most (up to 50%) of canine spinal tumors are extradural, and the majority of these are primary or secondary bone tumors, such as osteosarcoma and multiple myeloma (Figure 5-26). Other tumors, such as fibrosarcoma, chondrosarcoma, hemangiosarcoma, and liposarcoma, are less common. These tumors rarely invade through the dura. Lymphoma is usually extradural, but can be intradural,[30,31] and is usually associated with systemic disease. Intradural-extramedullary spinal neoplasms are most likely to be meningiomas or neurofibrosarcomas; these are most common in the cervical spinal cord.

Intramedullary tumors are rare in dogs. They are most commonly astrocytomas but occasionally can be metastatic lesions or part of a systemic disease, particularly lymphoma or hemangiosarcoma.[30]

Spinal tumors are more common in large-breed dogs (from 67% to 90% of dogs with spinal tumors[32]). There is no gender predisposition. The average age of affected dogs is 5 to 6 years.[32] In one study, more than 25% of the dogs with spinal tumors were younger than three years of age.[32] Intramedullary tumors are more common in young animals.

Clinical Presentation and History

In animals with extradural spinal tumors, the first sign is pain that results from the destruction of bone and compression of nerve roots. For both extradural and intradural-extramedullary spinal tumors, ataxia and paresis usually develop slowly, although rapid progression may occur and produce acute onset of paresis or plegia. Neurofibromas usually arise from dorsal nerve roots. The pain initially felt develops into paresis as the tumors slowly grow within the spinal canal and through the intervertebral foramen along peripheral nerves. Meningiomas cause similar signs; however, these tumors may invade the dura. Signs of intramedullary tumors usually progress rapidly (<2 weeks), whereas signs of other spinal tumors normally have a mean duration of one to two months.[32] Most extradural tumors occur at the thoracolumbar junction. Most intradural-extramedullary tumors occur in the cervicothoracic spine.

Staging and Diagnosis

Myelography is useful for distinguishing extradural, intradural-extramedullary, and intramedullary tumors. Histopathology is needed for definitive diagnosis, but decisions regarding the possible success of treatment often can be made using myelographic information alone. Extradural tumors compress the dura and cord, obstructing the flow of dye in the column, whereas intramedullary tumors cause diverging myelographic lines on both lateral and dorsoventral views. For intradural-extramedullary tumors, the mass may be outlined by contrast media, creating a "golf-tee" appearance[33] (Figure 5-27).

Cerebrospinal fluid analysis is not usually helpful in specifically diagnosing spinal tumors; spinal tumors rarely exfoliate (with the exception of some, but not all, spinal lymphomas).[30,31,34]

MANAGEMENT OF SPECIFIC DISEASES

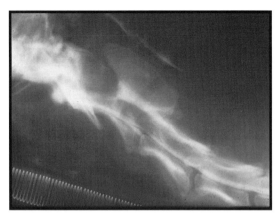

Figure 5-27: *An intradural-extramedullary neurofibrosarcoma is outlined by myelography to show a classic "golf-tee" appearance. (Courtesy A.S. Tidwell)*

Treatment

Surgery is the treatment of choice for most extradural tumors; the exception is extradural lymphoma, which may respond to chemotherapy or radiation therapy. In dogs with extensive bone lysis of the vertebra, removal of the vertebra may be the only option; however, vertebral removal does not often result in complete resection. Removal of extradural tumors is usually confined to tumors that have not yet damaged the vertebra structurally. The exception to this is multiple myeloma of the vertebrae, for which chemotherapy with prednisone and alkylating agents is the treatment of choice (see the chapter on Plasma Cell Tumors). Intradural-extramedullary tumors that have not invaded the spinal cord may be operable. Surgery was performed on 9 of 13 dogs with spinal meningioma and neurologic improvement was seen in six dogs.[35] Surgery was complicated by the friable nature of these tumors and by numerous adhesions to surrounding structures, even in the absence of cord invasion. Spinal cord invasion was present in 8 of 32 spinal meningiomas[35]; invasive tumors often are not operable. Although these tumors are benign and surgical resection can potentially

be curative, ventral location or location at an intumescence is associated with poor surgical outcome. Five of nine dogs that underwent surgery lived more than six months, and one dog was free of disease three years after surgery.[35] Intramedullary tumors usually are not operable.

Radiation may delay recurrence of an incompletely excised extradural or intradural-extramedullary tumor. Most published data in the veterinary literature is, however, indirectly extrapolated from data derived from treatment of brain tumors. One dog with intradural-extramedullary meningioma was treated by surgery and had a local recurrence 15 months later.[36] Treatment with megavoltage (^{60}Co) radiation therapy alone prolonged that remission by 19 months.

Corticosteroids (e.g., prednisone, 1 mg/kg BID) have been palliative for some intramedullary tumors,[30] but this presumably is a result of indirect effects on edema rather than of direct effects on the tumor. Because of the blood–brain barrier, chemotherapy is of little use in treating spinal tumors. Intrathecal chemotherapy with cytosine arabinoside (ara-C) was used in three dogs with spinal lymphoma in conjunction with craniospinal irradiation to a total dose of 30 Gy. Responses were dramatic but short-lived (6, 14, and 84 days), and were probably due to radiation rather than to chemotherapy.[31]

TUMORS OF THE FELINE SPINE
Incidence, Signalment, and Etiology

The most common spinal neoplasm in the cat is lymphoma; only meningioma of the brain is more common in the feline central nervous system. Most lymphomas are extradural (43 of 51 in two series)[37,38] and may be found in the cervical, thoracolumbar, and sacral regions. The tumor occasionally may invade the vertebra and rarely invades the dura and spinal cord. Most feline lymphomas are systemic at diagnosis, and these cats test positive for FeLV virus antigen (16 of 17 cats evaluated in one study).[38] In addition, up to 85% of cats with spinal lymphoma

> **KEY POINT:**
>
> *Myelography or CT scans are useful to distinguish extradural, extramedullary, and intramedullary tumors.*

MANAGEMENT OF SPECIFIC DISEASES

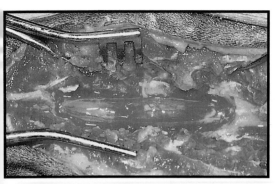

Figure 5-28: Surgery does not have a therapeutic role in the treatment of feline spinal lymphoma because of tumor involvement at multiple sites as shown above. The treatment of choice is chemotherapy; radiation therapy is a possible adjunct. (Courtesy J. Berg)

have lymphomatous infiltrates in the bone marrow.[18] Spinal lymphoma occurs in young cats (median age = 3 years; range = 7 months to 17 years). In one study, 14 (67%) of 21 cats were in the 1- to 5-year age range.[18] There was no obvious breed predisposition. A higher proportion of male cats were affected, consistent with the epidemiology of FeLV-related diseases.

Clinical Presentation and History

Spinal lymphoma is probably the most common cause of spinal dysfunction in cats. Clinical signs usually develop acutely and progress rapidly. Signs are typically present for only one week prior to presentation. These signs most commonly include spastic or flaccid paresis of the hindlimbs but may vary depending on the region of the cord affected by the tumor. Other causes of paresis are rare in cats. Some cats have signs referable to anemia or other cytopenias that are presumably secondary to bone marrow involvement with systemic lymphoma. These findings, however, are nonspecific for spinal lymphoma.

Staging and Diagnosis

Radiography of the spine should be performed to rule out obvious

KEY POINT:

Cats with spinal lymphoma are frequently FeLV positive and have bone marrow infiltration with lymphoblasts.

traumatic injury, but radiographically apparent bone invasion is rare in spinal lymphoma. Myelography may help to delineate the tumor, but definitive diagnosis requires demonstration of malignant tumor cells. Cerebrospinal fluid analysis is usually unremarkable. Bone marrow aspiration or core biopsy may provide a rapid and relatively noninvasive diagnosis. When malignant cells are found on bone marrow cytology, a myelogram is usually unnecessary. If a bone marrow sample does not provide a diagnosis, myelography and fluoroscopically guided fine-needle aspiration can provide a definitive diagnosis.[39]

Complete staging should also include a hemogram, biochemical profile, urinalysis, and FeLV antigen test as well as thoracic radiographs and abdominal ultrasound to identify other systemic evidence of lymphoma.

Treatment

Surgery is rarely indicated for feline lymphoma because of the multicentric nature of this disease. In addition, spinal lymphoma usually involves multiple vertebral bodies at multiple levels of the spinal cord; thus, destabilization of the spinal column is a risk of surgical intervention (Figure 5-28).

Radiation therapy is likely to reduce the tumor rapidly and thus improve neurologic function. Systemic chemotherapy is still necessary, however, because of the multicentric nature of this disease. Of a series of 23 cats with spinal lymphoma, three were treated with spinal irradiation and chemotherapy (i.e., L-asparaginase, vincristine, and prednisone)[38]; two cats improved and one continued to deteriorate. Another cat received the same chemotherapy after surgical debulking and improved neurologically. Three cats relapsed within 3 months; one was alive 13 months after treatment.

Chemotherapy rapidly resolves clinical signs of feline lymphoma. In a series of 21 cats with spinal lymphoma, nine were treated with chemotherapy and one with surgical

MANAGEMENT OF SPECIFIC DISEASES

decompression and chemotherapy.[39] Of six cats receiving the combination of vincristine, cyclophosphamide, and prednisone (COP), three attained complete remission (median = 14 weeks; range = 5 to 28 weeks) and three attained a partial remission (median = 6 weeks; range = 4 to 10 weeks). Three cats were given only prednisone: one failed to respond, and two had a partial remission for 4 and 10 weeks, respectively. One cat treated with surgical decompression and COP chemotherapy had a complete remission for 62 weeks; when the patient relapsed, treatment with doxorubicin (30 mg/m^2 IV) produced another complete remission.

Chemotherapy is, therefore, the treatment of choice for feline lymphoma. Surgical decompression is rarely warranted. Radiation therapy may result in rapid tumor shrinkage and is a useful adjuvant to chemotherapy.

TUMORS OF PERIPHERAL NERVES
Incidence, Signalment, and Etiology

Neurofibrosarcoma is the most common tumor of peripheral nerve tissue in the dog. It is sometimes termed *schwannoma, neurilemmoma, perineural fibroblastoma,* and *nerve-sheath tumor.* This neoplasm arises from the fibrous nerve sheath and most commonly occurs in the brachial plexus. Neurofibrosarcomas are classified as soft tissue sarcomas and are also discussed in the chapter on Tumors of the Skin. They are prone to regrowth and are invasive but rarely metastasize. As for all soft tissue sarcomas, the clinical behavior is similar regardless of whether the diagnosis is neurofibroma or neurofibrosarcoma.

Middle-aged dogs (median = 7 years; range = 4 to 9 years) are predisposed to cervical neurofibrosarcomas; there is no obvious breed or gender predilection. Large-breed dogs are most often affected.[40] Neurofibrosarcomas also occur in the thoracolumbar region as intradural-extramedullary tumors (see previous section).

The most common tumor of the peripheral nerves in cats is lymphoma, although neurofibrosarcomas have been described; both are rare in cats.[24]

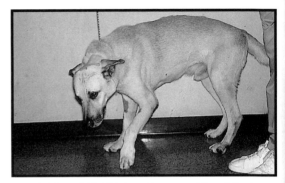

Figure 5-29: This dog with a tumor of the peripheral nerves in the brachial plexus demonstrates forelimb lameness with severe muscle atrophy over the scapula. (Courtesy J. Berg)

Clinical Presentation and History

The most common clinical sign of nerve sheath tumor in dogs is forelimb lameness that progresses slowly. Neurologic deficits are minimal, but severe muscle atrophy, particularly of the scapular musculature, is common (Figure 5-29). Depending on the nerves involved, Horner's syndrome may be present. The tumors occasionally extend through the intervertebral foramen to compress the spinal cord, resulting in neurologic deficits in the ipsilateral pelvic limb. The history of lameness is usually chronic, extending over many months.[40] A large mass may be palpated deep within the axilla, but small tumors may not be detectable on palpation.

Staging and Diagnosis

After a general health screen is performed and other causes of lameness and muscle wasting are ruled out, if a tumor of the peripheral nerves is suspected, staging should include the following. Myelography should be performed before treating brachial plexus neurofibrosarcomas because of their propensity for invasion of the intervertebral foramen, even if the dog shows no hindlimb signs. CT scanning or MRI may more accurately image these tumors.

One dog that had two surgical resections of a brachial plexus neurofibrosarcoma developed pulmonary metastases 20 months after the first surgery,[40] but this is rare.

Treatment

Peripheral nerve tumors are locally invasive and rarely metastasize; thus, the treatment of choice is surgical excision. For small tumors that involve only one or two nerves, excision of affected nerves close to the intervertebral foramen may allow complete resection. For large tumors that involve multiple nerves, or for dogs with severe neurologic deficits in the forelimb, amputation should be considered. If the tumor extends into the spinal canal, prognosis is guarded, as surgical excision (even with laminectomy) is unlikely to be complete. The owner of an animal that has any neurofibrosarcoma should be warned that excision may not be complete and that local recurrence is possible.

There are no published reports of the efficacy of adjunctive radiation therapy for brachial plexus neurofibrosarcomas, although responses similar to those reported for other soft tissue sarcomas are likely. Remission durations for dogs with soft tissue sarcomas treated with radiation therapy largely depend on the dose of radiation delivered. For one group of dogs, a total dose of 45 Gy controlled tumor growth in 48% of dogs for 1 year, whereas 67% of dogs treated with 50 Gy experienced similar control.[41] With higher doses of radiation and with accelerated fractionation (i.e., more frequent treatments), response rates for soft tissue sarcoma have improved. In a study using a megavoltage (^{60}Co) radiation total dose of 63 Gy to the surgical site of incompletely excised soft tissue sarcomas, only 4 of 21 dogs had tumor recurrence in the radiation field. Radiation doses of greater than 60 Gy seem to be effective in controlling soft tissue sarcoma in dogs.[42] Radiation therapy is probably the adjunctive therapy of choice in the treatment of soft tissue sarcomas in dogs and cats; however, irradiation of the spinal cord may limit the dose of radiation able to be safely delivered to neurofibrosarcomas.

Chemotherapy for brachial plexus neurofibrosarcoma is rarely justified. Local control is better achieved by surgery or radiation therapy, and metas-

> ## KEY POINT:
>
> *Nerve sheath tumors commonly affect the brachial plexus to cause forelimb lameness.*

tasis is rare. Chemotherapy for other soft tissue sarcomas is covered in more detail in the chapter on Tumors of the Skin.

Treatment for feline peripheral nerve lymphoma is as outlined for feline spinal lymphoma. However, peripheral nerve involvement is rare in cats.

REFERENCES

1. Heidner GL, Kornegay JN, Pager RL, et al: Analysis of survival in a retrospective study of 86 dogs with brain tumors. *J Vet Intern Med* 5:219–226, 1991.
2. Foster ES, Carrillo JM, Patnaik AK: Clinical signs of tumors affecting the rostral cerebrum in 43 dogs. *J Vet Intern Med* 2:71–74, 1988.
3. Palmer AC, Malinowski W, Barnett KC: Clinical signs including papilloedema associated with brain tumors in twenty-one dogs. *J Small Anim Pract* 15:359–386, 1974.
4. Davidson MG, Nasisse MP, Breitschwerdt EB, et al: Acute blindness associated with intracranial tumors in dogs and cats: Eight cases (1984–1989). *JAVMA* 199:755–758, 1991.
5. Kipperman PS, Feldman EC, Dybal NO, Nelson RW: Pituitary tumor size, neurologic signs, and relation to endocrine test results in dogs with pituitary-dependent hyperadrenocorticism: 43 cases (1980–1990). *JAVMA* 201:762–767, 1992.
6. Smith MO, Turrell JM, Bailey CS, Cain GR: Neurologic abnormalities as the predominant signs of neoplasia of the nasal cavity in dogs and cats: Seven cases (1973–1986). *JAVMA* 195:242–245, 1989.
7. Kornegay JN: Imaging brain neoplasms. Computed tomography and magnetic resonance imaging. *Vet Med Report* 2:372–390, 1990.
8. Schulman FY, Ribas JL, Carpenter JL, et al: Intracranial meningioma with pulmonary metastasis in three dogs. *Vet Pathol* 29:196–202, 1992.
9. Schmidt P, Geyer C, Hafner A, Bise K, et al: Malignes meningeom mit lungenmetastasen bei einem Boxer. *Tierarztl Prax* 19:315–319, 1991.
10. Turrel JM, Higgins RJ, Child G: Prognostic factors associated with irradiation of canine brain tumors. *Proc 6th Ann Conf Vet Cancer Soc*, 1986.
11. LeCouteur RA, Gillette EL, Dow SW: Radiation response of autochthonous canine brain tumors. *Int J Radiat Oncol Biol Phys* 13:166, 1987.
12. Iwamoto KS, Normal A, Freshwater DB, et al: Diagnosis and treatment of spontaneous canine brain

MANAGEMENT OF SPECIFIC DISEASES

tumors with a CT scanner. *Radiother Oncol* 26:76–78, 1993.

13. Evans SM, Dayrell-Hart B, Powlis W, et al: Ortho-voltage radiation therapy of canine brain masses. *Proc 10th Ann Conf Vet Cancer Soc*:80–81, 1990.

14. Feder BM, Fry TR, Kostolich M, et al: YAG laser cytoreduction of an invasive intracranial meningioma in a dog. *Prog Vet Neurol* 4:3–9, 1993.

15. Fulton LM, Steinberg HS: Preliminary study of lomustine in the treatment of intracranial masses in dogs following localization by imaging techniques. *Semin Vet Med Surg (Small Anim)* 5:241–245, 1990.

16. Hamilton TA, Cook JR, Scott-Moncreif C, et al: Carmustine chemotherapy for canine brain tumors. *Proc 11th Ann Conf Vet Cancer Soc*:43–44, 1991.

17. Dimski DS, Cook JR Jr: Carmustine-induced partial remission of an astrocytoma in a dog. *JAAHA* 26:179–182, 1990.

18. Sarfaty D, Carrillo JM, Peterson ME: Neurologic, endocrinologic, and pathologic findings associated with large pituitary tumors in dogs: (1976–1984). *JAVMA* 193:854–856, 1988.

19. Nelson RW, Ihle SL, Feldman EC: Pituitary macroadenomas and macroadenocarcinomas in dogs treated with mitotane for pituitary-dependent hyperadrenocorticism: 13 cases (1981–1986). *JAVMA* 194:1612–1617, 1989.

20. Davidson MG, Nasisse MP, Breitschwerdt EB, et al: Acute blindness associated with intracranial tumors in dogs and cats: Eight cases (1984–1989). *JAVMA* 199:755–758, 1991.

21. Boujon CE, Ritz U, Rossi GL, Bestetti GE: A clinico-pathological study of canine Cushing's disease caused by a pituitary carcinoma. *J Comp Pathol* 105:353–365, 1991.

22. Dow SW, LeCouteur RA: Radiation therapy for canine ACTH-secreting pituitary tumors, in Kirk RW, Bonaguara JD (eds): *Current Veterinary Therapy X*. Philadelphia, WB Saunders, 1989, pp 1031–1034.

23. Dow SW, LeCouteur RA, Rosychuk AW, et al: Response of dogs with functional pituitary macroadenomas and macrocarcinomas to radiation. *J Small Anim Pract* 31:287–294, 1990.

24. Carpenter JL, Andrews LK, Holzworth J: Tumors and tumor-like lesions, in Holzworth J (ed): *Diseases of the Cat. Medicine and Surgery*. Philadelphia, WB Saunders, 1987, pp 406–596.

25. Nafe LA: Meningiomas in cats: A retrospective clinical study of 36 cases. *JAVMA* 174:1224–1227, 1979.

26. Schrenzel MD, Higgins RJ, Hinrichs SH, et al: Type C retroviral expression in spontaneous feline olfactory neuroblastomas. *Acta Neuropathol* 80:547–553, 1990.

27. Gordon LE, Thacher C, Matthiesen DT, Joseph RJ: Results of craniotomy for the treatment of cerebral meningioma in 42 cats. *Vet Surg* 23:94–100, 1994.

28. Gallagher JG, Berg J, Knowles KE, et al: Prognosis after surgical excision of cerebral meningiomas in cats: 17 cases (1986–1992). *JAVMA* 203:1437–1440, 1993.

29. LeCouteur RA: Brain tumors of dogs and cats: Diagnosis and management. *Vet Med Rep* 2:332–342, 1990.

30. Waters DJ, Hayden DW: Intramedullary spinal cord metastasis in the dog. *J Vet Intern Med* 4:207–215, 1990.

31. Couto CG, Cullen J, Pedroia V, Turrel JM: Central nervous system lymphosarcoma in the dog. *JAVMA* 184:809–813, 1984.

32. Luttgen PJ, Braund WR Jr, Vandevelde M: A retrospective study of twenty-nine spinal tumors in the dog and cat. *J Small Anim Pract* 21:207–215, 1980.

33. Luttgen PJ: Spinal neoplasia: Diagnosis and treatment. *Semin Vet Med Surg (Small Anim)* 5:246–252, 1990.

34. Rosin A: Neurologic disease associated with lymphosarcoma in ten dogs. *JAVMA* 181:50–53, 1982.

35. Fingeroth JM, Prata RG, Patnaik AK: Spinal meningiomas in dogs: 13 cases (1972–1987). *JAVMA* 191:720–726, 1987.

36. Bell FW, Feeney DA, O'Brien TJ, et al: External beam radiation therapy for recurrent intraspinal meningioma in a dog. *JAAHA* 28:318–322, 1992.

37. Zaki FA, Hurvitz AI: Spontaneous neoplasms of the central nervous system of the cat. *J Small Anim Pract* 17:773–782, 1976.

38. Lane SB, Kornegary JN, Duncan JR, Oliver JE Jr: Feline spinal lymphosarcoma: A retrospective evaluation of 23 cats. *J Vet Intern Med* 8:99–104, 1994.

39. Spodnick GJ, Berg J, Moore FM, Cotter SM: Spinal lymphoma in cats: 21 cases (1976–1989). *JAVMA* 200:373–376, 1992.

40. Bradley RL, Withrow SJ, Shyder SP: Nerve sheath tumors in the dog. *JAAHA* 18:915–921, 1982.

41. McChesney SL, Withrow SJ, Gillette EL, et al: Radiotherapy of soft tissue sarcomas in dogs. *JAVMA* 194:60–63, 1989.

42. Mauldin GN, Meleo KA, Burk RL: Radiation therapy for the treatment of incompletely resected soft tissue sarcomas in dogs: 21 cases. *Proc Vet Cancer Soc 13th Ann Conf*:111, 1993.

CLINICAL BRIEFING: OCULAR AND RETROBULBAR TUMORS

Tumors of the Eye in Dogs

Common Clinical Presentation	Glaucoma, uveitis, hyphema, or visible mass
Common Histologic Types	Melanoma; less commonly, epithelial tumors of the ciliary body
Epidemiology and Biological Behavior	Melanomas and epithelial tumors have low potential for metastasis; old dogs are affected
Prognostic Factors	High mitotic index may indicate potential for metastasis in melanoma
Treatment Surgery	Enucleation is usually curative, even after failure of local excision; other treatment modalities not required

Tumors of the Eye in Cats

Common Clinical Presentation	Buphthalmos, poor vision, iris pigment change, and glaucoma
Common Histologic Types	Melanoma; less commonly, ocular sarcoma
Epidemiology and Biological Behavior	Melanomas are malignant and have high metastatic potential; old cats usually affected; no association with breed, gender, or FeLV status. Sarcomas (often preceded by ocular trauma) are highly malignant
Prognostic Factors	None identified

Treatment
   Surgery
 	
   Radiation Therapy
	Should be performed early in course of disease for melanoma; increasing degree of ocular involvement is associated with poorer survival
	 May improve local control, but melanoma and ocular sarcoma have high metastatic rates

MANAGEMENT OF SPECIFIC DISEASES

Retrobulbar Tumors in Dogs

Common Clinical Presentation	Exophthalmos, nictitans protrusion, and deviation of globe
Common Histologic Types	Multiple types; osteosarcoma, fibrosarcoma, mast cell tumors, and lymphoma are most common
Epidemiology and Biological Behavior	Most tumors are locally aggressive; metastatic rate varies with tumor type
Prognostic Factors	None identified

Treatment
  Surgery
  Radiation Therapy
 	
  Chemotherapy
	
	Orbitectomy may be curative for small tumors
	Should be useful as an adjunct to surgery for all tumor types but is still under investigation
	May be useful for lymphoma; cisplatin can be an adjunct to local modalities for treatment of osteosarcoma and osteochondrosarcoma

Retrobulbar Tumors in Cats

Common Clinical Presentation	Exophthalmos or enophthalmos
Common Histologic Types	Primary retrobulbar tumors are rare; extension of oral squamous cell carcinoma; nasal tumors and lymphoma
Epidemiology and Biological Behavior	Old cats; behavior varies with tumor type
Prognostic Factors	None identified

Treatment
  Surgery
 	
  Radiation Therapy
 	
  Chemotherapy
	
	Rarely useful as a primary modality, as most tumors have grown by extension from other sites; oral squamous cell carcinoma is unresponsive to surgery
	May be a useful adjunct for squamous cell carcinoma when used in combination with mitoxantrone chemotherapy (see the chapter on Tumors of the Oral Cavity) or for nasal tumors
	May be useful for retrobulbar lymphoma, with or without radiation therapy

MANAGEMENT OF SPECIFIC DISEASES

TUMORS OF THE EYE IN DOGS
Incidence, Signalment, and Etiology

Melanoma is the most common ocular tumor in dogs. In one study of 147 primary tumors, more than half were melanoma.[1] Ciliary body adenomas (n = 21) or ciliary adenocarcinomas (n = 37) were the next most common tumor types. Less frequently diagnosed tumors were medulloepitheliomas, sarcomas, and hemangiomas. Lymphoma was the most common secondary or metastatic tumor.[1]

Melanoma of the globe reportedly affects limbus, choroid, iris, and other areas of the uvea.[2,3] Ocular melanoma occurs primarily in old dogs. Although affected dogs range in age from 2 months to 17 years, 70% are 7 years of age or older.[4] Dogs with limbal tumors may be somewhat younger; most are younger than 7 years of age.[5,6] Most studies have not ascribed any breed predisposition for ocular melanoma,[4,7] although German shepherds accounted for 15 of 30 affected dogs in one study.[6] In another study, German shepherds and boxers were overrepresented compared with the general population.[5] One author suggested that primary acquired melanosis, which occurs in some brachycephalic breeds and as a consequence of pannus in German shepherds, may be a premalignant change for ocular melanoma.[8] This hypothesis, however, requires further exploration.

Melanoma should be distinguished clinically from uveal cysts. Uveal cysts are pigmented and usually free-floating in the anterior chamber; they are common in retrievers of any age.[9] If it is not possible to distinguish a uveal cyst from melanoma, the dog should be re-examined at a later date to check for growth of the lesion. Uveal cysts can be removed by fine-needle aspiration using a 25-ga needle.[9]

Benign hemangiomas or angiokeratomas occur on the conjunctiva,[10] nictitans,[11,12] and ciliary body[10,13] and may be more common in English setters.[11,13] There is no age or gender predilection.

Clinical Presentation and History

The most common reasons for presentations of dogs with ocular melanoma are the presence of a mass, glaucoma, uveitis, and hyphema. Less common reasons are corneal edema, epiphora, and hyperemic conjunctivae. In 48 (67%) of 72 dogs with melanoma, an intraocular or scleral mass was visible, and in 34 (47%) of these dogs, the mass was the only abnormality detected.[4] In contrast, nearly one third of dogs with glaucoma due to ocular melanoma have no visible tumor. The eye of any dog with unilateral glaucoma should be carefully examined for the presence of a mass.[7] Even when tumors are noticed, they may remain static for one year or more prior to definitive diagnosis.[5,6]

Staging and Diagnosis

Most melanomas arising from the uvea and corneoscleral limbus in dogs are not likely to metastasize; however, they may exhibit expansive growth patterns. Out of 229 dogs[3,7,8,14,15] (including 190 dogs in one study[7]), ocular melanomas metastasized in only 10 cases (4%). Metastasis usually occurred between 2 and 5 months after enucleation.[4,8,14] When it occurs, metastasis is widespread and has occurred to the lungs, liver, kidney, spleen, adrenal gland, heart, and mandibular lymph nodes.

Many criteria are proposed as possible predictors of malignant behavior; however, most histologic features, such as necrosis, inflammation, degree of pigmentation, and growth pattern of cells, have no prognostic value.[4] The most valuable indicator of malignancy is the mitotic index of the tumor. In one study of 61 dogs with ocular melanomas, nine dogs (15%) had a mitotic index of greater than 4, and four of these nine dogs developed metastases.[4] It should be noted that not all tumors with high mitotic indices metastasize[3,4,7]; overall, ocular melanoma should be considered a benign tumor in dogs, although staging procedures should be used to establish the good health of the patient prior to treatment.

Epithelial tumors of the ciliary

> **KEY POINT:**
>
> *Ocular melanoma in dogs should almost always be considered a benign tumor that can be cured by enucleation.*

body, whether adenomas or adenocarcinomas, also metastasize infrequently.[16] Similarly, squamous cell carcinoma of the cornea or corneoscleral limbus does not seem to metastasize.[5,17]

Prognostic Factors

As stated previously, melanomas with a mitotic index of greater than 4 may exhibit metastatic behavior, and a more guarded prognosis is warranted for dogs with this histologic finding.[4]

Treatment

Ocular melanoma in dogs is usually benign; therefore, observation alone may be a reasonable option for small, well-circumscribed lesions.[7,18] If the tumor grows, surgical resection of the tumor by enucleation should be curative.

Local excision is an option, particularly for tumors of the limbus.[4] Partial iridectomy[4] and lamellar keratectomy[6] also can achieve local removal. Recurrence rates after local excision range from 30% to 40%[4,6]; however, enucleation after recurrence is usually curative. Cryosurgery may reduce the chance of local recurrence after excision, but overzealous freezing can cause ocular damage. Other methods of local treatment have been reported, including the unsuccessful use of a synthetic polytetrafluoroethylene graft[19] and partial regression of some presumed melanomas after neodymium:YAG laser treatment.[15] Enucleation is curative for dogs whose tumors are not controlled by local excision or dogs that have ocular involvement and extensive tumor growth; after enucleation, more than 95% of dogs have no recurrence or metastases for one to five years.[4,5]

Enucleation is usually curative for epithelial tumors of the eye, including ciliary-body adenomas and adenocarcinomas.[16] Local excision of squamous cell carcinoma followed by nitrous oxide cryosurgery gave long-term control in two dogs for one year or longer.[17,20] One of these two dogs had recurrence of a squamous cell carcinoma years after the first treatment; the tumor recurred 9 months after a second treatment, but it did not metastasize.[20] An adenocarcinoma of the third eyelid did not recur within one year after excision.[21]

Local excision of hemangiomas of the nictitans or conjunctiva appears curative in most cases,[10-12] although one dog had a recurrence 28 months after surgery.[11] Enucleation is curative for intraocular lesions.

TUMORS OF THE EYE IN CATS
Incidence, Signalment, and Etiology

Melanoma is the most common ocular tumor in cats, but is less common than in dogs. There are few case series for this tumor, and information regarding its behavior is often conflicting. Ocular melanoma most often affects domestic shorthairs or domestic longhairs, although Persian[22-24] and Siamese[24,25] are occasionally affected. Cats with ocular melanoma are usually old, having a mean age of 10 to 11 years.[22,24] There is no gender predilection.[22,24-26] Feline sarcoma virus (FeSV) may cause ocular melanoma after experimental inoculation,[27] but the virus requires feline leukemia virus (FeLV) for replication. Only three (15%) of 19 tested cases[23-26] have been positive for FeLV antigen.[23,25] Therefore, it seems unlikely that FeSV plays any role in the natural development of ocular melanoma.

Ocular sarcoma has been reported in a number of cats. Histologically, these tumors are usually fibrosarcoma; however, osteosarcomas may occur.[28,29] These tumors are often associated with a history of trauma (13 [50%] of 26 reported cases) or chronic ocular disease (11 [40%] of 26 reported cases) that may have occurred 5 months to 12 years prior to tumor development.[28-31] Most affected cats are old; ages range from 7 to 15 years. Male cats may be more frequently affected.[30] Five cats that were tested for FeLV antigenemia were negative.[29-31] Ocular lymphoma may occasionally occur as part of systemic involvement (Figure 5-30).

Clinical Presentation and History

The ocular changes that are most frequently noticed by owners in association with ocular melanoma include buphthalmos, ophthalmitis, and, occasionally, poor vision.[25] Glaucoma accompanies melanoma in approximately 25% of cases[22]; in one

MANAGEMENT OF SPECIFIC DISEASES

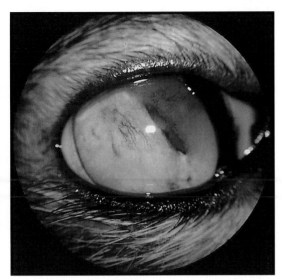

Figure 5-30: *A 15-year-old cat with intraocular lymphoma associated with multicentric disease. Complete resolution was attained with combination chemotherapy.*

study of the causes of glaucoma in 128 cats, 38 (30%) had iridal melanoma.[32] Of these 38 cats, glaucoma was the only recognizable abnormality and the tumor was not clinically detectable in 15 cats. Owners often observe a change in iris color; this change may precede tumor detection by 6 to 9 months.[23,26] Change of eye color was also a common presenting sign for cats with ocular sarcoma.[28,29,31] Buphthalmos and inflammatory ocular disease that is not responsive to medical treatment may occur.[30] Unilateral glaucoma or iridal pigment change in cats warrants careful ocular examination.

Staging and Diagnosis

The metastatic potential for ocular melanoma in cats is controversial. Early studies found that the metastatic rate for this tumor was low, and two recent studies described metastases as occurring in only 4 (11%) of 37 cases.[22,33] This rate is believed by some to reflect delayed growth of metastasis rather than a low rate of

metastasis,[26] and metastases have sometimes been detected up to 32 months after diagnosis.[26] In a recent study, only 1 of 16 cats (6%) showed metastases at diagnosis,[24] but another nine cats developed metastases an average of five months after treatment. In the same study, all three cats with palpebral melanoma developed widespread metastases, producing an overall metastatic rate of 70%. These metastases are usually to the mandibular lymph nodes (8 of 10 cases),[24] but they may be widespread and affect the lungs, liver, kidney, spleen, pericardium, or skeletal system.[22,24,26] Ocular sarcomas often exhibit aggressive growth, invading other ocular structures, crossing the sclera, and involving the optic nerve.[28,30] In one study, only 4 (30%) of 13 tumors were still localized at the time of diagnosis.[30] The metastatic potential for these tumors is high; eight (30%) of 28 cases metastasized. Most metastasized to local lymph nodes,[30,31] but some metastasized systemically.[28,30]

Both ocular melanoma and ocular sarcoma have a high potential for metastasis in cats, and careful staging by mandibular lymph node palpation and biopsy, thoracic radiographs, and (possibly) abdominal ultrasonography is warranted prior to definitive treatment.

Treatment

Observation alone is rarely warranted for feline ocular melanoma, although one cat had no change in a limbal lesion for 36 months after initial detection.[25] In another cat, glaucoma was treated medically for 20 months before enucleation was performed; however, this cat developed metastases one year later.[26] Local excision, with or without cryosurgery, of limbal tumors gave control in excess of 30 months in two cats.[25]

Early enucleation is the treatment of choice for feline ocular melanoma. Prognosis varies depending on the extent of involvement within the eye. Three of six cats with a tumor localized to the iris developed metastases an average of 301 days after surgery, while three of six cats

> **KEY POINT:**
>
> *Changes in iris color may be the first sign of an ocular tumor noted by the owner of a cat.*

MANAGEMENT OF SPECIFIC DISEASES

with tumors involving sclera, cornea, and chambers developed metastases an average of 144 days after surgery. Four cats with extensive tumors involving the entire globe developed metastases an average of 57 days after surgery. Three cats with palpebral melanoma developed metastases an average of 409 days after enucleation.[24] The average survival for 14 cats treated with enucleation was five months. Four cats were still alive an average of nine months after surgery.

Enucleation is the treatment of choice for feline ocular sarcoma. The metastatic potential for this tumor is high, however, and local invasion is often extensive, making complete excision difficult. Of 25 reported cases treated by enucleation, 16 cats died as a result of recurrent disease—which often extended along the optic nerve to involve the brain—or of metastatic disease.[28,30,31] Four cats were still alive 8, 12, 12, and 52 weeks after surgery.[28–30] Thus, prognosis is poor for cats with these tumors.

Adjunctive radiation therapy may reduce the local recurrence rate for nonmetastatic tumors, although no results have been reported. Radiation for soft tissue sarcomas of other sites appears to improve local control rates (see the chapter on Tumors of the Skin).

RETROBULBAR TUMORS IN DOGS
Incidence, Signalment, and Etiology

Many tumor types occur in the retrobulbar (orbital) space. In one survey, 22 of the 23 tumors were malignant.[34] In order of prevalence, the most common tumors were osteosarcoma, fibrosarcoma, mast cell tumors, and lymphoma. Most tumors were primary; however, tumors (e.g., nasal tumors) occasionally invaded the retrobulbar space. Most affected dogs were old (average age = 8 years), but dogs with lymphoma were young.[34] There were no gender or breed predilections. Tumors of the optic nerve

> ## KEY POINTS:
>
> *Enucleation may be curative in cats with melanoma if performed early in the disease process. Advanced tumors have a high metastatic rate.*
>
> ―――――――
>
> *Ultrasonographic guidance is very useful for obtaining retrobulbar biopsy specimens or aspirates.*

include gliomas,[35] ganglioneuroblastomas,[36] meningiomas[37,38] and osteochondromas.[39]

Clinical Presentation and History

Dogs with tumors of the retrobulbar space usually present with exophthalmos, deviation of the eye, and nictitans protrusion. On physical examination, it is difficult to retropulse the globe; however, animals rarely show pain on palpation, unlike dogs with retrobulbar infections or abscesses. Ocular examination may reveal loss of direct and consensual pupillary light reflexes, and the eye may not be visual.

Staging and Diagnosis

Any retrobulbar mass should be imaged by radiography, ultrasonography, or CT to determine the site of origin and to guide a biopsy. Staging should also include thoracic radiographs. Most retrobulbar tumors are aggressively invasive, and these tumors have the potential for metastasis.

Radiography is rarely helpful in delineating either the nature of the mass or the origin or extent of orbital involvement[34] unless the tumor is mineralized.[39] Ultrasonography is more helpful in delineating the extent of retrobulbar disease, but it is not able to provide a definitive diagnosis.[40] It may be difficult to distinguish neoplastic from inflammatory changes; however, ultrasonographic guidance is very successful in obtaining biopsy samples or needle aspirates for cytology and microbiology (Figure 5-31).

If the exophthalmos is mild and space for biopsy is limited, then CT provides more accurate guidance than ultrasonography (Figure 5-32). CT scans also provide information on the origin and extent of retrobulbar tumors.

Retrobulbar meningioma is rare in dogs. It may be imaged by ultrasonography[37] or CT.[38] Although this tumor grows primarily by extension along the optic

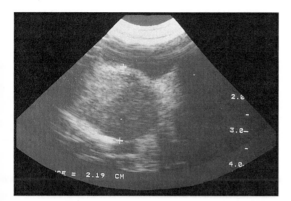

Figure 5-31: *Ultrasonography of a retrobulbar mass. The globe is closest to the transducer and is compressed concavely by a 2-cm mass. (Courtesy D.G. Penninck)*

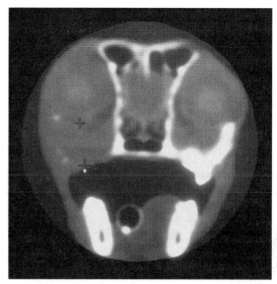

Figure 5-32: *Computed tomography (CT) allows assessment of the retrobulbar space and is superior to both radiography and ultrasonography in assessing destruction and invasion of normal structures. CT also provides accurate guidance for needle biopsy of the lesion. In this image, the left eye is displaced by a mass that has destroyed adjacent bone. (Courtesy A.S. Tidwell)*

nerve, it may metastasize, particularly if definitive treatment is delayed.[37,38]

Treatment

Orbital exenteration is the treatment of choice for all retrobulbar tumors. Exenteration, however, is rarely curative because of the infiltrative and destructive nature of these tumors. Even benign tumors may recur after surgery.[34]

A dog with a retrobulbar mast cell tumor was treated by exenteration and radiation therapy and was alive with no evidence of recurrence four years later.[34] Radiation therapy may be a useful adjunct to surgery for other tumor types, such as osteochondrosarcoma, but there are few reports of this approach.[41]

Early resection by orbital exenteration may be curative for orbital meningioma.[37] Although this tumor grows slowly, it is aggressive; therefore, delays in therapy may lead to incomplete excision. Recurrence and metastasis are rare and often occur long after surgery.[38]

RETROBULBAR TUMORS IN CATS
Incidence, Signalment, and Etiology

Primary neoplasms of the orbit were not common in one group of

> **KEY POINT:**
>
> *Extension of oral squamous cell carcinoma is the most common cause of a retrobulbar tumor in cats.*

21 cats with retrobulbar tumors.[42] Primary tumors, although rare, include fibrosarcoma, carcinoma, and hemangioma. The most common retrobulbar tumor is squamous cell carcinoma, which involves the orbit by extension, usually from the oral cavity.[43,44] Nasal carcinoma and chondroma also involve the orbit by extension. Lymphoma involved the orbit as part of the multicentric disease.[42] Bilateral parosteal osteomas were described in one cat.[45] Most affected cats, including those with lymphoma, were old, and 7 of 21 cats were Siamese. There was no gender predilection.

Clinical Presentation

Although most cats with a retrobulbar tumor display exophthalmos, it is relatively common for cats to present with enophthalmos.[42,46]

MANAGEMENT OF SPECIFIC DISEASES

Enophthalmos presumably results from tissue contracture and loss of retrobulbar fat.[46] Unlike retrobulbar infections, tumors are usually not associated with pain on palpation or opening of the mouth.

Staging and Diagnosis

Retrobulbar tumors in cats are most likely to grow by extension from the oral or nasal cavity. The imaging modalities used for dogs are also applicable for cats. Although metastasis from a retrobulbar tumor is rare,[45] affected cats should have a careful oral examination, skull radiographs, ultrasonography, or CT to look for signs of extension from an oral or nasal tumor as well as thoracic radiographs. Cats with retrobulbar lymphoma should be assessed for evidence of systemic lymphoma.

Access to the retrobulbar space is limited in cats, and radiology may be helpful if the tumor is mineralized[45] or if there is marked bony destruction.[42] Ultrasonography can be used to guide fine-needle aspiration of a localized mass, which is particularly helpful in making a diagnosis of lymphoma but may not be as helpful for other tumor types.[42]

Ultrasound-guided biopsy is most useful in cats with exophthalmos. Similarly, CT-guided biopsy is most likely to be successful when there is an obvious mass. Lateral orbitotomy may be required to obtain a definitive diagnosis, although the high rate of secondary retrobulbar tumors—especially oral squamous cell carcinoma—means that a biopsy specimen can often be obtained from the oral or nasal cavities.

Treatment

In one series of 21 cats, five cats were treated with ^{60}Co teletherapy. Surgical excision was performed in three cats.[45] Of the five cats treated with radiation, three cats with carcinomas, one cat with fibrosarcoma, and one cat with lymphoma died due to recurrence (lymphoma) or metastasis. The longest survival time was 12 months (median = 4 months). Surgery was even less successful; no cat survived more than four months. Owing to the high incidence of invasive oral squamous cell carcinoma in the retrobulbar space, radiation therapy should still be considered as an adjunct to surgery; however, high doses of radiation are required in conjunction with chemotherapy and surgery.[47] Radiation therapy may be useful for nasal carcinomas and could be used in combination with chemotherapy for retrobulbar lymphoma.

REFERENCES

1. Trucksa RC, McLean IW, Quinn AJ: Intraocular canine melanocytic neoplasms. *JAAHA* 21:85–88, 1985.
2. Dubielzieg RR, Aguirre GD, Gross SL, Diters RW: Choroidal melanomas in dogs. *Vet Pathol* 22:582–585, 1985.
3. Collinson PN, Peiffer RL Jr: Clinical presentation, morphology and behavior of primary choroidal melanomas in eight dogs. *Prog Vet Comp Ophthalmol* 3:158–164, 1993.
4. Wilcock BP, Peiffer RJ Jr: Morphology and behavior of primary ocular melanomas in 91 dogs. *Vet Pathol* 23:418–424, 1986.
5. Ryan AM, Diters RW: Clinical and pathologic features of canine ocular melanomas. *JAVMA* 184:60–67, 1984.
6. Diters RW, Ryan AM: Canine limbal melanoma. *Vet Med Small Anim Clin* 78:1529–1534, 1983.
7. Bussanich NM, Dolman PJ, Rootman J, Dolman CL: Canine uveal melanomas: Series and literature review. *JAAHA* 23:415–422, 1987.
8. Croxatto JO, Herrera HD, Lightowler CH: Malignant melanoma arising from primary acquired melanosis in a dog. *Canine Pract* 17:22–24, 1992.
9. Corcoran KA, Koch SA: Uveal cysts in dogs: 28 cases (1989–1991). *JAVMA* 203:545–546, 1993.
10. Murphey CJ, Bellhorn RW, Buyukmihci NC: Bilateral conjunctival masses in two dogs. *JAVMA* 195:225–228, 1989.
11. George C, Summers BA: Angiokeratoma: A benign vascular tumor of the dog. *J Small Anim Pract* 31:390–392, 1990.
12. Peiffer RL Jr, Duncan J, Terrell T: Hemangioma of the nictitating membrane in a dog. *JAVMA* 172:832–833, 1978.
13. Read RA: Ciliary body haemangioma in a dog with secondary glaucoma. *J Small Anim Pract* 34:405–408, 1993.
14. Minami T, Patnaik AK: Malignant anterior uveal melanoma with diffuse metastasis in a dog. *JAVMA* 201:1894–1896, 1992.
15. Nasisse MP, Davidson MG, Olivero DK, et al: Neodymium:YAG laser treatment of primary canine intraocular tumors. *Prog Vet Comp Ophthalmol* 3:152–157, 1993.
16. Peiffer RL, Gwin RM, Gelatt KN, et al: Ciliary body

epithelial tumors in four dogs. *JAVMA* 1728:578–583, 1978.

17. Latimer KS, Kaswan RL, Sundberg JP: Corneal squamous cell carcinoma in a dog. *JAVMA* 190:1430–1432, 1987.

18. Weisse I, Frese K, Meyer D: Benign melanoma of the choroid in a beagle: Ophthalmological, light and electron microscopical investigations. *Vet Pathol* 22:586–591, 1985.

19. Wilkie DA, Wolf ED: Treatment of epibulbar melanocytoma in a dog, using full-thickness eyewall resection and synthetic graft. *JAVMA* 198:1019–1022, 1991.

20. Ward DA, Latimer KS, Askren RM: Squamous cell carcinoma of the corneoscleral limbus in a dog. *JAVMA* 200:1503–1506, 1992.

21. Grahn B, Wolfer J: Diagnostic ophthalmology. *Can Vet J* 23:683, 1992.

22. Schaffer EH, Gordon S: Das feline okulare melanom: Klinische und patholgisch-anatomische befunde von 37 fallen. *Teiraztl Prax* 21:255–264, 1993.

23. Schwink K, Betts DM: Malignant melanoma of the iris in a cat. *Compan Anim Pract* 2:35–41, 1988.

24. Patnaik AK, Mooney S: Feline melanoma: A comparative study of ocular, oral and dermal neoplasms. *Vet Pathol* 25:105–112, 1988.

25. Harling DE, Peiffer RL Jr, Cook CS, Belkin PV: Feline limbal melanoma: Four cases. *JAAHA* 22:795–802, 1986.

26. Bertoy RW, Brightman AH, Regan K: Intraocular melanoma with multiple metastases in a cat. *JAVMA* 192:87–89, 1988.

27. Shadduck JA, Albert DM, NieDerkon JY: Feline uveal melanomas induced with feline sarcoma virus: Potential model of the human counterpart. *J Natl Cancer Inst* 67:619–620, 1981.

28. Dubielzig RR, Everitt J, Shadduck JA, Albert DM: Clinical and morphologic features of post-traumatic ocular sarcomas in cats. *Vet Pathol* 27:62–65, 1990.

29. Miller WW, Boosinger TR: Intraocular osteosarcoma in a cat. *JAAHA* 23:317–320, 1987.

30. Peiffer RL, Monticello T, Bouldin TW: Primary ocular sarcomas in the cat. *J Small Anim Pract* 29:105–116, 1988.

31. Hakanson N, Shively JN, Reed RE, Merideth RE: Intraocular spindle cell sarcoma following ocular trauma in a cat: Case report and literature review. *JAAHA* 26:63–66, 1990.

32. Wilcock BP, Peiffer RL Jr, Davidson MG: The causes of glaucoma in cats. *Vet Pathol* 27:35–40, 1990.

33. Carpenter JL, Andrews LK, Holzworth J: Tumors and tumor-like lesions, in Holzworth J (ed): *Diseases of the Cat. Medicine and Surgery.* Philadelphia, WB Saunders, 1987, pp 406–596.

34. Kern TJ: Orbital neoplasia in 23 dogs. *JAVMA* 186:489–491, 1985.

35. Spiess BM, Wilcock BP: Glioma of the optic nerve with intraocular and intracranial involvement in a dog. *J Comp Pathol* 97:79–84, 1987.

36. Brooks DE, Patton CS: An ocular ganglioneuroblastoma in a dog. *Prog Vet Comp Ophthalmol* 1:299–302, 1991.

37. Paulsen ME, Severin GA, LeCouteur RA, Young S: Primary optic nerve meningioma in a dog. *JAAHA* 25:147–152, 1989.

38. Dugan SJ, Schwarz PD, Roberts SM, Ching SV: Primary optic nerve meningioma and pulmonary metastasis in a dog. *JAAHA* 29:11–16, 1993.

39. Groff JM, Murphy CJ, Pool RR, et al: Orbital multilobular tumor of bone in dog. *J Small Anim Pract* 33:597–600, 1992.

40. Morgan RV: Ultrasonography of retrobulbar diseases of the dog and cat. *JAAHA* 25:393–399, 1989.

41. Straw RC, LeCouteur RA, Powers BE, Withrow SJ: Multibular osteochondrosarcoma of the canine skull: 16 cases (1978–1988). *JAVMA* 195:1764–1769, 1989.

42. Gilger BC, McLaughlin SA, Whittey RD, Wright JC: Orbital neoplasms in cats: 21 cases (1974–1990). *JAVMA* 201:1083–1086, 1992.

43. Cook CS, Peiffer RL Jr, Stine PE: Metastatic ocular squamous cell carcinoma in a cat. *JAVMA* 185:1547–1549, 1984.

44. Murphy CJ, Koblik P, Bellhorn RW, et al: Squamous cell carcinoma causing blindness and ophthalmoplegia in a cat. *JAVMA* 195:965–968, 1989.

45. Cottrill NB, Carter JD, Pechman RD, et al: Bilateral orbital parosteal osteoma in a cat. *JAAHA* 23:405–408, 1987.

46. Pentlarge VW, Powell-Johnson G, Martin CL, et al: Orbital neoplasia with enophthalmos in a cat. *JAVMA* 195:1249–1251, 1989.

47. Ogilvie GK, Moore AS, Obradovich JE, et al: Toxicoses and efficacy associated with the administration of mitoxantrone to cats with malignant tumors. *JAVMA* 202:1839–1844, 1993.

CLINICAL BRIEFING: TUMORS OF THE RESPIRATORY SYSTEM

Nasal Tumors in Dogs

Common Clinical Presentation	Unilateral epistaxis, facial deformity, and epiphora
Common Histologic Type	Adenocarcinoma
Epidemiology and Biological Behavior	Most common in old dogs; no breed or sex predisposition; tumor is locally invasive and rarely metastasizes to distant sites until late in the course of the disease
Prognostic Factors	Brain involvement is a poor prognostic sign

Treatment
  Surgery
  Radiation Therapy
 	
  Chemotherapy
	
	Contraindicated unless it is combined with radiation therapy
	Radiation, with or without surgery, is the treatment of choice; median survival rates vary from 8 to 23 months
	Cisplatin is reported to be effective

Nasal Tumors in Cats

Common Clinical Presentation	Epistaxis, sneezing, facial deformity, and epiphora
Common Histologic Types	Carcinoma and lymphoma
Epidemiology and Biological Behavior	Old males (8 to 10 years of age); locally invasive and rarely metastasizes to distant sites until late in the course of the disease
Prognostic Factors	None identified

Treatment
  Radiation Therapy
 	
  Chemotherapy
	
	Treatment of choice; survival time for nonhematopoietic malignancies is 20 to 27 months; median survival time for cats with nasal lymphoma approaches 16 months
	Recommended for nasal lymphoma due to systemic disease

MANAGEMENT OF SPECIFIC DISEASES

Lung Tumors in Dogs

Common Clinical Presentation	Chronic nonproductive cough, dyspnea, lethargy, lameness (hypertrophic osteopathy), and weight loss; some dogs are asymptomatic
Common Histologic Type	Adenocarcinoma
Epidemiology and Biological Behavior	Old, large-breed dogs; passive smoking and urban pollution may increase risk of developing primary lung tumor; metastasizes within lung and to regional lymph nodes
Prognostic Factors	Normal regional lymph nodes are associated with significantly longer survival than enlarged lymph nodes (345 versus 60 days); increasing size and presence of metastases are also negative prognostic signs
Treatment **Surgery**	Lung lobectomy is the treatment of choice

Lung Tumors in Cats

Common Clinical Presentation	Persistent cough, dyspnea, hemoptysis, lameness (metastasis), anorexia, lethargy, and malaise
Common Histologic Type	Adenocarcinoma
Epidemiology and Biological Behavior	Mean age is 11 years; tumors are likely to cause pleural effusion and respiratory stridor; metastases are common early in the course of the disease
Prognostic Factors	None identified
Treatment **Surgery**	Lung lobectomy is the treatment of choice

Other Tumors Reviewed

Tracheal and laryngeal tumors, canine lymphomatoid granulomatosis, and malignant histiocytosis of Bernese mountain dogs and other breeds

MANAGEMENT OF SPECIFIC DISEASES

Although malignant nasal tumors are the most common cause of unilateral epistaxis and facial deformity and epiphora in aged dogs and cats, other diagnostic differentials must be considered.[1,2] In each case, the definitive diagnosis is based on signalment, history, physical examination, radiographs, and histologic evidence of malignant neoplasia. Many treatment options exist for nasal tumors, but radiation therapy, with or without surgery, has been the most effective.

NASAL TUMORS IN DOGS
Incidence, Signalment, and Etiology

Tumors involving the nasal cavity and nearby sinuses are rare in dogs[3-5] and most often affect old animals (median age = 10 years), with no specific gender or breed distributions.[3-7] Carcinomas, especially adenocarcinoma, represent at least 66% of all tumors in the canine nasal cavity[1,2] but nonetheless are relatively rare in dogs.[3-5] Sarcomas, such as fibrosarcoma, chondrosarcoma, osteosarcoma, and undifferentiated sarcoma are less common.

Clinical Presentation and History

A range of different diseases within the nasal and paranasal sinuses cause problems that produce many identical clinical signs.[4,6,7] Dogs with nasal tumors frequently have facial deformity, epiphora, and unilateral epistaxis.[1,2] This epistaxis may become bilateral as the disease progresses. Less specific clinical signs include a purulent or mucoid nasal discharge, dyspnea, coughing, sneezing, ocular discharge, prolapse of the third eyelid, and neurologic signs.[4,6,7] These clinical signs persist for months. Owners often report that antibiotic therapy alleviates clinical signs transiently, probably due to the decrease in secondary bacterial infections that are often associated with most nasal tumors. Diagnostic differentials that must be considered include bacterial, allergic, or fungal rhinitis; foreign bodies; nasal para-

sites; bleeding disorders; and trauma. *Aspergillus* is the most common cause of fungal rhinitis.

Staging and Diagnosis

Diagnosis of a nasal tumor begins with a good history and physical examination. A definitive diagnosis can be confirmed only by histology. Supportive data can be obtained with rhinoscopy, plain radiographs, and computed tomography (CT) imaging. For fungal rhinitis, serology or mycotic cultures are indicated. Bacterial cultures are rarely of value. Before rhinoscopy, radiographs, or biopsy procedures are considered, routine screening tests to eliminate the possibility of bleeding disorders are recommended. These tests include a CBC, biochemical profile, urinalysis, clotting profile, and blood-pressure measurements (if indicated). Serology may determine the presence of such diseases as ehrlichiosis.

Nasal radiographs can determine the extent and location of the disease, which is useful for directing biopsy procedures and planning treatment.[8] As a general rule, the most valuable views are the frontal sinus and dorsoventral views. With the ventrodorsal open-mouth view, a high-resolution detail screen is placed as far caudal in the nasal cavity as possible. The open-mouth view shows the caudal nasal cavity and cribriform plate. Destruction and proliferation of bone and soft tissue densities within the nasal cavity suggest neoplasia.[4,7-10]

Thrall et al[11] demonstrated that CT is more accurate than radiographs in differentiating unilateral versus bilateral nasal cavity disease and in identifying tumor extension into nearby structures, such as the hard palate, pterygopalatine fossa, and cranial cavity (Figures 5-33 and 5-34). CT also enables more accurate tumor staging, which improves both the ability to predict treatment-related complications and to plan surgery and radiation therapy.[10,11] When brain involvement is suspected on the basis of history, physical examina-

> **KEY POINT:**
>
> *Dogs with nasal tumors often have unilateral epistaxis, epiphora, and facial deformity. Some clinical signs may resolve transiently with antibiotic therapy.*

MANAGEMENT OF SPECIFIC DISEASES

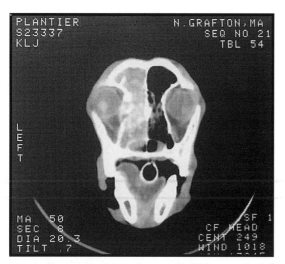

Figure 5-33: *Computed tomography (CT) image of a skull of a dog with a nasal adenocarcinoma filling the entire left side of the the nasal cavity. CT is an ideal imaging modality for determining the extent of disease in dogs and cats with nasal tumors.*

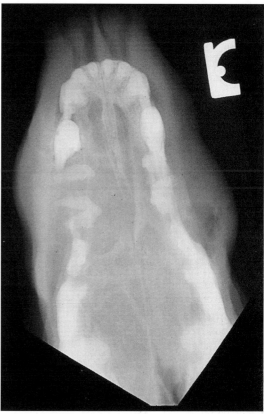

Figure 5-34: *Open-mouth radiographs of a dog with a nasal cavity tumor of the right nasal passage. Note the bone destruction and soft tissue density of the tumor. Open-mouth radiographs are often ideal for delineating the location of the tumor in a private practice setting.*

tion, or radiographic findings, an iodinated contrast agent should be injected intravenously before performing CT. If the blood–brain barrier is broken, the iodinated contrast agent will extend into the brain and surrounding tissue and will be noted on the CT as an area of increased radiodensity (contrast enhancement), which is a grave prognostic sign.

The cornerstone for diagnosis of nasal tumors is obtaining adequate tissue for histopathology. In most cases, the dog can be biopsied while it is anesthetized for radiography or other concurrent diagnostic tests. The simplest, cheapest, and most accurate method of obtaining adequate tissue in the dog without resorting to surgery is a transnostril core-sampling procedure[2] (see the Biopsy section). Alternatively, a bone curette can be used. If nonsurgical approaches do not work, then rhinotomy may be considered to obtain tissue for definitive diagnosis. A trephine is used to gain entry into the nasal cavity or sinus, and a curette is then used to scoop out tumor tissue. Rhinoscopy and nasal flushings can help to determine the extent of disease and support a diagnosis, but they are less effec-

tive than previously mentioned procedures. Rhinoscopy can be performed using a flexible bronchoscope or rigid cystoscope[1]; either allows direct visualization of the nasal cavity and surrounding structures. When a flexible endoscope is used, the caudal nasopharynx should be examined for neoplastic tissue by extending the endoscope through the oral cavity and then retroflexing the endoscope over the soft palate. The endoscope should then be directed toward the nares to locate any tumor or other abnormalities in the most caudal aspect of the nasopharyngeal area. Biopsy specimens can be taken concurrent-

MANAGEMENT OF SPECIFIC DISEASES

ly through the endoscope, although it may be prudent to follow this procedure with a transnasal core-biopsy procedure. Removal of foreign bodies and identification of nasal parasites can be accomplished easily by an experienced operator. Nasal washings or flushes reportedly have mixed results. One investigator reported a 50% success rate by flushing the nasal cavity and examining the resultant fluid cytologically, but others believe that the yield is much lower with the flushing procedure.[4,7] At the time of initial diagnosis, approximately 10% of lymph node biopsy specimens or aspirates contain tumor cells; thus, biopsies should be considered in cases with regional lymphadenopathy.[1,2] Metastatic disease to regional lymph nodes occurs in approximately 41% of cases during late stages of the disease.[2,6] Although thoracic radiographs are recommended as part of a standard staging scheme, they frequently fail to identify evidence of metastatic disease.[1,2] Metastasis has also been reported to occur to the brain and liver.[6] Metastatic rate is lowest among nonepithelial tumors.[6]

Treatment

Because nasal tumors rarely metastasize, therapy is directed at controlling localized disease. Surgical excision alone is not considered effective for treating nasal tumors in dogs because bone invasion occurs early in the pathogenesis of the disease and because the tumor is often located near the brain and eyes, which makes it impossible to obtain tumor-free surgical margins. Indeed, surgery alone is associated with prevalence of acute and chronic morbidity without significant extension of life.[4,7] Therefore, surgery is generally indicated only when combined with radiation therapy.

Radiation therapy, with or without surgical debulkment, is the only

KEY POINTS:

The simplest, cheapest, and most accurate method of obtaining adequate tissue for diagnosis in dogs without resorting to surgery is the transnostril core-sampling procedure.

Radiation therapy, with or without surgical debulkment, is the only treatment modality that increases survival time of dogs with nasal tumors. Cisplatin chemotherapy may be helpful in some cases.

treatment modality that increases survival time of dogs with nasal tumors.[7,12–14] Surgical debulking is necessary prior to orthovoltage radiotherapy to reduce tumor volume; this allows adequate delivery of radiation to the nasal cavity. Orthovoltage radiotherapy dosages of 40 to 50 Gy delivered in 10 to 12 fractions result in a median survival of 16 to 23 months, which is slightly better than megavoltage alone.[12–14] With orthovoltage radiotherapy, one- and two-year survival rates were 57% and 43%, respectively.[13]

Although the previously reported median survival for nasal tumors in dogs treated with megavoltage radiation alone was approximately eight months,[15] a recent report cited a median and mean survival of 12.8 and 20.7 months, respectively.[14] One- and two-year survival rates in this recent report were 59% and 22%, respectively. Dogs received from 41.8 to 54.0 Gy on a Monday/Wednesday/Friday schedule, using 10 to 12 fractions over 4 weeks. The improvement in survival over that reported previously was attributed to the use of CT for tumor localization and treatment plans. No prognostic variables were identified, and survival time did not differ significantly between carcinomas and sarcomas. Cytoreductive surgery did not significantly alter survival when megavoltage radiation was used.[14,15] Radiation therapy always produces some acute adverse effects, including oral mucositis, rhinitis, moist desquamation, and alteration of pigment and hair color.

Chemotherapy is not usually effective in treating canine nasal tumors, although cisplatin may be effective in some cases.[16]

NASAL TUMORS IN CATS
Incidence, Signalment, and Etiology

Tumors involving the nasal cavity and nearby sinuses are rarer in cats than in dogs. Affected cats are generally old males; the mean age of affected animals is 8 to 10 years.[17–20] The most common histopathologic diagnoses for feline nasal tumors are adenocarcinoma, undifferentiated carcinoma, olfactory neuroblastoma, lymphoma, fibrosarcoma, chondrosarcoma, and chondroma.[1,2,17–20] Other nonneoplastic differentials are similar to those of dogs. Viral rhinitis and cryptococcosis should be added to the list of diagnostic differentials for cats. Lymphoma of the nasal cavity occurs more commonly in cats than in dogs and is rarely associated with FeLV antigenemia.

Clinical Presentation and History

Unilateral or bilateral epistaxis, facial deformity, and epiphora are common in cats with nasal tumors.[1,2]

Staging and Diagnosis

Metastatic disease is rare. Staging and diagnostic procedures are essentially the same as for dogs, with minor differences. Each cat suspected of having a nasal tumor should have a minimum data base (e.g., CBC, biochemical profile, and urinalysis), chest radiographs, regional lymph node assessment by palpation and fine-needle aspiration cytology, radiographs, and biopsy of the nasal cavity. Open-mouth radiographs with nonscreen film and radiographs of the frontal sinuses are valuable for making an appropriate diagnosis and for directing a biopsy attempt. Computed tomography (CT) or magnetic resonance imaging (MRI) are considered superior to radiography, as brain invasion via the cribriform plate is common and has been reported in approximately 25% of cases.[17] Whenever lymphoma of the nasal cavity is suspected, a bone marrow aspirate and FeLV test should be performed in addition to the above procedures.[18,20] Cytology from nasal exudate, especially if examined with India ink, is ideal for identifying cryptococcosis. Routine histopathology, cytol-

> **KEY POINT:**
>
> *Biopsy of a suspected nasal tumor in a cat is performed by advancing a small bone curette through the nostril and into the nasal cavity of the anesthetized patient.*

ogy, and appropriate serologic titers for fungal or certain viral diseases are essential to confirm infection. Histopathology is required to make a definitive diagnosis of neoplasia. Obtaining tissue by rhinoscopy is not very successful in cats because of their small nasal cavities. One of the most effective methods of obtaining biopsy tissue in cats is by advancing a small bone curette through the nasal cavity while the cat is anesthetized. This methodology is described in detail in the Biopsy section of this manual.

Treatment

Cats with nasal tumors respond well to radiation therapy and in general have a better prognosis than dogs with nasal tumors. Cats that are treated with orthovoltage radiation after rhinotomy have mean and median survival times of 27.9 and 20.8 months.[13] Six cats with nasal carcinomas treated with megavoltage radiation alone had a mean survival time of 19 months; two cats were still alive at last report.[21] Localized nasal lymphomas in cats are ideally suited to local radiation therapy. Cats with intranasal lymphoma have disease-free intervals that last for more than 500 days.[18] Chemotherapy is recommended for cats with lymphoma to minimize the development of systemic lymphoma (see the chapter on Lymphoma).

TUMORS OF THE LARYNX AND TRACHEA
Incidence, Signalment, and Etiology

Tumors of the larynx and trachea are very rare in dogs and cats. There are few data concerning the prevalence of tumors of this site. Benign tracheal osteocartilaginous tumors are most common in young dogs with active osteochondral ossification. These tumors grow along with the rest of the musculoskeletal system.[2,22] Benign laryngeal oncocytomas also occur in young dogs. Other tumors of the canine larynx include osteosarcoma, chondrosarcoma, adenocarcinoma, melanoma, granular cell myoblastoma, undifferentiated carcinoma, fibrosarcoma, mast cell tumor, and squamous cell carcinoma.[2,22–24] In both dogs and cats, the most common tracheal tumors are lymphoma, chondrosarcoma, adenocarcinoma, squamous cell carcinoma, leiomyoma, polyp, and osteochondral tumors that arise from the tracheal rings.[2] In cats, lymphoma and squamous cell carcinoma predominate.

Clinical Presentation and History

Tracheal and laryngeal tumors may cause coughing, respiratory stridor, ptyalism, and voice change. These masses usually are not palpable.

Staging and Diagnosis

Endoscopy and radiography are usually required to determine the extent of the tumor. Because of the chance of metastatic disease and the increased risk of concurrent problems, such as bronchopneumonia, chest radiographs should be taken. Tissue should be obtained with endoscopy or during an open surgical biopsy. If lymphoma is suspected, chest and abdominal radiographs, CBC, biochemical profile, FeLV test (cats only), urinalysis, and bone marrow aspiration and cytology may be indicated to further stage the patient.

Treatment

Localized, relatively small tracheal tumors are treated effectively by removing the affected tracheal rings.[2]

Benign laryngeal tumors, such as oncocytomas, may be removed by a regional resection of the larynx.[2] In patients that require laryngectomy, permanent tracheostomies are indicated, but few clinical cases have been treated by this methodology.[22–24] Lymphoma of the larynx or trachea is best treated with chemotherapy and, in some cases, radiation therapy.[2]

PRIMARY LUNG TUMORS IN DOGS
Incidence, Signalment, and Etiology

Primary lung tumors are relatively rare in animals compared to hu-

mans.[25–27] The average age of a dog with primary lung tumor is 10.9 years (range = 2 to 18 years).[26] Male and female dogs are affected with equal frequency. Approximately 60% of dogs with primary lung tumors weigh between 20 and 30 kg.[25] Many investigators suggest that carcinogens in the environment may directly influence the incidence of lung tumors in dogs. In one study, 75% of dogs with primary lung tumors lived in urban environments.[25] There is a strong association between passive smoking and the prevalence of primary lung tumors in dogs. Brachycephalic dogs that are exposed to second-hand smoke have an increased risk of developing primary lung tumors compared to dolichocephalic dogs, presumably because of the increased filtration capacity of dolichocephalic dogs.[28] Adenocarcinoma is the most common type of lung tumor in dogs, followed by alveolar carcinoma, squamous cell carcinoma, and bronchial gland carcinoma.[26]

Clinical Presentation and History

The primary complaint noted by owners of dogs with primary lung tumors is chronic, nonproductive cough.[25,26] These and other clinical signs of primary lung tumors are listed in Table 5-8. Remarkably, many of these clinical signs do not directly relate to the pulmonary disease. Approximately 25% of dogs with primary lung tumors are asymptomatic at the time they are diagnosed.[25,26]

Compression of the anterior vena cava occasionally produces edema of the head and neck, which is known as anterior vena cava syndrome. It is seen with some mediastinal masses. Pleural effusion also occurs in some cases of primary and metastatic neoplasia. Dogs with pleural effusion frequently have dramatic signs of dyspnea. The most common paraneoplastic syndrome in dogs associated with primary and metastatic pulmonary neoplasia is hypertrophic osteopathy.[25,26] Dogs with this condition often present with lameness in one or more limbs. Radiographs reveal a characteristic periosteal proliferation

> **KEY POINT:**
>
> *Up to four tracheal rings can be removed with reasonable closure by an end-to-end anastomosis.*

MANAGEMENT OF SPECIFIC DISEASES

TABLE 5-8[25]
Clinical signs associated with primary lung tumors in dogs

Clinical Signs	Frequency
Cough	52.0%
Dyspnea	24.0%
Lethargy	18.0%
Weight loss	12.0%
Tachypnea	5.0%
Pyrexia	6.4%
Lameness	3.8%

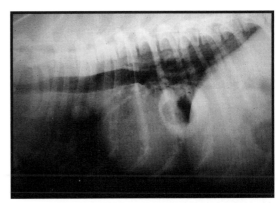

Figure 5-35: *Chest radiograph of a canine primary lung tumor that appears as a cavitated mass. Most primary lung tumors appear radiographically as a well-circumscribed solitary mass within the lung fields.*

perpendicular to the long shaft of the bone. Surgical resection of the pulmonary mass often causes rapid resolution of the condition. Lameness may rarely be due to metastatic spread of the lung tumor to the bones of the limbs. Other paraneoplastic syndromes include hypercalcemia, polyneuropathy, polymyopathy, fever, and ectopic production of ACTH, which causes hyperadrenocorticism.

Staging and Diagnosis

Thoracic radiography is the most important preoperative diagnostic tool for diagnosis of primary lung tumors.[25,26] Information gained from radiographic procedures directs subsequent diagnostic steps. The most common radiographic findings are airway obstruction, pleural extension, or regional lymph node enlargement. Most dogs have a solitary, well-circumscribed pulmonary mass that may cause airway obstruction. Invasion of pleura or regional pulmonary lymphatics by tumor cells can produce pleural effusion. When this occurs, details of thoracic structures may be obscured. The diagnostic potential of ultrasonography can be enhanced with pleural effusion and should be considered

KEY POINT:

Hypertrophic osteopathy is the most common paraneoplastic syndrome associated with primary lung tumor in dogs. Affected dogs are often lame.

when fluid is present. Otherwise, thoracic fluid should be drained to allow better visualization of the intrathoracic structures by radiography.

Pulmonary lymph node enlargement occurs in primary and metastatic neoplastic diseases as well as in infectious conditions and may be detected on plain radiographs. In the midwestern United States, fungal diseases must always be considered in dogs with pulmonary lymph node enlargement. Cavitation of pulmonary tissue secondary to primary lung tumors occasionally occurs, and abscess formation also can cause a cavitary lesion (Figure 5-35).

Although bronchoscopy may be used to visualize the airways, most dogs with lung tumors have compressive lesions that can be visualized only indirectly.[26] Tumors are often peripherally located and therefore inaccessible for visualization by bronchoscopy. If a bronchoscope is not available and it is necessary to obtain cells or fluid from the airways, a transtracheal aspirate can be performed in most awake animals. Culture and cytology of the material are mandatory. Carcinomas are more likely than sarcomas

MANAGEMENT OF SPECIFIC DISEASES

TABLE 5-9
Association of prognostic factors with remission and survival times[26]

Factor and Classification	Median Remission (days)	Median Survival (days)*
T_1: Solitary tumor surrounded by lung or pleura	270	224
T_2: Multiple tumors	120	120
T_3: Tumor invading neighboring tissues	60	45
N_0: No evidence of node involvement (at surgery)	450	345
N_1: Bronchial lymph node involvement (at surgery)	60	60
M_0: No metastases	150	180
M_1: Distant metastases	180	14

*Survival exceeds remission in some situations because survival data in this study include all dogs that were treated, whereas dogs that were rendered free of all evidence of tumor are in the remission group. Statistically, lymph node status (N_0 vs. N_1) was the most important prognostic variable for predicting outcome.

to exfoliate into the pulmonary airways.

Most pleural effusions associated with malignancies are exudates (total protein >3.0 g/dl; specific gravity >1.015). Some tumors do not exfoliate into the pleural fluid; therefore, lack of tumor cells in an exudative pleural effusion should not exclude a diagnosis of primary lung neoplasia.

A pulmonary mass that is not close to large, vascular structures can be aspirated safely. Most pulmonary masses are removed at surgery; therefore, it is not usually necessary to obtain tissue or cells prior to the definitive procedure. When performing a transthoracic aspirate, a 3-ml to 5-ml syringe with a 22-ga needle is directed into the mass while negative pressure is applied with the syringe. A quick "in-and-out" aspiration is done. There must be no negative pressure in the syringe when the needle is withdrawn from the mass and skin. This procedure has minimal risk. Possible complications include pneumothorax and hemoptysis. CT guidance improves the accuracy of this procedure.

As mentioned earlier, many dogs with primary lung tumors are diagnosed by excisional biopsy. This can elicit good long-term survival in many patients, especially if they do not have enlarged lymph nodes.

Because primary lung tumors tend to metastasize to other areas of lung and regional lymph nodes, special attention should be directed to obtaining and evaluating high-quality thoracic radiographs. If lameness is noted, radiographs of the affected area should be evaluated for hypertrophic osteopathy. Complete blood count, biochemical profile, and urinalysis are required to identify paraneoplastic syndromes or organ dysfunctions secondary to the neoplastic disease. Lymph node biopsy specimens are valuable in identifying the extent of primary disease and any metastasis.

Prognostic Factors (Table 5-9)

In one study, 54% of respiratory tumors were solitary,[1] 37% were multiple, and 5% invaded neighboring tissues. Enlarged lymph nodes were identified in 12% of the dogs with primary lung tumors.[1] Dogs with lymph nodes that are normal at the time of surgery have a significantly longer disease-free interval than dogs with enlarged nodes (345 days versus 60 days). The presence of enlarged lymph nodes is the most important prognostic factor (Figure 5-36), but increasing size of the malignant process and the presence of metastases can be important. The type of tumor did not influence survival times or the disease-free interval.

Treatment

Surgery is the treatment of choice for dogs with

MANAGEMENT OF SPECIFIC DISEASES

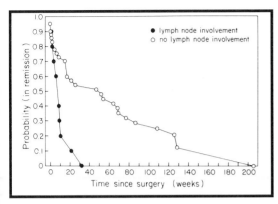

Figure 5-36: Probability curves demonstrating tumor-free interval for dogs with primary lung tumors, with and without large regional lymph nodes identified prior to surgical removal of the tumor. (From Ogilvie GK, Weigel RM, Haschek WM, et al: Prognostic factors for tumor remission and survival in dogs after surgery for primary lung tumors: 76 cases (1975–1985). JAVMA 195:109–112, 1989; with permission.)

primary lung tumors. For best results, the animal must be in relatively good health and have localized disease. A partial or complete lobectomy is the best choice. Automatic stapling devices reduce surgery time and patient morbidity (Figures 5-37 and 5-38). Dogs with neoplasms at the base of the lung lobe survive longer than dogs with tumors at the periphery.[26] In one study, 76 of 210 dogs diagnosed with a primary lung tumor had a therapeutic lobectomy. Twenty-three of the 76 dogs had enlarged lymph nodes.[26] Lymph nodes were biopsied in 13 of the dogs. Four lymph nodes were positive for tumor. Overall (treated and untreated) mean survival time was 120 days.

Although few reports document the efficacy of radiation therapy or chemotherapy to treat primary lung tumors in dogs, there is evidence that radiation therapy would signifi-

cantly extend the survival time of dogs with lung tumors. For optimum benefit, radiation should follow surgical debulkment. A linear accelerator or cobalt-radiation therapy unit is required to treat these tumors; however, radiation pneumonitis may be dose limiting. Cisplatin-based protocols may be the best chemotherapeutic option for this tumor.

PRIMARY LUNG TUMORS IN CATS
Incidence, Signalment, and Etiology

Primary lung tumors are much rarer in cats than in dogs.[29-31] Old cats (mean = 11 years) are more likely to be affected. No breed or sex predisposition has been noted. The most common tumor types are adenocarcinoma, bronchioalveolar carcinoma, and squamous cell carcinoma.[31]

Clinical Presentation and History

Clinical signs of affected cats include persistent cough, dyspnea, hemoptysis, anorexia, lethargy, malaise, and lameness. Although rare, hypertrophic osteopathy has been documented in cats with primary lung tumors and therefore must be considered as a cause in cats with lameness and a pulmonary mass.[29-31] Lameness is more commonly caused by metastasis to digits and skeletal muscles. Interestingly, cats may be presented for lameness or pain with no clinical signs attributable to the respiratory tract.[32]

Staging and Diagnosis

Cats with primary lung tumors should be staged with a CBC, biochemical profile, urinalysis, chest radiographs, and evaluation of any pleural effusion. Tracheal washes and transthoracic aspirates are useful in identifying malignant cells. When affected cats are staged, special attention should be directed at sites where metastases are likely. Metastatic lesions can be seen in up to 71% of

KEY POINTS:

Enlarged lymph nodes and the presence of tumor cells in regional lymph nodes are the most important prognostic factors influencing disease-free interval and survival.

Pleural effusion and dyspnea are more common in cats than in dogs with primary lung tumors.

MANAGEMENT OF SPECIFIC DISEASES

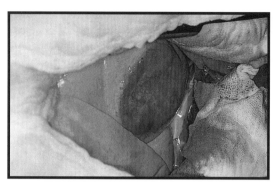

Figure 5-37: *Bronchogenic adenocarcinoma of the right caudal lung lobe exposed at surgery. (Courtesy J. Berg)*

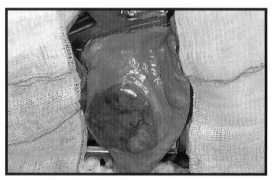

Figure 5-38: *The primary lung tumor is quickly and efficiently removed by using an automatic stapling device. Alternatively, the base of the lung can be clamped off and the tumor resected; the lung remnant is then sutured. Regional lymph nodes should be examined and biopsied during surgery, if possible. (Courtesy J. Berg)*

affected cats in many anatomic sites, including regional lymph nodes (34%), mediastinum (24%), pleura (32%), heart (13%), spleen (8%), and appendicular skeleton (5%).[31] This metastatic rate is higher than that in dogs.

Some radiographic changes associated with primary lung tumors are characteristic, whereas others are nonspecific. Primary adenocarcinomas are usually focal, solitary, well-circumscribed masses or consolidated regions of several pulmonary masses. Bronchioalveolar carcinomas and squamous cell carcinomas are more variable in appearance. More than half of the affected cats have a diffuse distribution of

tumor apparent on radiographs. Approximately 25% of affected cats have lobar consolidation; a smaller percentage has circumscribed masses.[31]

Diagnosis can be made by evaluating cytology obtained from bronchoscopy or from cytologic analysis of any fluid obtained from any pleural effusion. The simplest, cheapest, and most direct diagnosis is often made by a therapeutic thoracotomy to excise the entire mass. Histopathology is essential to differentiate this condition from granulomatous or metastatic disease.

Treatment

Surgery is the treatment of choice and should be considered for patients without metastatic disease. Survival times exceeding 18 months have been reported for cats with localized, completely excised primary lung tumors.[29] Prognosis is poor for cats with malignant pleural effusion or metastatic disease. There are few reports documenting the efficacy of chemotherapy or radiation therapy in this disease.

CANINE LYMPHOMATOID GRANULOMATOSIS
Incidence, Signalment, and Etiology

Canine lymphomatoid granulomatosis, also known as pulmonary lymphomatoid granulomatosis, is a rare neoplastic disease that affects young to middle-aged dogs. The etiology is not known.[33,34] The importance of this disease is that it resembles other malignant pulmonary diseases clinically, but it has a more favorable prognosis than most.

Clinical Presentation and History

Canine lymphomatoid granulomatosis produces diffuse or well-defined pulmonary masses that can induce significant pulmonary dysfunction. The most common clinical signs are abnormal lung sounds, coughing, dyspnea, anorexia, fever, weight loss, and lymphadenopathy.[33,34]

Staging and Diagnosis

Radiographic changes associated with lymphomatoid granulomatosis include lobar consolidation, poorly defined pulmonary masses, hilar lymphadenopathy, and pleural effusion.[1,33,34] Transthoracic fine-needle aspirates may reveal a sterile eosinophilic and neutrophilic inflammatory reaction. The most common laboratory abnormalities include basophilia, eosinophilia, and leukocytosis.[33,34] Most dogs test negative for heartworm disease. Tissues obtained at the time of thoracotomy or percutaneous biopsy are required for definitive diagnosis.

Treatment

Chemotherapy is the treatment of choice for lymphomatoid granulomatosis. Five dogs were given cyclophosphamide, vincristine, and prednisone (COP)[33]; three had clinical and radiographic resolution of their disease for 7, 12, and 32 months. One dog subsequently developed lymphoma, which suggests that this disease may be a preneoplastic condition. In another report,[34] various combinations of cyclophosphamide, vincristine, cytosine arabinoside, and prednisone were used to treat six dogs. The response to therapy was not favorable in these dogs. Survival times ranged from six days to four years; median survival was three months.

MALIGNANT HISTIOCYTOSIS IN BERNESE MOUNTAIN DOGS AND OTHER BREEDS
Incidence, Signalment, and Etiology

Malignant histiocytosis was first recognized in 10 male and one female Bernese mountain dogs.[35,36] This condition has been identified in other breeds, including golden retrievers. Most patients are middle-aged (mean = 7 years) (also see the chapter on Tumors of the Skin).

Staging and Diagnosis

Affected patients usually have large (>5 cm) and small pulmonary nodules. Most have widespread systemic disease; the most commonly affected sites are lymph node, liver, kidney, brain, and spinal cord.[35,36] Staging should include chest and abdominal radiographs as well as more specific imaging modalities, if indicated. Tissue must be obtained for histologic confirmation.

Treatment

There is no uniformly accepted method for treating this condition. Combination chemotherapy with doxorubicin, cyclophosphamide, and vincristine has been reported to cause measurable regression in the size of the tumors for as long as six months.[2]

REFERENCES

1. Ogilvie GK, LaRue SM: Canine and feline nasal and paranasal sinus tumors. *Vet Clin North Am Small Anim Pract* 22:1133–1144, 1992.
2. Withrow SJ: Tumors of the respiratory system, in Withrow SJ, MacEwen EG (eds): *Clinical Veterinary Oncology.* Philadelphia, JB Lippincott, 1989, pp 215–233.
3. Brodey RS: Canine and feline neoplasia. *Adv Vet Sci Comp Med* 14:309–354, 1970.
4. Madewell BR, Priester WA, Gillette EL, Snyder SP: Neoplasms of the nasal passages and paranasal sinuses in domesticated animals as reported by 13 veterinary colleges. *Am J Vet Res* 37:851–856, 1976.
5. Priester WA, McKay FW: *The Occurrence of Tumors in Domestic Animals.* Washington DC, National Institutes of Health, Monograph 54, November, 1980.
6. Patnaik AK: Canine sinonasal neoplasms: Clinicopathologic study of 285 cases. *JAAHA* 25:103–114, 1989.
7. Norris AM: Intranasal neoplasms in the dog. *JAAHA* 15:231–236, 1979.
8. Gibbs C, Lane JG, Denny HR: Radiographical features of intra-nasal tumor lesions in the dog: A review of 100 cases. *J Small Anim Pract* 20:515–535, 1979.
9. Harvey CE, Biery DN, Morello J, et al: Chronic nasal disease in the dog: Its radiographic diagnosis. *Vet Radiol* 20:91–98, 1979.
10. Park RD, Beck ER, LeCouteur RA: Comparison of computed tomography and radiology for detecting changes produced by malignant neoplasia in dogs. *JAVMA* 201:1720–1724, 1992.
11. Thrall DE, Robertson ID, McLeod DA, et al: A comparison of radiographic and computed tomographic findings in 31 dogs with malignant nasal cavity tumors. *Vet Radiol* 30:59–65, 1989.
12. Thrall DE, Harvey CE: Radiotherapy of malignant nasal tumors in 21 dogs. *JAVMA* 183:663–666, 1983.
13. Evans SM, Goldschmidt M, McKee LJ, Harvey CE: Prognostic factors and survival after radiotherapy for canine intranasal neoplasms: 70 cases (1974–1985). *JAVMA* 194:1460–1463, 1989.
14. McEntee MC, Page RL, Heidner GL, et al: A retrospective study of 27 dogs with intranasal neoplasms treated with cobalt radiation. *Vet Radiol* 32:135–139,

MANAGEMENT OF SPECIFIC DISEASES

1991.

15. Adams WM, Withrow SJ, Walshaw R, et al: Radiotherapy of malignant nasal tumors in 67 dogs. *JAVMA* 191:311–315, 1987.

16. Hahn KA, Knapp DW, Richardson RC, Matlock CL: Clinical response of nasal adenocarcinoma to cisplatin chemotherapy in 11 dogs. *JAVMA* 200:355–357, 1992.

17. Cox NR, Brawner WR, Powers RD, Wright JC: Tumors of the nose and paranasal sinuses in cats: 32 cases with comparison to a national database (1977 through 1987). *JAAHA* 27:339–347, 1991.

18. Elmslie RE, Ogilvie GK, Gillette EL, McChesney-Gillette S: Radiotherapy with and without chemotherapy for the control of localized lymphoma in cats: 10 cases (1983–1989). *Vet Radiol* 32:277–280, 1991.

19. Engle CG, Broday RS: A retrospective study of 395 feline neoplasms. *JAAHA* 5:21–31, 1969.

20. Elmslie RE, Ogilvie GK: Solitary extranodal lymphomas: Presentation and management, in August JR (ed): *Consultations in Feline Internal Medicine*, ed 2. Philadelphia, WB Saunders, 1993, pp 547–552.

21. Straw RC, Withrow SJ, Gillette EL, et al: Use of radiotherapy for the treatment of intranasal tumors in cats: Six cases (1989–1985). *JAVMA* 189:927–929, 1986.

22. Pass DA, Huxtable CR, Cooper BJ, et al: Canine laryngeal oncocytomas. *Vet Pathol* 17:672–677, 1980.

23. Wheeldon EB, Suter PF, Jenkeins T: Neoplasia of the larynx in the dog. *JAVMA* 180:642–647, 1982.

24. Saik JE, Toll SL, Diters RW, Goldschmidt MH: Canine and feline laryngeal neoplasia: A 10-year survey. *JAAHA* 22:359–365, 1986.

25. Ogilvie GK, Haschek WA, McKiernan B, et al: Classification of primary lung tumors in dogs: 210 cases (1975–1985). *JAVMA* 195:106–108, 1989.

26. Ogilvie GK, Weigel RM, Haschek WM, et al: Prognostic factors for tumor remission and survival in dogs after surgery for primary lung tumors: 76 cases (1975–1985). *JAVMA* 195:109–112, 1989.

27. Dorn CR, Taylor DON, Frey FL: Survey of animal neoplasms in Alameda and Contro Costa Counties, California. *J Natl Cancer Inst* 50:2295–2305, 1968.

28. Reif JS, Dunn K, Ogilvie GK, Harris CK: Passive smoking and canine lung cancer risk. *Int J Epidemiol* 135:234–239, 1992.

29. Mehlhalf CJ, Mooney S: Primary pulmonary neoplasia in the dog and cat. *Vet Clin North Am Small Anim Pract* 14:1061–1075, 1985.

30. Miles KG: A review of primary lung tumors in the dog and cat. *Vet Radiol* 29:122–133, 1988.

31. Barr IF, Gruffydd-Jones TJ, Brown PJ, et al: Primary lung tumors in the cat. *J Small Anim Pract* 28:1115–1125, 1987.

32. Moore AS, Middleton DJ. Pulmonary adenocarcinoma in three cats with non-respiratory signs only. *J Small Anim Pract* 23:501–509, 1982.

33. Postorino NC, Wheeler SL, Park RD, et al: A syndrome resembling lymphomatoid granulomatosis in the dog. *J Vet Intern Med* 3:15–19, 1989.

34. Berry CR, Moore PF, Thomas WP, et al: Pulmonary lymphomatoid granulomatosis in seven dogs (1976–1987). *J Vet Intern Med* 4:157–166, 1993.

35. Rosin A, Moore P, Debielzig R: Malignant histiocytosis in Bernese mountain dogs. *JAVMA* 188:1041–1045, 1986.

36. Moore PF: Systemic histiocytosis in Bernese mountain dogs. *Vet Pathol* 21:554–557, 1984.

CLINICAL BRIEFING: TUMORS OF THE ORAL CAVITY

Oral Tumors in Dogs

Common Clinical Presentation	Oral mass, halitosis, bleeding from the mouth, and dysphagia
Common Histologic Types	*Benign:* Fibromatous epulis; acanthomatous epulis (may invade bone) *Malignant:* Melanoma, squamous cell carcinoma, and fibrosarcoma
Epidemiology and Biological Behavior	*Melanoma:* High metastatic rate; old dogs *Squamous Cell Carcinoma:* Moderately metastatic; lingual and tonsillar types are highly metastatic; old dogs *Fibrosarcoma:* Low metastatic rate; young dogs *Epulides:* Do not metastasize; all ages
Prognostic Factors	*All Tumor Types:* Small tumors and rostral location have a better prognosis *Melanoma:* Low mitotic index is associated with better prognosis *Squamous Cell Carcinoma:* Dogs with maxillary tumors and young dogs have a better prognosis

Treatment
  Surgery
 	
  Radiation Therapy
 	
  Chemotherapy
 	
  Biological Response Modifiers
	
	Mandibulectomy or maxillectomy for local control of malignant tumors
	Curative for acanthomatous epulis; coarse fractionation may be useful for melanoma; adjunctive for squamous cell carcinoma and fibrosarcoma after surgery gives good control
	Platinum compounds best for melanoma, but still low efficacy; chemotherapy not usually required for other tumor types; cisplatin, mitoxantrone, and piroxicam may be effective for squamous cell carcinoma
	L-MTP-PE prolongs survival in dogs with melanoma

Oral Tumors in Cats

Common Clinical Presentation	Halitosis, bleeding from mouth, and dysphagia

MANAGEMENT OF SPECIFIC DISEASES

Common Histologic Types	Squamous cell carcinoma is most common, followed by fibrosarcoma and acanthomatous epulis
Epidemiology and Biological Behavior	Old cats; sublingual squamous cell carcinoma is more common than gingival squamous cell carcinoma
Prognostic Factors	None identified
Treatment	Surgery, radiation therapy, and mitoxantrone or carboplatin chemotherapy used in combination seem to give best control rates for oral squamous cell carcinoma; response to single modalities is poor

Salivary Gland Tumors in Dogs and Cats

Common Clinical Presentation	Cervical mass; anorexia or dysphagia is possible
Common Histologic Type	Adenocarcinoma
Epidemiology and Biological Behavior	May be diffuse oral tumor rather than a mass; metastasis may be more common in cats than dogs; old animals affected (median age is 10 years); poodles and Siamese cats are predisposed
Prognostic Factors	None identified

Treatment
  Surgery
  Radiation Therapy
	High rate of local recurrence in cats and dogs
	When used as an adjunct to surgery, radiation therapy seems to improve local control in dogs; presumably the same in cats

Before obtaining a biopsy or attempting surgical resection of an oral tumor, all dogs and cats should have their general good health confirmed with blood work and urinalysis. Thoracic radiographs should be obtained to rule out macroscopic pulmonary metastases. Fine-detail radiographs of the affected area provide information on the aggressiveness of the tumor. Any local lymphadenopathy should be further investigated by fine-needle aspiration or biopsy performed at the same time as tumor biopsy.

The first surgical excision is the most likely to result in tumor control. The tumor should not be scraped or peeled from underlying bone, as recurrence is certain and the tumor bed will be enlarged. A definitive aggressive first surgery, such as maxillectomy or mandibulectomy, should be performed.

MANAGEMENT OF SPECIFIC DISEASES

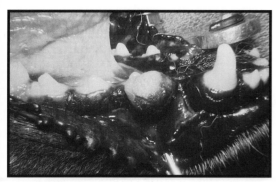

Figure 5-39: Epulides, like this fibromatous epulis in a 7-year-old dog, arise from the periodontal ligament; therefore, surgical excision at the level of the gingiva is not adequate. Acanthomatous epulis is an invasive variant of the epulides. (Courtesy G.H. Theilen)

TABLE 5-10
Distribution of 39 acanthomatous epulides in relation to dental groupings[3]

Location	Site	
	Maxilla	Mandible
Incisor	1	15
Canine	2	7
Premolar	2	2
Molar	2	8

Careful planning and wide margins are required for radiation therapy.

CANINE EPULIDES
Incidence, Signalment, and Etiology

There are three types of epulis. All arise from the periodontal ligament; therefore, despite their clinical appearance, they are intimately related to the dental arcade. Fibromatous epulides and ossifying epulides are benign, whereas acanthomatous epulides may act aggressively by destroying bone and surrounding tissue. Other terms used to described acanthomatous epulis include *adamantinoma* and *ameloblastoma*, although ameloblastoma may be a distinct tumor in young dogs.[1]

Epulides affect both sexes at equal rates.[2–4] Although most affected dogs are middle-aged, the age range is wide and epulides have been documented in dogs as young as 1 year[2,4] and as old as 15 years of age.[3] Although boxers may be predisposed to developing gingival hyperplasia, this breed does not seem to be at excessive risk for developing epulis.[2]

Clinical Presentation and History

Fibromatous and ossifying epu-

lides are slow growing, discrete masses that rarely exceed 2 cm in diameter. They are firm gingival tumors covered by oral epithelium. They may be single or multiple but are always discrete and located near teeth. Ossifying epulis differs from fibromatous only in osteoid production (Figure 5-39).[2]

Acanthomatous epulis is a more rapidly progressive tumor that has a high epithelial component and infiltrates readily into bone. It is usually found in the mandible (Table 5-10) but may occur in the maxilla.

Staging and Diagnosis

Staging should be performed as outlined on page 328. Fibromatous and ossifying epulides are not invasive; therefore, high-detail radiographs of the affected bone are unlikely to identify changes in bone. Such radiographs may be helpful in assessing the degree of bony destruction caused by acanthomatous epulides. In one series of 39 dogs with acanthomatous epulis, radiographic changes in bone were primarily osteolytic in 23 dogs and osteoblastic in only 8 dogs.[3] More than 50% of the bone must be replaced by tumor before lysis is evi-

KEY POINT:

Epulides arise from the periodontal ligament; therefore, excision at the level of the gingiva is incomplete, and the tumor will regrow.

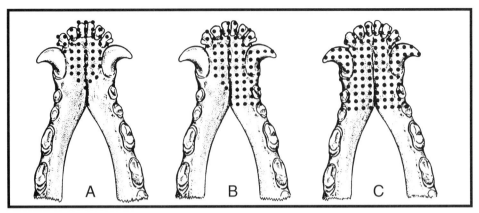

Figure 5-40: Diagram illustrating procedures for rostral mandibulectomy in dogs. (**A**) Partial, (**B**) unilateral, and (**C**) bilateral. (From White RAS: Mandibulectomy and maxillectomy in the dog: Long-term survival in 100 cases. J Small Anim Pract 32:69–74, 1991; with permission.)

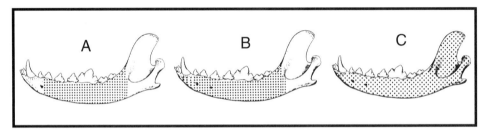

Figure 5-41: Diagram illustrating procedures for hemimandibulectomy in dogs. (**A**) Partial horizontal, (**B**) complete horizontal, and (**C**) total. (From White RAS: Mandibulectomy and maxillectomy in the dog: Long-term survival in 100 cases. J Small Anim Pract 32:69–74, 1991; with permission.)

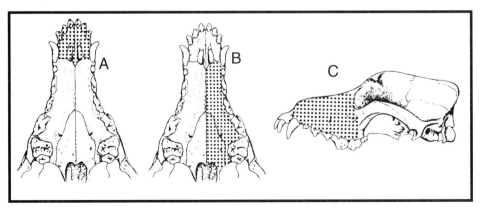

Figure 5-42: Diagram illustrating procedures for partial maxillectomy in dogs. (**A**) Rostral, (**B**) oral, and (**C**) nasal. (From White RAS: Mandibulectomy and maxillectomy in the dog: Long-term survival in 100 cases. J Small Anim Pract 32:69–74, 1991; with permission.)

dent radiographically; therefore, radiographs should not be relied on for surgical margins. Computed tomography (CT) may assist in delineating the margins of tumor involvement more accurately. Technetium-99m nuclide scans tend to overestimate tumor margins by imaging peripheral reactive bone.

Treatment

Local gingival excision of an epulis is rarely curative, as these tumors arise from the periodontal ligament and therefore readily regrow from subgingival tumor tissue in the tooth socket. Regrowth of fibromatous and ossifying epulides may be slow. The excision is curative if surgical margins include the affected tooth root, as with mandibulectomy or maxillectomy (Figures 5-40 to 5-42). Wide surgical margins that include a section of normal bone should be curative for acanthomatous epulis. For larger tumors, however, adequate margins may be difficult to obtain. In a series of 37 dogs surgically treated for acanthomatous epulis, only one had local recurrence and all lived more than one year.[5] Cryosurgery has been used for treatment of epulides, but recurrence is common, presumably because of poor ability to freeze bone and restricted periodontal space.[6] This modality should not be used if it will delay more definitive treatments.

Radiation therapy is very effective for the treatment of acanthomatous epulis. In a series of 39 dogs[3] that received between 20 and 70 Gy of orthovoltage radiation therapy on a 3-day-a-week schedule, 27 dogs achieved a complete remission. The majority (30 of 39) received 35 to 50 Gy. Even though 12 dogs did not have a complete regression of visible tumor, regrowth occurred in only three dogs at 8, 18, and 24 months after radiation. Two of these dogs had tumor that responded to re-irradiation. Overall survival ranged from 1 month to 102 months, with a median of 37 months. These dogs did not have surgery prior to radiation therapy. Possible adverse effects of orthovoltage radiation are osteonecrosis[3] and malignant transformation. Malignant transfor-

> **KEY POINT:**
>
> *Wide surgical excision or radiation therapy both have a high cure rate for acanthomatous epulis in dogs.*

mation, presumably as a consequence of radiation therapy, occurred in seven dogs at a median of 47 months after radiation.[3] More recent assessments of these data suggest that some of these tumors may have been initially misdiagnosed as epulides (D. Thrall, personal communication, 1994). In another series of 37 dogs with acanthomatous epulis, 85% were still free of tumor one year after ^{60}Co radiation therapy.[7] Malignant transformation was not observed.

In one young dog, an acanthomatous epulis regrew six weeks after receiving 50 Gy of orthovoltage radiation therapy. This dog had almost complete regression of the tumor after 10 treatment courses of doxorubicin (30 mg/m² IV every 3 weeks) and cyclophosphamide (50 mg/m² PO daily for 4 days every week) and remained stable for 20 months after starting chemotherapy.[4]

Treatment of acanthomatous epulis should take into account the findings just described. In young dogs, it may be prudent to offer surgery as the treatment of choice owing to the albeit low risk of radiation-induced tumorigenesis. For old dogs, radiation preserves the normal oral architecture and may be better tolerated than surgery, and the low risk of new tumor induction is unlikely to impact longevity.

Ameloblastomas are seen in young dogs. Although they arise from odontogenic tissue, they are distinct from acanthomatous epulides. Two dogs younger than one year of age with ameloblastoma were treated with surgery; tumors recurred in both dogs within six months. A second surgery resulted in a cure for one dog with no recurrence 105 months after surgery.[1]

ODONTOGENIC TUMORS IN CATS
Incidence, Signalment, and Etiology

Fibromatous epulis was the third most common feline oral tumor in one survey, accounting for 29 of 371 oral tumors (7.8%).[8] Some tumors had osseous components as is seen in dogs. Epulides occurred in cats of all ages (range = 1 to 17 years); the average age

MANAGEMENT OF SPECIFIC DISEASES

was 7.5 years. There were 13 male and 16 female cats in this group. Fibroameloblastomas are uncommon tumors that typically affect cats younger than one year of age. They are distinct from the epulides in that they histologically resemble embryonic connective tissue of the dental pulp.[1,9] These tumors are benign and grow by expansion rather than invasion. Complete surgical excision may be difficult if the tumor is large.

Staging and Diagnosis

Cats with oral tumors should be staged with fine-detail radiographs of the affected area as outlined on page 328. Thoracic radiographs rarely show evidence of metastasis from feline odontogenic tumors, which are considered to be benign.

Treatment

Surgery is the treatment of choice for feline fibroameloblastomas and is sometimes curative if adequate surgical margins are obtained. Of seven cats with fibroameloblastoma treated with surgery, one had recurrence of the tumor 42 months later; four cats had complete tumor control 6, 7, 24, and 36 months after surgery.[1] One cat had a second excision of a recurrent tumor and was tumor-free five years later.[9] Another cat had recurrence of the tumor after two surgeries and then again 10 months after radiation therapy. Although reports of treatment for fibromatous epulis in cats are not published, a prognosis similar to that of dogs should be expected after surgery or radiation therapy.

ORAL MALIGNANT MELANOMA IN DOGS
Incidence, Signalment, and Etiology

Oral melanoma is the most common oral malignancy in dogs[10,11] (Figure 5-43). Unlike cutaneous melanomas, which are often benign, canine melanomas of the oral cavity are uniformly malignant. Aggressive local growth and distant metastasis are usual. Even histologically benign melanomas of the oral cavity may act malignantly.[12] These tumors are most common in poodles, dachshunds, Scottish terriers, and golden retrievers.[10,13] In three large series

totalling 193 dogs with oral melanoma, there were 94 male and 99 female dogs.[13-15] This is a disease of old dogs. In one study, the median age of affected dogs was 11 years; ages ranged from 4 to 16 years.[14]

Clinical Presentation and History

Most melanomas arise in the gingiva.[14,15] In descending order of frequency, melanomas are also found on lips, tongue, and hard palate. A recent study found it most clinically relevant to describe tumors in relation to the underlying bone.[13] Of 41 dogs, 19 had tumors in the rostral maxilla, six in the caudal maxilla, seven in the rostral mandible, and seven in the caudal mandible. Two tumors were in the hard palate.

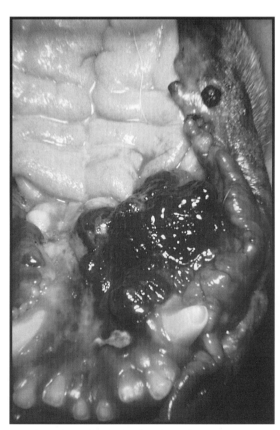

Figure 5-43: *Oral melanoma is the most common oral malignancy in dogs. It is usually heavily pigmented with melanin.*

MANAGEMENT OF SPECIFIC DISEASES

TABLE 5-11
Clinical stages of canine
oral melanoma (WHO)

| Clinical Stage | Criteria | | | |
	Tumor	Node	Metastasis	Percentage of Dogs[14]
Stage I	<2 cm	–	–	43
Stage II	2–4 cm	–	–	44
Stage III	>4 cm or any bone invasion	+	–	13
Stage IV	Any	Any	+	Not available

Owners may present dogs for an oral mass, or (more frequently) for persistent halitosis, bleeding from the mouth, and (occasionally) dysphagia. Tumors may be quite large, ranging in volume up to 64 cm³ in one study.[12] Although masses are frequently pigmented, amelanotic tumors are common. Oral melanomas are friable and invasive within the soft tissues of the mouth.[16] Because these tumors often surround the bony structures and invade bone, surgical excision is often difficult.

Staging and Diagnosis

Dogs with oral tumors of any type should be staged using blood work, radiographs, and cytology or histopathology, as outlined on page 328. Although histopathology is required for definitive diagnosis of oral melanoma, the index of suspicion for this tumor should be high in an old dog with a friable oral mass. The metastatic rate is very high for oral melanoma, but the time to metastasis varies. At diagnosis, the mandibular lymph nodes (both ipsilateral and contralateral) should be palpated and any enlarged node should have fine-needle aspiration performed for cytologic examination. In one study, only five (12%) of 41 dogs had metastatic disease in regional lymph nodes at diagnosis.[13] Aspiration cytology that is suspicious should be confirmed by surgical biopsy. Thoracic radiographs may indicate pulmonary metastasis

at the time of diagnosis. Pulmonary metastasis, however, frequently occurs late in the course of the disease. In one study, only three (7%) of 41 dogs had evidence of pulmonary metastasis at diagnosis,[13] but at the time of death, metastatic rate for this tumor approximated 80%.[17] Melanoma may also spread systemically, and metastasis is reported in kidney, myocardium, and brain[12] as well as other sites.

The World Health Organization (WHO) staging scheme for oral melanoma is summarized in Table 5-11.

Metastasis of tumors is probably an early event, occurring during clinical stages I and II; however, metastases are often not detected until long after the primary melanoma is resected. The growth rate of metastases may vary, and it is this variation, rather than the time that metastasis occurs, that determines survival time.

Some investigators have found that the WHO staging system provides prognostic information,[14] but an alternative staging system has been proposed that includes the WHO criteria and also uses the mitotic index from histopathology and location within the oral cavity (Figure 5-44). This staging system also offers prognostic information.

Current recommendations for staging oral melanoma therefore include lymph node evaluation by cytology or biopsy, thoracic radiographs, and tumor measurements as well as anatomic location

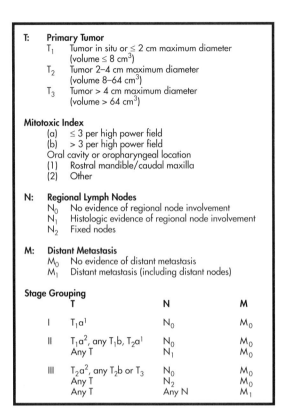

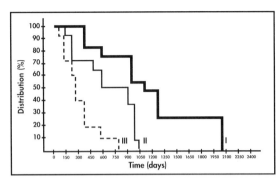

Figure 5-45: The staging scheme seen in Figure 5-44 influenced survival in 24 dogs with oral melanoma treated by surgery. Kaplan–Meier survival statistics showed a significant difference among the three melanoma stages when they were staged as stage I, stage II, or stage III. (From Hahn KA, DeNicola DB, Richardson RC, Hahn EA: Canine oral malignant melanoma: Prognostic utility of an alternative staging system. J Small Anim Pract 35:251–256, 1994; with permission.)

Figure 5-44: In dogs, a modified staging scheme has been proposed for oral melanoma that combines the traditional scheme with other criteria, such as the location of the tumor within the oral cavity and the mitotic index as seen on histopathology. (From Hahn KA, DeNicola DB, Richardson RC, Hahn EA: Canine oral malignant melanoma: Prognostic utility of an alternative staging system. J Small Anim Pract 35:251–256, 1994; with permission.)

stage I (small) tumors (median = 511 days) than for dogs with stage II or III tumors (median = 164 days).[14] Small melanomas were also associated with long survival times in another study.[7]

One study found that the location of the tumor was not prognostic,[14] but two other studies indicated that tumors of the rostral mandible and the caudal maxilla had longer remissions and survival after surgery.[7,13] Another study found longer survival times for dogs with tumors that had fewer than three mitotic figures per high-power field (Figure 5-45).[13]

Treatment

Surgery remains the mainstay of treatment for oral melanoma and should consist of mandibulectomy or maxillectomy. Radiation has a role in local tumor control. Chemotherapy with platinum compounds, perhaps combined with liposome-encapsulated muramyltripeptide-phosphatidyethanolamine (L-MTP-PE) immunotherapy, may offer the best adjunctive treatment for metastatic disease.

Oral melanomas in dogs have a

and evaluation of mitotic index as determined by histopathology.

Prognostic Factors

The ability of the WHO staging scheme to prognosticate accurately for dogs with oral melanoma has been controversial. Some studies found no utility for the scheme,[12,13] whereas other studies found significantly longer survival for dogs with

KEY POINT:

Dogs with rostrally located, small oral melanomas that have a low mitotic index probably have the best prognosis after treatment.

high metastatic rate, but metastases frequently are not observed until late in the course of disease, occasionally more than one year after local therapy.[18] Most dogs, therefore, are euthanatized because of progression or recurrence of local disease. If surgery is aggressive from the outset, it may prolong survival as well as provide palliation. Aggressive local therapy should include resection of underlying bone.[13] In one early study, 34 of 49 dogs had local recurrence of tumor,[12] and 33 dogs developed metastases. The recurrence rate of 84% probably reflects the less aggressive nature of the surgery, because more recent studies reported local recurrence rates of less than 15% for melanomas treated by mandibulectomy[5,16,19] to 48% for tumors treated by maxillectomy.[18] Both mandibulectomy and maxillectomy are tolerated well by dogs, with median hospitalization times ranging from two days for simple excision to eight days for total hemimandibulectomy.[16] In three studies, dogs treated with aggressive surgery had a median survival time of 7.3 to 9.1 months[15,16,18] compared with seven dogs that did not have surgery and survived a median of two months.[15] Mandibulectomy or maxillectomy should be the first surgery used to treat oral melanoma in dogs. Less aggressive surgeries do not prolong survival and make subsequent surgery more difficult.

Surgical excision was used to treat five dogs with melanoma of the tongue and achieved local control in three dogs, with survival times ranging from 3 months to 45 months (median = 19 months). Only one dog developed metastases.[20]

Metastatic disease occurs in the majority of patients and often occurs within six months of surgery,[16] although metastases may not be visible for longer than one year after surgery.[18,21] After metastases develop, dogs may still survive a long time, depending on the growth rate.[21] Dogs may tolerate pulmonary metastatic disease with very little apparent effect on their quality of life.

Radiation therapy has a role in the treatment of melanoma, particularly for small tumors. Thirty-three dogs with melanoma were treated with 48 Gy of ^{60}Co teletherapy.[7] Five dogs had local recurrence.

One dog had regional lymph node metastasis, and 14 developed distant metastasis. Dogs with rostrally located tumors and dogs with smaller tumors had longer remissions. Median progression-free survival was estimated to be 14 months.

Chemotherapy has very little effect on survival times in dogs with oral melanoma when used either as an adjunct to surgery or to treat gross metastatic disease. Drugs such as dacarbazine (DTIC) (1000 mg/m^2 IV every 3 weeks),[20,21] doxorubicin (30 mg/m^2 IV every 3 weeks), and melphalan (0.5 mg/kg IV every 4 weeks),[22] (D. Ruslander, personal communication, 1994) have not had repeatable success. Platinum compounds may be more efficacious; cisplatin (60 mg/m^2 IV every 3 weeks) provided partial response for a dog with metastatic disease,[23] and carboplatin (300 mg/m^2 IV every 3 weeks) appears to have some efficacy, although the response rate is still probably less than 25%.[24]

Immunotherapy has a role in treating melanoma in many species. Cimetidine, which appears to have its immunomodulating effect by inhibition of suppressor T cells, has been shown to cause regression of melanoma in some horses,[25] although its role in the treatment of the disease in dogs is not defined. Immunotherapy with interleukin-2 has been beneficial in treating humans with melanoma. Combined with tumor necrosis factor, this treatment might be useful for dogs.[26] This combination was administered to 13 dogs with measurable oral melanoma. Five dogs showed reduction in tumor size, although only two had durable responses. One of these dogs had a complete remission for more than three years.

Immunotherapy with heat-inactivated *Corynebacterium parvum* (0.1 mg/kg IV per week) was used as an adjunct to surgery in 42 dogs.[14] *Corynebacterium parvum* activates and increases production of macrophages, which enhances the antibody response. Immunotherapy with *C. parvum* was found to benefit dogs with small tumors (stage I).[14] A more specific macrophage activator, L-MTP-PE, improves survival in dogs treated after surgery for oral melanoma.[27] L-MTP-PE was administered to 24 dogs after surgery, and 26 dogs received a placebo. Only eight

MANAGEMENT OF SPECIFIC DISEASES

(30%) of the L-MTP-PE dogs had died at an interim analysis, whereas 14 of the placebo group had died, for a median survival of 8.2 months.

ORAL MELANOMA IN CATS
Incidence, Signalment, and Etiology

Oral melanoma is very rare in cats. Of eight reported cases, four were domestic shorthair, and one was Siamese. Six cats were female. The average age of affected cats was 12 years, with an age range of 8 to 16 years.[8,28]

Clinical Presentation and History

Cats with oral melanoma show signs of drooling and facial swelling. Tumors occur in gingiva, palate, and mandible.

Staging and Diagnosis

Any cat with an oral tumor should be staged by blood work, radiographs, and lymph node evaluation, as described on page 328. Metastasis of oral melanoma in cats is common, although it sometimes is late to occur. Metastasis occurred in all cats for which information was available; however, lymph-node metastasis in one cat occurred two years after surgery.[9,28]

Treatment

Surgical excision was performed on three cats. All three died because of metastatic disease within five months of surgery. Oral melanoma is an aggressive neoplasm, and without therapy adjunctive to surgery, a poor prognosis should be given.[28] No adjunctive therapy has been reported.

ORAL SQUAMOUS CELL CARCINOMA IN DOGS
Incidence, Signalment, and Etiology

Squamous cell carcinoma is the second most common oral malignancy in dogs. It is usually found in the gingival tissue, although the tongue and tonsils are frequently affected. Tumors of the tonsil behave very differently from other squamous cell carcinomas and are considered separately.

Squamous cell carcinoma usually occurs in older

TABLE 5-12
Distribution of nontonsillar oral squamous cell carcinoma in 33 dogs[29]

Location	Site		
	Maxilla	Mandible	Soft Tissue
Rostral	8	6	1
Caudal	7	—	3
Rostral and caudal	1	2	—
Tongue	—	—	5

dogs; the average age is nine years.[18,19,29] There is no apparent breed or gender predilection, although one study of squamous cell carcinoma of the tongue found that 43% of affected dogs had a white haircoat and 30% were poodles.[20] This finding has not been corroborated. Papillary squamous cell carcinoma occurs in dogs as young as two months of age.[30] Papillary squamous cell carcinoma is a progressive disease with a high rate of lytic bone involvement.

Clinical Presentation and History

Most oral squamous cell carcinomas are rostral within the mouth; the majority occur in the maxilla (Table 5-12).[29] Affected dogs show the same signs as do dogs with other oral tumors. The most common signs are drooling, halitosis, and (occasionally) dysphagia. Most dogs have shown signs for three months or less, but some dogs may show signs for six months to one year before diagnosis.[20]

Staging and Diagnosis

As with most oral tumors, biopsy is required to differentiate squamous cell carcinoma from amelanotic melanoma, ulcerated fibrosarcoma, or less common tumors. Staging should be performed as outlined on page 328. Squamous cell carcinoma is highly invasive; high-detail radiographs of the skull often reveal extensive bony lysis.[29] Bony lysis alone should not be relied on for surgical margins or radiotherapy field size, as

MANAGEMENT OF SPECIFIC DISEASES

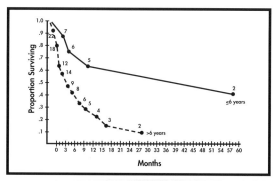

Figure 5-46: *Survival curves according to age at diagnosis of dogs with nontonsillar squamous cell carcinoma after treatment with radiation therapy. Young dogs tended to survive for longer periods after radiation therapy. (From Evans SM, Shofer F: Canine oral nontonsillar squamous cell carcinoma: Prognostic factors for recurrence and survival following orthovoltage radiation therapy.* Vet Radiol *29:133–137, 1988; with permission.)*

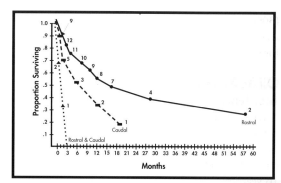

Figure 5-47: *Survival curves of the same dogs as in figure 5-46, comparing tumors that were located rostral to the second premolar, caudal to that point, and tumors that involved both rostral and caudal areas of the gingiva. (From Evans SM, Shofer F: Canine oral nontonsillar squamous cell carcinoma: Prognostic factors for recurrence and survival following orthovoltage radiation therapy.* Vet Radiol *29:133– 137, 1988; with permission.)*

this underestimates tumor size. CT scanning is recommended, particularly if radiation therapy is planned.

Metastasis of gingival squamous cell carcinoma is uncommon, and metastasis to the lungs at time of diagnosis is rare.[31] Regional lymph nodes are frequently enlarged at diagnosis and should be biopsied for cytology or histopathology; however, they usually do not contain metastases. In one study, 11 of 33 dogs had lymphadenopathy, and only three of these dogs had metastatic disease.[29] After therapy, regional lymph node metastasis is still uncommon. It was documented in five (20%) of 24 dogs in three case series.[16,18,19] In contrast, squamous cell carcinoma of the tongue seems more aggressive[5,20]; nine (43%) of 21 dogs in one study developed metastasis to lymph nodes, lung, or bone.[20]

Prognostic Factors

In one report,[29] dogs with maxillary tumors had a longer average response to radiation therapy (12 months) than did dogs with mandibular (3.4 months) or soft tissue tumors (1.8 months). In the same study, survival was influenced

by position within the oral cavity, size of the radiation field, and age of the dog. Eight dogs that were younger than six years of age lived for a median of 58 months after radiation; older dogs lived for a median of six months (Figure 5-46).[29] Dogs with rostrally located tumors live longer than dogs with caudal tumors, whereas dogs with tumors that extend both rostrally and caudally have significantly shorter survival times.[7,29] Therefore, larger tumors (and concomitantly larger radiation fields) are associated with shorter survival[7,29] (Figure 5-47).

Treatment

The relatively low metastatic rate of rostral gingival squamous cell carcinoma makes this malignancy a good candidate for local therapies, such as surgery and radiation. Aggressive surgery is necessary to obtain adequate surgical margins. Maxillectomy and mandibulectomy have been used to treat this tumor. In 53 dogs from seven reports,[5,16,18,19,21,31,32] median survival ranged from 9[19] to 18 months.[18,31] Recurrence was more frequent than

> **KEY POINT:**
>
> *For oral squamous cell carcinomas, small rostral tumors (particularly of the maxilla) seem to have the best prognosis.*

MANAGEMENT OF SPECIFIC DISEASES

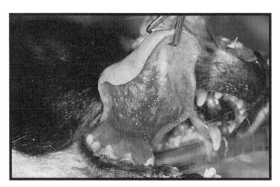

Figure 5-48: *Squamous cell carcinoma of the tongue is more likely to metastasize than gingival squamous cell carcinoma.*

metastasis after surgery. Incomplete surgical resection is commonly associated with recurrence, which emphasizes the importance of early diagnosis and obtaining wide surgical margins by mandibulectomy or maxillectomy at the first surgery. Adjunctive radiation therapy may also be useful.

Orthovoltage radiation therapy without surgery was used to treat 33 dogs to a total dose of approximately 40 Gy. Overall average survival was approximately 14 months; however, size and location of tumor and age of dog influenced these figures (see Prognostic Factors, page 337).[29] There was recurrence in 15 dogs, metastasis in three, and serious complications (e.g., bone necrosis) from radiation in two dogs. In another series, 31 dogs with squamous cell carcinoma were treated with 48 Gy of ^{60}Co teletherapy.[7] Eight dogs had local recurrence, two dogs developed metastases to regional lymph nodes, and four dogs had distant metastases. Dogs with rostrally located tumors and dogs with smaller tumors had longer remissions. Median progression-free survival was approximately 17 months.

A combination of radiation and surgery gives the best control for gingival squamous cell carcinoma, and postsurgical radiation should be considered for dogs with large tumors or for dogs with tumors that have "dirty" margins on histopathology. One dog treated in this way had no evidence of disease 16 months after treatment.[18] Clearly, this combined modality approach warrants more investigation.

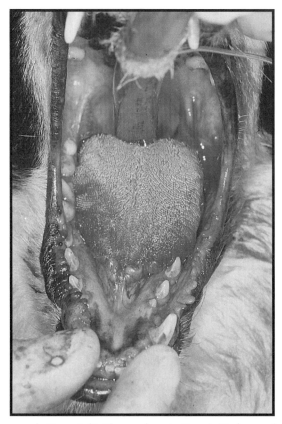

Figure 5-49: *The same dog as in Figure 5-48 after rostral linguectomy. Even after such radical procedures and adjuvant radiation therapy, local recurrence may be a problem. Dogs tolerate linguectomy surprisingly well.*

Squamous cell carcinoma of the tongue is a more aggressive tumor than gingival squamous cell carcinoma, and metastatic disease often determines survival. Surgery has variable results, and recurrence is common unless wide surgical margins are obtained. In some cases, complete removal of the tongue is indicated. Surprisingly, dogs adapt to this well (Figures 5-48 and 5-49). In one study,[20] five dogs with small tumors were treated with surgery alone and had a median survival time of eight months. Three of these dogs had local recurrence. Recurrence of tongue tumors is also common after radiation therapy. Larger tumors in 10 dogs were treated with radiation therapy, and the dogs survived for a median of four months; 9 of 10 dogs had recurrence.[20] The one dog that received radiation after surgery survived 26 months with no recurrence. A combined modality approach for larger tumors seems warranted for local control, although metastasis occurs in approximately 50% of the cases.[20] Chemotherapy should be considered for these tumors as an adjuvant to surgery.

Papillary squamous cell carcinoma in young dogs is a progressive disease. Conservative surgery alone is unlikely to be curative because of the high rate of bone involvement and the young age of the patient.[30] Radiation therapy has a good success rate, although disruption of normal bone growth in young dogs may produce facial malformations. Radiation therapy to a total dose of 40 Gy was used to treat three puppies with this disease. There was no evidence of disease in any dog 39, 32, and 10 months after treatment, respectively; one dog had malformation of the affected jaw.

Chemotherapy is rarely warranted for rostral gingival squamous cell carcinoma in dogs because of the low metastatic rate for this tumor. Chemotherapy may be indicated for squamous cell carcinoma of the tongue, tonsil, and caudal location of the mouth because of the high metastatic rate of such tumors. Subcutaneous bleomycin treatment[33] as well as doxorubicin, cyclophosphamide, and chlorambucil treatment[18] failed to induce responses in two dogs with oral squamous cell carcinoma. Cisplatin has caused responses in dogs with metastatic subungual squamous cell carcinoma[34]; however, no responses occurred in five dogs with oral squamous cell carcinoma (including one tongue and one tonsillar tumor).[35] In another report, cisplatin caused a partial response in three of five dogs with squamous cell carcinoma for 2, 10, and 15 weeks, respectively.[36] Cisplatin has yet to be fully evaluated for oral squamous cell carcinoma; however, it may be useful in combi-

nation therapy for this disease. Mitoxantrone (5 to 6 mg/m^2 every 3 weeks) caused objective responses in four (45%) of nine dogs with squamous cell carcinoma of various sites, including the oral cavity, for between 6 and 21 weeks.[37]

TONSILLAR SQUAMOUS CELL CARCINOMA IN DOGS
Incidence, Signalment, and Etiology
Tonsillar squamous cell carcinoma is considerably more aggressive than either gingival or lingual squamous cell carcinoma. This tumor occurs in dogs of a median age of 9 to 11 years.[33,38,39] There seems to be a male predisposition to developing tonsillar squamous cell carcinoma. No breed predisposition has been described. Tonsillar squamous cell carcinoma occasionally may occur bilaterally.[17]

Clinical Presentation and History
Most dogs with tonsillar squamous cell carcinoma present with dysphagia, anorexia, and pain, and owners may have noticed a cervical swelling, which is usually lymph node metastasis rather than primary tumor. In fact, the primary tumor may be quite small but lymphadenopathy may be marked. Most dogs have shown these signs for one month or less, although some dogs may show signs for up to three months before presentation.[39]

Staging and Diagnosis
A dog with a large cervical mass should have a thorough examination of both tonsils; aspiration cytology of the lymph node may confirm metastatic carcinoma. If no diagnosis can be reached, biopsy of the tonsil and the regional lymph node is warranted. Thoracic radiographs should be taken, although metastasis is unlikely to be seen at the time of diagnosis. If treatment is undertaken, radiographs should be repeated at regular intervals to screen for metastasis. In view of the high reported rate of intra-abdominal

KEY POINT:

Owners may notice lymphadenopathy due to metastasis from tonsillar squamous cell carcinoma long before a tonsillar tumor is suspected.

MANAGEMENT OF SPECIFIC DISEASES

metastases in one study,[38] abdominal radiographs and ultrasonography should be performed prior to any definitive treatment. They also may be useful for monitoring the patient for metastases after treatment.

Lymphadenopathy caused by metastasis from tonsillar carcinoma is common. In one group of 22 dogs, all had lymphadenopathy as well as infiltrative primary tumors at the time of diagnosis.[39] Despite early spread to the lymph nodes, pulmonary metastases are rarely noted at diagnosis. After treatment, nine (33%) of 27 dogs had evidence of distant metastases.[38,39] In two earlier studies, 77 (85%) of 91 dogs with tonsillar squamous cell carcinoma had metastasis to regional lymph nodes at necropsy.[17] Systemic metastases were less common; they occurred in the lung, spleen, liver, and thyroid gland. In a smaller group of dogs, metastasis to the spleen and liver occurred more often than to the lungs.[38]

Treatment

Surgery alone is not generally effective for treating tonsillar squamous cell carcinomas because of their high metastatic rate, which manifests early in the course of the disease. A combination of surgery and radiation provided good local control at radiation doses of 35 Gy to 42.5 Gy; six of eight dogs showed a complete response, and one dog showed a partial response.[38] Recurrence was seen in only two of the seven responding dogs, although metastatic disease to the spleen, liver, bone, and lungs was seen or suspected in all seven. Survival ranged from 44 to 631 days, with a median of 109 days.

In an attempt to improve this survival, dogs were treated with a combination of surgery, orthovoltage radiation therapy, and chemotherapy that alternated doxorubicin (30 mg/m^2 IV every 3 weeks) with cisplatin (60 mg/m^2 IV every 3 weeks).[39] Of six dogs receiving this protocol, five achieved a complete response with a median of 240 days. Four of these dogs developed tumor recurrence and metastatic disease. In comparison, 16 dogs had no response to treatment with this chemotherapy protocol (or combinations of doxorubicin, vinblastine, cisplatin, and cyclophosphamide), when it was administered with-

out radiation therapy.[39] Median survival for these 16 dogs was 105 days.

Clearly, the best results for this tumor can be obtained only if aggressive surgery and radiation therapy are combined with doxorubicin and cisplatin chemotherapy; even then, tumor progression is difficult to control. The prognosis for dogs with tonsillar squamous cell carcinoma is very poor.

ORAL SQUAMOUS CELL CARCINOMA IN CATS
Incidence, Signalment, and Etiology

Squamous cell carcinoma is the most common oral tumor in cats and accounts for approximately 60% of all oral tumors.[8] The tumor is most common in old cats that average 11 to 12 years of age; however, cats as young as three years of age may be affected.[8,9] No gender or breed predilection has been noted.[8]

Most squamous cell carcinomas occur at the base of the tongue and involve the frenulum (Figure 5-50). The extensive grooming habits of the cat possibly cause the species to contact carcinogens on its haircoat, thereby predisposing the tongue to development of neoplasia.[9]

Clinical Presentation and History

Squamous cell carcinomas are characterized by mucosal ulceration, necrosis, and severe suppurative

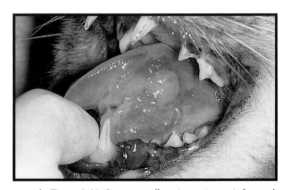

Figure 5-50: *Squamous cell carcinoma in cats is frequently found sublingually and is usually very advanced at the time of diagnosis. This is an aggressive tumor that is best treated by radiation and chemotherapy; however, tissue necrosis and ischemia are common, limiting the effectiveness of therapy.*

inflammation. Cats with this tumor usually present with dysphagia, halitosis, and drooling of rope-like saliva. In the early stages, differentiating squamous cell carcinoma from gingival proliferation and dental disease may be difficult, so any old cat with these symptoms should be biopsied. Cats are usually presented within three weeks of the onset of these signs; when the interval between onset and presentation is longer, tumors may be quite advanced.[41]

Gingival tumors are as likely to arise on the mandible as on the maxilla. Bone invasion is common with gingival tumors.[8] Some squamous cell carcinomas arise primarily within the mandible, causing enlargement of the jaw due to bony proliferation.[41] These tumors should be differentiated from deep-seated osteomyelitis generated by severe dental disease[42] and from other malignant tumors, such as osteosarcoma.[43,44] Feline tonsillar tumors are comparatively rare, but they are very aggressive locally and may metastasize to lymph nodes and lungs.

Staging and Diagnosis

Staging of any cat with an oral tumor should be performed as outlined on page 328. High-detail radiography of the skull provides information on bony lysis caused by gingival tumors.[31] As stated previously, however, radiographic appearance of lysis does not occur until more than 50% of the bone has been demineralized; therefore, radiography is a poor indicator of tumor margins. Biopsy is required for definitive diagnosis and should be considered in any old cat with severe gingival disease.

Metastasis is rare, although mandibular lymph nodes may be involved and should be evaluated by cytology or histopathology. Although lymphaden-

KEY POINTS:

Squamous cell carcinoma may cause an intense reaction in the mandible with massive bony proliferation. This lesion should be differentiated from osteomyelitis or osteosarcoma.

Placement of a gastrotomy tube is essential for any cat undergoing oral surgery or radiation and should be considered as a routine part of patient management for oral squamous cell carcinoma.

opathy is usually assumed to signal possible metastatic disease, two studies found that less than 50% of cats with enlarged lymph nodes had histologic evidence of metastatic disease.[40,41] Lymph node metastasis was seen in 8 of 59 cats in these two studies.[40,41] One author suggested that metastatic disease may occur late in the course of the disease,[45] or perhaps metastases are slow to progress. This is further supported by one cat that had no evidence of metastatic progression 16 months after lymph node metastasis was detected.[40] Other authors speculate that the low rate of metastatic disease may be caused by limited lymphatic drainage from the gingivae.[8]

Treatment

Mandibular resection alone was not very successful in maintaining a remission in five cats with squamous cell carcinoma.[31] Recurrence occurred in four cats within 5 to 12 months of surgery despite aggressive surgical technique. These tumors were all large (between 2 and 4 cm diameter), and all invaded bone. In another study, surgery alone resulted in a median survival of six weeks for seven cats.[40] Anecdotally, small tumors, particularly those located rostrally on the mandible, are amenable to complete surgical excision (Figures 5-51 and 5-52). The results of radiation therapy used alone are not promising. Radiation therapy (orthovoltage, 52 Gy) as a single modality was used to treat 11 cats with oral squamous cell carcinoma.[46] Treatment included ethanidazole, which is a hypoxic cell sensitizer that was injected intratumorally. Eight cats were evaluated for response. Four died from complications of therapy, which included tissue necrosis and ischemia of the tongue, between 45 and 341 days after radiation (median = 114 days). The other four

MANAGEMENT OF SPECIFIC DISEASES

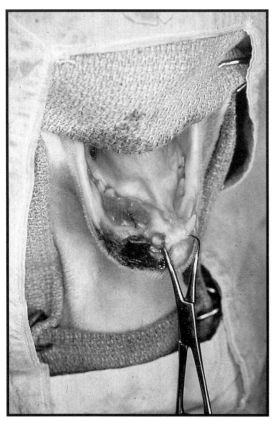

Figure 5-51: *Mandibular squamous cell carcinomas, particularly those located rostrally, can be treated by hemimandibulectomy. Most other oral squamous cell carcinomas in cats are not amenable to surgery. (Courtesy J. Berg)*

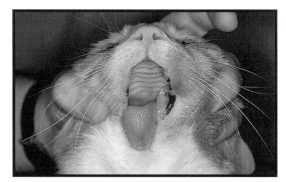

Figure 5-52: *Complete right and partial left mandibulectomy was performed one year before in this 15-year-old cat. Mandibulectomy is well tolerated by cats, and although enteral feeding by gastrotomy tube may be necessary until cats learn to eat, recovery is usually rapid.*

cats had tumor recurrence at 125 to 331 days after radiation (median = 170 days). No cats were alive one year after treatment. Overall median survival was 132 days. In another study, radiation alone or in combination with chemotherapy or with hyperthermia resulted in a median survival of 10 weeks for 45 cats.[40]

More successful outcome followed combined treatment with mandibulectomy followed by external beam radiation to a dose of 40 Gy to 45 Gy starting 10 to 15 days after surgery.[41] Six of seven cats had tumor recurrence between 3 and 36 months after treatment (median = 12.5 months). One cat died but showed no evidence of disease 14 months after com-

pleting radiation therapy. Complications were minor and included mandibular "drift," drooling after eating and messy eating habits.

Placement of a gastrotomy tube by endoscopy at the time of surgery may prolong survival in cats with squamous cell carcinoma.[40] The tube allows enteral feeding of the cat during recovery while allowing the mouth to heal. Gastrotomy tubes can remain in place after surgery until the cat is able to eat normally.

Although squamous cell carcinoma has a low metastatic rate, the paucity of other treatment options has led to trials of chemotherapeutic agents. Mitoxantrone at doses up to 6.5 mg/m^2 IV every 3 weeks caused one complete remission and three partial remissions for 21 to 60 days in 32 cats.[47] Even though this is not a startling efficacy, it prompted investigation of combined mitoxantrone chemotherapy and radiation therapy. Seven cats received mitoxantrone (5 mg/m^2 IV every 3 weeks) during and following megavoltage radiation therapy.[48] Radiation was delivered as a "shrinking field," whereby the tumor and mandibular lymph node received 39.6 to 46.2 Gy, the mandible received 49.5 to 51 Gy, and the gross tumor received 59.4 to 61.2 Gy in daily 3-Gy fractions. The median survival for these cats was 180 days. Thirty percent of the cats were alive one year after radiation therapy. Carboplatin may have efficacy against this disease and is currently being investigated.

The best therapy for oral squamous cell carcinoma in cats has not been determined. A combination of surgery, radiation therapy, and chemotherapy probably offers the best chance of success. Preoperative radiation and chemotherapy may cause tumor shrinkage and allow surgical margins to be more easily attained.

ORAL FIBROSARCOMA IN DOGS
Incidence, Signalment, and Etiology

Fibrosarcomas are the third most common oral tumor in dogs. They occur in young dogs more commonly than melanoma or squamous cell carcinoma.[17] The average age of dogs with oral fibrosarcoma is seven years,[16–18,21,49] although these tumors have been reported in dogs as young as six months of age.[16,17,49] There do not seem to be any breed predilections for dogs with this tumor, although four of 10 affected dogs in one study were golden retrievers.[49] There is an apparent male predilection for developing oral fibrosarcoma,[17,50] although this is not consistent in all studies.[49]

Clinical Presentation and History

Fibrosarcomas arise most commonly in the gingiva and are equally likely to be located around the maxilla or the mandible.[50] The hard palate is not commonly involved except by extension of a maxillary tumor. Tumors are usually large, with diameters of greater than 4 cm.[17,50]

Staging and Diagnosis

Before biopsy, dogs should be staged using blood work, thoracic radiographs, lymph node evaluation, and fine-detail skull radiographs as outlined on page 328. Fibrosarcomas frequently invade bone[17,50] and may extend much farther than is obvious by external viewing. In addition, all soft tissue sarcomas have "tendrils" of tumor cells that extend deep into normal surrounding tissues, making complete excision very difficult without wide margins.

Prior to attempting such a surgery, particularly when the tumor involves maxilla, high-detail skull radiographs should be obtained to gain a better appreciation of tumor borders. Radiographs are superior to clinical examination in determining tumor borders but do not allow imaging of bony lysis until more than 50% of the bone has been destroyed (demineralized). Therefore, radiographs usually underestimate tumor margins. CT scanning is a more accurate method of assessing fibrosarcoma margins. A CT scan provides a spatial assessment of the tumor that may be useful for planning surgery as well as either presurgery or postsurgery radiation therapy. CT scanning may also indicate whether a surgery is impossible, thereby protecting the animal from a poorly planned procedure.

Histologic reports of these tumors should be interpreted cautiously. Occasionally, a tumor may be termed a *fibroma*, which implies that the process is benign. In fact, all soft tissue sarcomas embrace a spectrum of disease and fibromas of the oral cavity should be treated as aggressively as fibrosarcomas. A recent report described 25 dogs with tumors that were histologically labelled as either fibromas, nodular fascitis, or granulation tissue. Although all of these lesions are considered benign, they invaded bone and metastasized in five dogs.[51] Bony invasion should be interpreted as a sign of malignancy regardless of the pathology report.

Metastasis is uncommon in fibrosarcoma, particularly at the time of diagnosis.[17,50] Especially in young dogs, however, mandibular lymph nodes should be palpated and (if enlarged) subjected to fine-needle aspiration or biopsy. Young dogs apparently have more aggressive tumors than old dogs. In eight series totalling 107 dogs, metastasis was reported in 23 (21%) dogs.[5,16–18,21,50] In most cases, metastasis was to regional lymph nodes[16,21,50]; it is rare for oral fibrosarcoma to metastasize to lungs.[17] Thoracic radiographs should, however, be performed prior to definitive surgery. Metastases often appear many months after surgery,[16] and it is possible that earlier reports with less effective therapies may have underestimated the metastatic rate, because dogs died from inadequate local tumor control before metastasis occurred.

MANAGEMENT OF SPECIFIC DISEASES

Treatment

The treatment of choice for fibrosarcoma of the oral cavity is complete surgical excision. Local excisions lead to rapid recurrence.[21] Radical surgical techniques such as maxillectomy and mandibulectomy are well tolerated by dogs and are necessary to obtain adequate surgical margins. In five series totalling 54 dogs treated for oral fibrosarcoma with aggressive surgery, the median survival was 12 months[5,16,18,19,21] and ranged from 1.5 weeks to 33 months.[18]

Even after mandibulectomy or maxillectomy, local recurrence was a problem in 20 of 54 dogs (37%). Tumor recurrence varied, however, depending on the study (and therefore the surgeon) from 20%[16] to nearly 60%[21] and occurred soon after surgery in studies with the highest rates of recurrence. In three dogs in one study,[18] recurrence was treated by a second surgery (2 dogs) or surgery plus radiation therapy (1 dog), for second remissions of 2 months, 15 months, and 2 years, respectively.

Pretreatment with 50 to 56 Gy of radiation seemed to improve control rates in one study, although few dogs were involved.[21] Early results of radiation therapy as a single treatment modality were disappointing for canine oral fibrosarcoma, but this may have reflected the source and dosage of radiation. Control of fibrosarcoma improves only at high doses of 50 Gy or more.[50,53] Of 17 dogs treated with 40.0 to 54.5 Gy of orthovoltage, four died during or soon after radiation therapy. Survival times in the remaining 13 dogs ranged from 2 months to more than 27 months, with a median survival of 6 months. Tumors recurred in 12 dogs at a mean time of 3.9 months after radiation was complete.[50] In another study, radiation therapy without surgery was able to control tumor growth in three of 13 dogs.[53] Megavoltage radiation may be more efficacious than orthovoltage in controlling oral fibrosarcomas. Seventeen dogs with fibrosarcoma were treated with 48 Gy of ^{60}Co teletherapy.[7] Seven dogs had local recurrence, and one dog developed distant metastasis. Dogs with rostrally located tumors and dogs with smaller tumors had longer remissions. Median progression-free survival was estimated to be 23 months.

When used in combination with radiation, interstitial hyperthermia provides better local control rates than those achieved by radiation alone. Ten dogs that received between 32 and 48 Gy of orthovoltage also received interstitial hyperthermia to a temperature of either 50°C or 43°C for 30 seconds.[49] Complete remissions were obtained in nine of 10 dogs, and overall median survival was 12.9 months, which is comparable to survival times for dogs that undergo surgery. Tumors recurred in four dogs between 38 days and 378 days after radiation. Complications of this combined modality include fistula formation and sepsis following tissue necrosis.[49]

Chemotherapy has little application in the treatment of oral cavity fibrosarcomas, although doxorubicin has been noted occasionally to produce objective responses in soft tissue sarcomas. Low doses of doxorubicin (10 mg/m² IV every 7 days) appear to act as a "radiation sensitizer" and improve tumor response at lower radiation therapy dosages.

Intratumoral injections of cisplatin and bovine collagen matrix were given every week during a 48 Gy course of ^{60}Co teletherapy to five dogs with oral fibrosarcoma. Complete remission was seen in three dogs, and partial remission was seen in one dog for a median duration of 14 weeks. There was tumor recurrence in three of these dogs.[54] In these and other dogs treated with radiochemotherapy, recurrences often took place at the periphery of the chemotherapy site but still within the radiation field, implying that the combination is synergistic or additive in its effect on the tumor.

The optimum treatment for oral fibrosarcoma probably involves combined surgery and radiation therapy

> ## KEY POINT:
>
> *A histologic diagnosis of fibroma, nodular fascitis, or granulation tissue for an oral lesion, particularly if bony invasion is present, should be interpreted as fibrosarcoma and treated appropriately.*

to dosages that exceed 50 Gy. Intralesional chemotherapy is investigational but may improve tumor control. Control rates similar to those seen with soft tissue sarcomas could be expected with this combined approach (see the chapter on Tumors of the Skin).

ORAL FIBROSARCOMA IN CATS
Incidence, Signalment, and Etiology

Fibrosarcoma is the second most common oral tumor in cats. It is still uncommon compared to squamous cell carcinoma, accounting for only 13%[8] to 17%[45] of feline oral tumors. There is no obvious breed or gender predilection. Affected cats range from 1 to 21 years of age,[8] although fibrosarcoma is most common in old cats that average 10 years of age.

Clinical Presentation and History

As in dogs, feline fibrosarcoma is found mostly in the oral gingivae[45] but has no obvious predilection site.[8] It may be ulcerated, causing halitosis and drooling, and it is difficult to distinguish clinically from squamous cell carcinoma.

Staging and Diagnosis

Staging procedures should be performed as outlined on page 328. Fibrosarcomas usually arise in the submucosa, causing tissue destruction and occasionally invading bone or muscle. On histopathology, these fibrosarcomas often have a high mitotic index; however, metastatic potential appears low.[8]

Treatment

There are few reports of treatment for oral fibrosarcoma in cats, and, as in dogs, results of aggressive surgery are mixed. Two cats were treated with hemimandibulectomy or premaxillectomy and were free of disease 11.5 months[31] and 24 months[21] after surgery. Another cat treated with hemimandibulectomy had recurrence in two months, and one cat failed to eat and was euthanatized.[55] A gastrotomy tube should be placed in all cats undergoing oral surgery.

Vincristine (0.5 mg/m^2 IV per week) caused complete regression of an oral fibrosarcoma in one cat when treated for 30 weeks.[56] Other chemotherapy for this tumor has not been described, although doxorubicin reportedly causes regression of fibrosarcoma at other sites in cats.

Because of the encouraging results of radiation therapy in cats with other soft tissue sarcomas (including fibrosarcoma), this modality in combination with surgery may offer the best chance of tumor control in cats, as it does in dogs.

SALIVARY GLAND TUMORS IN DOGS
Incidence, Signalment, and Etiology

These tumors occur in old animals (median age = 10 years) with no obvious gender predilection. Poodles are at higher risk for developing this disease than other breeds.[57,58] Malignant salivary gland tumors are considerably more common than benign tumors and account for more than 95% of reported cases.[57,58]

Carcinomas are the most common tumor type, although salivary glands occasionally are invaded by fibrosarcomas or mast cell tumors.[57,58] Enlargement of the salivary gland in a dog is more likely to be an inflammatory process than a tumor.[57]

Clinical Presentation and History

Most owners notice a swelling or mass in the neck; however, signs may also include anorexia, dysphagia, and pain on opening the mouth.[58]

Staging and Diagnosis

Lymph node metastasis may occur,[58] and dogs with enlarged nodes should have a biopsy or a fine-needle aspiration. Pulmonary metastases are rare, and thoracic radiographs should be taken as part of a general health screen in old animals rather than with the expectation of seeing metastases.

In one survey, the mandibular glands were more likely to be affected than the parotid gland. In many cases, tumor was dispersed throughout the salivary tissue in the submucosa of the oral cavity, tongue, and oropharynx.[57] Surgical excisional biopsy is warranted for localized tumors; however, more diffuse tumors may require incisional biopsy prior to a definitive procedure.

MANAGEMENT OF SPECIFIC DISEASES

Treatment

In two dogs, surgical excision resulted in local recurrence within six months.[58,59] One of these dogs and two other dogs received 45 Gy of orthovoltage radiation to the surgical site, and none of the three dogs had developed local recurrence or metastasis 12, 25, and 40 months after treatment.[59] Radiation therapy should be considered as an adjunct to surgery for salivary gland tumors.[60]

SALIVARY GLAND TUMORS IN CATS
Incidence, Signalment, and Etiology

Malignant salivary gland tumors are more common than benign tumors, and most tumors are carcinomas.[57,58] Enlargement of a salivary gland in cats is more likely to signal a tumor than inflammation or any other condition.[57] The median age of affected cats is 10 years, and there is no gender predilection. Siamese cats are at higher risk for developing salivary gland tumors; seven (26%) of 27 cats were Siamese in one survey.[58]

Clinical Presentation and History

A mass in the cervical region is often noticed by the owner and may be accompanied by other signs, such as anorexia, dysphagia, and salivation due to secondary infections and ulceration.[9,58]

Staging and Diagnosis

There is little information on the metastatic rate of salivary gland carcinomas in cats; however, most reported cats have regional lymph node metastases, and one cat developed lung metastases five months after surgery.[9,58] Careful palpation of regional lymph nodes followed by fine-needle aspiration or biopsy of enlarged nodes as well as thoracic radiographs should precede any definitive treatment for these tumors.

Treatment

Surgery alone led to recurrence or metastasis within six months in one study.[58] There are no reports of adjunctive radiation therapy, but limited success in dogs suggests that this therapy may be worthwhile to reduce the risk of local recurrence. The metastatic rate of salivary adenocarcinoma in cats implies that regional lymph nodes should also be irradiated, but distant metastasis may still be a problem. There are no reports of chemotherapy for this tumor.

REFERENCES

1. Poulet FM, Valentine BA, Summers BA: A survey of epithelial odontogenic tumors and cysts in dogs and cats. *Vet Pathol* 29:369–380, 1992.
2. Dubietzig RR, Goldschmidt MH, Brodey RS: The nomenclature of periodontal epulides in dogs. *Vet Pathol* 16:209–214, 1979.
3. Thrall DE: Orthovoltage radiotherapy of acanthomatous epulides in 39 dogs. *JAVMA* 184:826–829, 1984.
4. Gorman NT, Bright RM, Calderwood-Mays MB, Thrall DE: Chemotherapy of a recurrent acanthomatous epulis in a dog. *JAVMA* 184:1158–1160, 1984.
5. White RAS: Mandibulectomy and maxillectomy in the dog: Long term survival in 100 cases. *J Small Anim Pract* 32:69–74, 1991.
6. Werner RE Jr: Canine oral neoplasia: A review of 19 cases. *JAAHA* 17:67–69, 1981.
7. Theon AP, Rodriquez C, Madewell BR: Canine oral tumors treated with megavoltage irradiation: Analysis of prognostic factors in 140 dogs. *JAVMA*, 1994, in press.
8. Stebbins KE, Morse CE, Goldschmidt MH: Feline oral neoplasia: A ten year survey. *Vet Pathol* 26:121–128, 1989.
9. Carpenter JL, Andrews LK, Holzworth J: Tumors and tumor-like lesions, in Holzworth J (ed): *Diseases of the Cat. Medicine and Surgery*. Philadelphia, WB Saunders, 1987, pp 406–596.
10. Goldschmidt MH: Benign and malignant melanocytic neoplasms of domestic animals. *Am J Dermatopathol* 7:203–212, 1985.
11. Delverdier M, Guire F, Harverbeke Van G: Les tumeurs de la cavite buccale du chien: Etude anatomoclinique a partir de 117 cas. *Revue Med Vet* 142:811–816, 1991.
12. Bostock DE: Prognosis after surgical excision of canine melanomas. *Vet Pathol* 16:32–40, 1979.
13. Hahn KA, DeNicola DB, Richardson RC, Hahn EA: Canine oral malignant melanoma: Prognostic utility of an alternative staging system. *J Small Anim Pract* 35:251–256, 1994.
14. MacEwen EG, Patnaik AK, Harvey HJ, et al: Canine oral melanoma: Comparison of surgery versus surgery plus *Corynebacterium parvum*. *Cancer Invest* 4:397–402, 1986.
15. Harvey HJ, MacEwen EG, Braun D, et al: Prognostic

criteria for dogs with oral melanoma. *JAVMA* 178: 580–582, 1981.

16. Salisbury SK, Lantz GC: Long-term results of partial mandibulectomy for treatment of oral tumors in 30 dogs. *JAAHA* 24:285–294, 1988.

17. Todoroff RJ, Brodey RS: Oral and pharyngeal neoplasia in the dog: A retrospective study of 361 cases. *JAVMA* 175:567–571, 1979.

18. Wallace J, Matthiesen DT, Patnaik AK: Hemimaxillectomy for the treatment of oral tumors in 69 dogs. *Vet Surg* 21:337–341, 1992.

19. Schwarz PD, Withrow SJ, Curtis CR, et al: Mandibular resection as a treatment for oral cancer in 81 dogs. *JAAHA* 27:601–610, 1991.

20. Beck ER, Withrow SJ, McChesney AE, et al: Canine tongue tumors: A retrospective review of 57 cases. *JAAHA* 22:525–532, 1986.

21. Salisbury SK, Richardson DC, Lantz GC: Partial maxillectomy and premaxillectomy in the treatment of oral neoplasia in the dog and cat. *Vet Surg* 15:16–26, 1986.

22. Ruslander DM, Price GS, McEntee MC, et al: Intravenous melphalan: Phase II evaluation in dogs with malignant melanoma. *Proc Vet Cancer Soc 13th Ann Conf.*82, 1993.

23. Guptill L, Knapp DW, Hank K, et al: Retrospective study of cisplatin treatment for canine malignant melanoma. *Proc Vet Cancer Soc 13th Ann Conf.*65–66, 1993.

24. Kraegel SA, Page RL: Advances in platinum compound chemotherapy, in Kirk RW, Bonagura JD (eds): *Current Veterinary Therapy XII.* Philadelphia, WB Saunders, 1992, pp 395–399.

25. Goetz TE, Boulton CH, Ogilvie GK: Clinical management of progressive multifocal benign and malignant melanomas of horses with oral cimetidine. *Proc Am Assoc Equine Pract.*431–438, 1989.

26. Moore AS, Theilen GH, Newell AD, et al: Preclinical study of sequential tumor necrosis factor and interleukin-2 in the treatment of spontaneous canine neoplasms. *Cancer Res* 51:233–238, 1991.

27. MacEwen EG: Update on macrophage activation to prevent metastasis. *Proc 12th Ann Conf ACVIM* 11:862–864, 1994.

28. Patnaik AK, Mooney S: Feline melanoma: A comparative study of ocular, oral and dermal neoplasms. *Vet Pathol* 25:105–112, 1988.

29. Evans SM, Shofer F: Canine oral nontonsillar squamous cell carcinoma: Prognostic factors for recurrence and survival following orthovoltage radiation therapy. *Vet Radiol* 29:133–137, 1988.

30. Ogilvie GK, Sundberg JP, O'Banion K, et al: Papillary squamous cell carcinoma in three young dogs. *JAVMA* 192:933–935, 1988.

31. Bradley RL, MacEwen EG, Loar AS: Mandibular resection for removal of oral tumors in 30 dogs and 6 cats. *JAVMA* 184:460–463, 1984.

32. Withrow SJ, Nelson AW, Manley PA, Biggs DR: Premaxillectomy in the dog. *JAAHA* 21:45–55, 1985.

33. Buhles WC, Theilen GH: Preliminary evaluation of bleomycin in feline and canine squamous cell carcinoma. *Am J Vet Res* 34:289–291, 1973.

34. Himsel CA, Richardson RC, Craig JA: Cisplatin chemotherapy for metastatic squamous cell carcinoma in two dogs. *JAVMA* 189:1575–1578, 1986.

35. Knapp DW, Richardson RC, Booney PL, Hahn K: Cisplatin therapy in 41 dogs with malignant tumors. *J Vet Intern Med* 2:41–46, 1988.

36. Shapiro W, Kitchell BE, Fossum TW, et al: Cisplatin for treatment of transitional cell and squamous cell carcinomas in dogs. *JAVMA* 193:1530–1533, 1988.

37. Ogilvie GK, Obradovich JE, Elmslie RE, et al: Efficacy of mitoxantrone against various neoplasms in dogs. *JAVMA* 198:1618–1621, 1991.

38. MacMillan R, Withrow SJ, Gillette EL: Surgery and regional irradiation for treatment of canine tonsillar squamous cell carcinoma: Retrospective review of eight cases. *JAAHA* 18:311–314, 1982.

39. Brooks MB, Matus Re, Leifer CE, et al: Chemotherapy versus chemotherapy plus radiotherapy in the treatment of tonsillar squamous cell carcinoma in the dog. *J Vet Intern Med* 2:206–211, 1988.

40. Postorino Reeves NC, Turrel JM, Withrow SJ: Oral squamous cell carcinoma in the cat. *JAAHA* 29:438–441, 1993.

41. Hutson CA, Willauer CC, Walder EJ, et al: Treatment of mandibular squamous cell carcinoma in cats by use of mandibulectomy and radiotherapy: Seven cases (1987–1989). *JAVMA* 201:777–781, 1992.

42. Heymann SJ, Diefender DL, Goldschmidt MH, Newton CD: Canine axial skeletal osteosarcoma. A retrospective study of 116 cases (1986 to 1989). *Vet Surg* 21:304–310, 1992.

43. Kapatkin AS, Marretta SM, Patnaik AK, et al: Mandibular swelling in cats: prospective study of 24 cats. *JAAHA* 27:575–580, 1991.

44. Quigley PJ, Leedale AH: Tumors involving bone in the domestic cat: A review of fifty-eight cases. *Vet Pathol* 20:670–686, 1983.

45. Liu SK, Dorfman HD, Patnaik AK: Primary and secondary bone tumors in the cat. *J Small Anim Pract* 15: 141–156, 1974.

46. Cotter SM: Oral pharyngeal neoplasms in the cat. *JAAHA* 17:917–920, 1981.

47. Evans SM, LaCreta F, Helfand S, et al: Technique, pharmacokinetics, toxicity, and efficacy of intratumoral etanidaxole and radiotherapy for treatment of

spontaneous feline oral squamous cell carcinoma. *Int J Radiat Oncol* 20:703–708, 1991.

48. Ogilvie GK, Moore AS, Obradovich JE, et al: Toxicoses and efficacy associated with the administration of mitoxantrone to cats with malignant tumors. *JAVMA* 202:1839–1844, 1993.

49. LaRue SM, Vail DM, Ogilvie GK, et al: Shrinking-field radiation therapy in combination with mitoxantrone chemotherapy for the treatment of oral squamous cell carcinoma in the cat. *Proc 11th Ann Conf Vet Cancer Soc*:99, 1991.

50. Brewer WG Jr, Turrel JM: Radiotherapy and hyperthermia in the treatment of fibrosarcomas in the dog. *JAVMA* 181:146–150, 1982.

51. Thrall DE: Orthovoltage radiotherapy of oral fibrosarcomas in dogs. *JAVMA* 179:159–162, 1981.

52. Ciekot PA, Powers BE, Withrow SJ, et al: Histologically low grade yet biologically high grade fibrosarcomas of the mandible and maxilla of 25 dogs (1982 to 1991). *JAVMA* 204:610–615, 1994.

53. McChesney SL, Withrow SJ, Gillette EL, et al: Radiotherapy of soft tissue sarcomas in dogs. *JAVMA* 194:60–63, 1989.

54. McChesney SL, Gillette EL, Dewhirst MW, Withrow SJ: Influence of WR 2721 on radiation response of canine soft tissue sarcomas. *Int J Radiat Oncol* 12:1957–1963, 1986.

55. Theon AP, Madewell BR, Ryu J, Casto J: Concurrent irradiation and intratumoral chemotherapy with cisplatin: A pilot study in dogs with spontaneous tumors. *Int J Radiat Oncol Biol Phys* 29:1027–1034, 1994.

56. Bradley RL, Sponenberg DP, Martin RA: Oral neoplasia in 15 dogs and 4 cats. *Semin Vet Med Surg (Small Anim)* 1:33–42, 1986.

57. Hahn KA: Vincristine sulfate as single-agent chemotherapy in a dog and a cat with malignant neoplasms. *JAVMA* 197:796–798, 1990.

58. Spangler WL, Culbertson MR: Salivary gland disease in dogs and cats: 245 cases (1985–1988). *JAVMA* 198:465–469, 1991.

59. Carberry CA, Flanders JA, Harvey HJ, Ryan AM: Salivary gland tumors in dogs and cats: A literature and case review. *JAAHA* 24:561–567, 1988.

60. Evans SM, Thrall DE: Postoperative orthovoltage radiation therapy of parotid salivary gland adenocarcinoma in three dogs. *JAVMA* 182:993–994, 1983.

CLINICAL BRIEFING: GASTROINTESTINAL TUMORS

Stomach Tumors in Dogs

Common Clinical Presentation	Chronic vomiting, weight loss, and inappetence
Common Histologic Types	Adenocarcinoma; less commonly, leiomyoma; most common in lower two thirds of stomach
Epidemiology and Biological Behavior	Old, male dogs; tumors cause ulceration and commonly metastasize to perigastric lymph nodes or viscera
Prognostic Factors	None identified
Treatment Surgery	Tumors are usually diffuse and have metastasized at the time of diagnosis; therefore, aggressive surgery is rarely successful; no reports of other therapies

Intestinal Tumors in Dogs

Common Clinical Presentation	*Duodenum–Jejunum:* Vomiting, melena *Jejunum–Ileum:* Weight loss and diarrhea *Colon–Rectum:* Tenesmus and hematochezia
Common Histologic Types	Adenocarcinoma; less commonly, leiomyosarcoma and lymphoma; leiomyosarcoma common in the cecum
Epidemiology and Biological Behavior	Old, male dogs; adenocarcinoma more likely to metastasize than leiomyosarcoma, usually to regional lymph nodes
Prognostic Factors	*Colorectal:* Dogs with annular lesions have poor survival; other types of lesions have a better prognosis
Treatment Surgery	Little information for adenocarcinoma; average survival for dogs with colorectal adenocarcinoma is 15 months after surgery; median survival >1 year for leiomyosarcoma

MANAGEMENT OF SPECIFIC DISEASES

Radiation Therapy	Rectal adenocarcinoma may be controlled by high-dose fractions; median control is 6 months
Cryotherapy	Small, minimally invasive tumors of the rectum and distal colon
Chemotherapy	No reports; doxorubicin is investigational

Intestinal Tumors in Cats

Common Clinical Presentation	*Small Intestine:* Vomiting, weight loss, and anorexia *Large Intestine:* Hematochezia
Common Histologic Type	Adenocarcinoma; other tumors are rare
Epidemiology and Biological Behavior	Old cats; mean age is 11 years; Siamese predisposed; tumors usually cause annular constriction, and metastasis to peritoneal surfaces is common
Prognostic Factors	None identified
Treatment Surgery	Surgical resection results in 15-month average survival; some cats live more than 2 years; lymph node metastasis at surgery does not always influence survival; no adjunctive therapy has been reported

Anal Sac Adenocarcinoma

Common Clinical Presentation	Dyschezia, perianal mass, and polyuria and polydipsia due to hypercalcemia
Epidemiology and Biological Behavior	Old, female dogs; production of PTH-like hormone causes hypercalcemia; metastasis to regional lymph nodes is common
Prognostic Factors	Dogs with hypercalcemia or with detectable metastases have shorter survival times
Treatment Surgery	May require local excision of tumor and sublumbar lymph nodes; surgery usually resolves hypercalcemia

MANAGEMENT OF SPECIFIC DISEASES

Chemotherapy	Cisplatin may be useful as an adjunct to surgery

Other Tumors Reviewed
Stomach tumors in cats

STOMACH TUMORS IN DOGS
Incidence, Signalment, and Etiology

The most common tumor of the stomach in dogs is gastric adenocarcinoma, and most reports emphasize this neoplasm. The proportions of dogs affected by different tumor types were studied.[1-3] In 89 dogs with stomach tumors, 51 (60%) had an adenocarcinoma, and nine (10%) had adenoma. Leiomyoma (19 dogs [20%]) was more common than leiomyosarcoma (4 dogs [5%]). Lymphoma, either as a primary tumor or as part of systemic disease, occurred in six dogs (5% of total).

Most carcinomas occur in the lower two thirds of the stomach, particularly the pylorus. The lesser curvature is not usually affected except in Belgian shepherds.[4,5] Most affected dogs are old; the median age is 10 years. All studies report a male predominance ranging from 2:1 to 3:1.[5] One study suggested that males were affected with gastric carcinoma up to seven times more often than females, depending on the histologic subtype.[6] Females may have gastric adenomas more often than male dogs.[2]

Belgian shepherds in Italy (of the Groenendael type)[4,5] and rough collies[7] are apparently at high risk for gastric adenocarcinoma. Although gastric carcinomas can be experimentally induced in dogs by various compounds, there are no epidemiologic studies to support a role for these compounds in naturally occurring disease.

Clinical Presentation and History

Gastric tumors are consistently associated with vomiting, weight loss, and inappetence. Vomiting is often chronic and rarely associated with eating.

Hematemesis occurs in 20%[7] to 50%[4] of dogs. Other signs include polydipsia, abdominal pain, melena, and anemia.[1,3,4,7] Occasionally, ascites occurs as a result of carcinomatosis. Clinical signs, such as vomiting, are often chronic for 2 weeks to 18 months prior to presentation[3,7]; the median duration is two months.

Staging and Diagnosis

Gastric adenocarcinomas often involve a large area of the stomach wall, making them unresectable. These tumors arise in the mucosa, but most extend to or through the serosa.[5] Ulceration is common and often deep and crater-like, causing hematemesis or melena.[1,7,8] Contrast radiography, particularly with fluoroscopy, may give indications of gastric tumor, but these indications are rarely definitive.[7] Endoscopy can determine the location of most tumors, except when neoplasia is diffusely infiltrative, and may reveal tumor ulceration. Although endoscopy can be definitive,[7] it can also be inconclusive[5]; multiple biopsy specimens should be obtained, and deep biopsy specimens should be taken if the mucosa is not obviously involved. Endoscopy is ideal for evaluating the stomach itself, but ultrasonography should be used to assess epigastric lymph nodes and other abdominal viscera for evidence of metastasis. Ultrasonography also can be used to define the borders of localized tumors and to identify ulcerations and diffuse infiltration.[8] Ultrasound-guided microcore biopsy has a high diagnostic sensitivity.[9,10] When the aforementioned modalities are unsuitable, exploratory laparotomy can be used to obtain biopsy specimens from affected sites. A therapeutic excisional

MANAGEMENT OF SPECIFIC DISEASES

TABLE 5-13
Distribution of 108 intestinal tumors and
78 colorectal adenocarcinomas in dogs

Small Intestine Tumors[2,15,17]		Large Intestine Tumors[2]		Colorectal Adenocarcinomas[18]	
Location	Percentage	Location	Percentage	Location	Percentage
Jejunum	44%	Colon	50%	Distal rectum	27%
Duodenum	37%	Rectum	36%	Midrectum	49%
Ileum	19%	Cecum	14%	Proximal rectum	12%
				Colon	12%

biopsy may be possible for small localized tumors; however, incisional biopsy should be performed on larger tumors.

Gastric adenocarcinoma often metastasizes, particularly to perigastric lymph nodes and viscera.[1,5–7] Extension of gastric adenocarcinoma through the serosa creates an intense scirrhous reaction in the mesentery and omentum, which may cause ascites.[11]

Histology of gastric adenocarcinomas varies, and "intestinal" types of tumors (e.g., papillary, acinar, or solid) are less common than diffuse types (e.g., undifferentiated or glandular).[6] No differences in biological behavior have been ascribed to these different tumor types; all gastric adenocarcinomas are aggressive malignancies.

Treatment

The advanced stage of gastric adenocarcinomas at diagnosis, their diffuse nature, and their high rate of metastasis usually make surgery unsuccessful. Most tumors are too large or invasive for complete resection.[3,4] Wide resection often requires gastroduodenostomy (Billroth I procedure); however, most dogs die within four months of surgery from local recurrence and metastases.[1,12–14] Earlier diagnosis occasionally allows successful surgical resection and

long-term freedom from recurrence and metastasis.[4]

Photodynamic therapy with rhodamine dye was not successful in treating an unresectable tumor.[4] Results of chemotherapy for adenocarcinoma have not been reported.

INTESTINAL TUMORS IN DOGS
Incidence, Signalment, and History

In dogs, adenocarcinomas are the most common tumor in the intestine and the stomach. Leiomyosarcomas are less common than adenocarcinoma and occur more frequently in the intestine than in the stomach. Intestinal leiomyomas are uncommon. All reported cecal tumors have been of smooth muscle origin (i.e., leiomyosarcoma or leiomyoma). Epithelial and smooth-muscle tumors both occur in other areas of the intestinal tract. Lymphoma may be found anywhere within the gastrointestinal tract but is usually associated with systemic disease.[15,16] Table 5-13 summarizes canine intestinal tumor location and type as compiled from various studies. Less common tumor types include neurolemmoma, carcinoid,[2,19] and fibrosarcoma.[17]

Intestinal tumors occur in old dogs; the median age is 11 to 12 years, although the average age of dogs with lymphoma is younger.[16] There is no obvious breed predilection. Males are

> **KEY POINT:**
>
> *Adenocarcinoma of the stomach is usually large or diffuse, making complete surgical excision difficult.*

more frequently affected by intestinal tumors than females,[2,16-18] although this trend is most marked for adenocarcinoma and is less obvious for smooth-muscle tumors.[2,15,20-22]

Clinical Presentation and History

Clinical signs give very little indication as to the type of neoplasm in a dog with an intestinal tumor. Symptoms may, however, direct the clinician to a particular area of the intestinal tract. For example, vomiting is most often associated with tumors of the duodenum or jejunum, whereas weight loss and diarrhea are usually seen in dogs with jejunal or ileal tumors.[23] Tenesmus or hematochezia most often occurs with colonic or rectal tumors.[17,18,23] Distal rectal tumors are mostly palpable as a single pedunculated mass; tumors located rostrally are more likely to be multiple ("cobblestone appearance") or appear as an annular constriction.[18] Dogs with rectal leiomyomas may be asymptomatic, presumably owing to slow growth of these tumors; however, these tumors may become very large (up to 12 cm in one study).[22] Anorexia, depression, and lethargy may accompany tumors in any location. Hypochromic anemia is a less common sign; it may be due to melena and iron deficiency.[23,24] Ascites, abdominal pain, and peritonitis from intestinal rupture may occur[15,20,21]; the last condition is mainly seen with cecal leiomyosarcomas.[20,21] Clinical signs have often been present for weeks to months,[15,25-27] although dogs that are vomiting are usually presented by their owners more rapidly.

On physical examination, an abdominal mass may be palpated, particularly if the tumor is in the upper small intestine.[17] Rectal examination may reveal stricture, mass, or irregular rectal wall in more than 60% of affected dogs.[18,22]

Staging and Diagnosis

In addition to routine blood work and urinalysis,

thoracic and abdominal radiographs and endoscopy and ultrasonography should be used to image the tumor and to identify metastasis. Plain radiographs may help delineate an abdominal mass[17] and may also reveal other abnormalities, such as gas-filled and fluid-filled dilated loops of bowel, which are suggestive of obstruction. Pneumoperitoneum may indicate tumor rupture or a septic peritonitis.[15,17] Contrast radiography most often shows an "apple-core" lesion for tumors of the small intestine,[15] but also may show irregular filling defects or leakage caused by perforation. Ultrasonography is a noninvasive and rapid means of identifying intestinal tumors and provides a guide for obtaining biopsy specimens as well as a method of staging for abdominal metastases.[8-10] Ultrasonography is the staging method of choice for dogs with intestinal tumors.

Endoscopy can be used to obtained biopsy specimens, which may provide a definitive diagnosis for duodenal or rectal tumors[18,28,29]; however, multiple biopsy specimens should be taken, as lesions deep to the mucosa may escape detection, and tumors that create ulcerated lesions may be obscured by inflammatory changes. In one study, endoscopic biopsy of intestinal lymphoma was confounded by the presence of inflammatory infiltrates in nearly 50% of the dogs.[16] Endoscopy of the entire large bowel is particularly important when a distal rectal tumor is palpated, as dogs may have additional proximal lesions that could otherwise remain undetected and continue to cause clinical signs after surgery.

Metastasis is more commonly described for intestinal adenocarcinoma than for leiomyosarcoma.[17,23] In 22 (70%) of 31 dogs with small intestine adenocarcinoma, there was evidence of metastases to regional lymph nodes.[23] In contrast, metastasis occurred to liver and lung in four (13%) each of 31 dogs.[23] Metastasis of colorectal adenocarcinoma is considerably less common. There was no evidence of metas-

MANAGEMENT OF SPECIFIC DISEASES

tasis in 78 dogs with this disease even after long survival times following surgery.[18]

Leiomyosarcoma does not usually metastasize; metastases occur in less than 30% of affected dogs,[21,24,25] often long after definitive surgery.[21,25] *Carcinoid* is a term used to describe intestinal tumors of neuroendocrine derivation that may be hormonally active. Of five reported intestinal carcinoids, all had metastases to regional lymph nodes and liver at the time of diagnosis and there were additional sites of metastasis in two dogs.[19,23] Biopsy of small intestinal tumors often requires exploratory laparotomy, but rectal tumors may be biopsied via proctoscopy or by prolapsing the rectum manually or with stay sutures.[18]

Prognostic Factors

In one study of colorectal adenocarcinomas, dogs with annular tumors had the shortest average survival (1.6 months). Dogs with tumors that comprised multiple "cobblestone" nodules had an average survival of 12 months. Dogs with a single pedunculated polyp had the longest survival (32 months) after surgery.[18] These prognostic factors are probably related to the ease with which complete surgical excision may be performed.

Treatment

There is little information regarding survival after surgical resection of small intestinal adenocarcinomas. Four dogs with small intestinal tumors that had not metastasized at the time of surgery had survival times of three days, six months (2 dogs), and two years.[15] In another study, five dogs with surgically treated cancer of the small intestine had an average survival of 55 days.[17]

Surgical excision of intestinal or cecal leiomyosarcoma carries a better prognosis (Figure 5-53). Thirteen (55%) of 23 dogs with leiomyosarcoma survived the perioperative period and had median survivals of 8 to 13 months (ranging from 2 months to 7 years). Only three of these 13 dogs developed metastases.[21] One dog had evidence of metastasis at the time of surgery and without explanation survived three years

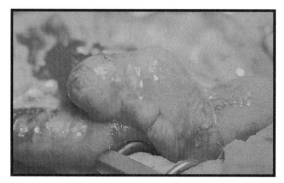

Figure 5-53: *Cecal leiomyosarcomas in dogs are unlikely to metastasize, and complete resection may give long survival. (Courtesy J. Berg)*

without adjuvant therapy.[21] Cecal rupture may occur and lead to death in some dogs as a result of peritonitis. Perioperative mortality was 60% in 10 dogs in one study.[20] Four dogs survived for 19 months, 28 months, 36 months, and 48 months. Two of these dogs died due to recurrence (28 months) or metastases (36 months).[20]

The median survival after surgical resection of colorectal leiomyoma was 26 months. Only one of five affected dogs died from tumor-related causes.[22] Colorectal adenocarcinomas have a low rate of metastasis, and treated dogs may have long survival times following diagnosis. In one study, dogs with this disease that were treated palliatively with stool softeners lived an average of 15 months.[18] Of multiple-treatment modalities, local excision gave the longest average survival (22 months) with the lowest complication rate.[18,19] Recurrence after local excision of a solitary mass occurred in 11 (50%) of 21 dogs.[18] In contrast, radical surgical excision of annular colorectal adenocarcinoma resulted in wound dehiscence and septic peritonitis in all four dogs treated.

Cryosurgery prolonged survival in 11 dogs with colorectal adenocarcinoma (average survival of 24 months). Recurrence was similar to that after local excision; however, additional complications, including stricture (5 of 11 dogs), rectal prolapse, and perineal hernia followed treatment.[18] Other techniques, such as electrocoagulation[18] and Nd:YAG laser-assist-

MANAGEMENT OF SPECIFIC DISEASES

ed surgery,[30] provide control similar to that of local excision.

Radiation therapy using a single high dose (15 Gy to 25 Gy) of orthovoltage teletherapy may provide reasonable control for recurrent distal rectal adenocarcinomas. In six dogs, median tumor control duration was six months, and no complications were reported.[31] In another group of dogs, one dog treated with radiation therapy suffered a rectal perforation and died from peritonitis two months after treatment.[18] Results of chemotherapy have not been reported for intestinal tumors in dogs.[18]

STOMACH TUMORS IN CATS

Stomach tumors are rare in cats. Most that do occur are lymphoma. Adenocarcinomas and leiomyosarcomas are rare.[32,33] Gastric thickening is common in cats with gastric lymphoma and is often substantial enough to palpate. Ultrasound-guided biopsy or fine-needle aspiration facilitates diagnosis (Figure 5-54). Endoscopic biopsy is useful in superficial lesions but is not as helpful for submucosal lymphoma. Lymphoma is rarely confined to the stomach and is best treated with chemotherapy. Responses of cats with gastrointestinal lymphoma to vincristine, cyclophosphamide, and prednisone are poor; treated cats have a median survival of less than two months (see the chapter on Lymphoma).

INTESTINAL TUMORS IN CATS
Incidence, Signalment, and Etiology

Adenocarcinoma is by far the most common non-hematopoietic tumor of the intestinal tract in cats; sarcomas are rarely described.[33] Intestinal adenocarcinoma is more common in cats than in dogs.[33] Hematopoietic neoplasms, primarily lymphoma (but also mast cell tumors) are more common in cats than in dogs; they are described in more detail in the appropriate chapters. The majority of intestinal adenocarcinomas occur in the small intestine of affected cats. The ileum or jejunum is most often affected.[32,33] The duodenum is rarely involved. Adenocarcinoma of the large intestine is less common and usually involves the colon, although the cecum and, rarely, rectum may be affected.[32-34]

Intestinal adenocarcinoma primarily affects old cats; the mean age of affected cats is 10 to 11 years,[32-37] although they may be as young as 2 years of age. The vast majority of affected cats are Siamese, which constitute 152 (70%) of 225 reported cases.[17,32-36] Other purebreds are rarely affected.[33] In one study, all 22 adenocarcinomas of the large intestine occurred in domestic shorthairs,[32] although no other study addressed this association. Cats with colonic adenocarcinoma typically are older, with a mean age of 16 years.[32] There seems to be no gender predilection for intestinal adenocarcinoma with the exception of one report in which male cats predominated.[34] FeLV is unlikely to play a role in this disease. Only two studies reported the FeLV status of affected cats; all 28 cats studied tested negative for FeLV antigenemia.[17,36]

Although benign tumors of the intestinal tract are rare and the duodenum is not usually affected, 18 cats with adenomatous polyps of the duodenum have been described.[38] Signalment was similar to that in cats with adenocarcinoma, in that older, primarily Oriental-breed cats are most often affected. The cats in this study were predominantly castrated males. Most cats were tested for FeLV and feline immunodeficiency virus (FIV), and all had negative results.[38] All polyps occurred within 1 cm of the pylorus. Cats with duodenal adenomatous polyps usually present with a history of acute or chronic vomiting.[38] Vomitus contains blood only in acutely affected cats.

Clinical Presentation and History

The most frequent presenting signs in cats with intestinal adenocarcinoma reflect involvement of the proximal small intestine. In decreasing order of frequency, vomiting, weight loss, and anorexia predom-

MANAGEMENT OF SPECIFIC DISEASES

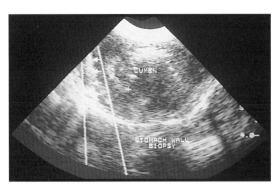

Figure 5-54: *Ultrasonography is particularly useful for obtaining needle biopsy specimens of the intestinal tract in both cats and dogs. The biopsy of this cat's stomach wall revealed lymphoma. Ultrasonography was used to monitor tumor regression following chemotherapy. (Courtesy D.G. Penninck)*

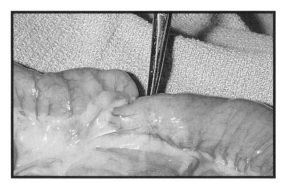

Figure 5-55: *A constrictive lesion in the ileum of a cat due to adenocarcinoma. (Courtesy J. Berg)*

inate.[33–36] Hematochezia is occasionally described in cats with colonic or rectal tumors. Clinical signs often have been present for a considerable time (median = 2 months, but up to 2 years).[33,35,36] Cats with tumors involving more proximal intestinal tract tend to present more rapidly (1 month) than cats with tumors of the lower small intestine (3.5 months) or large intestine (4.5 months),[35] presumably because owners perceive the more critical nature of vomiting and anorexia.

On physical examination, affected cats with intestinal tumors are often cachectic and usually dehydrated and an abdominal mass is frequently palpable. Peritoneal carcinomatosis is common and may produce marked ascites.[34]

Staging and Diagnosis

Cats with an intestinal tumor should have a contrast radiographic study and abdominal ultrasonography performed prior to thoracic radiographs, as metastatic disease is usually abdominal.

Intestinal adenocarcinomas in cats spread by intramural (rather than intraluminal) extension and thus generate an annular ("napkin ring") constriction rather than a mass lesion (Figure 5-55). Constriction of the intestinal tract causes obstruction. Abdominal radiographs may confirm the presence of a palpable abdominal mass, and plain or barium contrast radio-

graphs may reveal evidence of obstruction of the small intestine.[36] Osseous metaplasia may cause the intestinal tumor to mineralize.[33] Endoscopy may help identify lesions of the upper intestinal tract (although duodenal tumors are rare) or of the rectum and colon.[38] Ultrasonography provides a simple and reliable method to biopsy intestinal tumors in cats as well as imaging abdominal structures for evidence of metastasis.[9,10] Because of the localized and obstructive nature of the lesion, however, exploratory laparotomy followed by a resection and anastomosis is often both diagnostic and therapeutic.

Ascites from peritoneal metastases is common, and cytology of ascitic fluid may reveal malignant cells.[32,34] Different histopathologic descriptions have been used to classify intestinal adenocarcinomas as tubular, mucinous, or undifferentiated, but the prognostic significance of these subclassifications is negligible; all types have a high metastatic rate.[33]

Metastasis occurs to the peritoneum, mesentery, omentum, and regional lymph nodes in approximately 50% of affected cats.[32–35,37] Less common sites of metastasis are the liver, spleen, uterine stump or uterus, urinary bladder, and other areas in the intestinal tract. Metastasis to the lung is rarely reported.[17,32–35,37]

Treatment

Resection of the intestinal mass is the only reported treatment for intestinal adenocarcinoma in cats, and there is only one report of a cat that was treated with adjuvant therapy. That cat received levamisole (5 mg/kg PO three days per week) for 2 months and lived 28 months before developing widespread metastases.[39] The contribution of this treatment to survival is doubtful, because similar long survival times have been reported following surgery alone. Early studies that included some cats that died perioperatively had median survival times of 5 weeks[33] and 10 weeks[35]; however, both studies included some cats that lived for 2 years. In more recent studies, the average survival ranged from 6 to 15 months[32,36] and some cats lived more than 4 years. These figures are significant because seven cats with confirmed lymph node metastasis at the time of surgery lived for an average of 12 months,[32,36] and two cats with carcinomatosis lived 4.5 and 28 months.[36] The finding of metastatic disease at surgery should not be a disincentive to treat cats surgically for intestinal adenocarcinoma.

Resection of duodenal adenomatous polyps is predictably associated with a good surgical outcome, although anorexia is a postoperative complication in more than half of feline patients.[38] The role of adjuvant chemotherapy for feline intestinal adenocarcinoma has not been explored or reported.

ADENOCARCINOMA OF THE APOCRINE GLANDS OF THE ANAL SAC IN DOGS
Incidence, Signalment, and Etiology

Anal sac adenocarcinoma overwhelmingly occurs in old, female dogs, whether they are intact or neutered.[40–43] The age of affected dogs ranges from 5 to 17 years, with an average age of 10.5 years. In most reports, there is no obvious breed predilection and both crossbred and purebred dogs are affected equally; however, one European study reported that five of eight affected dogs were long-haired or wire-haired German shorthair pointers.[44]

> **KEY POINT:**
>
> *The presence of metastatic disease is not, in itself, a poor prognostic sign for cats with intestinal adenocarcinoma, and long survival times after surgical resection are possible.*

A characteristic feature of this tumor is production of a parathyroid hormone-related protein[45] that causes hypercalcemia and hypophosphatemia.

Clinical Presentation and History

Affected dogs are often presented to veterinarians because of an unrelated problem; because the owner notices a swelling in the perineum; or because there is dyschezia, tenesmus, or ribbon-like stools.[40,43] Tenesmus may be due either to the primary tumor or to sublumbar lymphadenopathy, which may be palpable rectally. Signs may be present for up to one year before presentation.[41] In 40% to 60% of dogs in reported series, the tumor was an incidental finding on rectal examination[40,41] or was found only after hypercalcemia had been identified.[43] This emphasizes the importance of including a rectal palpation in routine physical examinations. The tumor mass is usually between 1 and 10 cm in diameter; smaller primary masses that are difficult to palpate may be present.[40,42] Because the tumor may be bilateral, it is important to palpate both anal sacs.[40,41,43]

Other clinical signs are pruritus, ulceration and bleeding, decreased appetite, weight loss, and weakness or paresis. Polydipsia and polyuria are common in hypercalcemic dogs. The identification of hypercalcemia on a biochemical profile warrants careful palpation of the anal sacs.[43]

Staging and Diagnosis

If anal sac adenocarcinoma is suspected in a dog, routine blood chemistries should be performed to identify hypercalcemia and any secondary renal damage. Abdominal radiography or (preferably) ultrasonography should be performed to look for metastatic disease before taking thoracic radiographs, as pulmonary metastases are uncommon.

Hypercalcemia is common in dogs with apocrine gland adenocarcinoma of the anal sacs and may occur

MANAGEMENT OF SPECIFIC DISEASES

in both males and females.[43] In one study, serum calcium was elevated in 25%[40] of affected dogs to an average of 14.6 mg/dl.[40] In another study, 90% of dogs with anal sac adenocarcinoma had elevated serum calcium levels to an average of 16.1 mg/dl.[43] Hypophosphatemia occurred concurrently with hypercalcemia in some, but not all, affected dogs.[43]

This neoplasm is highly malignant and metastasizes early in the course of the disease to the sublumbar and iliac lymph nodes. In one study, approximately 50% of the dogs developed lymph node metastases[40]; in two other studies, 94% of the dogs had metastases to these sites.[43,44] Lateral abdominal radiographs are useful in identifying sublumbar lymphadenopathy,[40] but ultrasonography may be more accurate in disclosing the extent of lymph node involvement than radiographs or digital rectal palpation.

Less frequent sites of metastasis are the lungs, which may show a nodular or diffuse pattern radiographically,[40] and (rarely) the lumbar vertebrae, liver, and kidneys.[40,44] Metastasis may occur when the primary tumor is very small, and clinical signs relating to the primary tumor may not be obvious.[40] Definitive diagnosis is made by surgical biopsy, although a high index of suspicion for this disease should follow detection of a perianal mass in an old, female dog with hypercalcemia.

Prognostic Factors

In one study, hypercalcemic dogs had a median survival of 6 months after surgical excision of the tumor, compared with 11.5 months for normocalcemic dogs.[40] Dogs with metastases detected at surgery predictably had shorter median survival times (6 months) than did dogs without metastases (15.5 months).

Treatment

Surgical excision of the primary tumor is often difficult because of the large size of these tumors and their invasive growth characteristics.

Local recurrence occurs in approximately 25% of dogs.[40,41] Even with incomplete surgical excision, however, most dogs that are hypercalcemic become normocalcemic after surgery. Hypercalcemia presumably reflects some critical tumor mass, as even dogs with metastases may not show recurrence of hypercalcemia until those metastases become large.[44]

Complications of surgery reflect the difficulties encountered in any surgical procedure involving the perineal area. Fecal incontinence can follow surgery in up to 20% of dogs and may be permanent.[40] Wound infection can occur and cause sepsis.

Local recurrence is a problem with some dogs, and others develop recurrence in the regional lymph nodes. If the sublumbar nodes are enlarged at diagnosis, it may be possible to remove them surgically; however, tumor-invaded nodes are frequently friable and invade around the vessels and nerves in this area (Figure 5-56). The nodes were well encapsulated in 80% of dogs treated surgically in one study, but they were also well vascularized; thus, the surgeon should be prepared to encounter bleeding.[40] In this study, complications during lymph node surgery caused the death of one third of the dogs; almost one third of the survivors developed transient urinary incontinence, presumably as a result of neurologic trauma. Overall, 6 of 27 dogs died within 2 weeks after undergoing surgery for removal of either the primary tumor or its metastases.[40] Median survival for the remaining dogs was 8.3 months; the range of survival was 6 weeks to 39 months. Five dogs were still alive at 14 months after surgery. This moderate success rate was corroborated in another study in which 50% of the dogs died between 2 and 22 months after surgery, with an average survival of 8.8 months.[43]

Chemotherapy might be promising as adjuvant therapy for this tumor, but relatively little has been reported. Three dogs treated with

> ## KEY POINTS:
>
> *If hypercalcemia is detected on routine blood chemistry, palpation of the anal sacs for the presence of a tumor should be performed.*
>
> ---
>
> *Even with incomplete tumor excision, most dogs that are hypercalcemic become normocalcemic.*

MANAGEMENT OF SPECIFIC DISEASES

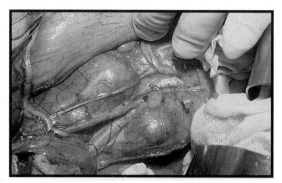

Figure 5-56: *Exploratory laparotomy reveals metastasis of an anal sac adenocarcinoma to the sublumbar nodes. These nodes are easily visualized with ultrasonography, and dogs with this tumor should be routinely examined for metastatic spread prior to definitive treatment. (Courtesy J. Berg)*

doxorubicin and cyclophosphamide, either alone or in combination with prednisone, vincristine, and L-asparaginase (for concurrent lymphoma), had survival times of 1, 2, and 14 months.[40] Another tumor did not respond to treatment with melphalan and cyclophosphamide.[41] Anecdotally, cisplatin has caused complete regression of metastatic lesions in some dogs with this disease (A.S. Moore, personal observations). Recent investigations suggest that surgical excision of the primary tumor and sublumbar lymph nodes followed by intraoperative and external beam radiation therapy combined with chemotherapy provides clinical remission times of more than one year (G.K. Ogilvie, personal observations).

Dogs with anal sac adenocarcinomas should be treated surgically in an attempt to achieve complete excision of the primary mass. Sublumbar lymph nodes should be removed if they are enlarged, although this is a technically demanding surgery. Adjuvant radiation therapy and chemotherapy using cisplatin should be considered, although the role of chemotherapy is still being defined.

REFERENCES

1. Murray M, Robinson PB, McKeating FJ, et al: Primary gastric neoplasia in the dog: A clinico-pathological study. *Vet Rec* 120:79–83, 1987.
2. Patnaik AK, Hurvitz AI, Johnson GF: Canine gastrointestinal neoplasms. *Vet Pathol* 14:547–555, 1977.
3. Saulter JH, Hanlon GF: Gastric neoplasms in the dog: A report of 20 cases. *JAVMA* 166:691–696, 1975.
4. Fonda D, Gualtieri M, Scanziani E: Gastric carcinoma in the dog: A clinicopathological study of 11 cases. *J Small Anim Pract* 30:353–360, 1989.
5. Scanziani E, Giusti AM, Gualtieri M, Fonda D: Gastric carcinoma in the Belgian shepherd dog. *J Small Anim Pract* 32:465–469, 1991.
6. Patnaik AK, Hurvitz AI, Johnson GF: Canine gastric adenocarcinoma. *Vet Pathol* 15:600–607, 1978.
7. Sullivan M, Lee R, Fisher EW, et al: A study of 31 cases of gastric carcinoma in dogs. *Vet Rec* 120:79–83, 1987.
8. Penninck DG, Nyland TG, Kerr LY, Fisher PE: Ultrasonographic evaluation of gastrointestinal diseases in small animals. *Vet Radiol* 31:134–141, 1990.
9. Penninck DG, Crystal MA, Matz ME, Pearson SH: The technique of percutaneous ultrasound guided fine-needle aspiration biopsy and automated microcore biopsy in small animal gastrointestinal diseases. *Vet Radiol Ultrasound* 34:433–436, 1993.
10. Crystal MA, Penninck DG, Matz ME, et al: Use of ultrasound-guided fine-needle aspiration biopsy and automated core biopsy for the diagnosis of gastrointestinal diseases in small animals. *Vet Radiol Ultrasound* 34:438–444, 1993.
11. Roth L, King JM: Mesenteric and omental sclerosis associated with metastases from gastrointestinal neoplasia in the dog. *J Small Anim Pract* 31:28–31, 1990.
12. Dorn AS, Anderson NV, Guffy MM, et al: Gastric carcinoma in a dog. *J Small Anim Pract* 17:109–117, 1976.
13. Sinclair CJ, Jones BR, Verkerk G: Gastric carcinoma in a bitch. *N Z Vet J* 27:16–18, 1979.
14. Elliott GS, Stroffregen DA, Richardson DC, et al: Surgical, medical and nutritional management of gastric adenocarcinoma in a dog. *JAVMA* 185:98–101, 1984.
15. Gibbs C, Pearson H: Localized tumors of the canine small intestine: A report of twenty cases. *J Small Anim Pract* 27:507–519, 1986.
16. Couto CG, Rutgers HC, Sherding RG, Rojko J: Gastrointestinal lymphoma in 20 dogs: A retrospective study. *J Vet Intern Med* 3:73–78, 1989.
17. Birchard SJ, Couto CG, Johnson S: Nonlymphoid intestinal neoplasia in 32 dogs and 14 cats. *JAAHA* 22:533–537, 1986.
18. Church EM, Mehlhaff CJ, Patnaik AK: Colorectal adenocarcinoma in dogs: 78 cases (1973–1984). *JAVMA* 191:727–730, 1987.
19. Coughlin A: Carcinoid in canine large intestine. *Vet Rec* 499–500, 1992.
20. Gibbons GC, Murtaugh RJ: Cecal smooth muscle

MANAGEMENT OF SPECIFIC DISEASES

neoplasia in the dog: Report of 11 cases and literature review. *JAAHA* 25:191–197, 1989.

21. Kapatkin AS, Mullen HS, Matthiesen DT, Patnaik AK: Leiomyosarcoma in dogs: 44 cases (1983–1988). *JAVMA* 201:1077–1079, 1992.

22. McPherron MA, Withrow SJ, Seim HB III, Powers BE: Colorectal leiomyomas in seven dogs. *JAAHA* 28: 43–46, 1992.

23. Patnaik AK, Hurvitz AI, Johnson GF: Canine intestinal adenocarcinoma and carcinoid. *Vet Pathol* 17:149–163, 1980.

24. Comer KM: Anemia as a feature of primary gastrointestinal neoplasia. *Compend Contin Educ Pract Vet* 12: 13–19, 1990.

25. Bruecker KA, Withrow SJ: Intestinal leiomyosarcomas in six dogs. *JAAHA* 24:281–284, 1988.

26. Chen HHC, Parris LS, Parris RG: Duodenal leiomyosarcoma with multiple hepatic metastases in a dog. *JAVMA* 184:1506, 1984.

27. Watson DE, Mahaffey MB, Neuwirth LA: Ultrasonographic detection of duodenojejunal intussception in a dog. *JAAHA* 27:367–369, 1991.

28. Leib MS, Fallin EA, Johnston SA: Endoscopy case of the month: Abnormally shaped feces in a dog. *Vet Med* 762–766, 1992.

29. Henroteaux M: L'adenocarcinoma du colon chez le chien. *Med Vet Quebec* 20:79–80, 1990.

30. Thompson JP, Christopher MM, Ellison GW, et al: Paraneoplastic leukocytosis associated with a rectal adenomatous polyp in a dog. *JAVMA* 201:737–738, 1992.

31. Turrel JM, Theon AP: Single high-dose irradiation for selected canine rectal carcinomas. *Vet Radiol* 27:141–145, 1986.

32. Carpenter JL, Andrews LK, Holzworth J: Tumors and tumor-like lesions, in Holzworth J (ed): *Diseases of the Cat. Medicine and Surgery*. Philadelphia, WB Saunders, 1987, pp 406–596.

33. Turk MAM, Gallina AM, Russell TS: Nonhematopoietic gastrointestinal neoplasia in cats: A retrospective study of 44 cases. *Vet Pathol* 18:614–620, 1981.

34. Patnaik AK, Liu S-K, Johnston GF: Feline intestinal adenocarcinoma: A clinicopathologic study of 22 cases. *Vet Pathol* 13:1–10, 1976.

35. Cribb AE: Feline gastrointestinal adenocarcinoma: A review and retrospective study. *Can Vet J* 29:709–712, 1988.

36. Kosovsky JE, Matthiesen DT, Patnaik AK: Small intestinal adenocarcinoma in cats: 32 cases (1978–1985). *JAVMA* 192:233–235, 1988.

37. Lingeman CH, Garner FM: Comparative study of intestinal adenocarcinomas of animals and man. *J Natl Cancer Inst* 48:325–346, 1972.

38. MacDonald JM, Mullen HS, Moroff SD: Adenomatous polyps of the duodenum in cats: 18 cases (1985–1990). *JAVMA* 202:647–651, 1993.

39. Patnaik AK, Johnson GF, Greene RW, et al: Surgical resection of intestinal adenocarcinoma in a cat, with survival of 28 months. *JAVMA* 178:479–481, 1981.

40. Ross JT, Scavelli TD, Matthiesen DT, Patnaik AK: Adenocarcinoma of the apocrine glands of the anal sac in dogs: A review of 32 cases. *JAAHA* 27:349–355, 1991.

41. Goldschmidt MH, Zoltowski C: Anal sac gland adenocarcinoma in the dog 14 cases. *J Small Anim Pract* 22:119–128, 1981.

42. Berrocal A, Vos JH, Ingh van den TSGAM, et al: Canine perineal tumors. *JAVMA* 36:739–749, 1989.

43. Meuten DJ, Cooper BJ, Capen CC, et al: Hypercalcemia associated with an adenocarcinoma derived from the apocrine glands of the anal sac. *Vet Pathol* 18:454–471, 1981.

44. Rijnberk A, Elsinghorst ThAM, Koeman JP, et al: Pseudohyperparathyroidism associated with perirectal adenocarcinomas in elderly female dogs. *Tijdschr Diergeneesk* 103:1069–1075, 1978.

45. Rosol TJ, Capen CC, Danks JA, et al: Identification of parathyroid hormone-related protein in canine apocrine adenocarcinoma of the anal sac. *Vet Pathol* 27:89–95, 1990.

CLINICAL BRIEFING: HEPATIC AND PANCREATIC NEOPLASIA

Liver Tumors in Dogs

Common Clinical Presentation	Nonspecific lethargy and weight loss; dogs may be asymptomatic and may have a palpable mass
Common Histologic Type	Primary hepatocellular carcinoma
Epidemiology and Biological Behavior	Old dogs; large solitary lesions have low metastatic rate, but the majority have multiple nodular or diffuse involvement
Prognostic Factors	Dogs with solitary hepatocellular carcinoma, regardless of size, have a good prognosis after resection
Treatment **Surgery**	Treatment of choice

Liver Tumors in Cats

Common Clinical Presentation	Nonspecific lethargy and anorexia; cats often have a palpable mass
Common Histologic Type	Intrahepatic bile duct tumors (more than half are benign); hepatocellular carcinoma is next most common
Epidemiology and Biological Behavior	Most cats >10 years of age; intrahepatic bile duct tumors may progress from benign to malignant; benign tumors usually involve a solitary lobe; carcinomas often metastasize
Prognostic Factors	None identified
Treatment **Surgery**	Treatment of choice for benign tumors; however, carcinomas are usually diffuse, and prognosis is poor

MANAGEMENT OF SPECIFIC DISEASES

Exocrine Pancreatic Tumors in Dogs	
Common Clinical Presentation	Nonspecific anorexia and weight loss
Common Histologic Type	Exocrine pancreatic carcinoma
Epidemiology and Biological Behavior	Old dogs (mean age is 9 years); cocker spaniels may be predisposed; high metastatic rate
Prognostic Factors	None identified
Treatment Surgery	May not to be beneficial due to high metastatic rate; other modalities unreported

PRIMARY LIVER TUMORS IN DOGS
Incidence, Signalment, and Etiology

In a study of 110 hepatic neoplasms, slightly more than 50% were primary hepatocellular tumors.[1] This type of tumor is the predominant nonhematopoietic, nonvascular liver tumor.[2] Cholangiocellular carcinomas and bile-duct cystadenomas are diagnosed less frequently. Dogs with liver tumors are old; the average age of affected dogs is 11 to 12 years.[1-3] In a study of primary hepatocellular tumors, the male-to-female ratio was 1.7:1.0.[1] Another study found that female dogs were more likely to have a cholangiocellular carcinoma.[3]

Clinical Presentation and History

Clinical signs associated with liver tumors are often nonspecific. Lethargy, weakness, anorexia, polyuria, polydipsia, and vomiting are most common and occur in up to 65% of animals.[1-3] Weight loss, seizures, ascites, diarrhea, jaundice, and hematochezia are less common signs. Infrequently, hypoglycemia will accompany very large tumors, inducing seizures.[1,3] In one study, 5 of 18 dogs with liver tumors were asymptomatic. On physical examination, most dogs have abdominal distension and palpable hepatomegaly.[1-4]

Staging and Diagnosis

Radiographs can be helpful when attempting to confirm a diagnosis of a hepatic tumor. The most common radiographically detected abnormality is a right cranioventral abdominal mass that displaces the gastric shadow caudally and to the left and displaces the small intestine caudally (Figure 5-57).[2,3] Peritoneal fluid from carcinomatosis may obscure radiographic detection of the mass.[3] Ultrasonography is more precise than radiography in detecting the site of origin of an abdominal mass and provides important information as to the extent of disease; however, the ultrasonographic appearance of a mass lesion is not helpful in determining the cell type of a neoplasm[5,6] and will not help to distinguish neoplastic from nonneoplastic lesions.[5] Ultrasound-guided biopsy with a Tru-Cut® needle usually provides a definitive diagnosis and is the diagnostic procedure of choice. Before performing a biopsy, however, a coagulation profile should be obtained, especially if liver function is abnormal.

Blood chemistry panels are rarely useful in diagnosing liver tumors, as changes in alanine aminotransferase (ALT), alkaline phosphatase (ALP), and aspartate aminotransferase (AST) are elevated in between 60% and 90% of dogs[1] but are not specific for liver tumor. ALP is the most commonly elevated

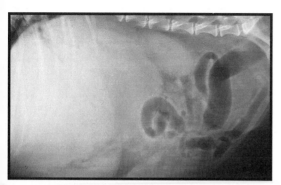

Figure 5-57: Abdominal radiography may delineate a cranial abdominal mass, as shown in this 11-year-old dachshund; however, ultrasonography or exploratory laparotomy usually is required to confirm that a mass arises from the liver.

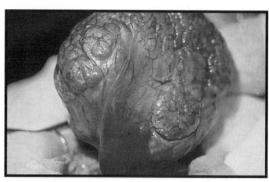

Figure 5-58: This large solitary liver tumor is a hepatocellular carcinoma. If no other lobes are involved with the disease, a good prognosis can be given after surgery. (Courtesy J. Berg)

parameter in dogs with liver tumors.[1,2,7,8] Fasting serum bile-acid concentrations do not assist in detecting neoplasia.[7,8] An enzymatic kit to detect α-fetoprotein (Tandem-E AFP ImmunoEnzMetric Assay, Hybritech, San Diego, CA) was used to distinguish different liver tumor types prior to biopsy.[7] Levels of α-fetoprotein were highest in dogs with cholangiocarcinoma and hepatocellular carcinoma; nevertheless, a biopsy of the lesion should be performed whenever possible in preference to this test.[7]

Thirty of 49 dogs (61%) with hepatocellular carcinoma had a massive lesion involving one hepatic lobe; however, 80% of these 30 dogs also had lesions in other lobes.[1] A mass lesion also was the most common presenting sign for hepatocellular carcinoma in two other studies.[2,3] Metastasis is common for all liver tumor types regardless of the histopathologic appearance of the tumor.[1] Metastasis occurred in 35 of 57 dogs (60%) in one study, most frequently to regional lymph nodes or to lungs (40% of dogs each). Metastasis also occurred to the peritoneal surfaces in approximately 20% of dogs.[1] Metastasis to the lungs was less common in another study and occurred in only two of 13 dogs with hepatocellular carcinoma and cholangiocellular carcinoma.[3] Large solitary hepatocellular carcino-

mas are less likely to metastasize than are multiple lesions. In one study, 13 (93%) of 14 dogs with either multiple or diffuse lesions developed metastasis, whereas only 11 of 30 dogs (37%) with solitary massive lesions developed metastasis.[1] The size of a solitary lesion apparently has little influence on prognosis. Dogs with primary liver tumors that are solitary mass lesions are probably the best candidates for treatment. Prior to surgery, thoracic radiographs should be performed and abdominal ultrasonography should be used to detect hepatic lymphadenopathy, other organ involvement, or lesions in multiple lobes. Dogs with lesions in multiple liver lobes have a poor prognosis.

Treatment

Dogs with hepatocellular carcinoma that involves a single liver lobe, or possibly two lobes, should be treated by lobectomy or partial hepatectomy. Such dogs have a good prognosis (Figure 5-58). Hepatocellular carcinoma was resected in 18 dogs.[2] In eight dogs that died, survival ranged from 1 to 548 days, with a median of 377 days. Five dogs died because of other disease. Of the 10 dogs that survived, one had recurrence at 240 days, and the remaining dogs were still alive at between 195

> ### KEY POINT:
>
> *Dogs with large solitary liver tumors usually have a good prognosis after surgery.*

MANAGEMENT OF SPECIFIC DISEASES

and 1025 days (median = 354 days).[2]

The success of treatment for other types of hepatic neoplasms is less defined. In one report, one dog with cholangiocellular carcinoma and one dog with adenocarcinoma had tumor recurrence six months after partial hepatectomy.[4] A hepatic mesenchymoma treated by excision recurred four months after surgery in another dog.[9] Chemotherapy is not useful for treatment of human patients with primary liver tumors. This is likely the case for dogs, but there are no reports of adjunctive chemotherapy to determine this.

PRIMARY LIVER TUMORS IN CATS
Incidence, Signalment, and Etiology

In contrast to dogs, the most common primary liver tumors in cats arise from the intrahepatic biliary tree. In 107 cats with nonvascular, nonhematopoietic liver tumors, 57 had intrahepatic bile duct tumors; 34 (60%) of these tumors were benign.[10,11] The majority of cats with intrahepatic bile duct tumors were old; affected cats ranged upward in age from 6 years.[11,12] In one study, all affected cats were older than 10 years of age.[12] In another study, male cats were overrepresented,[12] but the opposite was true in a different study.[11] Both studies found that intrahepatic bile duct tumors were more common in domestic shorthairs than in Siamese.[11,12] Feline leukemia virus (FeLV) does not seem to play a role in non-hematopoietic liver tumors.[13] Tumors arising from the extrahepatic bile ducts (9 of 107) or gall bladder (4 of 107) are usually malignant.[10,11] Hepatocellular carcinoma is less common in cats than in dogs and accounted for 25% of primary feline liver tumors.[10,11] The median age of affected cats is 11 years.[11] Males are most frequently affected (11 of 17 [65%]), and the tumor occurs mainly in domestic shorthairs. Hepatic myelolipomas consisting of adipose tissue and bone marrow elements have been associated with diaphragmatic hernias in cats and may be associated with chronic hypoxia or trauma to the liver.[14,15]

> ### KEY POINT:
>
> *More than one third of cats with a solitary liver tumor have a benign tumor that can be cured at surgery.*

Clinical Presentation and History

Cats with liver tumors usually show nonspecific signs of anorexia, lethargy, and weakness; vomiting, diarrhea, polydipsia, and ascites are less common signs.[11,12] Most cats have easily palpable hepatomegaly or an obvious mass in the anterior abdomen.

Staging and Diagnosis

Intrahepatic bile duct tumors in cats can progress from benign to malignant lesions; a mixed cellular pattern is often noted.[10] Benign lesions are usually cystic and multilocular, whereas malignant tumors frequently involve multiple lobes. In one study, 8 of 16 bile duct adenomas involved multiple lobes, and 7 of 9 bile duct carcinomas were widespread.[10] Metastasis is common in bile duct carcinomas. The most common sites of metastasis are the lungs, abdominal serosa, and hepatic lymph nodes. Metastases can occur to the thoracic nodes, diaphragm, spleen, urinary bladder, intestine, and bone.[10,11] Hepatocellular carcinoma may be less likely to metastasize than biliary carcinomas; only five (25%) of 18 cats with hepatocellular carcinoma had metastases to either regional lymph nodes or spleen and lung.[11] Unlike dogs, cats with liver tumors rarely have elevated ALP levels, probably because of its short serum half-life. Elevations in ALT and AST are not specific for neoplasia.[12] Abdominal radiographs and abdominal ultrasonography have the same utility and limitations as they do in dogs for diagnosing and staging of these tumors. Ultrasonography is useful in obtaining guided needle core biopsy of lesions in the liver and for detecting involvement of multiple lobes and other abdominal sites. When a solitary tumor is diagnosed in a cat, surgery should be considered.

Treatment

Benign biliary cystadenomas predominate in cats (35%); therefore, long-term remission after resection

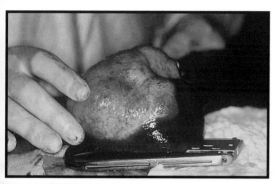

Figure 5-59: This hepatobiliary adenoma in a domesticated cat is amenable to removal by lobectomy, either by finger-fracture or, as in this case, stapling. (Courtesy J. Berg)

is often possible (Figure 5-59). One cat with a cystadenoma that involved both the left medial and lateral lobes of the liver that was treated by lobectomy was still alive with no tumor recurrence 18 months later.[16] Similarly, a 16-year-old cat lived 27 months after surgical excision of a myelolipoma and had no tumor recurrence.[14]

TUMORS OF THE EXOCRINE PANCREAS

Tumors of the exocrine pancreas are rare in both dogs and cats. Insulinoma, a rare tumor of the islet cells of the pancreas, is discussed in the chapter on Tumors of the Endocrine System.

Incidence, Signalment, and Etiology

Exocrine pancreas tumors show no obvious gender predilection. They are most common in old dogs, with a mean age of about 9 years.[17–20] In one report, cocker spaniels accounted for 3 of 14 dogs.[17] Only spaniel breeds were affected in another study.[18]

Clinical Presentation and History

Clinical signs are often nonspecific and include weight loss, depression, and anorexia. Although pancreatic tumors are commonly believed to cause emesis, vomiting is actually

uncommon[18,19] and is a late, often terminal, occurrence.[17,20] A mass in the anterior abdomen may be palpable, and ascites may occur.[17] In three dogs, clinical signs related to panniculitis caused subcutaneous swellings and shifting lameness over a period of months.[18] In these dogs, pancreatic carcinoma was an incidental necropsy finding and no clinical signs directly attributable to the tumor were noted before death.

Staging and Diagnosis

After performing a general health screen with blood work, urinalysis, and thoracic radiographs, ultrasonography of the abdomen should be considered. Pancreatic tumors are a solitary mass in 50% of affected dogs.[17] The remaining dogs may have numerous nodules throughout the pancreas. Metastases in the liver were present in 12 of 13 dogs, in the omentum and mesentery in 6 of 13 dogs, and in regional lymph nodes in 4 of 13 dogs.[17] Other visceral sites are less frequently affected.[17,19,20] One dog with diabetes insipidus had metastasis to the pituitary gland.[19] No metastases were seen in one series of three dogs even though all three had a long history of panniculitis. One of these dogs had no signs referable to pancreatitis despite marked elevations in serum lipase and amylase.[18] Serum lipase levels may be extremely elevated in dogs with this disease, and a level 25 times greater than normal is probably diagnostic for exocrine pancreatic carcinoma.[21] Pancreatic carcinoma, both metastatic and localized, has been reported in association with diabetes mellitus in two cats.

Ultrasonography can be useful in detecting a pancreatic mass,[22] although the pancreas is difficult to image because of shadowing from gas-filled gastrointestinal structures. Liver metastases may also be detected, although definitive diagnosis requires biopsy.

Treatment

Treatment has not been described for this tumor, and surgical resection usually requires a Billroth II proce-

> **KEY POINT:**
>
> *Contrary to common belief, vomiting is rarely reported with exocrine pancreatic tumors in dogs.*

dure. Chemotherapy is rarely helpful in human patients and has not been described in cats or dogs.

REFERENCES

1. Patnaik AK, Hurvitz AI, Lieberman PH, Johnson GF: Canine hepatocellular carcinoma. *Vet Pathol* 18:427–438, 1981.
2. Kosovsky JE, Manfra-Marretta S, Matthiesen DT, Patnaik AK: Results of partial hepatectomy in 18 dogs with hepatocellular carcinoma. *JAAHA* 25:203–206, 1989.
3. Evans SM: The radiographic appearance of primary liver neoplasia in dogs. *Vet Radiol* 28:192–196, 1987.
4. Fry PD, Rest JR: Partial hepatectomy in two dogs. *J Small Anim Pract* 34:192–195, 1993.
5. Voros K, Vrabely T, Papp L, et al: Correlation of ultrasonographic and pathomorphological findings in canine hepatic diseases. *J Small Anim Pract* 32:627–634, 1991.
6. Feeney DA, Johnston GR, Hardy RM: Two-dimensional, gray-scale ultrasonography for assessment of hepatic and splenic neoplasia in the dog and cat. *JAVMA* 184:68–80, 1984.
7. Lowseth LA, Gillett NA, Ghang I-Y, et al: Detection of serum α-fetoprotein in dogs with hepatic tumors. *JAVMA* 199:735–741, 1991.
8. Center SA, Baldwin BH, Erb NH, Tennant BC: Bile acid concentrations in the diagnosis of hepatobiliary disease in the dog. *JAVMA* 187:935–940, 1985.
9. McDonald RK, Helman RG: Hepatic malignant mesenchymoma in a dog. *JAVMA* 188:1052–1053, 1986.
10. Patnaik AK: A morphologic and immunocytochemical study of hepatic neoplasms in cats. *Vet Pathol* 29:405–415, 1992.
11. Carpenter JL, Andrews LK, Holzworth J: Tumors and tumor-like lesions, in Holzworth J (ed): *Diseases of the Cat. Medicine and Surgery.* Philadelphia, WB Saunders, 1987, pp 406–596.
12. Post G, Patnaik AK: Nonhematopoietic hepatic neoplasms in cats: 21 cases (1983–1988). *JAVMA* 201:1080–1082, 1992.
13. Feldman BF, Strafuss AC, Gabbert N: Bile duct carcinoma in the cat: Three case reports. *Fel Pract* 6:33–39, 1976.
14. McCaw DL, Curiel da Silva JMA, Shaw DP: Hepatic myelolipomas in a cat. *JAVMA* 197:243–244, 1990.
15. Schuh JCL: Hepatic nodular myelolipomatosis (myelolipomas) associated with a peritoneo-pericardial diaphragmatic hernia in a cat. *J Comp Pathol* 97:231–235, 1987.
16. Peterson SL: Intrahepatic biliary cystadenoma in a cat. *Feline Pract* 14:29–32, 1984.
17. Anderson NV, Johnson KH: Pancreatic carcinoma in the dog. *JAVMA* 150:286–295, 1967.
18. Brown PJ, Mason KV, Merrett DJ, et al: Multifocal necrotizing steatitis associated with pancreatic carcinoma in three dogs. *J Small Anim Pract* 35:129–132, 1994.
19. Davenport DJ, Chew DJ, Johnson GC: Diabetes insipidus associated with metastatic pancreatic carcinoma in a dog. *JAVMA* 189:204–205, 1986.
20. Xu F-N: Ultrastructural examinations as an aid to the diagnosis of canine pancreatic neoplasms. *Austral Vet J* 62:197–198, 1985.
21. Fineman L, DeNicola D, Bruyette D, et al: Serum lipase concentrations in dogs with pancreatic carcinoma. *Proc 14th Ann Vet Cancer Soc:* 16–17, 1994.
22. Love NE, Jones C: What's your diagnosis? *JAVMA* 195:1285–1286, 1989.

CLINICAL BRIEFING: HEMANGIOSARCOMA

Splenic Hemangiosarcoma in Dogs

Common Clinical Presentation	Palpable abdominal mass; hemoperitoneum; anemia; shock; and, possibly, collapse
Epidemiology and Biological Behavior	Average age is 10 years; German shepherds predisposed; metastasis may be confined to abdominal cavity if no concurrent right atrial lesion exists
Prognostic Factors	Clinical stage

Treatment
  Surgery
  Chemotherapy
 	
  Immunotherapy
	
	Palliative without gross metastases, but survival is short
	Doxorubicin and doxorubicin/vincristine/cyclophosphamide are still investigational but may prolong survival
	Therapy with biological response modifier L-MTP-PE prolongs survival in dogs with micrometastatic disease

Cardiac Hemangiosarcoma in Dogs

Common Clinical Presentation	Collapse and cardiac tamponade; hindlimb paresis; and right atrial mass
Epidemiology and Biological Behavior	Average age is 10 years; German shepherds predisposed; metastasis may be widespread, commonly to lungs
Prognostic Factors	None identified

Treatment
  Surgery
  Chemotherapy
	
	Palliative in dogs with resectable lesions
	Role of doxorubicin and doxorubicin/vincristine/ cyclophosphamide is being defined

Cutaneous Hemangiosarcoma in Dogs

Common Clinical Presentation	Raised, red lesion often in skin that is lightly pigmented
Epidemiology and Biological Behavior	Average age is 10 years; whippets and other dogs with glabrous skin are predisposed; metastasis is uncommon

MANAGEMENT OF SPECIFIC DISEASES

Prognostic Factors	Histopathologic evidence of solar elastosis adjacent to tumor is good prognostic sign Tumors within epidermis and dermis have a good prognosis
Treatment **Surgery** **Chemotherapy**	May be curative in majority of cases Role undecided due to low metastatic rate and resultant lack of need for adjuvant therapy

Nonlymphoid, Nonangiogenic Splenic Tumors in Dogs

Common Clinical Presentation	Abdominal swelling and weakness; palpable abdominal mass
Common Histologic Types	Leiomyosarcoma, osteosarcoma, and fibrosarcoma
Epidemiology and Biological Behavior	Average age is 11 years; no breed or gender predilection; metastasis commonly occurs to abdominal sites
Prognostic Factors	None identified
Treatment **Splenectomy** **Chemotherapy**	May be palliative; survival is often shortened by metastases Unknown

Hemangiosarcoma in Cats

Common Clinical Presentation	Intra-abdominal and cutaneous tumors occur with similar frequency as in dogs
Epidemiology and Biological Behavior	Cutaneous hemangiosarcoma may be sunlight-induced in areas of unpigmented skin
Prognostic Factors	Hemangiosarcomas of spleen and mesentery are highly metastatic; tumors of skin and (perhaps) liver are not
Treatment **Surgery** **Radiation Therapy** **Chemotherapy**	Excision of cutaneous tumors is potentially curative if wide margins are obtained Unknown Unknown

MANAGEMENT OF SPECIFIC DISEASES

SPLENIC HEMANGIOSARCOMA IN DOGS

Incidence, Signalment, and Etiology

The spleen is the most common primary site for hemangiosarcoma in dogs. The tumor is characterized by rapid growth and widespread metastasis, presumably due to its tissue of origin, the vascular endothelium, and its resultant ready access to systemic circulation.

Old dogs are affected by this disease (average age = 9 to 11 years). German shepherds are predisposed.[1-3] There is no clear gender predilection, as male dogs are overrepresented in some studies[1,4] and females in others.[3,5] Splenic hemangiosarcoma can occur in conjunction with hemangiosarcoma of the right atrium, which may represent synchronous primary tumors rather than metastatic disease.[5] No etiologic agent has been identified in dogs; in humans, exposure to vinyl chloride appears to be a high risk factor.[6]

Clinical Presentation and History

Between one[3,5] and two thirds[7] of all splenic masses are malignant tumors, and the majority of malignant tumors are hemangiosarcoma. It is critical to differentiate splenic hemangiosarcoma from other possible diagnoses, which include splenic hematoma, hyperplastic nodules, and leiomyosarcoma. The important differential diagnosis for a dog presented with a palpable splenic mass is the combination of splenic hematoma and hyperplastic nodules, which are as common as hemangiosarcoma on surgical biopsy and necropsy surveys.[3,5,8] It is impossible to differentiate these conditions on the basis of gross appearance using radiology or ultrasonography or at surgery. Certain clinical signs may help to distinguish the conditions before a definitive histopathologic diagnosis is obtained.

Collapse, hemoperitoneum, and anorexia are more common in dogs with splenic hemangiosarcoma than in dogs with splenic hematoma or other tumors of the spleen. In one study, however, such signs as lethargy, enlarged abdomen, sensitive abdomen, vomiting, and diarrhea[3] were as common in dogs with hematoma and hemangiosarcoma of the spleen. Both diseases occur in a similar size and age group of dogs, and both are most common in German shepherds. The distinction is critical, however, as survival times differ greatly among the various diseases (e.g., average is 19 days for hemangiosarcoma versus 340 days for hematoma) (Figure 5-60).[3] Other signs noted on clinical examination are pale mucous membranes and general weakness owing to anemia, which results from chronic bleeding either into the tumor or abdomen. Hematologic data from dogs with splenic hemangiosarcoma may be a useful diagnostic feature. Red blood cell morphologic changes, such as acanthocytes, schistocytes, and nucleated red blood cells are common in splenic hemangiosarcoma. Schistocytes are associated with red cell fragmentation, microangiopathy, and disseminated intravascular coagulopathy (DIC) in dogs; they may reflect an inability of the diseased spleen to remove them normally from circulation.

Staging and Diagnosis

Staging for a dog with a suspected hemangiosarcoma should include a complete blood count and serum chemistry profile and urinalysis as well as more definitive procedures, such as radiography and ultrasonography. Ultrasonography may be effective for examining an enlarged spleen in a dog, identifying peritoneal effusion, and detecting sites of abdominal metastasis. In one study,[9] a splenic mass was easily identified, although ultrasonographic findings ranged from anechoic to hyperechoic areas throughout the same lesion. These findings are not helpful in distinguishing splenic hemangiosarcoma from splenic hematoma or nodular hyperplasia. Ultrasonography aided in the detection of metastases in the liver and peri-

> **KEY POINT:**
>
> *Approximately one to two thirds of splenic masses are malignant; however, collapse and hemoperitoneum seem to be more common in dogs with splenic hemangiosarcoma.*

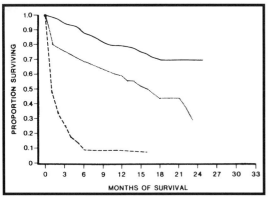

Figure 5-60: *Survival duration for 59 dogs with splenic hemangiosarcoma* (dashed line), *125 dogs with splenic hematoma* (dotted line), *and 84 matched control dogs* (solid line). *(From Prymak C, McKee LJ, Goldschmidt MH, Glickman LT: Epidemiologic, clinical, pathologic, and prognostic characteristics of splenic hemangiosarcoma and splenic hematoma in dogs: 217 cases (1985).* JAVMA 193:706–712, 1988; with permission.)

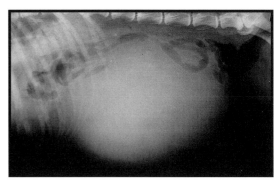

Figure 5-61: *Abdominal radiographs confirm the presence of a mass in a dog with abdominal swelling. The mass is suspected of being splenic on the basis of dorsal, cranial, and caudal displacement of intestinal loops, but confirmation requires ultrasonography or exploratory laparotomy. (Courtesy J. Berg)*

toneum.[9] Care must be taken to distinguish hepatic regenerative nodules from metastases (which may be difficult). Overall, ultrasonography is more useful than abdominal radiography in detecting a primary lesion and its metastases. Abdominal fluid from bleeding may complicate a radiographic diagnosis (Figure 5-61).

Up to 25% of dogs with splenic hemangiosarcoma may also have a right atrial hemangiosarcoma[10]; therefore, it is important to examine the right atrial appendage by ultrasonography for presence of a mass prior to making firm recommendation for surgery or adjunctive therapy. Pulmonary metastases are much more common in dogs with both sites involved than in dogs in which the spleen is the only site of hemangiosarcoma at presentation. Splenic hemangiosarcoma and associated metastases almost always are confined to the peritoneal cavity.[10] This has important implications for monitoring of dogs after treatment for splenic hemangiosarcoma, as tho-

racic radiographs would be expected to have a low yield. Abdominal ultrasonography, therefore, may be the imaging modality of choice. In 19 dogs with splenic hemangiosarcoma without right atrial involvement, 15 (79%) had metastases to the liver (n = 13), omentum (n = 8), and mesentery (n = 7). Metastases also occurred to the kidney, urinary bladder, small intestine, diaphragm, adrenal gland, and mesenteric lymph nodes.[10] In a review of dogs with splenic hemangiosarcoma without right atrial involvement, only 14 (25%) of 55 dogs developed metastases outside the abdominal cavity.[10]

Definitive diagnosis of hemangiosarcoma requires histopathologic examination of surgically obtained biopsy specimens. Aspiration cytology and needle biopsy specimens are rarely useful because of the heterogeneous nature of the neoplasm. The tumor contains mixed areas consisting of hematomas, fibrotic areas, and areas of extramedullary hematopoiesis,[11] which means aspiration or needle biopsy rarely provides a definitive diagnosis. In addition, the risk of bleeding is high in these patients after such procedures are performed.

> **KEY POINT:**
>
> *Metastases associated with splenic hemangiosarcoma are mostly confined to the peritoneal cavity.*

MANAGEMENT OF SPECIFIC DISEASES

Prognostic Factors

Some believe that clinical staging is of prognostic benefit. Stage I hemangiosarcomas are tumors confined to the spleen with no evidence of metastasis, whereas dogs with stage II disease may have a ruptured spleen, with or without regional lymph node involvement. Stage III tumors are large, invasive tumors with distant metastases.[12]

Treatment
Surgery

Surgery is the treatment of choice for splenic hemangiosarcoma. Surgery relieves abdominal distention caused by a large tumor and may provide palliation by stopping bleeding from the primary tumor (Figure 5-62). Surgery, however, does little to prolong survival because of rapid growth of metastases. Survival-time data are distorted by the high rate of intraoperative euthanasia and perioperative mortality. The literature assessing the role of surgery in this disease has usually included dogs that receive adjuvant chemotherapy and immunotherapy[4]; therefore, the true impact of surgery as a single treatment modality in dogs with less advanced disease has been difficult to assess.

A group of 32 dogs (with stage I or II splenic hemangiosarcoma) that survived at least two weeks after surgery and received no further treatment was found to have a median survival of 83 days (mean = 116 days; range = 14 to 470 days), and only two dogs were alive one year after surgery. Metastatic disease was the overwhelming cause of death in all dogs. Interestingly, such factors as whether the spleen had ruptured (stage I versus stage II), the presence of either anemia or postoperative arrhythmias, and whether the dog received a blood transfusion failed to affect survival in these dogs.[13]

Dogs undergoing splenectomy should be monitored electrocardiographically before, during, and after surgery. In a series of 59 dogs undergoing splenectomy for hemangiosarcoma, 14 developed ventricular arrhythmia after surgery. None of these dogs had pre-existing cardiac disease. Anemia was believed to cause these arrhythmias by decreasing

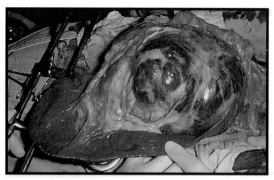

Figure 5-62: *The same dog shown in Figure 5-61. A vascular splenic mass has not ruptured, and micrometastases are not visible at surgery. The liver, however, should be examined for evidence of gross metastatic disease. (Courtesy J. Berg)*

myocardial oxygenation; only one dog developed arrhythmias that were not attributed to anemia. In another series, metastatic myocardial disease was seen in 12 of 18 dogs, although only three of these dogs developed ventricular arrhythmias.[14] Treatment of arrhythmias with such drugs as lidocaine and procainamide, along with continuous monitoring, should resolve the arrhythmias within one to five days.

Chemotherapy

The effect of chemotherapy on such malignancies as osteosarcoma raised hopes that drug therapy may also improve survival for dogs with hemangiosarcoma. Splenic hemangiosarcoma would appear to be very likely to respond positively to adjunctive therapy, as the disease burden is often low after splenectomy. Thus far, however, the true impact of chemotherapy has been difficult to assess. In a series that included eight dogs with splenic hemangiosarcoma that received vincristine (0.75 mg/m² IV), doxorubicin (30 mg/m² IV), and cyclophosphamide (100–150 mg/m² IV) followed by chlorambucil (20 mg/m² PO) and methotrexate (2.5 mg/m² PO), overall median survival was 164 days (range = 10 to 1084+ days).[12] In another group of dogs that received doxorubicin (30 mg/m² IV) and cyclophosphamide (50 to 75 mg/m² PO), the median survival time was

179 days.[8] Many of these dogs had metastatic disease.[8,12] Toxicities in both studies included neutropenia and gastrointestinal signs that were severe enough to necessitate hospitalization in 7 of 15 and 3 of 16 dogs, respectively. One dog in each study (2 of 31 dogs) died of sepsis as a result of chemotherapy-induced neutropenia, and two dogs died of cardiomyopathy, presumably doxorubicin-induced.[8,12]

In another study, 46 dogs with metastatic (stage III) hemangiosarcoma (splenic = 14, cardiac = 5, subcutaneous = 9, and other sites = 18) had the tumor and accessible metastatic disease surgically resected and then were treated with doxorubicin (30 mg/m² IV every 3 weeks for up to 5 total treatments). The average survival time for dogs in which all visible disease was resected was 267 days, whereas dogs that did not have complete resection lived an average of 67 days.[15]

The effect of chemotherapy on this disease is, therefore, investigational at this time. Future investigations of newer chemotherapeutics may provide more substantial improvements in survival. The confinement of metastatic disease to the abdominal cavity in the majority of these dogs has led some investigators to suggest that intracavitary chemotherapy may be a logical approach to splenic hemangiosarcoma.[10] Intracavitary chemotherapy provides high levels of chemotherapy to the abdominal, visceral, and parietal surfaces as well as to the hepatic circulation, where splenic hemangiosarcoma most frequently metastasizes.

Biological Response Modifiers and Chemotherapy

An early study found trends in survival that suggested dogs with splenic hemangiosarcoma may benefit from chemotherapy and treatment with biological response modifiers after splenectomy.[4] The most impressive improvement in survival for dogs with splenic hemangiosarcoma that has not metastasized results from postoperative treatment with doxorubicin and cyclophosphamide followed by treatment with liposome-encapsulated muramyl-tripeptide-phosphatidyethanolamine (L-MTP-PE).

L-MTP-PE activates macrophages, enhancing their tumoricidal ability. The median survival was 273 days in 12 dogs that were treated with L-MTP-PE, which was significantly higher than the median survival of 144 days seen for dogs treated with chemotherapy alone.[16]

CARDIAC HEMANGIOSARCOMA IN DOGS

Incidence, Signalment, and Etiology

The right atrium is the third most common site of occurrence for hemangiosarcoma, accounting for three of 104 tumors,[4] 15 of 134 tumors,[1] and 31 of 61 tumors[17] in three separate studies. Two series of dogs with cardiac hemangiosarcoma (totalling 69 dogs)[17,18] indicated that German shepherds are at high risk for developing this disease and account for 20% to 30% of affected dogs. The average age of affected dogs in both studies were 10 years, ranging from 2 to 15 years; all but one dog was 5 years of age or older. There was no obvious gender predilection. Epidemiology of visceral hemangiosarcoma, therefore, appears fairly constant, regardless of the site of origin. Most hemangiosarcomas of the right atrium are solitary, but they can be multiple within the atrium and auricle. Some are very large and invasive. Erosion of the endocardium may result in rupture of the atrial wall and subsequent cardiac tamponade. Sudden death follows in some dogs.

Clinical Presentation and History

Most dogs are presented after a short duration of signs, which range from acute collapse and cardiac tamponade to nonspecific lethargy and generalized weakness. Weakness is common and frequently affects the hindlimbs.[17]

In one study, one third of the dogs with pericardial effusion were found to have right atrial hemangiosarcoma; this condition in an old dog should increase suspicion for this tumor.

Staging and Diagnosis

In addition to staging procedures outlined for dogs with splenic hemangiosarcoma, thoracic radiographs

MANAGEMENT OF SPECIFIC DISEASES

and cardiac evaluation using ultrasonography will provide valuable information. Abdominal ultrasound should also be performed to identify dogs with other organ involvement.

Primary cardiac hemangiosarcoma has a very high rate of pulmonary metastases compared to splenic and cutaneous hemangiosarcoma. In two studies, pulmonary metastases were found at the time of presentation in 37 (62%) of 60 dogs.[17,18] Metastases in the liver and spleen are less common. Metastases to abdominal viscera, skin, and brain are observed in some dogs.

Cardiac masses may be very difficult to see on thoracic radiographs, although findings of pericardial effusion, right heart, or specific right atrial enlargement may be suggestive of this condition. In one survey, this condition was recognized radiographically in less than 50% of dogs with cardiac hemangiosarcoma. Pulmonary metastases were less frequently overlooked in the same study, but because these metastases are small and miliary in distribution, both right and left lateral views are recommended to improve the chances for detection.[19]

Two-dimensional echocardiography is a noninvasive technique to examine the right atrium and auricle; when it is used by a skilled operator, it can be helpful in detecting masses in this area.[20] In one study, pneumopericardiography successfully outlined masses in the right atrium in seven of 12 dogs.[18] Cytology of pericardial fluid is rarely diagnostic for right atrial hemangiosarcoma.[17] Definitive diagnosis usually requires thoracotomy and surgical biopsy, but in an older dog with a right atrial mass and a hemorrhagic pericardial effusion, any diagnosis other than hemangiosarcoma is unlikely.

Treatment

Most reported animals with cardiac hemangiosarcoma either die or are euthanatized at or shortly after diagnosis because of the high rate of metastasis.

> **KEY POINT:**
>
> *Right atrial hemangiosarcoma is a common cause of pericardial effusion; ultrasonography should be used in these dogs to identify any suspicious mass.*

Surgery

Surgical resection of right atrial hemangiosarcoma was attempted in nine dogs that lacked evidence of pulmonary metastasis on radiographs.[18] In six of these dogs, the tumor was confined to the right auricle and was completely resected. In three dogs, the tumor was more extensive, and excision was incomplete. One of the latter dogs died in the perioperative period, and two other dogs that showed evidence of metastases at the time of surgery did not survive long. Survival times for all nine dogs ranged from 2 days to 8 months (mean = 4 months); all dogs developed disseminated metastatic disease. In another study, all three dogs that underwent a similar surgery died within 13 weeks of surgery[21] (Figures 5-63 and 5-64).

Chemotherapy

Reports of chemotherapy for cardiac hemangiosarcoma are rare and largely anecdotal. One dog received doxorubicin (30 mg/m² IV), cyclophosphamide (100 mg/m² IV), and vincristine (0.5 mg/m² IV) for 105 days. The size of the primary tumor was reduced, but pulmonary metastases developed during chemotherapy.[20] The dog developed cardiomyopathy, presumably because of the doxorubicin therapy, and died 140 days after starting chemotherapy. Three dogs with disseminated hemangiosarcoma that included the right atrium were treated with surgery (1 dog) and chemotherapy as just described. The three dogs lived 172, 173, and 218 days; the longest survivor died of cardiotoxicity.[12]

Chemotherapy for cardiac hemangiosarcoma has not been proved to result in definitive improvement in survival and quality of life. Doxorubicin alone may be as effective as combination chemotherapy.

CUTANEOUS HEMANGIOSARCOMA IN DOGS (see also the chapter on Tumors of the Skin)

Incidence, Signalment, and Etiology

Cutaneous hemangiosarcoma occurs in old dogs

MANAGEMENT OF SPECIFIC DISEASES

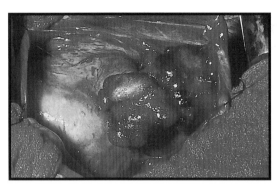

Figure 5-63

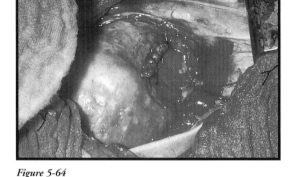

Figure 5-64

Figures 5-63 and 5-64: A hemangiosarcoma of the right auricle may be clearly visible at exploratory thoracotomy. The auricle may be resected with little morbidity to the dog; however, survival times are short. (Courtesy J. Berg)

(average age = 10 years) and is most common in females. Unlike those with hemangiosarcoma of other sites, dogs with lightly haired, poorly pigmented skin are predisposed; whippets, salukis, bloodhounds, and English pointers are at increased risk.[22] In one study, a colony of 991 beagles developed 48 cutaneous hemangiosarcomas.[23] Tumors in these breeds are often found in skin that shows evidence of solar dermatosis, which is a sunlight-induced (actinic) change. These findings suggest that cutaneous hemangiosarcoma is an actinic tumor in many dogs. Actinic dermatosis may precede tumor development by many years, and dogs may develop hemangiomas long before malignancy is detected. Cutaneous hemangiosarcoma may also be metastatic from systemic hemangiosarcoma, as found in one study with a high rate of metastatic skin involvement from visceral sites[24] (Figure 5-65).

Clinical Presentation and History

Dogs may have cutaneous hemangiomas and hemangiosarcomas concurrently, and these may be clinically indistinguishable. Hemangiosarcomas are more likely to affect the dermis than the subcutis[22] and have a predilection for the ventral abdominal skin. Forty-two of 48 dogs had tumors in their abdominal skin.[22] The overlying epidermis is frequently thickened and ulcerated; it may be raised and

red in appearance. Tumors below the dermis tend to be larger, possibly due to later detection by owners.[25]

Staging and Diagnosis

Cutaneous hemangiosarcoma may represent a metastasis from visceral sites; therefore, a thorough staging procedure should be performed. Careful abdominal palpation to identify organomegaly, followed by abdominal ultrasonography, may help to eliminate the possibility of a splenic tumor. In addition, echocardiography to detect right atrial hemangiosarcoma should be performed. Thoracic radiographs with both right and left lateral views along with a ventrodorsal image should be taken as well as routine blood work and urinalysis. If the skin is the primary site of the hemangiosarcoma, the prognosis is still guarded but considerably better than for visceral hemangiosarcoma. This assumption is alluded to in many studies, in which cutaneous hemangiosarcoma is frequently staged as stage I disease.[8,12] In one study, only 2 of 25 dogs developed distant metastases despite long survival times after surgery.[25]

In a series of 212 dogs with cutaneous hemangiomas or hemangiosarcomas, 11 dogs developed hemostatic defects that led to bleeding or petechiation and ecchymoses.[26] Six of these dogs had systemic hemangiosarcoma, and three had large unresectable tumors. The risk of developing DIC in dogs with pri-

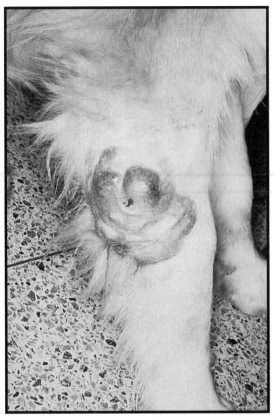

Figure 5-65: *Cutaneous and subcutaneous hemangiosarco-ma may arise as primary tumors or as a metastasis from a visceral primary tumor. (Courtesy G.H. Theilen)*

mary cutaneous hemangiosarcomas, therefore, seems to be low.

Prognostic Factors

Solar elastosis in the skin adjacent to hemangiosarcomas is related to long survival, implying that solar-induced cutaneous hemangiosarcomas may be less aggressive tumors than other hemangiosarcomas.[22]

Treatment
Surgery

Of 84 dogs with cutaneous hemangiosarcoma treated by surgical excision, only 11 had tumor recurrence at the site of surgery.[22] Twenty-five dogs died from hemangiosarcoma. Four dogs with hemangiosarcoma concurrent with solar elastosis died from their tumors. In two of these dogs, the tumor had been present for 1.2 and 2.7 years before surgical removal. In another group of 48 beagles with cutaneous hemangiosarcomas, 11 dogs developed metastases and died from them.[23] Primary cutaneous hemangiosarcoma, particularly if found in association with solar-induced changes, apparently is not as aggressive as hemangiosarcoma arising from other sites. In a series of 25 dogs, local recurrence after surgery was more common in dogs with subdermal tumors, and median survival for these dogs was significantly shorter than for dogs with dermal tumors (307 days versus 780 days).[25]

Chemotherapy

The lower metastatic potential for this tumor is reflected in studies involving chemotherapy for cutaneous hemangiosarcoma. In one study, six dogs received doxorubicin (30 mg/m² IV), cyclophosphamide (100 to 150 mg/m² IV), and vincristine (0.75 mg/m² IV) as well as chlorambucil and methotrexate. Survival times in three dogs that underwent surgical excision prior to chemotherapy were good, ranging from 277 days to more than 1046 days.[12] Responses in three dogs treated with chemotherapy alone were not as impressive; two of the dogs developed progressive disease and died 86 and 112 days after treatment began. One dog that maintained stable disease lived for 435 days. In another study, dogs with cutaneous hemangiosarcoma that were treated with doxorubicin (30 mg/m² IV) and cyclophosphamide (50–75 mg/m² PO for 4 days) had a median survival of 250 days, with a mean survival of 403 days.[8] In light of the long remissions that follow surgery alone for cutaneous hemangiosarcoma, the contribution of chemotherapy to survival times is difficult to assess.

> **KEY POINT:**
>
> *Cutaneous hemangiosarcoma affects dogs with glabrous skin and is often a sunlight-induced tumor.*

HEMANGIOSARCOMA OF OTHER SITES IN DOGS

Hemangiosarcoma most commonly arises in the spleen, skin, or right atrium, but as blood vessels are ubiquitous, primary hemangiosarcoma may arise in any organ. Primary hemangiosarcoma of the ribs[27] and the vertebrae[28] have been reported and were associated with rapid metastasis and short survival times. A primary prostatic hemangiosarcoma failed to respond to a course of radiation therapy and had metastasized widely at the time of euthanasia.[29]

Any dog with hemangiosarcoma should be staged (as previously described for cutaneous hemangiosarcoma) to ascertain that the affected site is not a metastasis from more commonly affected sites, such as the spleen or right atrium. With the exception of some cutaneous hemangiosarcomas, the prognosis for any dog with hemangiosarcoma is poor. Adjunctive chemotherapy is investigational.

OTHER SPLENIC TUMORS IN DOGS
Incidence, Signalment, and Etiology

The most common neoplasms affecting the canine spleen are hemangiosarcoma (see preceding section) and lymphoma (see Lymphoma chapter). Fifty-seven dogs were included in a series of nonvascular, nonlymphatous tumors of the spleen.[30] Sixteen dogs had leiomyosarcomas, 10 had osteosarcomas, seven had fibrosarcomas, three had liposarcomas, two had myxosarcomas, and 15 had undifferentiated sarcomas. In three dogs, the tumor had mixed histogenesis with myxosarcomatous, rhabomyosarcomatous, or chondrosarcomatous components predominating. One dog had a fibrous histiocytoma. The median age of all affected dogs was 11 years. There were no breed or gender predilections. Sarcomas predominate in the spleen of dogs and vary as to their mesenchymal differentiation.

Malignant fibrous histiocytoma was diagnosed in the spleen of six dogs.[31] These dogs were of a similar population to the dogs just described (median age = 12 years; no sex or breed predilection).

KEY POINT:

Histopathologic evidence of solar elastosis in the skin adjacent to cutaneous hemangiosarcoma may be associated with a low chance of metastatic spread.

Clinical Presentation and History

Clinical signs of splenic tumors are vague, consisting of lethargy, anorexia, weakness, weight loss, and abdominal distention in some dogs. Tumors are often large (>15 cm); therefore, physical examination will usually detect a splenic mass[31] and may reveal abdominal pain.

In one study, the duration of clinical signs was more than one week in 70% of the dogs and longer than one month in 20%.[30]

Staging and Diagnosis

A dog with a suspected splenic mass should be staged in the same way as outlined for splenic hemangiosarcoma, using blood work, radiography, and ultrasonography.

Thoracic radiographs were obtained in 53 of 57 dogs with different types of splenic tumors, and pulmonary metastases were present in four.[30] Pleural effusion (2 dogs) and enlarged sternal lymph nodes (1 dog) also were detected. Metastatic disease was documented at surgery or necropsy in 40 of the 57 dogs. Sites of metastasis varied; the liver was most commonly involved (35 dogs), but metastasis occurred in multiple visceral sites both within the abdomen and the lungs. Although one of six dogs with malignant fibrous histiocytoma was reported to have metastases, follow-up times were short.[31] This tumor seems to have high metastatic potential.

Abdominal radiographs were able to confirm the presence of a splenic mass but contributed little other information. Abdominal ultrasonography is better able to define the origin of a palpable abdominal mass; however, needle biopsies are often nondiagnostic, and definitive diagnosis usually follows exploratory laparotomy. Thoracic radiographs should be taken prior to any definitive treatment.

MANAGEMENT OF SPECIFIC DISEASES

Treatment

Splenectomy is the treatment of choice for all splenic tumors except lymphoma. Splenectomy was performed in 27 of 57 dogs with splenic tumors[30] and in six dogs with malignant fibrous histiocytoma.[31] Of the 27 dogs in the first series, 11 dogs had obvious metastatic disease at the time of surgery. Five dogs died perioperatively, emphasizing the importance of postsurgical monitoring for signs of shock, blood loss, coagulopathies, and ventricular arrhythmias. Only five dogs lived more than one year. Overall median survival was 2.5 months. The median survival improved to 9 months for dogs without evidence of metastasis at the time of surgery.

In a group of 16 dogs with splenic leiomyosarcoma, five dogs had evidence of multiple organ involvement at laparotomy and were euthanatized. Splenectomy was performed in 11 dogs that survived for a median of 8 months after surgery (range = 1 to 21 months). Nine of 11 developed liver metastases.[32]

One dog with malignant fibrous histiocytoma was treated with doxorubicin but developed hepatic metastases nine months after surgery.[31] Chemotherapy should be considered investigational for this tumor.

INTRA-ABDOMINAL HEMANGIOSARCOMA IN CATS
Incidence, Signalment, and Etiology

Feline hemangiosarcomas are rare tumors that seem equally likely to arise from abdominal organs or from the subcutis.[33,34] In two surveys, hemangiosarcoma arising from abdominal organs accounted for 15 of 31[33] and 25 of 56[34] feline cases. Sites of origin were spleen (16 of 40), mesentery (14), liver (5), intestines (4), and abdominal musculature (1).

Affected cats are usually old (average age = 10 years; range = 5 months to 17 years). There is no obvious gender predilection, although male cats were overrepresented in one study.[33] Most reported cases have been in domestic shorthairs.

Clinical Presentation and History

Most clinical signs are nonspecific and include anorexia, lethargy, and vomiting. More specific signs reported are abdominal distention and, rarely, collapse secondary to hypovolemic shock from bleeding. Most cats have a palpable abdominal mass and are anemic on routine blood work. Schistocytes have not been reported in cats with hemangiosarcoma.

Staging and Diagnosis

A cat with suspected hemangiosarcoma of the abdominal cavity should be staged using blood work, urinalysis, and thoracic radiographs, although clinically detectable pulmonary metastases are rare. Abdominal ultrasonography is recommended prior to definitive treatment to identify involved organs and to screen for metastases.

Hemangiosarcoma of the abdominal cavity apparently is highly metastatic, although at least one report suggested that hepatic hemangiosarcoma was less aggressive, with only two of nine cats showing metastasis.[33,34] Thoracic radiographs at the time of presentation showed no evidence of metastasis in any cat with abdominal hemangiosarcoma, although 9 of 15 cats had evidence of metastasis at necropsy.[33]

Ten of 14 cats with splenic hemangiosarcoma had metastasis either after surgery or at diagnosis. As with dogs, the most common sites of metastasis are the regional lymph nodes and liver.[33,34] Mesenteric hemangiosarcoma is similarly aggressive; 13 of 15 reported tumors metastasized, most often to the liver and other intra-abdominal sites but also to the lungs.[33,34]

Treatment

There are few reports of surgery for abdominal hemangiosarcomas in cats. Of five cats undergoing splenectomy for hemangiosarcoma, survival ranged from 6 to 35 weeks (median = 20 weeks), although four of these cats developed hepatic metastases. No

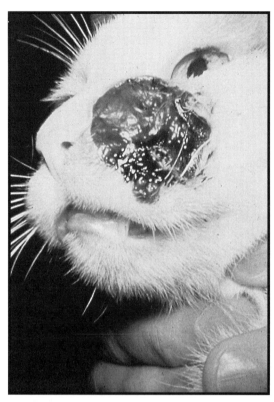

Figure 5-66: *Feline cutaneous hemangiosarcoma is a sunlight-induced (actinic) neoplasm that may be seen in the same location as squamous cell carcinoma in lightly pigmented cats. Cutaneous hemangiosarcoma is frequently proliferative. (Courtesy B.R. Madewell)*

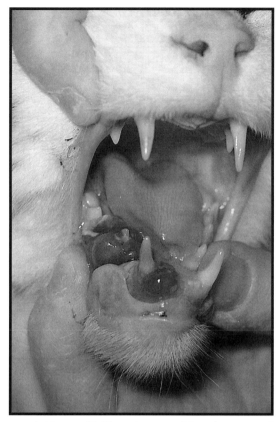

Figure 5-67: *Hemangiosarcoma of the oral cavity in a 6-year-old cat. The metastatic rate of this tumor in extra-abdominal sites is uncertain, but local excision is warranted as long as wide margins can be assured.*

adjuvant chemotherapy has been reported for feline hemangiosarcoma.

CUTANEOUS HEMANGIOSARCOMA IN CATS

Incidence, Signalment, and Etiology

In cats, hemangiosarcoma of the skin occurs with equal prevalence as hemangiosarcoma of all other sites. In two studies, cutaneous hemangiosarcoma accounted for 25 of 56[34] and 13 of 31[33] cases. Signalment for these cats was similar to that for cats with abdominal hemangiosarcoma. In one study, cutaneous hemangiosarcoma occurred in unpigmented skin, implicating solar exposure as a predisposing factor,[35] as is seen in dogs (Figure 5-66).

Clinical Presentation and History

In one study, 8 of 13 cutaneous tumors were located in the inguinal region.[35] In another study, most cutaneous hemangiosarcomas occurred on the head and particularly involved unpigmented skin on the pinnae.[35]

Staging and Diagnosis

Routine staging procedures are recommended as part of a general health screen and to ensure that the lesion is not metastatic from some visceral site.

Cutaneous hemangiosarcoma in cats behaves like a soft tissue sarcoma. It is an infiltrative tumor that rarely metastasizes but often recurs locally after surgery. It may invade adjacent structures, including bone.[33] One of 34 cats with cutaneous hemangiosarcoma[33–35] showed metastasis.[34]

Treatment

Reports of surgical excision have not been favorable, which may, in part, reflect inadequately aggressive surgeries. Aggressive surgery for cutaneous hemangiosarcoma is warranted in affected cats, as the metastatic rate is low. For complete excision, it is necessary to perform surgery with margins of up to 2 cm around the perceived tumor borders and to excise the same distance (or one fascial plane) beneath the tumor. In one study, tumors recurred in 22 of 29 cats.[33–35] Recurrences occurred an average of 16[33] to 34[35] weeks after excision, and some cats were treated with repeated excisions but did not develop distant metastases. Median survival time after surgery was 58 weeks in one study.[33] Adjuvant chemotherapy does not assist in treatment of this disease. Radiation therapy as an adjunct to surgery may assist in treatment, as it does for soft tissue sarcomas; however, there are no reports of its efficacy in treating hemangiosarcomas in cats.

HEMANGIOSARCOMA OF OTHER SITES IN CATS
Incidence, Signalment, and Etiology

Hemangiosarcoma of the right atrium is common in dogs but unreported in cats. Hemangiosarcomas have been reported in cats in the nasal cavity (3 of 87),[33,34] thoracic cavity and anterior mediastinum (3 of 87),[33,34] tongue (2 of 56)[34], and hard palate (1 of 56)[34] (Figure 5-67).

Clinical Presentation and History

Cats with intrathoracic hemangiosarcoma general-

KEY POINTS:

Cutaneous hemangiosarcoma in cats is locally invasive, but metastatic disease seems to be rare.

Hemangiosarcoma of the abdominal cavity in cats seems to be a highly metastatic tumor.

---

ly present with dyspnea arising from hemorrhagic pleural effusion. In one study, however, none of these tumors had metastasized to extrathoracic sites at the time of diagnosis.[33]

Cats with nasal hemangiosarcoma presented with epistaxis in another study.[34] None of the cats with nasal or oral hemangiosarcoma had evidence of metastasis, but there was considerable bony destruction from these tumors.

Treatment

Surgical excision is the treatment of choice for these tumors, although adequate margins in these locations are difficult to obtain. In view of the apparently low metastatic rate for hemangiosarcoma of these sites, external beam radiation therapy may be a consideration, although reports of its efficacy are lacking.

REFERENCES

1. Srebernik N, Appleby EC: Breed prevalence and sites of haemangioma and haemangiosarcoma in dogs. *Vet Rec* 129:408–409, 1991.
2. Ng CY, Mills JN: Clinical and haematological features of haemangiosarcoma in dogs. *Aust Vet J* 62:1–4, 1985.
3. Prymak C, McKee LJ, Goldschmidt MH, Glickman LT: Epidemiologic, clinical, pathologic, and prognostic characteristics of splenic hemangiosarcoma and splenic hematoma in dogs: 217 cases (1985). *JAVMA* 193:706–712, 1988.
4. Brown NO, Patnaik AK, MacEwen EG: Canine hemangiosarcoma: Retrospective analysis of 104 cases. *JAVMA* 186:56–58, 1985.
5. Spangler WL, Culbertson MR: Prevalence, type, and importance of splenic diseases in dogs: 1,480 cases (1985–1989). *JAVMA* 200:829–834, 1992.
6. Popper H, Thomas LB, Telles NC, et al: Development of hepatic angiosarcoma in man induced by vinyl chloride, thorotrast and arsenic. *Am J Pathol* 92:349–376, 1978.
7. Johnson KA, Powers BE, Withrow SJ, et al: Splenomegaly in dogs: Predictors of neoplasia and survival after splenectomy. *J Vet Intern Med* 3:160–166, 1989.

MANAGEMENT OF SPECIFIC DISEASES

8. Sorenmo KU, Jeglum KA, Helfand SC: Chemotherapy of canine hemangiosarcoma with doxorubicin and cyclophosphamide. *J Vet Intern Med* 7:370–376, 1993.

9. Wrigley RH, Park RD, Knode LJ, Lebel JL: Ultrasonographic features of splenic hemangiosarcoma in dogs: 18 cases (1980–1986). *JAVMA* 192:1113–1117, 1988.

10. Waters DJ, Caywood DD, Hayden DW, Klausner JS: Metastatic pattern in dogs with splenic haemangiosarcoma: Clinical implications. *J Small Anim Pract* 29:805–814, 1988.

11. O'Keefe DA, Couto CG: Fine-needle aspiration of the spleen as an aid in the diagnosis of splenomegaly. *J Vet Intern Med* 1:102–109, 1987.

12. Hammer AS, Couto CG, Filppi J, et al: Efficacy and toxicity of VAC chemotherapy (vincristine, doxorubicin, and cyclophosphamide) in dogs with hemangiosarcoma. *J Vet Intern Med* 5:160–166, 1991.

13. Wood CA, Moore AS, Gliatto JG, et al: Prognosis for dogs with stage I or stage II splenic hemangiosarcoma treated by splenectomy alone: 32 cases (1991–1993). *JAVMA*, in press.

14. Keyes ML, Rush JE, Autran de Morais HS, Couto CG: Ventricular arrhythmias in dogs with splenic masses. *Vet Emerg Crit Care* 3:33–38, 1994.

15. Ogilvie GK, Powers BE, Mallinckrodt CH, Withrow SJ: Doxorubicin chemotherapy and surgery for hemangiosarcoma in the dog. *Proc 14th Ann Vet Cancer Soc*:39–40, 1994.

16. MacEwen EG, Kurzman I, Vail DM, et al: Preliminary report of a randomized clinical trial on the efficacy of liposome-encapsulated muramyl tripeptide phosphatidylethanolamine (L-MTP-PE) immunotherapy for the treatment of splenic hemangiosarcoma in the dog. *Vet Cancer Soc Newsletter* 17:6–7, 1994.

17. Kleine LJ, Zook BC, Munson TO: Primary cardiac hemangiosarcomas in dogs. *JAVMA* 157:326–337, 1970.

18. Aronson M: Cardiac hemangiosarcoma in the dog. A review of 38 cases. *JAVMA* 187:326–337, 1985.

19. Holt D, Van Winkle T, Schelling C, Prymak C: Correlation between thoracic radiographs and postmortem findings in dogs with hemangiosarcoma: 77 cases (1984–1989). *JAVMA* 200:1535–1539, 1992.

20. Madrone DE, Helfand SC, Stebbins KE: Use of chemotherapy for treatment of cardiac hemangiosarcoma in a dog. *JAVMA* 190:887–891, 1987.

21. Berg RJ, Wingfield W: Pericardial effusion in the dog: A review of 42 cases. *JAAHA* 20:721–730, 1984.

22. Hargis AM, Ihrke PJ, Spangler WL, Stannard AA: A retrospective clinicopathologic study of 212 dogs with cutaneous hemangiomas and hemangiosarcomas. *Vet Pathol* 29:316–328, 1992.

23. Nikula KJ, Benjamin SA, Angleton GM, et al: Ultraviolet radiation, solar dermatosis, and cutaneous neoplasia in beagle dogs. *Radiat Res* 129:11–18, 1992.

24. Oksanen A: Hemangiosarcoma in dogs. *J Comp Pathol* 88:585–595, 1978.

25. Ward H, Fox LE, Calderwood-Mays MP, et al: Cutaneous hemangiosarcoma in 25 dogs: A retrospective study. *J Vet Intern Med* 8:345–348, 1994.

26. Hargis AM, Feldman BF: Evaluation of hemostatic defects secondary to vascular tumors in dogs: 11 cases (1983–1988). *JAVMA* 198:891–894, 1991.

27. Pirkey-Ehrhart N, Straw RC, Withrow SJ, et al: Primary rib tumors in 54 dogs. *JAAHA*, 1994, in press.

28. Parchman MB, Crameri FM: Primary veterbral hemangiosarcoma in a dog. *JAVMA* 194:79–81, 1989.

29. Hayden DW, Bartges JW, Bell FW, Klausner JS: Prostatic hemangiosarcoma in a dog: Clinical and pathological findings. *J Vet Diagn Invest* 4:209–211, 1992.

30. Weinstein MJ, Carpenter JL, Schunk-Mehlaff CJ: Nonangiogenic and nonlymphomatous sarcomas of the canine spleen: 57 cases (1975–1987). *JAVMA* 195:784–788, 1989.

31. Hendrick MJ, Brooks JJ, Bruce EH: Six cases of malignant fibrous histiocytoma of the canine spleen. *Vet Pathol* 29:351–354, 1992.

32. Kapatkin AS, Mullen HS, Matthiesen DT, Patnaik AK: Leiomyosarcoma in dogs: 44 cases (1983–1988). *JAVMA* 201:1077–1079, 1992.

33. Scavelli TD, Patnaik AK, Mehlaff CJ, Hayes AA: Hemangiosarcoma in the cat: Retrospective evaluation of 31 surgical cases. *JAVMA* 187:817–819, 1985.

34. Carpenter JL, Andrews LK, Holzworth J: Tumors and tumor-like lesions, in Holzworth J (ed): *Diseases of the Cat. Medicine and Surgery*. Philadelphia, WB Saunders, 1987, pp 406–596.

35. Miller MA, Ramos JA, Kreeger JM: Cutaneous vascular neoplasia in 15 cats: Clinical, morphologic, and immunohistochemical studies. *Vet Pathol* 29:329–336, 1992.

CLINICAL BRIEFING: TUMORS OF THE ENDOCRINE SYSTEM

Hyperadrenocorticism in Dogs

Common Clinical Presentation	Hypercortisolism, polydipsia, polyuria, and cutaneous changes; nervous system dysfunction with large pituitary tumors
Common Histologic Types	Pituitary adenomas of pars distalis in 80% of dogs; less commonly, adrenal gland tumors (usually carcinomas)
Epidemiology and Biological Behavior	Middle-aged to old dogs; poodles, dachshunds, and boxers at higher risk; no gender predilection; metastasis rare for pituitary tumors but common for adrenal tumors
Prognostic Factors	None identified

Treatment
  Surgery
  Medical Management
 	
  Radiation Therapy
	Treatment of choice for adrenal tumors
	For pituitary tumors, mitotane and ketoconazole offer good long-term palliation by their effects of adrenal cortical destruction and interference with steroid synthesis, respectively; L-deprenyl may also be a useful agent; mitotane (o,p'-DDD) may be a useful agent at high doses for adrenal tumors
	Provides good palliation for neurologic dysfunction caused by large pituitary tumors and gives moderate control of cortisol levels

Insulinoma in Dogs

Common Clinical Presentation	Hypoglycemia and hyperinsulinemia; tachycardia and neurologic signs may be intermittent; peripheral polyneuropathy may cause tetraparesis
Common Histologic Type	Carcinoma
Epidemiology and Biological Behavior	Old dogs with no gender predisposition; large-breed dogs more commonly affected; most tumors are highly metastatic

MANAGEMENT OF SPECIFIC DISEASES

Prognostic Factors	Dogs with tumors confined to pancreas have a longer symptom-free period and survival after surgery; dogs that only have lymph node metastases live longer than dogs with distant metastases

Treatment
    Surgery
    Medical Management
 	
    Chemotherapy
	Treatment of choice for localized tumors
	Prednisone, diazoxide, sandostatin (octreotide), and propanolol may control hypoglycemia
	Streptozocin and alloxan may be effective; however, both may be renal toxins in dogs

Thyroid Tumors in Dogs

Common Clinical Presentation	Mass in ventral neck; rarely, signs of hyperthyroidism
Common Histologic Type	Adenocarcinoma
Epidemiology and Biological Behavior	Old dogs; no gender predilection; beagles, golden retrievers, and boxers predisposed; local invasion is common; moderate metastatic rate
Prognostic Factors	Dogs with invasive tumors ("fixed" to underlying tissues) or large tumors have worse survival rates; not correlated with histologic type, age, breed, or gender

Treatment
    Surgery
 	
    Radiation Therapy
 	
    Chemotherapy
	Curative for adenomas; may provide long-term control for small, noninvasive carcinomas, but these have potential to metastasize
	External beam radiation may improve local control or reduce size of mass before surgery; radioactive iodine (^{131}I) may cause regression in active hormonal tumors (which are rarely seen in dogs)
	Cisplatin and doxorubicin both have antitumor activity in adenocarcinomas, and both may have an adjunctive role with surgery

Thyroid Tumors in Cats

Common Clinical Presentation	Hyperthyroidism with associated cardiac and hypermetabolic changes; peritracheal mass may be palpable

MANAGEMENT OF SPECIFIC DISEASES

Common Histologic Types	Adenoma; carcinomas are rare
Epidemiology and Biological Behavior	Old cats; no gender or breed predisposition
Prognostic Factors	None identified
Treatment **Supportive Treatment**	For example, propranolol and diltiazem, particularly for cardiac conditions
Medical Management	Methimazole and carbimazole reduce circulating thyroid hormone levels, but long-term use requires dosage increase
Surgery	As tumors are often bilateral, both glands should be removed; hypoparathyroidism or hypothyroidism may occur but is usually of short duration
Radiation Therapy	Radioactive iodine (^{131}I) gives good response with prolonged remissions and few side effects; may also palliate effects of thyroid carcinoma
Other Tumors Reviewed	
Gastrinoma, pheochromocytoma, parathyroid tumor, chemodectoma, and growth-hormone secreting tumors	

ENDOCRINE NEOPLASIA

The major effect of most neoplasms is functional impairment of an organ or structure. Tumors of the endocrine system also affect the host by producing hormones at elevated levels.

HYPERADRENOCORTICISM IN DOGS
Pituitary-Dependent Hyperadrenocorticism
Incidence, Signalment, and Etiology

Hyperadrenocorticism is the most common endocrinopathy in dogs. Affected dogs are middle-aged to old (>6 years of age). Neither sex is predisposed. Poodles, dachshunds, and boxers are at increased risk. Adenoma of the pars distalis of the pituitary is the most common tumor in this disease, although pars intermedia tumors also have been described.

Clinical Presentation and History

Eighty to 85% of dogs with hyperadrenocorticism have a secretory tumor of the pituitary gland that is usually a microadenoma. Dogs with hyperadrenocorticism show signs of polydipsia, polyuria, polyphagia, and biochemical abnormalities as well as cutaneous and haircoat changes. These signs are reviewed in detail elsewhere.[1] Occasionally, the tumor is large and clinical signs are complicated by tumor expansion into the hypothalamus. Dogs with pituitary macroadenomas or macroadenocarcinomas may show central nervous system signs of mental dullness, disorientation, ataxia, blindness, or convulsions.

Staging and Diagnosis

Hyperadrenocorticism can be confirmed by a low-dose dexamethasone-suppression (LDDS) test in which an injection of 0.01 or 0.015 mg/kg dexamethasone is given intravenously. Pretreatment and 4- and 8-hour posttreatment serum samples are collected for cortisol levels. Failure to suppress cortisol levels below 1.5 µg/dl indicates hyperadrenocorticism.

MANAGEMENT OF SPECIFIC DISEASES

Other tests helpful in diagnosing this disease are adrenocorticotropic (ACTH) hormone-response test, a high-dose dexamethasone-suppression (HDDS) test (1 mg/kg IV), plasma ACTH level, and urine cortisol-to-creatinine ratio.[1] Failure to suppress to a level less than 1.5 µg/dl in response to a HDDS test at 3 and 8 hours suggests pituitary-dependent hyperadrenocorticism. In addition to routine blood work and thoracic radiographs as a general health screen, abdominal radiographs should be obtained. Ultrasonography may be helpful in imaging bilateral adrenal hypertrophy. Macroadenoma of the pituitary gland can be confirmed by computed tomography (CT) scan or magnetic resonance imaging (MRI).

Treatment

Surgery. For pituitary-dependent hyperadrenocorticism, surgical hypophysectomy or bilateral adrenalectomy has been successful.[2] With either approach, excellent surgical skills, close postoperative monitoring, and lifelong hormonal supplementation are required; therefore, medical management is recommended.

Medical Therapy. Mitotane (o,p'-DDD; Lysodren®, Bristol-Myers, NJ) is selectively cytotoxic to the adrenal cortex. Mitotane is often administered in two phases: a high induction dose and a lower maintenance dose. For induction of remission, mitotane is given at 50 to 75 mg/kg PO in divided daily doses for 10 to 14 days. Prednisone (0.2 mg/kg/day) can be given concurrently to help reduce toxic side effects; however, the question of when and even whether to use prednisone is controversial. Anorexia, vomiting, and weakness are toxicoses that necessitate temporary cessation of mitotane therapy. ACTH-stimulation tests should be performed at 7- to 14-day intervals until serum cortisol levels fall to below 1.0 µg/dl. Prednisone is withheld on days when testing is performed because it would elevate cortisol values. A maintenance dose of mitotane at 100 to 200

> **KEY POINT:**
>
> *Ketoconazole can control signs of hyperadrenocorticism prior to surgery in dogs with an adrenal tumor.*

mg/kg/week is given in divided doses with periodic ACTH-response tests to monitor the effectiveness of treatment.[1] The disease is considered well controlled if ACTH-stimulation tests indicate that precortisol and postcortisol rates are at, or somewhat below, normal levels.

An alternative protocol suggests destroying the adrenal cortices with high-dose mitotane, after which hypoadrenocorticism requires lifelong glucocorticoid and mineralocorticoid supplementation.[3] With this protocol, recurrence of signs is uncommon. Investigators believed that it was superior to conventional mitotane therapy for symptom and toxicity control. The protocol was also useful for treatment of adrenal tumors (ATs) and occasionally resolved all evidence of grossly measurable tumor. The protocol is discussed below. Before starting treatment, however, the reader is advised to read the original article.[3] Briefly, mitotane (50–75 mg/kg) is given daily for 25 days in divided doses with meals. On the third treatment day, supplementation is started with cortisone acetate (2 mg/kg divided BID until 1 week after mitotane is stopped, then 1 mg/kg divided BID), fludrocortisone acetate (0.0125 mg/kg SID) and NaCl (0.1 mg/kg divided into two or three meals).[3] Strict owner compliance and good veterinary support is required, particularly in the early stages of mitotane therapy when the risk of hypoadrenocorticism is highest. A repeat ACTH-response test one week after mitotane therapy has ended, particularly for ATs, ensures that functional adrenal cortical tissue has been destroyed. Measurement of serum electrolytes should be made at this time and at least every three to six months thereafter.

Ketoconazole (Nizoral®, Janssen, NJ) is an antifungal agent that acts to block adrenal and gonadal steroid synthesis in dogs. Unlike mitotane, it is not cytotoxic and has been recommended to control the signs of hyperadrenocorticism in specific situations: (1) For medical management of dogs with ATs that are malignant or when surgery is not an

MANAGEMENT OF SPECIFIC DISEASES

option, (2) in dogs with hyperadrenocorticism that cannot be treated with mitotane because of drug toxicity, and (3) prior to surgery in dogs with an adrenal tumor. Ketoconazole is effective in rapidly reducing cortisol secretion (within 30 minutes of administration).

Ketoconazole is given at a dose of 5 mg/kg BID PO for one week. If side effects (e.g., hepatopathy) are absent, the dose is doubled. If there is no improvement in the ACTH-response test after 14 days, the dose may be increased to 15 mg/kg BID PO. The ACTH-response test should be started within 1 to 3 hours of the last ketoconazole dosage. In a series of 43 dogs, eight (20%) did not respond to ketoconazole therapy; however, toxicity was rare, and overdosage resulting in hypoadrenocorticism was unusual.[4] When overdosage occurred, ketoconazole was simply suspended and glucocorticoid supplementation was provided. The response was rapid, and within days, ketoconazole could be reinitiated.

L-deprenyl is a drug that indirectly acts to increase dopamine levels. At a dose of 2 mg/kg PO daily, this agent caused significant clinical and biochemical improvement in 30 dogs with pituitary dependent hyperadrenocorticism.[6]

Radiation Therapy. For dogs with confirmed macroadenoma of the pituitary, 40 to 45 Gy of megavoltage radiation to the tumor and 1 cm of surrounding normal tissue resolves neurologic signs within six months of therapy in all reported cases.[5] Resolution of signs of hyperadrenocorticism is more variable. Radiation alone decreased ACTH levels in some dogs to normal, whereas others required concurrent o,p'-DDD therapy. Hypopituitarism was not noted in any of the dogs treated (see the chapter on Tumors of the Nervous System).

Canine Adrenocortical Tumors
Incidence, Signalment, and Etiology

The majority of dogs with hyperadrenocorticism have a secretory pituitary tumor. In 15% to 20%, however, the cause of hyperadrenocorticism is adrenal tumors, of which approximately half are malignant carcinomas.

Clinical Presentation and History

Excessive cortisol produces classic signs of hyperadrenocorticism, including polydipsia, polyuria, cutaneous changes, and biochemical abnormalities. These abnormalities are reviewed in greater detail elsewhere.[1]

Staging and Diagnosis

Hyperadrenocorticism is confirmed by a low-dose dexamethasone-suppression test or an adrenocorticotrophic hormone-stimulation test (see previous section on pages 383–384). A high-dose dexamethasone-suppression (HDDS) test may suggest the presence of an adrenal tumor if the serum cortisol is not suppressed (i.e., remains above 1.5 μg/dl at 3 and 8 hours post injection). It is equally likely, however, that a dog with cortisol levels unaffected by an HDDS test has nonsuppressible pituitary-dependent hyperadrenocorticism (PDH).[7] In dogs with ATs, measurement of plasma ACTH levels should be undetectable to low; however, ACTH is labile, and samples must be handled very carefully to ensure valid results.[1]

Adrenal masses may be difficult to image. A mineralized adrenal mass may be seen on radiographs in 25% to 50% of dogs with an adrenal tumor and can be associated with malignancy. In one study, an adrenal tumor was detected radiographically in only eight of 31 dogs.[7] Ultrasonography is a more sensitive, but nonspecific, diagnostic aid that may enable visualization of other abdominal organs for evidence of metastases. In one study, ultrasonography was successfully used to detect 6 of 13 adrenal masses.[7] Computed tomography (CT scan) was most successful in visualizing an adrenal mass and obtained a positive finding in 11 of 11 dogs[7] (Figure 5-68).

Metastasis is common from carcinomas. It usually occurs to the liver but can also affect the lungs; however, metastases may not be detectable clinically for months to years after initial diagnosis.[7] Screening dogs with ATs for metastatic disease prior to surgery or mitotane therapy requires thoracic radiographs and abdominal ultrasonography.

Treatment

Surgical removal is the treatment of choice for ATs.

MANAGEMENT OF SPECIFIC DISEASES

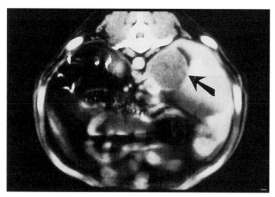

Figure 5-68: *Computed tomography (CT) is more successful than either ultrasonography or radiography in distinguishing an adrenal tumor. In this CT scan, a cystic right adrenal tumor is seen* (arrow). *(Courtesy A.S. Tidwell)*

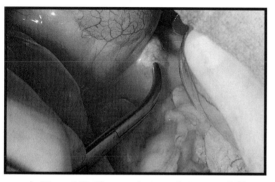

Figure 5-69: *If computed tomography is not available, surgical exploration may be necessary to demonstrate an adrenal mass, as pictured. The contralateral adrenal gland is usually atrophied as a result of cortisol secretion by the affected adrenal and therefore suppression of ACTH. (Courtesy J. Berg)*

Atrophy of the contralateral adrenal gland is a consistent finding with ATs (Figure 5-69). Exogenous glucocorticoids are required until the contralateral gland regains function.[8] On the morning before surgery, large doses of intravenous steroids should be given (5 mg/kg soluble hydrocortisone, 2.0 mg/kg prednisone sodium succinate, or 0.1 to 0.2 mg/kg dexamethasone). Just prior to surgery, dogs with ATs should be treated with 15 mg/kg of ketoconazole to normalize adrenocortical function and thereby

improve surgical outcome. Ketoconazole rapidly reduces cortisol secretion within 30 minutes of administration. After surgery, the preoperative dose of steroids should be repeated. On the first postoperative day, 0.5 mg/kg prednisolone or prednisone BID, 2.5 mg/kg cortisone BID, or 0.1 mg/kg dexamethasone every 24 hours should be given. The dose of steroids can be tapered to maintenance by 7 to 10 days and usually can be discontinued by 2 months after surgery. If both adrenal glands are enlarged, non–dexamethasone-suppressible PDH should be suspected, and biopsy of an adrenal gland should be performed to confirm the diagnosis.

In a recent review of 25 dogs undergoing surgery for an adrenal tumor, 50% of the dogs that were not euthanatized during surgery developed serious complications, including cardiac arrest, pneumonia, pulmonary artery thromboembolism, pancreatitis, and acute renal failure. In another review of 10 dogs with ATs,[9] however, complications following surgery were minimal. Surgical excision of adenomas is often curative. Surgery also may be curative for carcinomas if metastasis has not occurred.

Dogs with hyperadrenocorticism caused by ATs are generally more resistant to mitotane than those with pituitary tumors.[10] Treatment with mitotane results in fair to good control of cortisol levels in dogs with adrenocortical adenomas. For dogs with small carcinomas, similar results can be achieved with mitotane but the duration of control is shorter. In dogs with large adrenocortical carcinomas or metastases, mitotane provides short-term palliation of signs; however, the high doses necessary to achieve these results are usually associated with unacceptable toxicity.[7] Mitotane was used to treat 32 dogs with ATs at doses that ranged from 27.5 mg/kg to 75.0 mg/kg (average 46.3 mg/kg) for 10 to 14 days. After two weeks, 14 of 32 dogs were still hyperadrenocorticoid and higher doses of mitotane were required for a further period (median = 30 days) to control their disease. Signs were controlled in 30 dogs for periods ranging from 24 days to 4.9 years (median = 10.5 months); it was more difficult to achieve control in dogs with metastatic disease.[7]

MANAGEMENT OF SPECIFIC DISEASES

HYPERADRENOCORTICISM IN CATS
Incidence, Signalment, and Etiology

This rare condition predominantly affects old, female cats.

Clinical Presentation and History

Affected cats are polydipsic and polyuric from glucocorticoid-induced hyperglycemia with subsequent glucosuria. Chronic or recurrent infections may occur. Polyphagia and hair loss affect the majority of cats with hyperadrenocorticism.

Staging and Diagnosis

The ACTH-response test is a useful screening test for cats, but the LDDS test appears unreliable. The HDDS test for hyperadrenocorticism in cats (1–2 mg/kg IV) is the best way to distinguish pituitary-based from adrenal disease.[11]

Treatment

Cats seem susceptible to mitotane toxicity because of their sensitivity to chlorinated hydrocarbons, and doses of mitotane low enough to avoid toxicity in cats are unable to suppress the adrenal cortex. Bilateral adrenalectomy followed by mineralocorticoid and glucocorticoid replacement seems better tolerated in cats than in dogs and may be the treatment of choice. No postoperative complications were reported in five cats treated in this manner.[11]

INSULINOMA IN DOGS

Insulinomas are functional, insulin-secreting β-cell tumors of the pancreas. Excessive insulin secretion by the tumor causes clinical signs of hypoglycemia.

Incidence, Signalment, and Etiology

The mean age of onset of clinical signs in dogs with insulinoma is between 8 and 10 years (range = 4–14 years).[12–14] There is no apparent gender predisposition. Although insulinomas are reported in all sizes and many breeds, large-breed dogs, such as Irish setters, golden retrievers, boxers, and German shepherds are most frequently afflicted.[12,13] The disease is rare in cats but is quite common in ferrets.

Clinical Presentation and History

Clinical signs of hypoglycemia fall into two categories: adrenergic and neuroglucopenic.[15] When glucose concentrations fall rapidly, increased sympathetic tone may produce such adrenergic signs as tachycardia, nervousness, tremors, and hunger. With a more gradual decrease in blood glucose, neuroglucopenic signs may include seizures, dullness, weakness, confusion, and hypothermia. Signs may be episodic and may be related to events such as fasting, eating, or exercise. Studies indicate no correlation between stage of disease and clinical signs.[12]

A syndrome of peripheral polyneuropathy associated with canine (as well as human) insulinoma has been described.[16] One dog was presented with tetraparesis/paralysis after at least eight months of documented symptomatic hypoglycemia.[17] The pathophysiology of this remains unclear. Current hypotheses explain this syndrome as (1) a metabolic defect of peripheral nerves that renders them susceptible to hypoglycemia, (2) an immune response arising from similarity between tumor and nervous-tissue antigens, and (3) toxic effects at peripheral nerves caused by tumor-produced substances.

Staging and Diagnosis

Insulinomas have been categorized as stage I (confined to pancreas), stage II (confined to pancreas and regional lymph nodes), and stage III (distant metastasis).[12] This staging system has some prognostic importance.

The only consistent abnormality seen on chemistry profiles is hypoglycemia; however, glucose concentrations may be within the normal range. Diagnosis is based on demonstration of excessive insulin secretion concurrent with hypoglycemia. Several methods demonstrate these findings. In normal, fasted animals,

> **KEY POINT:**
>
> *High doses of mitotane may be necessary to control signs in dogs with an adrenocortical carcinoma.*

MANAGEMENT OF SPECIFIC DISEASES

insulin levels decrease as glucose concentration falls. If initial testing for insulinoma fails to show simultaneous hypoglycemia and increased insulin levels, the animal is re-tested. Glucose levels are monitored periodically during fasting until glucose falls below a prescribed level, usually 60 mg/dl. At that time, serum insulin and glucose are measured.

Although controversial, results are interpreted in light of insulin:glucose, glucose:insulin, and/or amended insulin:glucose ratios. An insulin:glucose ratio of greater than 0.3 or a glucose:insulin ratio of less than 2.5 supports the diagnosis of insulinoma. The amended insulin:glucose ratio (AIGR) is calculated as follows:

$$(\text{Serum insulin } [\mu U/ml] \times 100) \div (\text{Serum glucose } [mg/\mu l] - 30) = AIGR$$

A result of greater than 30 indicates insulinoma.[14] The AIGR has been reported to be the most sensitive but least specific of these tests (i.e., it provides the fewest false-negative but the most false-positive results).[13] The test is particularly misleading when glucose concentrations are extremely low (less than 30). Therefore, the diagnosis of insulinoma should not be based solely on an abnormal AIGR. It is important to recognize that dogs with low blood glucose should have a low blood–insulin level; any other finding (normal to high insulin level) must be considered abnormal. Provocative tests of insulin release can be used but are not often necessary. In a fasted patient, glucose, glucagon, or tolbutamide are administered to release excess insulin from neoplastic cells. These tests are not without risk, however; tolbutamide, in particular, may cause severe and prolonged hypoglycemia and seizures.

Because tumors are small, ultrasonographic examination may not be revealing; however, ultrasonography may reveal metastases to lymph nodes or other abdominal viscera. CT scans in human patients are complementary to ultrasonography. In dogs, defini-

KEY POINT:

Prolonged hypoglycemia due to insulinoma may result in a peripheral polyneuropathy.

tive diagnosis is usually confirmed by exploratory laparotomy and histopathologic examination. Careful abdominal exploration, including abdominal lymph node palpation and gentle digital palpation of the pancreas, is important. Metastasis occurs in approximately half the cases, and pancreatic masses may not be readily visualized.[15]

Prognostic Factors

In several studies, mean survival for all dogs with insulinoma has been estimated at about 12 months. Young dogs have shorter survival times than old dogs. For 52 dogs treated by surgery, dogs with stage I tumors had mean hypoglycemia-free intervals of 14 months, which was significantly longer than dogs with either lymph node or distant metastases; dogs with stage II tumors also lived longer than dogs that had distant metastases at the time of surgery.[12] (Figure 5-70).

Treatment
Surgery

The treatment of choice is wide surgical excision (partial pancreatectomy) in conjunction with preop-

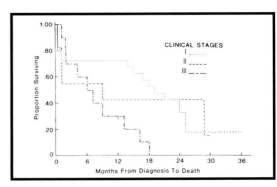

Figure 5-70: *Dogs with stage I insulinoma (confined to the pancreas) have longer symptom-free survival than dogs with metastases. Dogs with both stage I and stage II (regional node metastasis) insulinoma live longer than dogs with distant metastases (stage III). (From Caywood DD, Klausner JS, O'Leary TP, et al: Pancreatic insulin-secreting neoplasms: Clinical, diagnostic and prognostic features in 73 dogs. JAAHA 24:577–584, 1988; with permission.)*

erative and/or postoperative medical management. Mean survival is longer in dogs that undergo surgical resection than in dogs that receive medical management alone.[13] Masses are reportedly distributed equally between the two limbs of the pancreas (Figure 5-71). Metastasis most commonly occurs to regional lymph nodes and liver, although it has been reported in mesentery, spleen, duodenum, and spinal cord. One source recommends removing one half of the pancreas when tumor is not visualized at surgery, in an attempt to remove the portion that contains tumor.[14]

A 5% glucose solution should be infused intravenously during and after surgery to prevent hypoglycemia. Preoperative and postoperative glucocorticoid therapy is also important. Adequate fluid therapy perioperatively is necessary to prevent secondary pancreatitis, ensuring good circulation through the pancreatic microvasculature. A fluid rate of two times maintenance levels has been recommended.[15]

Postoperative complications include iatrogenic pancreatitis, diabetes mellitus that requires insulin therapy for variable intervals (up to 1118 days in one study),[13] hypoglycemia, and persistent seizures that continue despite resolution of hypoglycemia. Diabetes mellitus is believed to be caused by inadequate insulin secretion by atrophied normal β cells. Persistent seizures are attributed to cerebral laminar necrosis secondary to prolonged hypoglycemia.

Medical Management
Medical management is indicated if surgery does not eliminate the insulin-secreting tumor or if surgery is not performed. In some dogs, frequent feedings of small, high-protein, low-carbohydrate meals, in addition to exercise restriction, may control hypoglycemia. If this fails, drug therapy must begin.

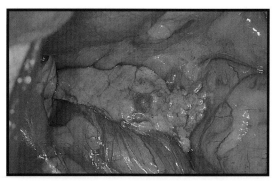

Figure 5-71: *Exploratory laparotomy is usually required to identify an insulinoma, as these tumors are frequently very small. Regional lymph nodes and the liver should be examined carefully for evidence of metastatic spread. (Courtesy J. Berg)*

KEY POINTS:

Dogs with low blood glucose should have a low blood insulin level; any other insulin level must be considered abnormal.

Dogs with insulinoma confined to the pancreas at surgery have longer survival times than dogs with metastasis to the lymph nodes or distant sites.

Diazoxide (Proglycem®, Pioneer Pharmaceuticals, NJ) is a nondiuretic, benzothiadiazine, antihypertensive drug with anti-insulin effects. It inhibits insulin secretion by blocking calcium mobilization, stimulates hepatic gluconeogenesis and glycogenolysis through stimulation of the β-adrenergic system, and decreases peripheral glucose utilization. In one study, diazoxide controlled hypoglycemia in 70% of dogs treated.[13] The recommended initial dose is 10 mg/kg/day PO three times a day; the dose may be increased gradually to 40 mg/kg/day.[13] The most common side effects are anorexia, vomiting, and diarrhea, which may be alleviated by administration with a meal.

Other drugs used to treat insulinomas include prednisone, somatostatin, octreotide, propranolol, alloxan, and streptozocin. If prednisone is used as the initial treatment, a dose of 0.5 mg/kg/day divided BID is used; this can be gradually increased to 4 to 6 mg/kg/day, if necessary. Prednisone can be administered in conjunction with diazoxide. Sandostatin® (Sandoz, NJ) is a somatostatin analogue that inhibits insulin synthesis and secretion. Octreotide is a long-acting somatostatin analogue that effectively controlled clinical signs in 5 dogs for 9 to 12 months at a dose of 10 to 20 µg BID–TID.[18] Propranolol (Propranolol®, Danbury Pharmaceutical, CT) suppresses the insulin response to glucose and has been used in humans to induce hyperglycemia. Chemotherapy with nitrosourea and streptozocin has been effective in human patients with insulinoma. Streptozocin (Zanosar®, Upjohn, MI) is selectively cytotoxic to β cells, although its clinical use in dogs has been limited by nephrotoxicity. Initial reports of toxicities of this drug were compromised by high dosages and lack of pretreatment hydration.[19,20] Further evaluation of this drug is warranted. Alloxan is also selectively cytotoxic to β cells. At a dose of 5 mg/kg administered once to normal dogs, 2 of 5 dogs developed hyperglycemia for many months.[21] Alloxan can be nephrotoxic. Other chemotherapeutic agents have not been evaluated in the treatment of canine insulinoma; however, L-asparaginase may reverse hypoglycemia by inhibition of protein (insulin) synthesis.[22]

THYROID TUMORS IN DOGS

Thyroid tumors are relatively uncommon and account for less than 2% of all canine tumors. Most of those reported are malignant (carcinomas), and approximately one third have radiographically detectable metastases at the time of diagnosis. Between 40% and 80% of thyroid carcinomas metastasize at some point in their clinical course.

Incidence, Signalment, and Etiology

Old dogs are most commonly affected (average age = 9.6 years). Beagles, boxers, and golden retrievers are at greater risk for developing thyroid carcinomas than other breeds.[23,24]

Clinical Presentation and History

Thyroid adenomas are rarely detected clinically and are usually an incidental necropsy finding. In contrast, thyroid carcinomas are usually recognized

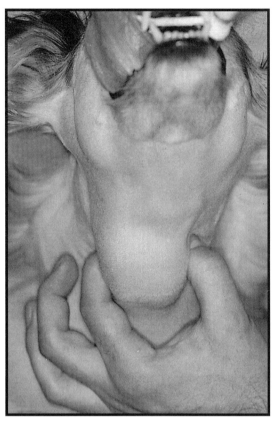

Figure 5-72: *A large palpable mass in the area of the thyroid should be suspected of being a thyroid carcinoma. Adenomas are rarely clinically detectable. (Courtesy J. Berg)*

by the owner as a mass in the ventral neck. This mass may be unilateral or, rarely, bilateral[23,24] (Figure 5-72). Occasionally, these masses may have been present for as long as two years.[24]

Most dogs with thyroid carcinoma are euthyroid, and some may be hypothyroid, presumably through inhibition of pituitary thyrotropin (TSH) secretion by tumor production of biologically inactive thyroid hormones or because the normal thyroid tissue is destroyed. Canine thyroid carcinomas can, rarely, be hyperfunctional. Clinical signs most commonly observed in dogs include polydipsia, polyuria, and weight loss despite adequate caloric intake. Restlessness, heat intolerance, and panting are less common signs.

MANAGEMENT OF SPECIFIC DISEASES

Staging and Diagnosis

Surgical biopsy and even fine-needle aspiration may cause considerable bleeding, so care should be taken when biopsying thyroid masses; the surgeon should be prepared to do a definitive resection if bleeding is excessive. Biopsy should be done via a midline approach through the sternothyroidohyoideus muscle to avoid "seeding" tumor cells into the tissue along the jugular furrow, where future excision would be difficult. Excisional biopsy is rarely complete, especially when the tumor is fixed (indicating invasion of associated structures). Pulmonary metastasis following invasion of the cranial and caudal thyroid veins occurs early in the course of the disease; this is followed by spread to regional lymph nodes (retropharyngeal or caudal cervical) and eventual invasion of the jugular veins and associated neck structures. Metastasis is clinically detectable in 30% to 40% of dogs with thyroid carcinoma at the time of diagnosis.[25,26] Histopathologic evidence of follicular patterns in thyroid carcinomas is associated with more aggressive behavior and metastasis than other tumor types. All types may metastasize, however.

Thyroid carcinomas may arise from ectopic mediastinal thyroid tissue and have been reported at the heart base.[27] Staging of the tumor should include thoracic radiographs (e.g., dorsoventral and right and left lateral), palpation of regional lymph nodes, and fine-needle aspiration of enlarged nodes. Radiographs of the cervical area are unlikely to be helpful. Nuclear scintigraphy of the thyroid may be useful in some cases. Thyroxine (T_4) and triiodothyronine (T_3) tests are also indicated prior to surgery. Dogs with thyroid neoplasms apparently are at higher risk of developing other primary tumors.[28] When staging dogs with thyroid carcinoma, the clinician should be aware that other tumor types may be encountered.

Canine functional thyroid carcinomas are rare. However, even when resting T_3 and T_4 levels are within normal range, the thyroid malignancy may still concentrate technetium pertechnetate (^{99m}Tc) and radioactive iodine (^{125}I, ^{123}I, and ^{131}I)[23] (Figure 5-73). Lung metastases occasionally may be seen on scintigraphy but not be radiographically apparent.[23] Scintigraphy with ^{99m}Tc imaged both benign and malignant thyroid tumors in 29 dogs regardless of their thyroid-hormone status (i.e., euthyroid versus hypothyroid versus hyperthyroid)[29]. Heterogeneous uptake was associated with histologic evidence of capsular invasion in most cases. Pertechnetate scintigraphy was as sensitive as thoracic radiographs in detecting metastasis; however, gross evidence of metastatic disease is uncommon at the time of diagnosis. Accumulation of pertechnetate by a thyroid tumor does not necessarily mean that the tumor will respond to treatment with radioactive iodine. Therefore, in dogs with thyroid tumors, a pertechnetate scan may not be of great benefit other than as a diagnostic tool or as a screening test to look for ectopic tumor tissue or an ancillary aid to diagnosis of a cervical mass. Radioactive iodine scans are more specific and provide more information regarding therapy; however, these studies require longer hospitalization because of the longer half-life of radioactive iodine compounds, and so create a radiation-exposure hazard for hospital personnel. Ectopic thyroid tissue at the thoracic inlet, mediastinum, or cardiac muscle[30] may require ultrasonography, CT scan, or radionuclide imaging for detection.

Prognostic Factors

Prognostic factors were evaluated in a series of 54 dogs treated surgically for thyroid carcinomas without evidence of metastases.[29] Histologic grading of the tumor, which took into account cellular and nuclear

KEY POINTS:

Most dogs with thyroid carcinoma are euthyroid or even hypothyroid.

Surgical biopsy or even fine-needle aspiration of a thyroid tumor may cause considerable bleeding. The surgeon should be prepared to do a resection if an incisional biopsy results in excessive bleeding.

MANAGEMENT OF SPECIFIC DISEASES

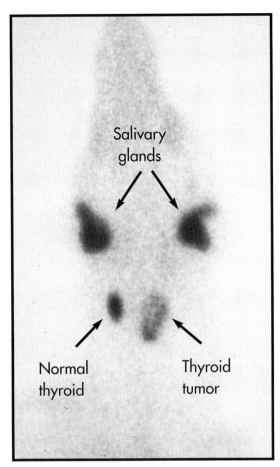

Figure 5-73: *Thyroid carcinomas in dogs are usually nonfunctional, and a technetium scan may demonstrate a unilateral area of decreased nuclide uptake, or a "cold" scan as seen above. The contralateral thyroid is frequently normal in these dogs. This is a dorsoventral scan of a dog's head and neck. (Courtesy C.R. Lamb)*

polymorphism, capsular and vascular invasion, and mitotic rate, was the most important prognostic factor for survival. There were no differences in survival among different breeds, genders, or ages of dogs or histologic types of tumors. Plasma T_4 level and results of thyroid scintigraphy failed to predict survival. Large tumor size has been related to poor survival in many studies and may be an indication that larger tumors are more likely to invade surrounding struc-

tures (i.e., have a higher histologic grade).

In summary, dogs with invasive or fixed tumors have a poor survival. Median survival of the 23 dogs able to undergo surgery (nonfixed tumors) in the study just described was 12 months; the longest survival time was 49 months.[29] In contrast, 9 of 15 dogs with tumors considered inoperable because of invasiveness and/or distant metastases were euthanatized within one week, and the remaining six dogs survived a median of 15 weeks (range = 2–38 weeks) with no treatment.

Treatment
Surgery

Complete surgical excision of thyroid adenomas should be curative. Surgery is important in management of canine carcinomas and should be performed when possible, especially if the tumor is moveable (i.e., noninvasive). If the tumor is localized and not fixed to underlying tissue, surgical excision has at least the potential for cure, particularly for tumors of low histologic grade. For more invasive tumors, it may be necessary to ligate and remove carotid arteries and jugular veins. Hypoparathyroidism and bleeding are serious, potentially life-threatening complications; patients must be carefully selected.

When bilateral thyroidectomy is performed, it is usually not possible to preserve the parathyroid glands; hypoparathyroidism is a frequent consequence. Hypocalcemia may cause signs of nervousness, irritability, panting, pyrexia, and, occasionally, convulsions or tetany. In a hypocalcemic crisis, intravenous 10% calcium gluconate should be administered at a dose of 1.0 to 1.5 ml/kg over 10 to 20 minutes and then 2.5 ml/kg as an intravenous infusion over 6 to 8 hours. In addition, oral vitamin D and calcium therapy should be started. Dihydrotachysterol may be administered at a loading dose of 0.05 mg/kg/day for 2 days and then 0.02 mg/kg/day for 2 days before starting maintenance therapy at a dose of 0.01 mg/kg/day. Calcium gluconate is given at a dose of 0.5 to 1.0 gram/kg in divided doses, and the dose is adjusted according to weekly serum calcium determinations. Hypothyroidism should be treated with L-thyroxine at a dose of 20 to 30 µg/kg SID.

MANAGEMENT OF SPECIFIC DISEASES

Radiation Therapy

Radioactive iodine therapy has been documented in only a few canine cases. Follow-up in many of these cases is poor, but palliation of signs and shrinkage of the treated tumor have been described.[31] In human patients with functional thyroid carcinoma, the treatment of choice is extensive surgical debulking followed by radioiodine therapy in an attempt to ablate remaining tumor tissue. Radioiodine alone is unlikely to be curative. The efficacy of ^{131}I therapy in dogs (compared to cats) is often compromised by the high doses required to treat their disease. If debulking of the tumor to reduce the required dose of radioactive iodine is not possible, hospitalization in isolation is often required for many weeks.[31]

For tumors that do not appear to have metastasized and cannot be completely excised, adjuvant therapy with external beam radiation therapy to the surgical site gives local control.[23] Distant metastases, however, may require additional treatment. The tumor is highly sensitive to radiation, as indicated by the response to radionuclide therapy in humans and some dogs. In some dogs, external beam radiation therapy may reduce the size of the tumor and form a fibrous capsule. Such a capsule enables surgery to be performed on a tumor once considered "inoperable."

Chemotherapy

In cases of metastatic thyroid carcinoma in which radionuclide imaging provides no evidence of increased function, chemotherapy is the treatment of choice. For these tumors, doxorubicin (30 mg/m^2 IV every 3 weeks) has been recommended, although there is little published evidence for this claim. Doxorubicin was given to 16 dogs with thyroid carcinoma; however, measurable disease was present in only nine dogs, three of which had a partial response.[32] Duration of response was not provided. In another study, 13 dogs with thyroid carcinoma received two doses of doxorubicin; one had a complete response and two showed partial responses.[33] Again, duration of response was not provided. In an anecdotal review of 64 cases from Colorado State University, doxorubicin following surgery may have improved survival com-

pared to surgery alone when the tumor was resected down to microscopic disease.[34] In another report, 10 dogs with thyroid carcinoma received mitoxantrone chemotherapy at various doses.[35] One dog had a short-term (21 days) partial response. Chemotherapeutics used as single agents in human patients with thyroid carcinoma include etoposide and cisplatin. Ten dogs with thyroid carcinoma were treated intravenously every 21 days with 60 mg/m^2 of cisplatin.[36] Six of these dogs had partial responses for a median of 143 days. Cisplatin and possibly doxorubicin are the drugs of choice for treatment of canine malignant thyroid tumors and may be useful as an adjuvant to surgery or radiation therapy.

Thyroid Supplementation

Sodium levothyroxine has been used postsurgically to reduce stimulation of residual tumor cells by TSH. No follow-up has been provided to assess the success of this type of therapy.

THYROID ADENOMATOUS HYPERPLASIA IN CATS

Incidence, Signalment, and Etiology

Hyperthyroidism in cats is most commonly associated with adenomatous hyperplasia of the thyroid glands, which usually involves both glands. Old cats (mean age = 12 years) are most frequently affected; there is no gender predisposition. Although no hard evidence has been cited, the increased frequency of diagnosis of this disorder since it was first described in 1980 has led to suggestions that high iodine concentrations in cat food or other environmental influences play an etiologic role in the disease.

Clinical Presentation and History

The most common presenting complaint is loss of weight, despite good appetite. The owner may note increased stool volume and diarrhea, periodic vomiting, polyuria and polydipsia, and increased activity. About 20% of cats have periods of anorexia between longer periods of increased appetite. Clinical signs are often chronic and have been observed for up to 15 months in one study.[37] Auscultation of cardiac mur-

MANAGEMENT OF SPECIFIC DISEASES

murs, altered rhythm, and tachycardia can indicate thyrotoxicosis-induced hypertrophic cardiomyopathy. Congestive heart failure may be the initial presenting sign for a cat with hyperthyroidism.

Staging and Diagnosis

Appropriate staging should include routine blood work and urinalysis as well as serum thyroxine (T_4) level. In addition, an electrocardiogram, echocardiogram, and thoracic radiographs should be obtained and nuclear scintigraphy of the thyroid glands should be performed. Thyroxine (T_4) levels are almost always elevated, whereas triiodothyronine (T_3) may be normal. A small percentage of cats that are clinically hyperthyroid have normal T_3 and T_4 values, but nuclear scans of these cats diagnose hyperthyroidism. Nonspecific elevations in liver enzymes and subtle alterations in some parameters on the CBC occur frequently and may distract the clinician from the primary problem of hyperthyroidism. Scintigraphic examination of cats with hyperthyroidism may identify hyperthyroid-accessory nodules, ectopic thyroid glands within the chest, and hyperthyroid glands that appear normal on clinical examination or palpation as well as metastatic lesions from malignant thyroid carcinomas (Figure 5-74). Cats are given a low dose (0.5 mCi) of sodium pertechnetate, which is taken up by the thyroid. A scintigraphic scan measures radioactivity, which is high in functional tissue but low in atrophied normal thyroid tissue. Technetium is excreted within 24 hours, so the entire scanning procedure is complete in 36 to 48 hours.

Treatment

Critical patients may require supportive therapeutic measures beyond definitive treatment for thyroid hyperplasia. In each case, the patient should be stabilized prior to definitive therapy. If cardiac manifestations, such as significant hypertrophy of the myocardium or supraventricular tachycardia are clinically apparent, propranolol or diltiazem may stabilize tachyarrhythmias and improve cardiac performance. Furosemide and other drugs may be indicated for cats in overt cardiac failure.

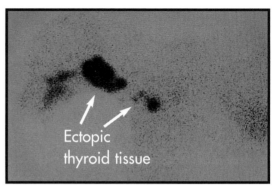

Figure 5-74: *A technetium scan may demonstrate ectopic active thyroid tissue in cats with hyperthyroidism, which would change the prognosis for surgery and may, as in this case, make the clinician suspicious of a malignant process rather than the more usual benign tumor. This lateral view of a cat's head, neck, and thorax demonstrates pertechnetate accumulation in a thyroid carcinoma. (Courtesy P.P. Kintzer)*

Antithyroid Drugs

Propylthiouracil (PTU) inhibits production of thyroid hormones by blocking iodine incorporation. The drug has been used at a dose of 50 mg PO three times daily prior to surgery to stabilize signs in hyperthyroid cats. Side effects include vomiting and anorexia as well as a variety of immune-mediated reactions that primarily affect red cells and platelets.[38] PTU is no longer appropriate for treatment of hyperthyroidism in cats because of hematologic side effects. Methimazole (Tapazole®, Eli Lilly, IN) (5 mg TID) also reduces circulating levels of T_3 and T_4, and fewer side effects have been reported with the use of this drug than with PTU.[39] Carbimazole is a methimazole derivative; in cats, it appears to require similar dosages to methimazole. Approximately 10% of treated cats in one study failed to respond to carbimazole treatment.[40] Strict scheduling of dosage (5 mg every 8 hours prior to a surgical resection of the thyroid or 5 mg every 12 hours for maintenance of an euthyroid state without surgery) is necessary to obtain optimal results.

Long-term maintenance of cats on these drugs diminishes their effects. Periodic thyroid hormone–level checks and appropriate dose adjustments are necessary to maintain euthyroid status.

MANAGEMENT OF SPECIFIC DISEASES

Surgery

Many veterinarians consider surgery to be the treatment of choice for feline hyperthyroidism. About 70% of hyperthyroid cats require a bilateral thyroidectomy. During surgery, the parathyroid gland should be identified and preserved, if possible.

Cats should be monitored after surgery for hypocalcemia, which occurs if the parathyroid glands are removed or destroyed. Very fine twitching is often the first clinical sign; it may progress to tetany, convulsions, and death. If hypocalcemia is life-threatening, 1.0 to 1.5 ml/kg of 10% calcium gluconate is *slowly* administered intravenously. After signs are controlled, 2 ml/kg of the same solution is administered over 6 to 8 hours. This is best done using an infusion pump. Oral medications are started as soon as possible. Total daily calcium dose should be 40 to 60 mg/kg/day of calcium lactate.

Vitamin D should be administered in one of two forms. Vitamin D_2 (Calciferol®, Kremers Urban, WI; Drisdol®, Winthrop, NY) is inexpensive, but its onset requires 4 weeks. As an alternative, loading doses of 4000 to 6000 units/kg/day of vitamin D_2 are given until serum calcium reaches 9 mg/dl; doses are then reduced to 1000 to 2000 units/kg/day. If hypercalcemia occurs, it may persist for days after vitamin D_2 is discontinued. Furosemide and 0.9% saline, therefore, should be used to induce caliuresis. Dihydrotachysterol is more expensive; however, serum calcium normalizes rapidly. Dosage is 0.03 mg/kg/day for 2 days, then 0.02 mg/kg/day for 2 days, and finally 0.01 mg/kg/day. 1,25 dihydroxyvitamin D (Rochaltrol®, Roche, NJ) has a rapid onset of action (2 to 4 days) at a dose of 0.03 to 0.06 µg/kg/day.

After bilateral thyroidectomy, thyroid hormone replacement may be needed, although accessory thyroid tissue will usually start to produce thyroid hormones if supplementation is delayed.

Radioactive Iodine

This treatment has been used in humans for hyperthyroidic conditions. It is widely used in cats. In a report of radioactive ^{131}I treatment for 265 hyperthyroid cats, 90% became euthyroid, 9% remained hyperthyroid, and 1% became hypothyroid. Of 17 hyperthyroid cats that were retreated, 15 became euthyroid. Disadvantages of this therapy are the need for prolonged hospitalization until radioactive iodine is excreted and the potential for human (handler) exposure during this period. Subcutaneous administration of ^{131}I reduces exposure of personnel, and one study found that it was just as effective as intravenous administration in treating hyperthyroid cats. Eighty-five percent of cats were euthyroid four years after treatment regardless of the route of administration.[37]

THYROID CARCINOMA IN CATS
Incidence, Signalment, and Etiology

In cats, thyroid malignancies are rare compared to adenomatous hyperplasia. In contrast to those in dogs, most feline carcinomas are functional. The mean age of affected cats is 12 to 13 years.

Clinical Presentation and History

In a series of 14 cats with hyperfunctional thyroid carcinomas, presenting signs were indistinguishable from those in cats with functional adenomatous hyperplasia.[41] Clinical examination was not helpful—multiple nodules were often not palpable, and only one cat had radiographic evidence of metastasis.

Staging and Diagnosis

Staging procedures for a cat with suspected thyroid carcinoma are identical to those for cats with benign thyroid hyperplasia. The most useful diagnostic aid for feline thyroid carcinoma is thyroid scintigraphy; it may reveal multiple nodular areas of high radionuclide uptake in the cervical region, thoracic inlet, or cranial mediastinum.

Treatment

Surgery is difficult because of dif-

KEY POINT:

Hypocalcemia may occur due to removal of parathyroid glands when bilateral thyroidectomy is performed. Cats should be monitored after surgery.

fuse distribution and location of the tumors. Therapy was successful in only a few of 14 cats treated with radioactive iodine.[41] Poor case selection and inadequate dosing may have contributed to lack of success.

OTHER ENDOCRINE TUMORS

Excepting the foregoing neoplasms, most other endocrine tumors are rare in dogs and cats. Therapy for these tumors is uncertain beyond surgery, and few, if any, reports of radiation therapy or chemotherapy exist in the veterinary literature.

GASTRINOMA

This tumor of the pancreas is notable for the production of gastrin and the resultant hypertrophic gastritis with peptic ulcers (Zollinger–Ellison syndrome). Like insulinomas, gastrinomas tend to be discrete and small within the pancreatic parenchyma. In the few documented cases, tumors were malignant, with metastasis to regional lymph nodes and liver. This tumor is very rare in cats and dogs.[42–45]

Treatment

The clinical course is often chronic, and H$_2$ histamine blockers appear to palliate human patients. One dog with a gastrinoma was treated with a somatostatin analogue (SMS201-995; Sandostatin®, Sandoz, NJ) at a subcutaneous dose of 10 μg three times daily; complete resolution of clinical signs was achieved for 20 months.[20] Attempts to discontinue therapy during this time resulted in recurrences of gastric ulceration and vomiting.

PARATHYROID TUMORS IN DOGS
Incidence, Signalment, and Etiology

Parathyroid tumors are rare in dogs. Affected animals are middle-aged to old (7 to 13 years). There is no gender predilection.[46] In one series of cases, keeshonds appeared overrepresented; these tumors were also observed in a litter of German shepherd puppies.[47] Most reported cases involve parathyroid adenomas, although carcinomas can occur. These tumors are usually found in the cervical region, although an ectopic parathyroid adenocarcinoma was

reported in the anterior mediastinum of one dog.[48]

Clinical Presentation and History

Hypercalcemia is a consistent finding in dogs with a parathyroid tumor. Dogs are usually presented for polyuria, polydipsia, listlessness, and muscle weakness. Parathyroid tumors are often small and, therefore, are rarely palpable on clinical examination.

Staging and Diagnosis

The most common cause of canine hypercalcemia is lymphoma. Dogs with elevated serum calcium should have their lymph nodes palpated and aspirated. Thoracic radiographs should be performed, and the abdomen should be imaged by ultrasonography to rule out this disease. In addition, a careful rectal examination should be performed to detect possible adenocarcinoma of the anal sac, another cause of hypercalcemia. Lytic bone lesions on radiographs or an elevated globulin level may indicate multiple myeloma. Once other neoplastic and metabolic causes have been eliminated, primary hyperparathyroidism can be considered, and either a cervical exploratory surgery is performed or a serum-parathormone level is obtained.

Treatment

Surgical excision of the affected gland or glands should cure parathyroid adenoma. After removal of a parathyroid tumor, the remaining normal parathyroid tissue will be atrophied from chronic hypercalcemia and the dog should be treated for hypoparathyroidism, as outlined in the section on thyroid tumors. Treatment usually is required for only 2 to 3 months until normal tissue regains function.[46]

PARATHYROID TUMORS IN CATS
Incidence, Signalment, and Etiology

Primary hyperparathyroidism in cats is rare. It was found in 7 cats among 3145 necropsies, and 9 cats among 3248 feline tumors.[49] Only 1 of these 16 cats had a parathyroid adenocarcinoma; the remainder had adenomas. A recent report described clinical findings in another seven cats with parathyroid tumors.[50] Parathyroid adenomas occurred in old cats with an average age of 13 years. More female cats were affected, and the tumor was more common in Siamese.

Clinical Presentation and History

Despite persistent hypercalcemia, only two cats were polydipsic (which is the most common sign in dogs with parathyroid tumors and hypercalcemia). Other signs were nonspecific and included anorexia and lethargy; some cats were asymptomatic. The abnormal parathyroid was palpable in two of seven affected cats.[50] Histopathology revealed a solitary parathyroid adenoma in five cats, one cat had bilateral parathyroid cystadenomas, and one had parathyroid adenocarcinoma. Serum calcium levels ranged from 13.3 mg/dl to 22.8 mg/dl (mean = 15.8 mg/dl).

Treatment

After surgical excision of the tumor tissue, the six cats with adenomas became normocalcemic within 24 hours and only two cats had transient but asymptomatic episodes of hypocalcemia. One of these cats developed parathyroid carcinoma approximately 1.5 years after a parathyroid adenoma was surgically removed.[50]

PHEOCHROMOCYTOMA
Incidence, Signalment, and Etiology

Pheochromocytomas are functional tumors of the adrenal medulla that secrete catecholamines. These tumors are very rare, having been described in only a few dogs and not at all in cats. Pheochromocytomas occur in old dogs with a median age of 10.5 years (range = 3 to 15 years). There is no obvious gender or breed predilection. Rarely, pheochromocytoma may be bilateral.[51,52]

Clinical Presentation and History

Increased circulating catecholamines cause hypertension that may occur episodically or paroxysmally and may be interspersed by asymptomatic periods that last from days to years. The resulting clinical signs may be vague; episodic panting, weakness, and restlessness are the predominate signs. Pheochromocytoma is frequently an incidental necropsy finding with no clinical history that would suggest its presence. In one study,

the diagnosis was retrospectively suspected in only 26 of 50 dogs.[51] Central nervous system abnormalities, such as seizures attributable to brain metastasis or paraparesis due to aortic thrombus, were less common. Approximately 25% of dogs had clinical signs for more than one month and up to three years.[51]

Staging and Diagnosis

Pheochromocytoma may obstruct the caudal vena cava and invade the vessel. In one study, thoracic radiographs showed nonspecific cardiovascular changes in many dogs. Although four dogs had pulmonary metastases, only two had radiographically detectable changes.[51] The tumor may be imaged by ultrasonography or renal caval contrast venography to outline venous thrombosis. Abdominal ultrasonography is more sensitive than radiography in detecting an abdominal mass in the renal and adrenal region, particularly if the mass is small or if abdominal fluid is present. On necropsy, distant metastases to lung, liver, spleen, kidney and other sites were more common (12 of 50 dogs) than lymph node metastases (6 of 50 dogs). There was local tumor invasion in 26 of 50 dogs.[51] High circulating levels of catecholamine and increased urinary excretion of their breakdown products are helpful in establishing the diagnosis.

Treatment

The treatment of choice for this rare tumor is surgery. Surgery is, however, technically demanding because of the invasion of many pheochromocytomas around caudal vena cava and periaortic tissues. This situation is further complicated because these patients are at high risk while undergoing anesthesia and surgery. Preoperatively, medical management to inhibit the effects of catecholamine is important and is also necessary for dogs that cannot undergo surgery. Phenoxybenzamine hydrochloride, an α-adrenergic–blocking agent, should be administered at a dosage of 0.2 to 1.5 mg/kg BID PO for 10 to 14 days prior to surgery, with dosing starting at the low end of the range and gradually increasing until the blood pressure is acceptable.

Care must be taken in selecting the anesthesia used

MANAGEMENT OF SPECIFIC DISEASES

for these dogs. Phenothiazines, such as acepromazine, should be avoided because they have α-blocking effects and could precipitate a hypotensive crisis. Narcotic agents may be used as preanesthetics. Because dogs with this tumor may show pronounced tachycardia after receiving atropine, its use should be avoided. Isofluorane mask induction and maintenance anesthesia is recommended because of its low arrhythmogenic properties. Central venous pressure should be monitored throughout the surgery, and hypertensive episodes should be treated with intravenous phentolamine (0.02–0.1 mg/kg). It is important to remember that these tumors may be found in association with other endocrine tumors (multiendocrine neoplasia) as well as with other, unrelated tumors. Chemotherapy for inoperable tumors in dogs has not been reported.

CHEMODECTOMA
Incidence, Signalment, and Etiology

The most common chemodectomas are aortic body tumors and carotid body tumors. These tumors are uncommon in dogs and are even more rare in cats.[53,54]

In dogs, most chemodectomas are aortic body tumors; carotid body tumors account for only 10% to 20% of this type.[55,56] Affected dogs are old (10–15 years of age). Boxers and Boston terriers are predisposed. Chronic hypoxemia is suspected of having a role in the etiology of chemodectomas, which would explain this predisposition in brachycephalic breeds. Male dogs are more likely to develop aortic body tumors, but there is no sex predilection for carotid body tumors.

Clinical Signs and History

Aortic body tumors may be extremely large (up to 13 cm or more) and may cause congestive heart failure. Dogs with carotid body tumors usually present with a neck mass, dysphagia, or dyspnea.

Staging and Diagnosis

Malignant tumors are rare. When they occur, carcinomas often are larger than adenomas and may metastasize widely to the lungs, myocardium, liver, kidney, brain, and bone. Local invasion by chemodectomas is common and may involve surrounding blood vessels. Local invasion into thoracic vertebrae has been reported.[57]

Canine chemodectoma seems to be associated with presence of such other endocrine tumors as pheochromocytoma. In one series of cases, thyroid tumors were present in 11 of 67 dogs with chemodectoma.[56]

Treatment

Treatment of chemodectoma has rarely been described in animals, and surgery is difficult due to the invasive nature of these tumors. Mobile masses in the neck may be amenable to successful surgical removal. In one series of 10 dogs with carotid body tumors, surgical excision was attempted and perioperative mortality was 40%.[58] Four surviving dogs received no adjunctive treatment and survived a median of 25.5 months (range = 12–45 months); two dogs that received postoperative radiation therapy lived 6 and 27 months. Three of these six dogs died of distant metastases. Radiation therapy has been anecdotally recommended for aortic body tumors, but side effects (e.g., pneumonitis) reduce its practicality.

ACROMEGALY IN CATS
Incidence, Signalment, and Etiology

Pituitary acidophil adenomas in cats may secrete excessive quantities of growth hormone. Growth hormone induces peripheral insulin resistance and resultant diabetes mellitus that requires high doses of exogenous insulin to be controlled, which is the most common sign in affected cats. Affected cats are middle-aged or older, and all reported cats have been mixed breeds. Male cats predominate; only 1 of 14 cats in one study was female.[59]

Clinical Presentation and History

Signs of diabetes mellitus predomi-

> **KEY POINT:**
>
> *Pituitary adenoma causing acromegaly should be suspected in any male cat with insulin-resistant diabetes.*

nate; polyuria, polydipsia, and polyphagia have been reported in all affected cats. Growth hormone excess results in hypertrophy of various organs, which is most commonly clinically detected as hepatomegaly, cardiomegaly, or renomegaly. Prognathia inferior (enlargement of the mandible) was seen in 10 of 14 cats.[59]

Central nervous system signs, such as stupor or seizures, may occasionally be seen when the pituitary tumor grows large enough to compress surrounding structures.

Staging and Diagnosis

Pituitary adenoma causing acromegaly should be suspected in any cat with diabetes mellitus that requires very large doses of insulin to control the disease or that is resistant to the effects of insulin, particularly if the cat is male and other signs of acromegaly are present.

The disease is confirmed by demonstrating increased circulating growth hormone (GH) concentrations. Computed tomography is the best method of detecting a mass in the region of the pituitary. In five of six scanned cats with acromegaly, an expansible mass was easily detected.[59] A CT scan is most useful if radiation therapy is planned for the pituitary tumor.

Treatment

Treatment of acromegaly in cats mainly attempts to manage the signs secondary to GH excess, rather than directing attention at the primary tumor itself. Severe insulin-resistant diabetes mellitus may be reasonably controlled by using large doses of insulin in divided daily doses. Cats with cardiac disease seem to respond well to diuretic therapy; however, congestive heart failure or renal failure is often the cause of death in these cats.

Megavoltage radiation therapy (48 Gy) was used to treat two cats with central nervous system signs due to a pituitary mass. One cat responded well for six months, but the other cat failed to respond. In four cats, a somatostatin analogue, octreotide, failed to reduce GH secretion.[59]

REFERENCES

1. Feldman EC, Nelson RW: *Canine and Feline Endocrinology and Reproduction.* Philadelphia, WB Saunders, 1987, pp 375–398.
2. Nelson RW, Ihle SL, Feldman EC: Pituitary macrodenomas and macroadenocarcinomas in dogs treated with mitotane for pituitary-dependent hyperadrenocorticism: 13 cases (1981–1986). *JAVMA* 194:1612–1617, 1989.
3. Rijnberk AD, Belshaw BE: o,p'-DDD treatment of canine hyperadrenocorticism: An alternative protocol, in Kirk RW, Bonagura JD (eds): *Current Veterinary Therapy XI.* Philadelphia, WB Saunders, 1992, pp 345–349.
4. Feldman EC, Nelson RW: Use of ketoconazole for control of canine hyperadrenocorticism, in Kirk RW, Bonagura JD (eds): *Current Veterinary Therapy XI.* Philadelphia, WB Saunders, 1992, pp 349–352.
5. Dow SW, LeCouteur RA: Radiation therapy for canine ACTH-secreting pituitary tumors, in Kirk RW, Bonagura JD (eds): *Current Veterinary Therapy XI.* Philadelphia, WB Saunders, 1992, pp 1031–1034.
6. Bruyette DS, Ruehl WW, Smidberg TL: Canine pituitary-dependent hyperadrenocorticism: A spontaneous animal model for neurodegenerative disorders and their treatment with L-deprenyl, in *Progress in Brain Research*, Elsevier, Amsterdam, 1994, in press.
7. Kintzer PP, Peterson ME: Mitotane (o,p'-DDD) treatment of 32 dogs with cortisol secreting adrenocortical neoplasia. *JAVMA* 205:54–61, 1994.
8. Scavelli TD, Peterson ME, Matthiesen DT: Results of surgical treatment for hyperadrenocorticism caused by adrenocortical neoplasia in the dog. 25 cases (1980–1984). *JAVMA* 189:1360–1364, 1986.
9. Enns SG, Johnston DE, Eigenmann JE: Adrenalectomy in the management of canine hyperadrenocorticism. *JAAHA* 23:557–564, 1987.
10. Feldman EC, Nelson RW, Feldman MS, Farver TB: Comparison of mitotane treatment for adrenal tumor versus pituitary-dependent hyperadrenocorticism in dogs. *JAVMA* 200:1642–1647, 1992.
11. Zerbe CA: Feline hyperadrenocorticism, in Kirk RW (ed): *Current Veterinary Therapy X.* Philadelphia, WB Saunders, 1989, pp 1038–1042.
12. Caywood DD, Klausner JS, O'Leary TP, et al: Pancreatic insulin-secreting neoplasms: Clinical, diagnostic, and prognostic features in 73 dogs. *JAAHA* 24:577–584, 1988.
13. Leifer CE, Peterson ME, Matus RE: Insulin-secreting tumor: Diagnosis and medical and surgical management in 55 dogs. *JAVMA* 188:60–64, 1986.
14. Kruth SA, Feldman EC, Kennedy PC: Insulin-secreting islet cell tumors: Establishing a diagnosis and the

clinical course for 25 dogs. *JAVMA* 181:54–58, 1982.

15. Rogers KS, Luttgen PJ: Hyperinsulinism. *Compend Contin Educ Pract Vet* 7:829–840, 1985.

16. Braund KG, Steiss JE, Amling KA, et al: Insulinoma and subclinical peripheral neuropathy in two dogs. *J Vet Intern Med* 1:86–90, 1987.

17. Schraumen E: Clinical peripheral neuropathy associated with canine insulinoma. *Vet Rec* 128:211–212, 1991.

18. Lothrop CD: Medical treatment of neuroendocrine tumors of the gastroenteropancreatic system with somatostatin, in Kirk RW, Bonagura JD (eds): *Current Veterinary Therapy XI.* Philadelphia, WB Saunders, 1992, pp 1020–1024.

19. Meyer DJ: Temporary remission of hypoglycemia in a dog with an insulinoma after treatment with streptozotocin. *Am J Vet Res* 38:1201–1204, 1977.

20. Meyer DJ: Pancreatic islet cell carcinoma in a dog treated with streptozotocin. *Am J Vet Res* 37:1221–1223, 1976.

21. Rossini AA, Arungel MA, Cahill CF: Studies of alloxan toxicity on the beta cell. *Diabetes* 24:516–523, 1975.

22. Sadoff L: Control of hypoglycemia with L-asparaginase in a patient with islet cell cancer. *J Clin Endocrinol Metab* 36:334–337, 1973.

23. Mitchell M, Jurov LI, Troy GC: Canine thyroid carcinomas clinical occurrence, staging by means of scintiscans, and therapy of 15 cases. *Vet Surg* 8:112–118, 1979.

24. Brodey RS, Kelly DF: Thyroid neoplasms in the dog. A clinicopathologic study of fifty-seven cases. *Cancer* 22:406–416, 1968.

25. Mitchell M, Hurov LI, Troy GC: Canine thyroid carcinomas: Clinical occurrence, staging by means of scintiscans, and therapy in 15 cases. *Vet Surg* 8:112–118, 1979.

26. Harari J, Patterson JS, Rosenthal RC: Clinical and pathologic features of thyroid tumours in 26 dogs. *JAVMA* 188:1160–1164, 1986.

27. Walsh KM, Diters RW: Carcinoma of ectopic thyroid in a dog. *JAAHA* 20:665–668, 1982.

28. Hayes MM, Fraumeni JF: Canine thyroid neoplasms: Epidemiologic features. *J Natl Cancer Inst* 55:931–934, 1975.

29. Verschueren CP, Rutteman GR, Dijk van JE, et al: Evaluation of some prognostic factors in surgically-treated canine thyroid cancer, in *Clinico-pathological and Endocrine Aspects of Canine Thyroid Cancer.* Utrecht, Netherlands, C.P.L.J. Verschueren Proefschrift Faculteit Diergeneeskunde Rijksuniversiteit, 1992, pp 11–25.

30. Ware WA, Merkley DF, Riedesel DH: Intracardiac thyroid tumor in a dog: Diagnosis and surgical removal. *JAAHA* 30:20–23, 1994.

31. Peterson ME, Kinter PP, Hurley JR, Becker DV: Radioactive iodine treatment of a functional thyroid carcinoma producing hyperthyroidism in a dog. *J Vet Intern Med* 3:20–25, 1989.

32. Jeglum KA, Whereat A: Chemotherapy of canine and thyroid carcinoma. *Compend Contin Educ Pract Vet* 5:96–98, 1983.

33. Ogilvie GK, Reynolds HA, Richardson RC, et al: Phase II evaluation of doxorubicin for treatment of various canine neoplasm. *JAVMA* 195:1580–1583, 1989.

34. Wheeler SL: Endocrine tumors, in Withrow SJ, MacEwan EG (eds): *Clinical Veterinary Oncology.* Philadelphia, JB Lippincott, 1989, pp 253–282.

35. Ogilvie GK, Obradovich JE, Elmslie RE, et al: Efficacy of mitoxantrone against various neoplasms in dogs. *JAVMA* 198:1618–1621, 1991.

36. Hamilton TA, Morrison WB, Vonderhaar MA, et al: Cisplatin chemotherapy for canine thyroid carcinoma. *Proc 11th Ann Conf Vet Cancer Soc*:97, 1991.

37. Theon AP, VanVechten MK, Feldman E: A prospective randomized comparison of intravenous versus subcutaneous administration of radioiodine for treatment of feline hyperthyroidism: A study of 120 cats. *Am J Vet Res*, 1994, in press.

38. Peterson ME, Hurvitz AI, Leib MS, et al: Propylthiouracil-associated hemolytic anemia, thrombocytopenia and antinuclear antibodies in cats with hyperthyroidism. *JAVMA* 184:806, 1984.

39. Peterson ME, Kintzer PP, Hurvitz AI: Methimazole treatment of 262 cats with hyperthyroidism. *J Vet Intern Med* 2:150, 1988.

40. Thoday KL, Mooney CT: Medical management of feline hyperthyroidism, in Kirk RW, Bonagura JD (eds): *Current Veterinary Therapy XI.* Philadelphia, WB Saunders, 1992, pp 338–345.

41. Turrel JM, Feldman EC, Nelson RW, Cain GR: Thyroid carcinoma causing hyperthyroidism in cats: 14 cases (1981–1986). *JAVMA* 193:359–364, 1988.

42. Happe HP, Gaag Van Der I, Lamers GRHW: Zollinger–Ellison syndrome in three dogs. *Vet Pathol* 17:177–186, 1980.

43. Jones BR, Nicholls MR, Badman R: Peptic ulceration in a dog associated with an islet cell carcinoma of the pancreas and an elevated plasma gastrin level. *J Small Anim Pract* 17:593–598, 1976.

44. Middleton DJ, Watson ADJ: Duodenal ulceration associated with gastrin-secreting pancreatic tumor in a cat. *JAVMA* 183:461–462, 1983.

45. Straus E, Johnson GF, Yalow RS: Canine Zollinger–Ellison syndrome. *Gastroenterology* 72:380–381, 1977.

46. Berger B, Feldman EC: Primary hyperparathyroidism in dogs: 21 cases (1976–1986). *JAVMA* 191:350–356, 1987.

47. Thompson KG, Jones LP, Smylie WA: Primary hyperparathyroidism in German shepherd dogs: A disorder of probable genetic origin. *Vet Pathol* 21:370–376, 1984.

48. Patnaik AK, MacEwen EG, Erlandson RA: Mediastinal parathyroid adenocarcinoma in a dog. *Vet Pathol* 15:55–63, 1978.

49. Carpenter JL, Andrews LK, Holzworth J: Tumors and tumor-like lesions, in Holzworth J (ed): *Diseases of the Cat. Medicine and Surgery*. Philadelphia, WB Saunders, 1987, pp 406–596.

50. Kallet AJ, Richter KP, Feldman EC, Brum DE: Primary hyperparathyroidism in cats: Seven cases (1984–1989). *JAVMA* 199:1767–1771, 1991.

51. Gilson SD, Withrow SJ, Wheeler SL, Twedt DC: Pheochromocytoma in 50 dogs. *J Vet Intern Med* 8:228–232, 1994.

52. Wheeler SL: Canine pheochromocytoma, in Kirk RW (ed): *Current Veterinary Therapy IX*. Philadelphia, WB

53. Buergelt CD, Das KM: Aortic body tumor in a cat, a case report. *Pathol Vet* 5:84–90, 1968.

54. Collins DR; Thoracic tumor in a cat. *Vet Med Small Anim Clin* 59:459, 1964.

55. Hayes HM: An hypothesis for the aetiology of canine chemoreceptor system neoplasms, based upon an epidemiological study of 73 cases among hospital patients. *J Small Anim Pract* 16:337–343, 1975.

56. Patnaik AK, Liu SK, Hurvitz AI, et al: Canine chemodectoma (extra-adrenal paragangliomas)—A comparative study. *J Small Anim Pract* 16:785–801, 1975.

57. Blackmore J, Gorman NT, Kagan K, et al: Neurologic complications of a chemodectoma in a dog. *JAVMA* 184:475–478, 1984.

58. Obradovich JE, Withrow SJ, Powers BE, Walshaw R: Carotid body tumors in the dog. Eleven cases (1978–1988). *J Vet Intern Med* 6:96–101, 1992.

59. Peterson ME, Taylor RS, Greco DS, et al: Acromegaly in 14 cats. *J Vet Intern Med* 4:192–201, 1990.

Saunders, 1986, pp 977–981.

CLINICAL BRIEFING: TUMORS OF THE URINARY TRACT

Renal Tumors in Dogs

Common Clinical Presentation	Often no clinical signs; hematuria with transitional cell carcinoma
Common Histologic Types	Carcinomas and adenocarcinomas
Epidemiology and Biological Behavior	Old dogs, usually males; nephroblastoma in young dogs; German shepherds may have cystoadenocarcinomas and nodular dermatofibrosis on an inherited basis
Prognostic Factors	None identified

Treatment
   Surgery
 	
   Chemotherapy
	
	High metastatic rate for carcinomas makes cure unlikely; early removal of nephroblastoma may be curative
	Only reported for nephroblastoma; vincristine, doxorubicin, and actinomycin D may be palliative

Lower Urinary Tract Tumors in Dogs

Common Clinical Presentation	*Mimic Infection:* Hematuria, stranguria, and pollakiuria; often have secondary infections
Common Histologic Type	Transitional cell carcinoma
Epidemiology and Biological Behavior	Old dogs, usually females; insecticidal "dips" and obesity may be associated with development of bladder tumors
Prognostic Factors	None identified

Treatment
   Surgery
   Radiation Therapy
   Chemotherapy
	
	Palliative only; most tumors involve trigone of bladder
	Local control, but fibrosis of bladder may occur as late effect
	Palliative; best results with cisplatin, piroxicam, and doxorubicin and cyclophosphamide

MANAGEMENT OF SPECIFIC DISEASES

Renal Tumors in Cats

Common Clinical Presentation	Nonspecific; hematuria rare
Common Histologic Types	Lymphoma, then adenocarcinoma
Epidemiology and Biological Behavior	Old cats; no gender or breed predisposition; nephroblastoma can occur in young cats but is rare
Prognostic Factors	None identified
Treatment Surgery Chemotherapy	Rarely reported; carcinomas may have high metastatic rate Renal lymphoma may respond to combination chemotherapy; see lymphoma section for details

Lower Urinary Tract Tumors in Cats

Common Clinical Presentation	Hematuria, mucoid vaginal discharge, and other signs of bladder inflammation
Common Histologic Type	Transitional cell carcinoma
Epidemiology and Biological Behavior	Old cats, except lymphoma and rhabdomyosarcoma
Prognostic Factors	None identified
Treatment Surgery Chemotherapy	Recurrence is common unless surgery is aggressive; cats more amenable to surgery than dogs May be helpful for lymphoma, otherwise few reports; cisplatin is contraindicated in cats

RENAL TUMORS IN DOGS

Nephroblastomas seem to have a unique biological behavior and response to treatment and will therefore be discussed separately.

Incidence, Signalment, and Etiology

Renal tumors are rare in dogs. The majority of affected dogs are old (average = 8–9 years of age) males.[1-14] German shepherds are the only breed known to be at increased risk; they develop renal cystadenocarcinomas and multifocal nodular dermatofibrosis.[7,8] These dogs seem to have an inherited tumor susceptibility, which is probably autosomal dominant.[8]

MANAGEMENT OF SPECIFIC DISEASES

The most common tumor types are carcinomas and adenocarcinomas, which constituted more than 60% of 243 tumors in three extensive studies.[3,5,14] Other tumor types reported are fibrosarcomas, fibromas (also called interstitial cell tumors[12]), adenomas, hemangiosarcomas, and neurofibromas.[2] Tumors of the renal pelvis are most often squamous cell carcinomas, transitional cell carcinomas (TCCs), papillomas, and fibrosarcomas.

Clinical Presentation and History

For many renal tumors, particularly such benign tumors as fibromas,[2] adenomas, and papillomas,[5] there are no clinical signs noted other than the presence of a palpable abdominal mass.[2,5,9] Some dogs with malignant tumors also are free of signs.[14] In a series of 31 dogs with renal carcinoma, 14 had a palpable abdominal mass that was often quite large (ranging from 1 to 22 cm diameter) but was usually between 10 to 20 cm in diameter.[5] Some dogs present with weight loss, and a few dogs present with hematuria.

Hematuria is more common in dogs with TCCs of the renal pelvis.[5] It is rarely described in other tumor types,[4,8,10,13] as are other signs referable to the urinary tract, such as dysuria[1] and pollakiuria.[5] Renal failure is uncommonly described in dogs with renal tumors, except in German shepherds that have renal cystadenocarcinomas. Eight of 17 dogs were azotemic in one study of this tumor type.[8] Dogs with renal cystadenocarcinomas usually present with numerous, very firm skin nodules. These dogs also show abdominal distension, enlarged and irregular kidneys, and, often, nonspecific signs that may have a duration of weeks to months. Two dogs with renal tubular adenocarcinoma had extreme paraneoplastic neutrophilic leukocytosis (128,000 to 238,000 cells/µl), presumably as a result of tumor-derived colony-stimulating factors.[11,13] Polycythemia may also occur, pre-

KEY POINTS:

Renal failure is rare in dogs with renal tumors, and dogs with tumors other than transitional cell carcinomas rarely show hematuria.

———————

German shepherds may have concurrent multifocal nodular dermatofibrosis and renal cystadenocarcinomas as a hereditary disorder.

sumably as a result of tumor-induced erythropoietin secretion[15] (see the section on Paraneoplastic Syndromes). Dogs with bone metastases may present with lameness and stiff gait.[1,11]

Staging and Diagnosis

In staging dogs with renal tumors, abdominal ultrasonography should be used to evaluate both kidneys and to look for visceral metastases. Thoracic radiographs should be obtained. Routine blood work should be performed as outlined at the beginning of this section, although azotemia due to renal tumors is rarely encountered.

Renal tumors are often large and therefore may be obvious on abdominal palpation. For smaller tumors, plain radiography may outline an irregular kidney. Contrast studies, such as arteriography and excretory urography, may outline an abnormal area but do not distinguish cystic structures from soft tissue densities.[8,10] Ultrasonography enables examination of renal architecture and guided-needle biopsy of suspected renal masses and of intraabdominal viscera that may contain metastases. Ultrasonography therefore is the diagnostic tool of choice.[4,14]

In two larger studies, almost half of dogs with renal carcinoma had metastases. Renal tumors most commonly metastasize to the lungs, liver, and serosal surfaces.[14] Tumors that spread through lymphatics commonly spread to para-aortic and cranial–sternal lymph nodes,[8] but popliteal lymph nodes may be affected.[1] Metastases to bone are rare[1,4,11,14]; however, vertebrae may be involved by local extension.[11] Ten of 11 female German shepherds with renal cystadenocarcinomas and nodular dermatofibrosis also had multiple uterine leiomyomas.[8] Renal carcinomas are usually histologically classified as tubular, papillary, or solid and commonly contain more than one histologic pattern; however, histologic pattern fails to correlate with biological behavior.[5]

MANAGEMENT OF SPECIFIC DISEASES

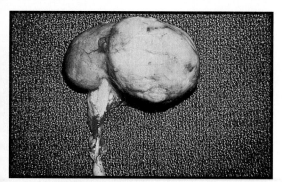

Figure 5-75: *Solitary renal adenocarcinoma is best treated by nephrectomy; however, the high metastatic rate means that even with complete excision, the possibility of a cure is remote. (Courtesy J. Berg)*

Treatment

Surgical excision of renal tumors is rarely reported (Figure 5-75). One dog with a spindle cell sarcoma[9] and one with a hemangioma[9] were both free of disease nine months after nephrectomy. Another dog with renal fibrosarcoma was free of disease 20 months after surgery.[15] Two dogs with renal tubular adenocarcinoma were treated with nephrectomies.[13] One dog with apparently localized disease died nine months later due to unknown causes after resolution of its leukemoid response. The second dog had evidence of bone metastases and was treated with ^{60}Co palliatively; however, there was no response and the dog died seven weeks after surgery.

Nephrectomy was performed in 29 dogs, of which 11 died in the immediate postoperative period. For 15 dogs that survived the first 3 weeks, survival times ranged from 1 to 25 months.[14] The high metastatic rate for carcinomas, which are the most common tumor type, makes surgery alone unlikely to be curative; however, no reports of successful adjunctive chemotherapy exist. In human patients, this tumor is commonly resistant to chemotherapy.

NEPHROBLASTOMA IN DOGS
Incidence, Signalment, and Etiology

Nephroblastoma (or embryonal nephroma) is rare in dogs. This kidney tumor is unilateral, congenital,

and often very large. The tumor is mostly described in young dogs with a mean age of 11 months,[4,5,16–23] although it may occur in old dogs.[4,14,24] Male dogs seem to be predisposed.[5] This is a congenital tumor, but there is no evidence that it is hereditary, although most reported cases have occurred in purebred dogs.

Clinical Presentation and History

Some dogs are presented for hematuria,[5,23] but most owners observe abdominal swelling.[5] One dog with hypertrophic osteopathy and polycythemia due to nephroblastoma was presented for lameness.[20]

Staging and Diagnosis

Complete staging of dogs with a renal tumor is outlined on page 404. Nephroblastoma should be suspected in young dogs with a large unilateral tumor. Nephroblastoma can be highly invasive locally and often grows large. Postsurgical follow-up examinations of dogs with nephroblastoma often document metastases. Metastases are primarily to the liver, mesentery, and lungs; however, metastases to the mesenteric, mediastinal, and bronchial lymph nodes have also been observed. The contralateral kidney, adrenal gland, thyroid, urinary bladder, and bone are also commonly affected.

Treatment

Surgical excision of nephroblastoma has been reported in a few dogs. Of four dogs treated with surgery alone, two developed metastases and were euthanatized one month and six months after surgery.[18,19] The other two had no evidence of recurrence 6 months and 14 months after surgery.[20,25] Adjuvant treatment was prescribed for four dogs that were discovered to have either metastases or grossly unresectable tumors at surgery.[24] One dog received 21 Gy of radiation to the surgical site and chemotherapy with actinomycin D. Treatment was continued intermittently even after metastases were discovered 40 weeks after surgery. The dog died 69 weeks after surgery. Another dog received actinomycin D, vincristine, and doxorubicin after an incomplete surgery and remained stable until chemotherapy was discon-

MANAGEMENT OF SPECIFIC DISEASES

tinued.[22] The dog had widespread metastases and was euthanized 16 weeks after surgery. A third dog was treated with mithramycin after developing pulmonary metastases six weeks after surgery.[19] There was partial regression of lung metastases; however, the dog died as a result of drug-induced myelosuppression. The fourth dog failed to have any response to vincristine and cyclophosphamide chemotherapy.[26] It seems that unless surgical excision is performed early in the course of the disease, surgery alone is unlikely to be curative. Chemotherapy, particularly with vincristine, doxorubicin, and actinomycin D, should be considered for incompletely resected or metastatic tumors. This, however, is still under investigation.

RENAL TUMORS IN CATS
Incidence, Signalment, and Etiology

By far, the most common renal tumor in cats is lymphoma of the kidney. Other renal tumors are rare, and the literature contains only case reports and mentions such tumors in general surveys of feline neoplasms. Renal carcinomas constituted the largest group of reported feline renal tumors after lymphoma.[27] Benign tumors are rare. Nephroblastomas occasionally have been reported. With the exception of nephroblastoma, feline renal tumors occur in old cats (average age = 9 years). There is no obvious gender or breed predilection, although tricolors may have been overrepresented in one series.[27] Mixed cell tumors of the kidney have been reported.[28]

Clinical Presentation and History

Clinical signs for cats with renal tumors are nonspecific and include weight loss, lethargy, and inappetence. Hematuria is uncommon, as are other signs referable to the urinary system. Azotemia is rare unless the contralateral kidney shows chronic inflammation or both kidneys have tumors. In cats with renal lymphoma, both kidneys often contain tumor; this also was report-

> **KEY POINT:**
>
> *When a nephroblastoma is small, nephrectomy may be curative. Large tumors, however, have frequently metastasized, and adjuvant chemotherapy should be considered.*

ed in one cat with TCC.[27] On physical examination, an enlarged or irregular kidney may be palpated, although tumors may be small and overlooked on palpation.

Staging and Diagnosis

Complete staging of a cat with a renal tumor should follow the same guidelines used for dogs. Thoracic radiography, excretory urography, routine blood work, and abdominal ultrasonography give information regarding tumor location and the presence of metastases and also guide biopsy by micro-core techniques. From the few reported cases, it is difficult to assess the frequency of metastasis for different tumor types. In one group of 18 cats with different tumor types,[27] metastases were found in eight cats with TCC and one cat with squamous cell carcinoma. No metastases occurred in six cats with renal cell carcinomas or in two with undifferentiated sarcoma. One cat with a renal sarcomatoid carcinoma had developed metastasis by the time of diagnosis.[28] In all cats with metastases, sites were widespread within the abdominal cavity; in some cases, lungs, pleura, and meninges were also involved.[27,28]

Treatment

Because of either direct extension or metastases, many cats with renal tumors have progressed beyond the point where surgery can be beneficial by the time a definitive diagnosis is made. In old cats, it is important to ensure that the remaining kidney is functional before offering surgery. Reports of the success of nephrectomy are few; however, two cats with nephroblastoma had long survival times after removal of the tumor, and another cat lived seven months after a renal adenoma was removed.[27,29,30]

BLADDER AND URETHRAL TUMORS IN DOGS
Incidence, Signalment, and Etiology

Tumors of the lower urinary tract are more com-

MANAGEMENT OF SPECIFIC DISEASES

TABLE 5-14
Tumors of the lower urinary tract in 422 dogs[31-34]

Epithelial Tumors	Number of Dogs	Mesenchymal Tumors	Number of Dogs
Transitional cell carcinoma	278	Leiomyosarcoma	11
Squamous cell carcinoma	20	Leiomyoma	13
Adenocarcinoma	23	Fibrosarcoma	7
Papilloma	30	Fibroma	5
Undifferentiated carcinoma	18	Hemangiosarcoma	4
Adenoma	1	Hemangioma	3
		Rhabdomyosarcoma	1
		Undifferentiated sarcoma	8

mon in dogs than renal neoplasia. In five series of 453 dogs with primary tumors of the bladder and urethra,[31-35] the vast majority (90%–97%) were epithelial tumors; of these, most were TCCs. Bladder and urethral tumors are most likely to be malignant. In one series of dogs, only 3% of tumors were benign,[32] and benign tumors, such as fibromas and papillomas, are often associated with chronic urinary tract disease and calculi.[33,36] Most tumors originate in the bladder urothelium, but some tumors arise from the urethra. The point of origin is not clinically significant, as these tumors frequently involve multiple areas of the urinary tract.

Female dogs are predisposed to developing TCC, perhaps because they urinate less frequently than males, thereby maintaining contact between the bladder wall and any carcinogens that are excreted in the urine.[31,33,37] Many such carcinogens have been identified in experimental studies, but their role in the natural disease is uncertain. Two other studies have not found any gender predilection,[32,34] although neutered animals seemed at increased risk of tumor formation.[32] In one study, males outnumbered females 11:2 in the development of urethral TCC, and the prostatic urethra was a predilection site.[38] These dogs were beagles, and this breed is considered to be predisposed to development of lower urinary tract tumors, thus confounding the gender issue.[31]

Other breeds at high risk are Scottish terriers,[31,32] Shetland sheepdogs, collies, and Airedales.[31] In one study, dogs that weighed less than 10 kg were at higher risk for developing bladder tumors.[32] Rhabdomyosarcomas can occur in the urinary bladder, and most occur in young dogs (1 to 2 years of age). In one report, four of seven rhabdomyosarcomas occurred in Saint Bernards.[39] For other bladder tumors, affected dogs are older (average age = 9.5 years).[32-34] In one study, only 2 of 114 dogs with tumors were younger than 2 years of age.[32]

Other epidemiologic factors increasing the risk for bladder cancer in dogs include the application of insecticidal "dips" (but not powders, sprays, or collars). Dogs that were "dipped" once or twice a year had 1.6 times the risk of developing a bladder tumor; the risk rose to 3.5 times for dogs that were treated more than twice a year.[40] Dogs that live near marshes were also at high risk. It was postulated that this resulted from insecticidal spraying for mosquitoes. Risks were higher in overweight or obese animals,[40] although only nine (13%) of 70 dogs in one survey of bladder tumors were categorized as obese.[41] There is a tenuous association between cyclophosphamide treatment and the development of TCC in dogs.[41]

Tumor types diagnosed in a group of 422 tumors[31-34] are found in Table 5-14.

MANAGEMENT OF SPECIFIC DISEASES

Clinical Presentation and History

In dogs with renal tumors, signs referable to the urinary tract are rare, but they are common with tumors of the lower urinary tract. Most presenting signs are identical to those in animals with infections or inflammatory conditions of the bladder or urethra, which may occur at the same time as a tumor. Dogs with tumors of the lower urinary tract may show clinical improvement when treated with antibiotics but then show a relapse of clinical signs. The most common presenting signs are hematuria, stranguria, and pollakiuria for both malignant[32,33] and benign[36] tumors. Less common signs are polyuria and polydipsia, urinary incontinence, and tenesmus. Signs can occur in affected dogs for up to 1 to 2.5 years before definitive diagnosis,[32,33] but for most dogs, signs have been present for 4 weeks.[32] Occasionally, a dog with bony metastasis presents with lameness,[31,32] but this is rare. Pulmonary metastases are rarely associated with dyspnea despite diffuse involvement of lungs.[31,41]

Physical examination may not be rewarding. In one group of dogs, 35 of 115 had no obvious abnormalities.[31] More commonly, however, rectal or vaginal examination reveals a urethral mass or urethral thickening, prostatomegaly, and (possibly) a distended bladder. A mass in the region of the urinary bladder may be palpated abdominally.

Staging and Diagnosis

Dogs with suspected urinary bladder cancer should have routine blood work and urinalysis performed. Abdominal ultrasonography should be performed to examine the entire urinary tract as other sites are frequently involved. Thoracic radiographs should be obtained prior to definitive diagnosis.

Routine blood work is helpful to establish a baseline for anesthesia, surgery, and chemotherapy. Urinalysis may reveal hematuria and an active inflammatory sediment. Neoplastic cells may be seen on urinalysis; however, the yield is 30% or less.[31] Extreme care should be taken in interpreting cytology of sediment, as severe chronic inflammatory changes in transitional epithelium may be difficult to distinguish from neoplastic changes.[32,42]

A closed biopsy technique that uses a urinary catheter and negative pressure while moving the catheter in a suspicious area may result in a better diagnostic yield than sediment cytology. Accuracy for this technique approaches 80%; there are occasional false-positive diagnoses.[31,34] Aspiration cytology was diagnostic in over 90% of cases in one study[31] and is preferred to cytology of urethral washes or urine sediment. Surgical biopsy should be performed if a definitive diagnosis is required. Rarely, fine-needle aspiration has been associated with "seeding" of tumor cells along the biopsy tract,[43] as has surgical biopsy.[44]

Abdominal plain radiographs may reveal prostatomegaly, sublumbar lymphadenopathy, and (occasionally) evidence of vertebral body metastasis.[31] Double-contrast cystography is helpful in outlining irregularities or mass lesions in the bladder or urethra. In two studies, this method assisted in making a diagnosis in nearly all of affected dogs.[32,33] (Figure 5-76). Care is necessary in interpreting radiographs, particularly for urethral lesions, where chronic urethritis may be difficult to distinguish from neoplasia on the basis of urethrography alone.[35] Abdominal ultrasonography provides a noninvasive method of examining the urinary bladder, cranial urethra, and prostate gland and is useful in obtaining needle-guided biopsy specimens or aspirates and measurements to assess efficacy of treatment modalities (Figure 5-77). Abdominal ultrasonography also allows examination of regional lymph nodes and other abdominal organs for presence of metastases or tumor extension. Extension of the primary tumor to involve other areas of the urinary tract is common with TCC, and dogs may present with involvement of bladder, urethra, and

> **KEY POINT:**
>
> *In one study, obesity and insecticidal dipping were shown to increase the risk of developing bladder cancer in dogs.*

MANAGEMENT OF SPECIFIC DISEASES

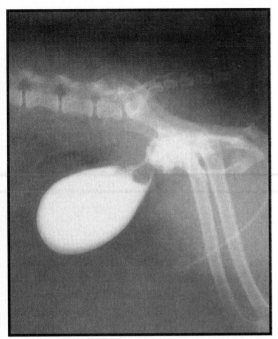

Figure 5-76: Transitional cell carcinoma of the bladder is frequently trigonal in location and is well visualized on contrast cystography. (Courtesy D.G. Penninck)

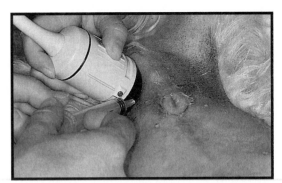

Figure 5-77: Ultrasonography may be used to guide either needle biopsy or fine-needle aspiration of the primary tumor or suspected lymph node metastasis, as in this West Highland white terrier.

vagina[46] or with ureteral and renal involvement. Careful evaluation of the entire urinary tract is warranted before definitive treatment is undertaken.

Metastasis occurs in over 50% of dogs at diagnosis,[32] and a further 25% are diagnosed at necropsy. Thoracic radiographs occasionally show evidence of metastasis at the time of diagnosis.[32] Pulmonary metastatic pattern has been described as interstitial nodular and as diffuse unstructured interstitial opacity and may appear similar to chronic aging changes. Metastases have been described as a "semidense, diffuse, lacelike haze" by one author.[42] Metastasis to the lumbar vertebrae and pelvis has been described, and regional lymph node metastasis is observed in up to 40% of dogs.[33,34] Regional lymph nodes are iliac/sublumbar nodes, but other nodes reported to be affected are sternal, mediastinal, tracheobronchial, hepatic, retropharyngeal, and popliteal nodes.[38,42] In one study, 22% of dogs with bladder or urethral tumors had a second, third, or fourth primary malignancy.[32]

Treatment

The trigonal location of most tumors of the bladder and urethra means that surgical excision is impossible unless the ureters are sacrificed or translocated. In an early study, 44 dogs were diagnosed with TCC; only four dogs lived more than 4 months, and only one was alive 7 months after surgery.[33] In contrast, 11 dogs with benign bladder tumors had postsurgical survivals of 6 months to more than 5 years.[33] Similarly, 41 of 43 dogs with surgically removed fibromas were free of symptoms for 3 to 52 months. In 10 of these 43 dogs, there was local recurrence.[36] Surgery for benign bladder tumors is potentially curative.

For urethral tumors, a sagittal pubic osteotomy was performed and surgical tumor excision included a section of the urethra.[37] Three of 10 dogs died perioperatively. The median survival for all dogs was 5.5

> **KEY POINT:**
>
> *Metastases from urinary bladder transitional cell carcinomas are present at diagnosis in more than 50% of affected dogs.*

MANAGEMENT OF SPECIFIC DISEASES

months. Local recurrence, metastasis, and incontinence were reasons for euthanasia. Aggressive surgical techniques, including trigonal colonic anastomosis[47] and ureterocolonic anastomosis,[48,49] have been used to allow removal of the bladder and urethra in dogs with TCC. Survival times ranged from 1 to 5 months,[47–49] but one dog lived 2.7 years.[47] Complications of these surgeries were hyperchloremic acidosis, which was controlled in some dogs with oral sodium bicarbonate (from 0.5 g to 1.0 g BID),[49] pyelonephritis (30% to 50% of dogs),[47,49] hydroureter, hydronephrosis, ureteral stenosis, and urinary incontinence. Despite these complications, most owners reported that their dogs had an acceptable quality of life.[49] Surgical complications were the cause of death or euthanasia in most cases, but local recurrence[48] and metastasis[49] also were common. Local therapies, such as surgery, are unlikely to improve survival unless the tumor is located in the bladder away from the trigone. In these animals, complete tumor resection is possible; one study found median survival of 12 months.[32] Surgical transplantation of tumor cells into the incision line has been reported in five dogs with TCC and was the cause of death in one dog[44]; therefore, care should be taken to "flush" the surgical area after surgery. A different instrument pack should always be used for laparotomy closure.

Localized radiation therapy has been used for bladder tumors. Intraoperative radiation using ^{137}Cs for a single treatment of 22 to 29 Gy (median = 27 Gy) was delivered to 11 dogs with nonmetastatic TCC, to one dog with rhabdomyosarcoma, and to one with leiomyosarcoma.[50] The latter two dogs lived 12 and 25 months, respectively; one dog was euthanatized because of incontinence and the other because of tumor recurrence. The median survival for dogs with TCC was 15 months, with a range of 3 to 67 months. Complications of radiation therapy included pollakiuria and incontinence in 50% of the dogs, cystitis in 40%, and stranguria in 15%—in other words—the same clinical signs that were associated with the tumor. Hydronephrosis due to ureteral fibrosis was common. Local recurrence occurred in six dogs (46%), and two of these dogs had distant

metastases. Two dogs had metastases without local recurrence. In an attempt to reduce local recurrence, nine dogs with TCC received a median of 30 Gy intraoperatively to the tumor bed and a further median of 30 Gy in fractions as external beam radiation using a 6 MeV linear accelerator.[51] Despite these high dosages, tumor recurrence was still common and occurred in seven of nine dogs; six of these dogs also had distant metastases. Most dogs become incontinent within a month of radiation therapy due to bladder fibrosis that renders the organ nondistensible. Survival was for a median of 4 months (range = 1 to 15 months). Nine dogs treated with surgery and radiation therapy as intraoperative and/or external beam radiation had a median survival of 3.5 months (range = 1 to 21 months).[32]

Complications of radiation therapy, the high rate of local recurrence, and the propensity of TCC to metastasize makes this an unlikely treatment modality even with adjuvant chemotherapy. A pilot study using ^{60}Co teletherapy and preradiation cisplatin chemotherapy (44 and 48 Gy external beam, 50 mg/m^2 divided into 3 doses before first 3 and last 3 radiation treatments) found a minor shrinkage in tumor volume. Survival times were 6 and 7 months.[52]

Chemotherapy has been used alone to treat TCC of the lower urinary tract. One dog failed to respond to low doses of cyclophosphamide,[43] and four dogs had tumor growth during cyclophosphamide treatment.[32] Other drugs used anecdotally without response include interferon, megestrol acetate, and doxorubicin.[32] In another trial, 11 dogs treated with doxorubicin and cyclophosphamide had longer survival times (mean = 259 days) than did 14 dogs treated with surgery alone (86 days) and six dogs treated with intravesicular thiotepa (57 days).[44,53] Intravesicular therapy is unlikely to be of significant benefit for large tumors.

Cisplatin has been one of the most active chemotherapeutic agents to date, causing one complete and two partial remissions in three dogs in one study.[32] In a more extensive study of 15 dogs, cisplatin (50 mg/m^2 IV every 4 weeks) caused no complete remissions but resulted in three partial remis-

MANAGEMENT OF SPECIFIC DISEASES

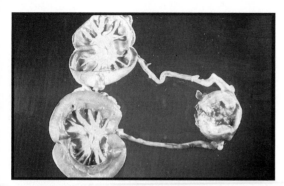

Figure 5-78: *Bilateral hydronephrosis may occur with advanced transitional cell carcinoma of the trigone due to ureteral compromise. Dogs with bladder tumors are at high risk of developing cisplatin nephrotoxicosis possibly due to subclinical renal dysfunction secondary to hydronephrosis. (Courtesy G.H. Theilen)*

sions for a median of 147 days. Three dogs had a minimal response to cisplatin. Median survival time was 6 months, and dogs with any tumor response had longer survival, implying that even minor tumor shrinkage may drastically improve clinical signs and therefore delay euthanasia.[54] Renal toxicity was more common in this series of dogs than for dogs with other tumor types treated with cisplatin, presumably because the subclinical renal disease in these dogs predisposed them to cisplatin-induced renal damage (Figure 5-78). Anecdotally, carboplatin, which is not a significant renal toxin, may have similar efficacy to cisplatin in the treatment of this disease.

One of six dogs with TCC treated with mitoxantrone chemotherapy had a partial remission for 63 days.[55] Piroxicam, a nonsteroid anti-inflammatory drug, given at a dose of 0.3 mg/kg SID PO, showed efficacy against canine TCC in 34 dogs.[56] Two dogs showed a complete remission, and four dogs showed partial remission for between 4 months and 11 months (median = 7 months). Concurrent misoprostol administration (6.5 µg/kg BID PO) may prevent gastrointestinal irritation. Subsequent

experience with mitoxantrone, with and without piroxicam, suggests that some patients have their tumors controlled for approximately one year (G.K. Ogilvie, personal observations, 1994). The most effective treatment for TCC has yet to be determined. For tumors located a distance from the trigone in which surgical margins are possible, surgical excision is the treatment of choice; the second choice would be adjuvant chemotherapy using cisplatin, carboplatin, mitoxantrone, or piroxicam. For large tumors, particularly those that involve the trigone, surgical debulking may be palliative but the primary treatment modality should be chemotherapy using one of the four drugs just mentioned.

URINARY BLADDER TUMORS IN CATS
Incidence, Signalment, and Etiology

Bladder tumors in cats are rare, and the only reports of tumors of the urethra are anecdotal.[27,57] There are four series of cats with bladder tumors in the veterinary literature, comprising a total of 76 cats[27,58-60] (two series reported the same animals[58,60]). Of the 76 reported cases, 65 tumors were malignant, and 44 were TCC.[27,59,60] Other tumor types included squamous cell carcinoma, adenocarcinoma, hemangiosarcoma, hemangioma, leiomyosarcoma, leiomyoma, rhabdomyosarcoma, and lymphoma.[27,59,60]

Affected cats are usually old; the average age is between 10 and 13 years (range = 3 to 18 years of age). Cats with lymphoma and rhabdomyosarcoma are young (3 to 5 years of age).[60] There is no obvious breed disposition.

In one study, 11 of 12 cats tested were negative for FeLV antigenemia. No epidemiologic factors have been identified for these rare tumors.

Clinical Presentation and History

Clinical signs for cats with bladder cancer are very similar to those reported for dogs. Hematuria predominates and may be concurrent with mucous discharge.[27,58] In addi-

> **KEY POINT:**
>
> *Even minor tumor shrinkage may drastically reduce clinical signs and therefore improve quality of life for dogs with bladder cancer.*

MANAGEMENT OF SPECIFIC DISEASES

tion, stranguria, pollakiuria, dysuria, and tenesmus are commonly seen. All signs may be present for a period ranging from two weeks to six months before presentation. Physical examination often reveals a palpable abdominal bladder mass.

Staging and Diagnosis

Cats with suspected bladder cancer should have routine blood work and urinalysis. Thoracic radiographs and abdominal ultrasonography should be performed prior to taking definitive diagnostic steps.

Urinalysis usually reveals hematuria; however, bacteriologic culture is rarely productive.[27] Azotemia is seen in some cats, presumably secondary to postrenal obstruction.[60] Abdominal radiographs showed calculi, bladder wall calcification, and thickened bladder wall in one group of cats.[60] In general, however, positive, negative, or double-contrast cystography is required to delineate a bladder mass. Irregular filling defects or diffuse bladder thickening are most common; in the latter case, the cystographic appearance may be difficult to distinguish from chronic cystitis.[27,60] Intravenous pyelography may reveal hydroureter and hydronephrosis. Ultrasonography is less invasive, gives similar information to contrast radiography, and allows visualization of other abdominal organs to check for spread and metastasis.

In two studies,[27,60] tumors were located in the apex of the bladder in 15 of 40 cats, in the ventral wall in seven cats, in the trigone in six cats, in the dorsal wall in four cats, and diffusely in seven cats. The urethra was involved in only one cat. This is in contrast to dogs, where bladder tumors are frequently in the trigonal region and often involve the urethra, either primarily or by extension. Bladder tumors infiltrated perivesicularly in five (20%) of 25 cats in one study,[27] and 10 (30%) of 34 carcinomas showed metastases to iliac lymph nodes, lungs, uterine stump, omentum, and abdominal wall.[27,60] Feline bladder tumors may be more amendable to surgical resection due to their location; however, metastases make curative surgery unlikely.

Treatment

Surgical resection is the only treatment reported for bladder tumors in cats. Carcinomas are prone to rapid recurrence. Six cats all had recurrence within 6 months of surgery (median = 4 months).[27,60,61] Mesenchymal tumors may have a better prognosis. Two cats with leiomyosarcoma had no recurrence at 4 months and recurrence at 7.5 months, respectively.[27,60] Two cats with leiomyoma had no recurrence at 7 years and recurrence at 6 months, respectively.[60] A cat with a bladder fibroma and one with hemangiosarcoma had no recurrence 18 months and 22 months after resection, respectively.[60] These data reinforce the importance of obtaining adequate surgical margins at surgery.

One cat with bladder lymphoma did not respond to chemotherapy with cyclophosphamide, vincristine, prednisone and L-asparaginase and died two months later.[60] Chemotherapy for TCC in cats has not been reported; however, cisplatin cannot be safely administered to cats.[62] Carboplatin is currently investigational.

REFERENCES

1. Arai C, Ono M, Une Y, et al: Canine renal carcinoma with extensive bone metastasis. *J Vet Med Sci* 53:495–497, 1991.
2. Zwicker GM, Cronin NS: Naturally occurring renal neurofibroma in a laboratory beagle. *Toxicol Pathol* 20:112–114, 1992.
3. Hayes HM Jr, Fraumeni JF Jr: Epidemiological features of canine renal neoplasms. *Cancer Res* 37:2553–2556, 1977.
4. Konde LF, Wrigley RH, Park RD: Sonographic appearance of renal neoplasia in the dog. *Vet Radiol* 26:74–81, 1985.
5. Baskin GB, Paoli De A: Primary renal neoplasms of the dog. *Vet Pathol* 14:591–605, 1977.
6. Picut CA, Valentine BA: Renal fibroma in four dogs. *Vet Pathol* 22:422–423, 1985.
7. Cosenza SF, Seely JC: Generalized nodular dermatofibrosis and renal cystadenocarcinomas in a German shepherd dog. *JAVMA* 189:1587–1590, 1986.
8. Llum B, Moe L: Hereditary multifocal renal cystadenocarcinomas and nodular dermatofibrosis in the German shepherd dog: Macroscopic and histopathologic changes. *Vet Pathol* 22:447–455, 1985.
9. Rudd RG, Whitehair JG, Leipold HW: Spindle cell sarcoma in the kidney of a dog. *JAVMA* 198:1023–1024, 1991.
10. Widmer WR, Carlton WW: Persistent hematuria in a

dog with renal hemangioma. *JAVMA* 197:237–239, 1990.

11. Madewell BR, Wilson DW, Hornof WJ, Gregory CR: Leukemoid blood response and bone infarcts in a dog with renal tubular adenocarcinoma. *JAVMA* 197:1623–1625, 1990.

12. Diters RW, Wells M: Renal interstitial cell tumors in the dog. *Vet Pathol* 23:74–76, 1986.

13. Lappin MR, Latimer KS: Hematuria and extreme neutrophilic leukocytosis in a dog with renal tubular carcinoma. *JAVMA* 192:1289–1292, 1988.

14. Klein MK, Cockerell GL, Harris CK, et al: Canine primary renal neoplasms: A retrospective review of 54 cases. *JAAHA* 24:443–452, 1988.

15. Gorse MJ: Polycythemia associated with renal fibrosarcoma in a dog. *JAVMA* 192:793–794, 1988.

16. Jones TL: Embryonal nephroma in a dog. *Can J Comp Med* 164:153–154, 1952.

17. Savage A, Isa JM: Embryonal nephroma with metastasis in a dog. *JAVMA* 124:185–186, 1954.

18. Medway W, Nielsen SW: Canine renal disorders II. Embryonal nephroma in a puppy. *North Am Vet* 920–923, 1954.

19. Coleman GL, Gralla EJ, Knirsch AK, Stebbons RB: Canine embryonal nephroma: A case report. *Am J Vet Res* 31:1315–1320, 1970.

20. Simpson RM, Gliatto JM, Casey HW, Henk WG: The histologic, ultrastructural, and immunohistochemical features of a blastema-predominant canine nephroblastoma. *Vet Pathol* 26:281–282, 1989.

21. Takeda T, Makita T, Nakamura N, Horie H: Congenital mesoblastic nephroma in a dog: A benign variant of nephroblastoma. *Vet Pathol* 26:281–282, 1989.

22. Frimberger AE, Moore AS, Schelling S: Treatment of nephroblastoma in a juvenile Bernese mountain dog. *JAVMA*, 1994, in press.

23. Caywood DD, Osborne CA, Stevens JB, Jessen CR, et al: Hypertrophic osteoarthropathy associated with an atypical nephroblastoma in a dog. *JAAHA* 16:855–865, 1980.

24. Sagartz JW, Ayers KM, Cashell IG, Robinson FR: Malignant embryonal nephroma in an aged dog. *JAVMA* 161:1658–1660, 1972.

25. Seibold HR, Hoerlein BF: Embryonal nephroma (nephroblastoma) in a dog. *JAVMA* 130:82–85, 1957.

26. Nakayama H, Hayashi T, Takahashi R, Fujiwara K: Nephroblastoma with liver and lung metastases in an adult dog. *Jpn J Vet Sci* 46:897–900, 1984.

27. Carpenter JL, Andrews LK, Holzworth J: Tumors and tumor-like lesions, in Holzworth J (ed): *Diseases of the Cat. Medicine and Surgery*. Philadelphia, WB Saunders, 1987, pp 406–596.

28. Britt JO, Ryan CP, Howard EB: Sarcomatoid renal adenocarcinoma in a cat. *Vet Pathol* 22:514–515, 1985.

29. Potkay S, Garman R: Nephroblastoma in a cat: The effects of nephrectomy and occlusion of the caudal vena cava. *J Small Anim Pract* 10:345–369, 1969.

30. Clark WR, Wilson RB: Renal adenoma in a cat. *JAVMA* 193:1557–1559, 1988.

31. Hayes HM Jr: Canine bladder cancer: Epidemiologic features. *Am J Epidemiol* 104:673–677, 1976.

32. Norris AM, Laing EJ, Valli VEO, et al: Canine bladder and urethral tumors: A retrospective study of 115 cases (1980–1985). *J Vet Intern Med* 6:145–153, 1992.

33. Burnie AG, Weaver AD: Urinary bladder neoplasia in the dog: A review of seventy cases. *J Small Anim Pract* 24:129–143, 1983.

34. Osborne CA, Low DG, Perman V, Barnes DM: Neoplasms of the canine and feline urinary bladder: Incidence, etiologic factors, occurrence and pathologic features. *Am J Vet Res* 29:2041–2055, 1968.

35. Moroff SD, Brown BA, Matthiesen DT, Scott RC: Infiltrative urethral disease in female dogs: 41 cases (1980–1987). *JAVMA* 199:247–251, 1991.

36. Esplin DG: Urinary bladder fibromas in dogs: 51 cases (1981–1985). *JAVMA* 190:440–444, 1987.

37. Davies JV, Read HM: Urethral tumours in dogs. *J Small Anim Pract* 31:131–136, 1990.

38. Nikula KJ, Benjamin SA, Angleton GM, Lee AC: Transitional cell carcinomas of the urinary tract in a colony of beagle dogs. *Vet Pathol* 26:455–461, 1989.

39. Kelly DF: Rhabdomyosarcoma of the urinary bladder in dogs. *Vet Path* 10:375–384, 1973.

40. Glickman LT, Schofer FS, McKee LJ, et al: Epidemiologic study of insecticide exposures, obesity, and risk of bladder cancer in household dogs. *J Toxicol Environ Health* 28:407–414, 1989.

41. Macy DW, Withrow SJ, Hoopes J: Transitional cell carcinoma of the bladder associated with cyclophosphamide administration. *JAAHA* 19:965–969, 1983.

42. Walter PA, Haynes JS, Feeney DA, Johnston GR: Radiographic appearance of pulmonary metastases from transitional cell carcinoma of the bladder and urethra of the dog. *JAVMA* 185:411–418, 1984.

43. Rozengaurt N, Hyman WJ, Berry A, et al: Urinary cytology of a canine bladder carcinoma. *J Comp Pathol* 96:581–585, 1986.

44. Gilson SD, Stone EA: Surgically induced tumor seeding in eight dogs and two cats. *JAVMA* 190:1427–1429, 1987.

45. Anderson WI, Dunham BM, King JM, Scott DW: Presumptive subcutaneous surgical transplantation of a urinary bladder transitional cell carcinoma in a dog. *Cornell Vet* 79:263–266, 1989.

46. Magrie ML, Hoopes PJ, Kainer RA, et al: Urinary tract carcinomas involving the canine vagina and vestibule. *JAAHA* 21:767–772, 1985.

47. Bovee KC, Pass MA, Wardley R, Biery D, et al: Trigonal-colonic anastomosis: A urinary diversion procedure in dogs. *JAVMA* 174:184–191, 1979.

48. Montgomery RD, Hankes GH: Ureterocolonic anastomosis in a dog with transitional cell carcinoma of the urinary bladder. *JAVMA* 190:1427–1429, 1987.

49. Stone EA, Withrow SJ, Page RL, et al: Ureterocolonic anastomosis in ten dogs with transitional cell carcinoma. *Vet Surg* 17:147–153, 1988.

50. Walker M, Breider M: Intraoperative radiotherapy of canine bladder cancer. *Vet Radiol* 28:200–204, 1987.

51. Withrow SJ, Gillette EL, Hoopes PJ, McChesney SL: Intraoperative irradiation of 16 spontaneously occurring canine neoplasms. *Vet Surg* 18:7–11, 1989.

52. McCaw DL, Lattimer JC: Radiation and cisplatin for treatment of canine urinary bladder carcinoma: A report of two case histories. *Vet Radiol* 29:264–268, 1988.

53. Helfand SC, Hamilton TA, Hungerford L, et al: Comparison of three treatments for transitional cell carcinoma of the bladder in the dog. *JAAHA* 30:270–275, 1994.

54. Moore AS, Cardona A, Shapiro W, Madewell BR: Cisplatin (cisdiamminedichloroplatinum) for treatment of transitional cell carcinoma of the urinary bladder or urethra. A retrospective study of 15 dogs. *J Vet Intern Med* 4:148–152, 1990.

55. Ogilvie GK, Obradovich JE, Elmslie RE, et al: Efficacy of mitoxantrone against various neoplasms in dogs. *JAVMA* 198:1618–1621, 1991.

56. Knapp DW, Richardson RC, Chan TCK, et al: Piroxicam therapy in 34 dogs with transitional cell carcinoma of the urinary bladder. *J Vet Intern Med* 8:273–278, 1994.

57. Swalec KM, Smeak DD, Baker AL: Urethral leiomyoma in a cat. *JAVMA* 195:961–962, 1989.

58. Patnaik AK, Schwarz PD, Greene RW: A histopathologic study of twenty urinary bladder neoplasms in the cat. *J Small Anim Pract* 27:433–435, 1986.

59. Caywood DD, Osborne CA, Johnston GR: Neoplasms of the canine and feline urinary tracts, in Kirk RW (ed): *Current Veterinary Therapy VII*. Philadelphia, WB Saunders, 1988, pp 1203–1212.

60. Schwarz PD, Greene RW, Patnaik AK: Urinary bladder tumors in the cat: A review of 27 cases. *JAAHA* 21:237–245, 1985.

61. Brearley MJ, Thatcher C, Cooper JE: Three cases of transitional cell carcinoma in the cat and a review of the literature. *Vet Rec* 118:91–94, 1986.

62. Knapp DW, Richardson RC, DeNicola DB, et al: Cisplatin toxicity in cats. *J Vet Intern Med* 1:29–35, 1987.

CLINICAL BRIEFING: TUMORS OF THE REPRODUCTIVE SYSTEM

Ovarian Tumors in Dogs

Common Clinical Presentation	Abdominal mass or swelling; unexplained or abnormal estrus or bleeding
Common Histologic Types	Adenomas and adenocarcinomas
Epidemiology and Biological Behavior	Old dogs (median age is 10 years); teratomas occur in young dogs
Prognostic Factors	None identified

Treatment
   Surgery
   Chemotherapy
	Surgical excision curative for most tumors
	Adenocarcinomas may metastasize within the abdomen, causing carcinomatosis; cisplatin may be the drug of choice

Vaginal and Uterine Tumors in Dogs

Common Clinical Presentation	Vaginal mass; possibly, tenesmus
Common Histologic Types	Leiomyoma and fibroma
Epidemiology and Biological Behavior	More common than ovarian tumors; vagina most common site; old dogs (median age is 11 years)
Prognostic Factors	None identified
Treatment Surgery	Treatment of choice; most tumors are benign; therefore, complete excision may be curative

Transmissible Venereal Tumor in Dogs

Common Clinical Presentation	Bleeding mass on external genitalia

MANAGEMENT OF SPECIFIC DISEASES

Epidemiology and Biological Behavior	Spread by coitus and canine social behavior; females more susceptible than males; spontaneous regression in most cases after months, but not in immunosuppressed animals; rare metastasis
Prognostic Factors	None identified

Treatment
  Surgery
  Radiation Therapy
  Chemotherapy
	
	Curative if wide excision and localized tumor
	Low doses (10 Gy); may be curative if localized
	Vincristine (0.5 mg/m^2) is treatment of choice

Testicular Tumors in Dogs

Common Clinical Presentation	Palpable mass in normal or atrophic testis; many are *not* palpable; feminization changes with some Sertoli cell tumors and seminomas
Common Histologic Types	Seminomas, Sertoli cell tumors, and interstitial cell tumors
Epidemiology and Biological Behavior	Seminomas and Sertoli cell tumors have a high incidence in retained testes; old dogs; no breed predilection
Prognostic Factors	None identified

Treatment
  Surgery
  Radiation Therapy
 	
  Chemotherapy
	
	Usually curative as metastatic rate is low
	May achieve long-term control for metastatic seminoma to sublumbar nodes
	No reports of chemotherapy for metastatic tumors

Prostatic Tumors in Dogs

Common Clinical Presentation	Tenesmus, constipation, dyschezia, and (less commonly) dysuria and hematuria
Common Histologic Type	Adenocarcinoma
Epidemiology and Biological Behavior	Equal frequency in castrated and uncastrated dogs regardless of age at castration; old dogs (median age is 10 years)

MANAGEMENT OF SPECIFIC DISEASES

Prognostic Factors	May be more aggressive in castrated dogs (but highly malignant in both castrated and uncastrated)

Treatment
  Surgery
  Radiation Therapy
  Chemotherapy
  Hormonal Therapy
	Difficult because of anatomy of canine prostate
	Palliative only, due to high metastatic rate
	Has no proven efficacy
	Ineffective because of hormone independence of canine prostatic carcinoma

Ovarian Tumors in Cats

Common Clinical Presentation	Irregular or prolonged estrus
Common Histologic Type	Granulosa cell tumor
Epidemiology and Biological Behavior	Mainly domestic shorthairs; ovarian tumors are *rare* tumors
Prognostic Factors	None identified

Treatment
  Surgery
 	
  Radiation Therapy
  Chemotherapy
	Rarely curative because of high metastatic rate of all tumor types
	Unproven
	Unproven

Vaginal and Uterine Tumors in Cats

Common Clinical Presentation	Signs due to pelvic or urethral obstruction
Common Histologic Type	Leiomyoma and fibroma
Epidemiology and Biological Behavior	Rare tumors, usually benign; often associated with ovarian cysts and endometrial hyperplasia
Prognostic Factors	None identified
Treatment **Surgery**	May be curative for benign lesions

MANAGEMENT OF SPECIFIC DISEASES

TUMORS OF THE FEMALE REPRODUCTIVE TRACT IN DOGS
Ovarian Tumors
Incidence, Signalment, and Etiology

Ovarian tumors are rare in dogs, at least in part because of early neutering. Theses tumors tend to occur in old dogs (median age = 10 years). Teratomas are the exception and usually affect young dogs (median age = 4 years). Boston terriers, German shepherds, and (possibly) poodles have a higher incidence of ovarian neoplasia than other breeds.[1] In one study, the most common ovarian tumors were adenomas and adenocarcinomas, comprising 33 (46%) of 71 tumors.[1]

Most ovarian tumors are unilateral regardless of tumor type. Adenocarcinomas and Sertoli–Leydig tumors are bilateral in about 30% of cases, however.[1] Secondary cystic changes are sometimes seen in the contralateral ovary and in the endometrium in dogs with ovarian tumors, particularly sex-cord stromal tumors (e.g., granulosa cell tumors, Sertoli–Leydig tumors, and thecomas). Sex-cord stromal tumors are often associated with production of sex hormones.

Long-term treatment with mibolerone, a nonprogestational androgenic steroid, induces ovarian fibromas in dogs.[2]

Clinical Presentation and History

Ovarian tumors are often very large (up to 15,000 cm³ in one study). More than half of the dogs with ovarian germ cell tumors, ovarian adenocarcinoma, and granulosa cell tumors had a mass that was larger than 125 cm³ in volume.[1] Therefore, most ovarian tumors are palpable on careful physical examination.

Dogs with ovarian neoplasia, particularly of sex-cord stromal origin, may present with vaginal bleeding, pyometra, and/or unusual frequency of estrus.[3,4] This is not surprising, given the high rate of endometrial hyperplasia with these tumors. One report described episodic depression, anorexia, and extreme timidity that resolved after surgical resection of a granulosa theca cell tumor.[4] Rarely does a granulosa cell tumor produce sufficient estrogen over a prolonged period to cause bone marrow aplasia. These dogs may present with clinical signs, such as fever and sepsis due to neutropenia or bleeding due to thrombocytopenia.

Peritoneal carcinomatosis may occur following seeding from the primary tumor, and malignant ascites may accumulate, which is perceived by the owner as abdominal swelling. Visceral metastases outside the abdominal cavity are rare except with malignant teratomas.[1]

Staging and Diagnosis

Ovarian tumors rarely metastasize. In one study, however, three of six ovarian teratomas and 10 of 21 adenocarcinomas had metastases, usually in the form of carcinomatosis.[5] Distant metastasis was seen with teratomas and occurred in the kidneys, adrenal glands, lung, bone, and mediastinal lymph nodes.

Ultrasonography may help to determine the origin of a large abdominal mass and will disclose any ascites that might signal carcinomatosis.

Treatment

Surgery is the treatment of choice for dogs that show no evidence of metastasis, and survival following surgery is usually long. In the few clinical reports of surgical resection of ovarian tumors, the following results were reported. In two dogs with dysgerminoma, one dog survived 13 months and died of metastatic transitional cell carcinoma of the urinary bladder; the other dog survived 4 years.[5] Of seven dogs with teratoma, four survived more than one year. Two dogs were alive 2 and 6 years after surgery. Two dogs died of metastatic disease 1 and 5 months after surgery, and one dog died intraoperatively.[3,5,6] One dog with a granulosa theca cell tumor survived more than 2 years.[4]

Reports of therapy for metastatic

> **KEY POINT:**
>
> *Most ovarian tumors are unilateral; however, adenocarcinomas and Leydig cell tumors are bilateral in about 30% of cases.*

ovarian tumors are few. In humans with ovarian carcinomatosis, long-term remissions and cures are sometimes obtained with cisplatin therapy. One dog with ovarian carcinomatosis was treated three times with 50 mg/m² of cisplatin intraperitoneally and was still alive 5 years after treatment.[7] Similar anecdotal successes indicate that cisplatin by either intracavitary or possibly intravenous administration may give long-term control of ovarian carcinoma. Another dog treated with six intracavitary cisplatin treatments for a metastatic papillary adenocarcinoma survived 8 months.[8] This dog was macroscopically free of disease 6 months after surgery but died from hemoperitoneum 2 months after chemotherapy was discontinued. A dog with metastatic ovarian papillary cystadenoma with carcinomatosis was treated for 4 months with cyclophosphamide (50 mg/m² QOD PO), chlorambucil (8 mg/m² PO twice per week), and lomustine (CCNU) (90 to 130 mg/m² PO every 6 weeks). When fluid reaccumulated, intracavitary bleomycin (10 units/m² in 100 ml of 0.9% NaCl) was infused, and the dog had no evidence of tumor 10 months after surgery.[9] No reports of chemotherapy for other canine ovarian tumors were found.

Vaginal and Uterine Tumors
Incidence, Signalment, and Etiology

In dogs, tumors of the uterus, vulva, and vagina are rare but are more common than ovarian neoplasms.[10] Most tumors of the reproductive tract originate in the vulva and vagina; relatively few are in the uterus (11 of 90 reproductive tract tumors in one study[10]). This may reflect neutering practices in dogs. The most common tumors are benign and are derived from the supportive stroma of these structures; leiomyomas and fibromas accounted for 70 of 90 tumors in the same study.[10] Transmissible venereal tumor is the next most common tumor and is dealt with in a separate section. Malignant tumors are rare; leiomyosarcomas and squamous cell carcinomas are the most often diagnosed.[11]

> ### KEY POINT:
>
> *Intracavitary cisplatin chemotherapy may give long-term control of ovarian carcinomatosis.*

The mean age of affected dogs is 11 years (range = 5 to 16 years). There is no obvious breed predilection, although poodles accounted for 16 of 99 cases in one study.[11]

Clinical Presentation and History

Owners usually notice tumors that arise from the vestibule wall as protruding from the vulvar labia (Figure 5-79). Such tumors often produce a perineal mass, vulvar bleeding, and (occasionally) tenesmus and dysuria. Specific clinical signs in dogs with uterine and cervical carcinomas have not been reported,[12] although the abdomen of one dog had noticeably enlarged over several months as a result of a large adenomatous papilloma of the uterus.[13]

There is no reported association between the occurrence of leiomyomas and fibromas and abnormal estrous cycles in affected dogs; however, dogs that have been pregnant have a higher risk of developing these tumors. A tenuous association between exogenous hormonal therapy and development of endometrial carcinoma arose in a dog treated with ethinylestradiol, methyltestosterone, and megestrol acetate.[14]

Staging and Diagnosis

Routine staging with blood work, urinalysis, and thoracic radiographs will provide a general health

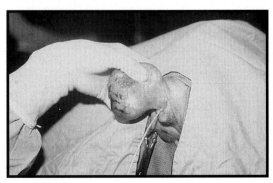

Figure 5-79: *The owner often first notes vaginal leiomyoma in a dog as a protruding mass. (Courtesy J. Berg)*

MANAGEMENT OF SPECIFIC DISEASES

screen for affected dogs. In addition, abdominal ultrasonography should be performed. Benign tumors are often slow growing and cause no clinical signs until they are very large. Malignant tumors vary in metastatic rate. Leiomyosarcomas are not reported to metastasize; however, carcinomas of the uterine horns in three dogs metastasized to the lungs and kidney. In one of these dogs, metastases were also found in the liver and adrenal and thyroid glands.[12] Definitive diagnosis is made by biopsy; however, clinical findings of a pedunculated vaginal mass are most consistent with a benign tumor. Ultrasonography may be useful in determining the site of origin for intra-abdominal tumors and whether metastasis has occurred.

Treatment

Surgery is the treatment of choice for benign and malignant tumors of the vagina and vestibule. For benign tumors, it is usually curative.[10] There are, however, few reports of surgery for malignant tumors. One dog with uterine leiomyosarcoma had a mass for 2 years prior to excision, and another dog with leiomyosarcoma of the vagina had four surgical excisions over a 2.5-year period.[10] Six dogs with vulvar leiomyosarcoma and two dogs with squamous cell carcinoma survived an average of 11.3 and 15.5 months, respectively, after surgery. Recurrence was noted in only one dog with each tumor type.[11] A dog with vaginal fibrosarcoma was treated with carbon dioxide laser ablation and two doses of doxorubicin (30 mg/m^2 IV) and had no evidence of disease when it died 20 months later.[15] Uterine carcinoma is a rare but highly metastatic tumor for which surgery is unlikely to be curative. As malignant tumors of the uterus, vagina, and vulva are rare, reports of adjunctive therapy to surgery are unlikely to be anything but anecdotal.

TRANSMISSIBLE VENEREAL TUMOR
Incidence, Signalment, and Etiology

Transmissible venereal tumor (TVT) is readily transmitted during coitus by transfer of cells from diseased to healthy dogs, but it also may be spread by social behavior, such as sniffing or licking of genitalia. Any breed may be affected. This tumor most often affects young, sexually active dogs. The tumor is most common in regions where many dogs are either feral or stray and without breeding management. Females are more susceptible to TVT than males. Tumor behavior was studied through 40 generations of dogs and implantation was found to occur in 68% of exposed animals.[16] The chromosomal complement of this tumor is constant worldwide, with 58 to 59 chromosomes found in the tumor (compared with 78 for cells of normal dogs).

Clinical Presentation and History

TVT may be solitary or multiple and nearly always involves the external genitalia as firm, soft, or friable masses prone to ulceration and bleeding. Secondary bacterial infection may follow deeper mucosal involvement, and either serosanguinous or pure hemorrhagic discharge results. Deformity of the genitalia, including marked swelling and ulceration, may follow. Dysuria or weakness occasionally occurs.[17]

Staging and Diagnosis

Metastasis is uncommon and occurs in less than 5% of reported cases, mainly in immunosuppressed dogs or in puppies inoculated with the tumor. The tumor may spread by extension from external genitalia to the uterus and oviducts in female dogs. The inguinal lymph nodes are the most likely site of lymphatic metastasis, and distant metastases have been seen in the abdominal viscera, skin, and central nervous system. In normal adult dogs, the tumor regresses after approximately two to four months of progressive growth after tumor infiltration by T lymphocytes.[18] Definitive diagnosis is made by biopsy, but cytologic preparations from fine-needle aspiration or impression smears from the tumor surface characterize TVT. Tumor cells are discrete ("round cell tumor") with nuclei that contain aggregated chromatin; the cytoplasm is pale blue or colorless with distinct clear vacuoles. Refer to the chapter on Clinical Cytology and Neoplasia in the Biopsy section for more information.

Treatment

Surgical excision of tumors was performed in 35 dogs with primary or metastatic (nongenital) lesions.[19] Of 23 dogs that only had genital lesions, the tumor recurred within six months in four dogs (locally in 1 dog and at other sites in 3 dogs). There was recurrence in 7 of 12 dogs with extragenital lesions. Surgery is not considered an effective treatment for this disease.

Canine TVT is responsive to radiation therapy; 100% "cure" is obtained with a single therapeutic dose of 10 Gy as long as metastasis has not occurred.[20] Owing to the risk of metastasis as well as the cost and limited availability of radiation therapy, chemotherapy is the treatment of choice for canine TVT.

Vincristine at a dosage of 0.025 mg/kg (to a maximum dose of 1 mg) was administered to 41 dogs with TVT and resulted in a complete remission in 39 dogs and a partial remission in one dog.[21] The dogs received between two and seven treatments (mean = 3.3). Five dogs (13%) experienced either vomiting (3 dogs) or transient leukopenia (2 dogs). All 20 dogs receiving vincristine at a dose of 0.5 mg/m² IV achieved complete remission; only one dog relapsed in a period of 12 months. Vincristine at a dose of 0.6 mg/m² intravenously resulted in complete remission in 138 of 140 dogs with TVT. These responses occurred within two to six weeks.[17] Animals older than five years of age were more likely to show gastrointestinal toxicities.

A comparison of single-agent treatment was made using either vincristine (0.5 mg/m² IV weekly [to 20 dogs]), methotrexate (2.5 mg/m² QOD PO for 6 weeks [to 8 dogs]), or cyclophosphamide (50 mg/m² PO for 4 days per week for 6 weeks [to 4 dogs] or 50 mg/m² IV for 4 days per week for 6 weeks [to 8 dogs]).[22] Two dogs treated with intravenous cyclophosphamide had partial responses, and tumors in all 20 dogs treated with vincristine completely resolved. Tumor progression occurred in all other dogs as well as in six untreated dogs. Vinblastine caused complete regression of TVT in seven of seven dogs.[23] Of two dogs in another study that failed to respond to vincristine, there was no response to combination chemotherapy, although one of the two dogs had a complete response to doxorubicin (30 mg/m² IV at 7-day intervals, which is a higher than normal dosage).[21] Single-agent vincristine is the treatment of choice for canine TVT, and combination chemotherapy seems to have no advantage (Figures 5-80 and 5-81).

TUMORS OF THE MALE REPRODUCTIVE TRACT IN DOGS
Testicular Tumors
Incidence, Signalment, and Etiology

There are three commonly diagnosed testicular tumors in dogs. Sertoli cell tumors and interstitial (Leydig) cell tumors are both sex-cord, gonadostromal tumors; seminomas are germ cell tumors. All types seem to occur with approximately equal frequency.[24–26] A more recent study, however, found that interstitial cell tumors account for approximately 40% of testicular tumors; seminomas and Sertoli cell tumors were the next most common.[27] Dogs may have tumors that contain more than one cell population[27] and may have more than one tumor type in the same or contralateral testis. Some tumors are bilateral.

Approximately 20% of all testicular tumors and 33% of all Sertoli cell tumors[26] occur in cryptorchid testes. This may result from the higher temperature at which undescended testes are maintained compared with scrotal testes (Figure 5-82).

An elevated incidence of seminomas has been observed in military working dogs stationed at Okinawa

KEY POINTS:

Vincristine chemotherapy has a cure rate of nearly 100% for TVT. Responses occur within 2 to 6 weeks.

Dogs with cryptorchid testes or inguinal hernia are 9 and 4 times more likely, respectively, to develop testicular tumors than dogs with normally descended testes.[28]

MANAGEMENT OF SPECIFIC DISEASES

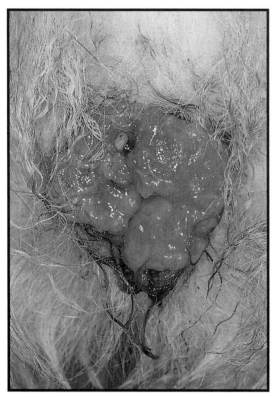

Figure 5-80: *Transmissible venereal tumor of the vulva in a 3-year-old mixed-breed dog before treatment with vincristine.*

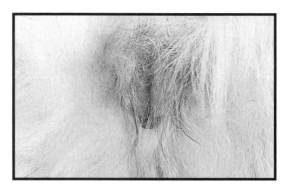

Figure 5-81: *The same dog as in Figure 5-80 after five weekly doses of vincristine at 0.5 mg/m² IV.*

and Vietnam, possibly due to tetracycline treatment or exposure to pesticides.[29] The incidence for all canine testicular tumors increases with age. The average age at diagnosis for dogs with all tumor types was between 9 and 11 years of age, although dogs with tumors in cryptorchid testes are often younger than those with tumors of scrotal testes. No breed prevalence has been described for any tumor type.

Clinical Presentation and History

Most interstitial cell tumors are small (<1 cm diameter) and are rarely palpable (Figure 5-83). There have been no reports of hormonal effects from these tumors on the dog as a whole or on the contralateral testicle.

Seminomas are larger than interstitial cell tumors

and may be palpable as a mass in an otherwise normal testis. They are commonly found in undescended testicles. Seminomas often occur in association with interstitial and Sertoli cell tumors. Feminization changes have been described in dogs with seminoma, but these may have been due to undetected Sertoli cell tumors.

Sertoli cell tumors produce signs of feminization in approximately 30% of affected dogs, and this syndrome is particularly common with tumors of cryptorchid testicles. Feminization may be concurrent with elevated serum estrogen levels in some dogs. These effects also may be associated with suppression of pituitary gonadotrophin secretion. Affected dogs often have atrophy of the contralateral testicle, prostatic hyperplasia, gynecomastia, and haircoat changes, including bilaterally symmetric alopecia and epidermal atrophy due to atrophy of hair follicles and sebaceous glands. Alopecic skin may be hyperpigmented. Prostatic hyperplasia due to squamous metaplasia may result in cyst and abscess formation. Affected dogs become attractive to other male dogs, who will attempt to mate with them. Sertoli cell tumors are often large, and the contralateral testicle and normal testicular tissue in the affected testicle are often atrophic.

Staging and Diagnosis

Routine staging and health screening should be

MANAGEMENT OF SPECIFIC DISEASES

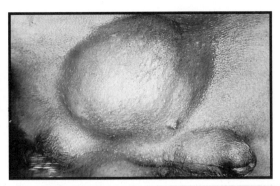

Figure 5-82: A 9-year-old miniature poodle with an inguinal Sertoli cell tumor in an undescended testicle. (Courtesy G.H. Theilen)

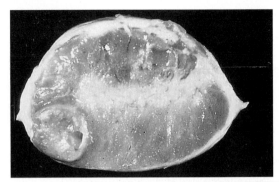

Figure 5-83: Interstitial cell tumors, as seen above, arise within the testicular parenchyma and are rarely palpable.

undertaken for all dogs with a testicular tumor. In certain cases, testicular and abdominal ultrasonography may be helpful.

Malignant interstitial cell tumors have not been described, but approximately half of these tumors occur bilaterally. Metastasis is seen in 5% to 10% of dogs with seminomas, primarily to the regional lymph nodes and occasionally to lungs or other viscera. Regional lymph nodes are the inguinal, iliac, and sublumbar nodes. Metastasis has been reported to occur to the brain and eyes.[30] Seminomas are bilateral in approximately 10% of cases.

Sertoli cell tumors are reported to metastasize at about the same rate as seminomas and are bilateral in about 10% of cases. Metastasis occurs first to regional lymph nodes (i.e., inguinal, iliac, and sublumbar nodes) but may continue to paraaortic and mesenteric nodes. Widespread metastasis to lungs and abdominal viscera may occur. Metastatic tumors may be functional and cause return or continuation of feminization signs in a dog that has had the primary tumor removed.

Ultrasonography and radiography of the abdomen may be useful diagnostic tools to look for a retained testicle or to evaluate abdominal lymph nodes and organs in a dog in which metastasis of either a seminoma or Sertoli cell tumor is suspected. In addition, ultrasonography of the testicle is useful to identify and evaluate small testicular tumors for biopsy in breeding dogs for which castration is not an option and to identify tumors in the contralateral testicle. The risk of pulmonary metastasis is low, but thoracic radiographs should be taken for completeness and as part of a health screen in old dogs.

Treatment

Surgical castration cures the majority of dogs with a testicular tumor. Unilateral castration may be an acceptable option for some dogs with Sertoli cell tumor or seminoma, as these tumors are rarely bilateral, and metastasis is rare. Bilateral castration, however, is preferred, particularly if the dog is not a valuable breeding animal and other diseases such as prostatic disease are present. Careful ultrasonography may help identify dogs with tumors in the contralateral testicle.

There are few reports of therapy for tumors that have metastasized. Four dogs with metastasis of a seminoma to the sublumbar lymph nodes but no other gross evidence of metastatic disease were treated with

> **KEY POINT:**
>
> *Interstitial cell tumors are bilateral in approximately 50% of cases, while seminomas and Sertoli cell tumors are bilateral in only 10% of cases.*

MANAGEMENT OF SPECIFIC DISEASES

[137]Cs radiation therapy to a total dose of 17 to 40 Gy.[31] Lymph node metastases regressed in all four dogs, and survival times of 37, 43, and 57 months were seen in three dogs that died of apparently unrelated causes. The fourth dog died because of transitional cell carcinoma of the urinary bladder with no evidence of seminoma six months after receiving radiation treatment. This tumor is radiation-sensitive; in dogs with metastatic seminoma localized to regional lymph nodes, radiation therapy may provide long survival.

There are no reports of chemotherapy for the treatment of widespread metastatic testicular tumors in dogs. In human patients, cisplatin is a useful agent; however, this activity has not been documented in dogs.

Prostatic Tumors
Incidence, Signalment, and Etiology

Prostatic neoplasia is uncommon in dogs but is much more common than in any other species except humans. Hyperplasia of the prostate is common in old dogs, but progression to tumor formation is rare. Prostatic tumors are always malignant; adenocarcinoma and undifferentiated carcinoma are the two histologic diagnoses.

Prostatic carcinoma is a disease of old dogs; 46 of 56 reported dogs were 8 years of age or older.[32–35] The median age in one study was 10 years,[36] and mean age was 10 years in another report.[37] The disease shows no apparent breed predilection.

Prostatic neoplasia traditionally has been believed to be a disease of old, sexually intact dogs. Recent evidence refutes this assumption, however. In two studies, castration was not found to reduce the incidence of prostatic carcinoma regardless of when surgery occurred.[36,37] In one survey of 43 dogs, 19 (45%) had been castrated at least three years prior to developing prostatic carcinoma, including seven dogs that were castrated at younger than one year of age.[37] In the other study, 10 (30%) of 31 dogs had been castrated

> ## KEY POINT:
>
> *Early castration of dogs does not seem to reduce the risk of developing prostatic adenocarcinoma.*

two or more years prior to developing prostatic malignancy.[36] These data imply that testosterone is unlikely to be an etiologic factor in the development of prostatic carcinoma in dogs.

Clinical Presentation and History

The most frequent presenting signs relate to the lower bowel and include tenesmus, constipation, and dyschezia. Dogs may show anorexia and weight loss and signs referable to the urinary tract, such as stranguria and hematuria. Urinary tract signs, particularly in a castrated dog, should raise suspicion for prostatic neoplasia.[36] Lumbar pain and hindlimb weakness or lameness have been described, often in association with metastasis to the lumbar spine.[38] Duration of signs varies widely from weeks to years, although most affected dogs have signs for less than one month.[35,36]

Prostatomegaly is usually noted on digital rectal examination. In one series, only 16 (50%) of 31 dogs had prostatic enlargement. In 10 of these dogs, it was asymmetric.[36] There were no differences in these findings between the group of castrated dogs and uncastrated dogs,[36] although prostatomegaly may be less frequently detected on digital rectal palpation in castrated dogs because of involution of normal prostatic tissue after castration. Approximately 30% of dogs show pain on rectal or abdominal palpation. The prostate tumor is often fixed to the floor of the pelvis and may cause narrowing of the pelvic canal[32] as well as invading surrounding bone in the pelvis and sacral spine.[38]

Staging and Diagnosis

Hematology and serum biochemistry are rarely helpful in establishing a diagnosis. Urinalysis often reveals pyuria and hematuria (in 60%–65% of dogs).[36] Despite these findings, secondary bacterial infections are rarely found on urine culture or on prostatic aspiration or massage.[36] In one group of 31 dogs with prostatic carcinoma, malignant cells were seen on urinalysis.[36]

MANAGEMENT OF SPECIFIC DISEASES

Radiography helps to identify prostatomegaly and changes in size or contour of the prostate. Prostatic mineralization is most frequently associated with neoplasia and occurred in approximately 40% of the dogs in one study[36]; however, mineralization may occur with chronic prostatitis.[39] A distension retrograde urethrocystogram may reveal distortion of the prostatic urethra and is a reliable indicator of neoplasia but does not distinguish between primary urethral and primary prostatic tumors. Thoracic radiographs should be taken, as pulmonary metastasis occurs in more than 60% of dogs at necropsy[32,36] and is identified radiographically in nearly half of the affected dogs.[36]

On ultrasonography, nearly 70% of dogs with prostatic neoplasia show multifocal areas of increased prostatic echogenicity. Although not specific for prostatic carcinoma, this finding is strongly suggestive of a neoplastic process. Prostatic cysts are most frequently associated with prostatitis or hyperplasia, but they also may be seen with prostatic carcinoma. Ultrasonography is useful for evaluation of the sublumbar lymph nodes and other organs, such as the liver. Metastasis occurs to both sites in about one third of cases.[36]

Bone metastasis of prostatic carcinoma occurs in between 15% and 40% of affected dogs[32,36,38]; the most common sites are the pelvis and lumbosacral spine.[38] Dogs with hindlimb weakness or lameness should be evaluated by radiographs or bone scintigraphy for evidence of bony metastases to the pelvis and lumbar vertebrae or to distant bones. Bone scintigraphy may be more sensitive than radiographs in detecting bony metastases from prostatic carcinoma.[38]

Definitive diagnosis is made by cytology or histopathology. Ultrasonographic guidance is very helpful in obtaining cytology samples by fine-needle aspiration. This method gives a high rate of positive diagnosis (80% in two studies[36,40]). False-negative results are more likely with such techniques as prostatic wash or prostatic massage via a urethral catheter, which does not direct the sampler to a suspicious lesion.[41] Transrectal biopsy with a Franzen transrectal needle guide rarely presents any complications.[36] The use of needle biopsy instruments transrectally is described in the Biopsy section. If ultrasonography is available, however, the transabdominal approach is probably preferable for fine-needle aspiration and needle biopsy.

Prognostic Factors

One study found a significantly higher rate of pulmonary metastasis for prostatic carcinoma arising in castrated dogs compared with intact dogs (100% versus 47%, respectively). There was no difference in overall metastatic rate, indicating that other metastatic sites are common.[36] This finding may correlate with the higher rate of poorly differentiated tumors in castrated dogs and implies that prostatic carcinoma is a more aggressive disease in castrated dogs.

Treatment

Surgery is the treatment of choice for many canine tumors but is not recommended for prostatic carcinoma because of technical difficulties and the high rate of metastasis. When surgical removal of the prostate was performed for six dogs with prostatic adenocarcinoma, five of the six dogs had survival times of less than 30 days, and the remaining dog died 60 days after surgery.[33] Metastasis was common.

Hormonal therapy in dogs has been limited to surgical castration and/or estrogen therapy. Neither approach has been useful, and these treatments give survival times of fewer than 30 days with no improvement in clinical signs.[33,35,36] Ketoconazole, which interferes with steroid synthesis, was used in two dogs in combination with external beam radiation therapy, with no effect.[36] The lack of effect of these hormonal manipulations is not surprising, given the lack of influence of castration on development of this disease.[36,37]

Radiation therapy may be palliative in the treatment of prostatic carcinoma, but the high rate of metas-

> **°KEY POINT:**
>
> *Half of the dogs with prostatic carcinoma do not have an enlarged prostate gland.*

tasis (85% to 100%[36]) means that, as for surgery, overall survival statistics are unlikely to be greatly affected. Orthovoltage radiation therapy was given intraoperatively to 10 dogs with prostatic carcinoma.[42] Doses of 15 to 30 Gy were delivered to the prostate alone in seven dogs that had disease macroscopically confined to the prostate, and the sublumbar nodes of three dogs received the same dose. Median survival was 114 days (range = 41 to 750 days) despite a complete response to radiation in five dogs. Two dogs died of unrelated disease, and one had no evidence of disease at the last follow-up examination. The remainder of the dogs died of complications of treatment or recurrent disease. In three dogs, ^{60}Co radiation therapy combined with a prostatectomy[36,43] (in addition to ketoconazole in two dogs[36]) gave survival times of 4, 3, and 4 months, respectively.

There are few reports of chemotherapy for this disease. Two dogs that underwent subtotal intracapsular prostatectomy received mitoxantrone (5 mg/m[2] IV every 3 weeks) for 2 and 3 treatments.[42] Survival times in these two dogs were 5 and 3 months, respectively. Two dogs that received intraoperative radiation also received cyclophosphamide (50 mg/m[2] QOD PO) and 5-fluorouracil (100 mg/m[2] IV weekly) chemotherapy, and one of these dogs also received doxorubicin (30 mg/m[2] IV every 3 weeks). Survival times from the start of chemotherapy were 120 and 80 days, respectively. Further investigation is needed to define the role of chemotherapy in the treatment of prostatic carcinoma.

TUMORS OF THE FEMALE REPRODUCTIVE TRACT IN CATS
Ovarian Tumors
Incidence, Signalment, and Etiology
Tumors of the feline ovary are rare, and there are few reports of cases in the literature. The rarity of these tumors probably reflects neutering practices rather than intrinsic resistance to tumor formation. The majority of reported cases have been in domestic shorthairs, but ovarian tumors occasionally occur in purebred cats.[44,45] Granulosa cell tumors are the most commonly diagnosed tumors. In 32 reported cases, ages of affected cats ranged from 6 months to 20 years of age (average = 9 years of age).[44,45] These tumors were unilateral in cases for which a location was known. Other tumors are rarely seen but include germ cell tumors (i.e., dysgerminoma and teratoma), interstitial cell tumors, and lymphoma. Epithelial tumors are rarely reported.

Clinical Presentation and History
Cats with granulosa cell tumors usually show prolonged or irregular estrous behavior due to the production of sex hormones. Abnormal behavior (aggression) has been noted and may resolve after surgery.[45] Feline ovarian tumors are rarely larger than 5 cm in diameter and may not be palpable on physical examination.

Staging and Diagnosis
Metastases to the lungs, liver and spleen, or kidney have been seen with granulosa cell tumors, and dysgerminomas have been reported to metastasize.[44] Epithelial tumors, although rare, are usually malignant and metastasize to the abdominal cavity with resulting carcinomatosis.[45] Any cat with an ovarian tumor should have abdominal ultrasonography performed and thoracic radiographs taken prior to a definitive surgery.

Treatment
Surgical resection of an affected ovary may be curative; however, it should be noted that most ovarian tumors in the cat are malignant and that the most common tumor types have been reported to metastasize. There are no reports of chemotherapy for these tumors. Although cisplatin seems to be an active agent in the treatment of human and canine ovarian carcinomatosis, it is contraindicated in cats.

Vaginal and Uterine Tumors
Incidence, Signalment, and Etiology
Tumors of the uterus and vagina in cats are extremely rare, and the majority are benign growths. As with dogs, the most common tumor types are leiomyomas and fibromas. These tumors may be single or multiple and are usually in the body of the uterus. Lower reproductive tract tumors are most common in cats 9 years

of age or older. Leiomyomas and fibromas seem to be hormonally influenced and may be found in association with such changes as ovarian cysts and cystic hyperplasia of the endometrium.

Malignant tumors are less common and are usually adenocarcinomas, although leiomyosarcomas can occur. Lymphoma has been described in association with multicentric disease. Vaginal tumors are less common than uterine tumors but are of the same histologic types.

Clinical Presentation and History

Large leiomyomas or fibromas may block the uterine lumen, and cats have presented with dystocia or pyometra. Malignant tumors may cause fluid accumulation in the uterus with signs very similar to those of pyometra. A large uterine mass may cause constipation as a result of its space-occupying effect.

Staging and Diagnosis

Metastasis has been reported with uterine and vaginal carcinomas and sarcomas. Metastasis usually is to the mesentery and omentum and may involve other intra-abdominal organs or structures. A leiomyosarcoma was reported to have metastasized to the lungs[45]; therefore, thoracic radiographs and abdominal ultrasonography should be performed prior to definitive treatment.

Treatment

Surgical excision by hysterectomy should be curative for benign lesions. Malignant tumors are often metastatic at the time of presentation, and no adjunctive therapy has been reported.

TUMORS OF THE MALE REPRODUCTIVE TRACT IN CATS
Testicular Tumors

Testicular tumors are extremely rare in cats, and there are few details regarding their behavior. A seminoma that occurred in a cryptorchid testicle in a 2-year-old cat metastasized to the sublumbar lymph nodes; this was the only site of metastasis at necropsy.[45] Sertoli cell tumors that were not apparently hormonally functional have been described in two cats.[45] A functional interstitial cell tumor that arose in the spermatic cord of an 11-year-old castrated cat has been described, but treatment was not attempted.[46]

Prostatic Tumors
Incidence, Signalment, and Etiology

Unlike in dogs, prostatic tumors are extremely rare in cats and seem to affect aged animals; the median age of 5 reported cats was 15 years with a range of 11 to 22 years.[45,47,48] All affected cats had been castrated. Adenocarcinomas were seen in four cats, and one cat had a fibroadenoma.[48]

Clinical Presentation and History

Common clinical signs are hematuria, dysuria, and incontinence, and affected cats may experience acute urethral obstruction. A palpable mass may be felt on the pelvic brim or during a rectal examination.

Treatment

Treatment was attempted in one cat with prostatic adenocarcinoma.[47] The prostate was surgically resected by urethral transection. Although there was no evidence of metastatic disease on thoracic radiographs or on histologic examination of the iliac lymph nodes, adjunctive doxorubicin (30 mg/m^2 IV) and cyclophosphamide (300 mg/m^2) every 4 weeks was given for four treatments. Local tumor recurrence and metastasis to the pancreas and lungs occurred 10 months after surgery.

REFERENCES
1. Patnaik AK, Greenlee PG: Canine ovarian neoplasms: A clinicopathologic study of 71 cases, including histology of 12 granulosa cell tumors. *Vet Pathol* 24:509–514, 1987.
2. Seaman WJ: Canine ovarian fibroma associated with prolonged exposure to mibolerone. *Toxicol Pathol* 13:177–180, 1985.
3. Jergens AE, Knapp DW, Shaw DP: Ovarian teratoma in a bitch. *JAVMA* 191:81–83, 1987.
4. Cheng N: Aberrant behavior in a bitch with a granulosa-theca cell tumor. *Aust Vet J* 70:71–72, 1992.
5. Greenlee PG, Patnaik AK: Canine ovarian tumors of germ cell origin. *Vet Pathol* 22:117–122, 1985.

MANAGEMENT OF SPECIFIC DISEASES

6. Wilson RB, Cave JS, Copeland JS, Onks J: Ovarian teratoma in two dogs. *JAAHA* 21:249–253, 1985.

7. Moore AS, Kirk C, Cardona A: Intracavitary cisplatin chemotherapy experience with six dogs. *J Vet Intern Med* 5:227–231, 1991.

8. Olsen J, Komtebedde J, Lackner A, Madewell BR: Cytoreductive treatment of ovarian carcinoma. *J Vet Intern Med* 8:133–135, 1994.

9. Greene JA, Richardson RC, Thornhill JA, et al; Ovarian papillary cystadenocarcinoma in a bitch: Case report and literature review. *JAAHA* 15:351–356, 1979.

10. Brodey RS, Roszel JF: Neoplasms of the canine uterus, vagina and vulva: A clinicopathologic survey of 90 cases. *JAVMA* 151:1294–1307, 1967.

11. Thacher C, Bradley RL: Vulvar and vaginal tumors in the dog: A retrospective study. *JAVMA* 183:690–692, 1983.

12. Vos JH: Uterine and cervical carcinomas in five dogs. *J Vet Med* 35:385–390, 1988.

13. Sailasuta A, Tateyama S, Yamaguchi R, et al: Adenomatous papilloma of the uterine tube (oviduct) fimbriae in a dog. *Jpn J Vet Sci* 51:632–633, 1989.

14. Payne-Johnson CE, Kelly DF, Davies PT: Endometrial carcinoma in a young dog. *J Comp Pathol* 96:463–467, 1986.

15. Peavy GM, Rettenmaier MA, Berns MW: Carbon dioxide laser ablation combined with doxorubicin hydrochloride treatment for vaginal fibrosarcoma in a dog. *JAVMA* 201:109–110, 1992.

16. Karlson AG, Mann FC: The transmissible venereal tumor of dogs: Observations on forty generations of experimental transfers. *Ann NY Acad Sci* 54:1197–1213, 1952.

17. Boscos C: Canine transmissible venereal tumor: Clinical observations and treatment. *Anim Famil* 3:10–15, 1988.

18. Yang TJ: Immunobiology of a spontaneously regressive tumor, the canine transmissible venereal sarcoma (review). *Anticancer Res* 8:93–96, 1988.

19. Amber EI, Henderson RA: Canine transmissible venereal tumor: Evaluation of surgical excision of primary and metastatic lesions in Zaire–Nigeria. *JAAHA* 1882:350–352, 1982.

20. Thrall DE: Orthovoltage radiotherapy of canine transmissible venereal tumors. *Vet Radiol* 23:217–219, 1982.

21. Calvert CA, Leifer CE, MacEwen EG: Vincristine for treatment of transmissible venereal tumor in the dog. *JAVMA* 181:163–164, 1982.

22. Amber EI, Henderson RA, Adeyanju JB, Gyang EO: Single-drug chemotherapy of canine transmissible venereal tumor with cyclophosphamide, methotrexate

23. Wasecki A, Mazur O: Zastosowaine preparatu vinblastin w leczeniu gozow stickera. *Medycyna Weterynaryjna* 33:142–143, 1977.

24. Nielson SW, Lein DH: Tumours of the testis. *Bull WHO* 50:71–78, 1974.

25. Hayes HM, Pendergrass TW: Canine testicular tumors. Epidemiologic features of 410 dogs. *Int J Cancer* 18:482–487, 1976.

26. Nieto JM, Pizarro M, Balaguer LM, Romano J: Canine testicular tumors in descended and cryptorchid testes. *DTW Dtsch Tierarztl Wochenschr* 96:186–189, 1989.

27. Patnaik AK, Mostofi FK: A clinicopathologic, histologic and immunohistochemical study of mixed germ cell-stomal tumors of the testis in 16 dogs. *Vet Pathol* 10:287–295, 1993.

28. Hayes HM, Wilson GP, Pendergrass TW, Cox VS: Canine cryptorchidism and subsequent testicular neoplasia: Case control study with epidemiologic update. *Teratology* 32:51–56, 1985.

29. Hayes HM, Tarone RE, Casey HW, Huxsoll DL: Excess of seminomas observed in Vietnam service U.S. military working dogs. *J Natl Cancer Inst* 82:1042–1046, 1990.

30. HogenEsch H, Whiteley HE, Vicini DS, Helper LC: Seminoma with metastases in the eyes and the brain in a dog. *Vet Pathol* 24:278–280, 1987.

31. McDonald RK, Walker M, Legendre AM, et al: Radiotherapy of metastatic seminoma in the dog: Case reports. *J Vet Intern Med* 2:103–107, 1988.

32. Leav I, Ling GV: Adenocarcinoma of the canine prostate. *Cancer* 22:1329–1345, 1968.

33. Hargis AM, Miller LM: Prostatic carcinoma in dogs. *Compend Contin Educ Pract Vet* 5:647–653, 1983.

34. O'Shea JD: Studies of the canine prostate gland. II. Prostatic neoplasms. *J Comp Pathol* 73:244–254, 1963.

35. Weaver AD: Fifteen cases of prostatic carcinoma in the dog. *Vet Rec* 109:71–75, 1981.

36. Bell FW, Klausner JS, Hayden DW, et al: Clinical and pathological features of prostatic adenocarcinoma in sexually intact and castrated dogs: 31 cases (1970–1987). *JAVMA* 199:1623–1630, 1991.

37. Obradovich J, Walshaw R, Goulland E: The influence of castration of the development of prostatic carcinoma in the dog: 43 cases (1978–1985). *J Vet Intern Med* 1:183–187, 1987.

38. Durham SK, Deitze AE: Prostatic adenocarcinoma with and without metastasis to bone in dogs. *JAVMA* 188:1432–1436, 1986.

39. Feeney DA, Johnston GR, Klausner JR, et al: Canine prostatic disease: Comparison of radiographic appearance with morphologic and microbiology findings in

30 cases (1981–1985). *JAVMA* 190:1018–1026, 1987.

40. Nickel RF, Teske E: Diagnosis of canine prostatic carcinoma. *Tijdschr Diergeneeskd* 117(Suppl):32S, 1992.
41. Barsanti JA, Finco DR: Evaluation of techniques for diagnosis of canine prostatic diseases. *JAVMA* 190:48–52, 1987.
42. Turrel JM: Intraoperative radiotherapy of carcinoma of the prostate gland in ten dogs. *JAVMA* 190:48–52, 1987.
43. Mann FA, Barrett RJ, Henderson RA: Use of a retained urethral catheter in three dogs with prostatic neoplasia. *Vet Surg* 21:342–347, 1992.
44. Gelberg HB: Feline ovarian neoplasms. *Vet Pathol*
22:572–576, 1985.

45. Carpenter JL, Andrews LK, Holzworth J: Tumors and tumor-like lesions, in Holzworth J (ed): *Diseases of the Cat. Medicine and Surgery*. Philadelphia, WB Saunders, 1987, pp 406–596.
46. Rosen DK, Carpenter JL: Functional ectopic interstitial cell tumor in a castrated male cat. *JAVMA* 202:1865–1866, 1993.
47. Hubbard BS, Vulgamott JC, Liska WD: Prostatic adenocarcinoma in a cat. *JAVMA* 197:1493–1494, 1990.
48. Cotchin E: Neoplasia, in Wilkinson GT (ed): *Diseases of the Cat and their Management*. Melbourne, Australia, Blackwell Scientific Public, 1983.

CLINICAL BRIEFING: MAMMARY NEOPLASIA

Mammary Tumors in Dogs

Common Clinical Presentation	Presence of a mass in the mammary chain
Common Histologic Types	Approximately 50% are benign (e.g., fibroadenomas, simple adenomas, and benign mixed mammary tumors); approximately 50% are malignant (e.g., solid carcinomas and tubular or papillary adenocarcinomas)
Epidemiology and Biological Behavior	Most common neoplasm in females; average age is 10–11 years; poodles, terriers, cocker spaniels, and German shepherds are overrepresented; early ovariohysterectomy protective; 50% of tumors are multiple; lungs and lymph nodes are most common sites of metastasis
Prognostic Factors	German shepherds have a poor prognosis; poor prognosis associated with increasing tumor size, ulceration, degree of invasion, increasing degree of malignancy, lymph node involvement, and lack of hormone receptors

Treatment
  Surgery
 	
  Chemotherapy
	
	Regional resection of tumor is as effective as mastectomy for localized tumor(s); removal of lymph node may be of prognostic value; ovariohysterectomy may not be of value for preventing recurrence
	Doxorubicin- or mitoxantrone-based protocols may be effective in some cases

Mammary Tumors in Cats

Common Clinical Presentation	Presence of a mass in the mammary chain
Common Histologic Type	Mammary adenocarcinoma
Epidemiology and Biological Behavior	Siamese may be at increased risk; most affected cats are 10–12 years of age; 70%–90% of tumors are malignant; >25% are ulcerated; >50% involve multiple glands; >80% have metastases at time of euthanasia

MANAGEMENT OF SPECIFIC DISEASES

Prognostic Factors	Increasing tumor size is associated with poor prognosis
Treatment Surgery	Mastectomy of the affected side is superior to regional resection; recurrence not likely to be reduced by ovariohysterectomy; recurrence of tumor should be treated with surgery whenever possible
Chemotherapy	Doxorubicin and cyclophosphamide reported to reduce metastatic disease; mitoxantrone may be helpful in some cases

MAMMARY TUMORS IN DOGS
Incidence, Signalment, and Etiology

Mammary tumors are the most common neoplasm in female dogs and account for approximately half of all neoplasms in the bitch.[1-3] In contrast, mammary neoplasms are rare in male dogs, accounting for less than 1% of these types of tumors. The incidence of mammary tumors is higher in dogs than any other domesticated animal and is three times the incidence in humans.[2,3] Approximately half of the tumors are malignant, and half of these have metastasized by the time they are initially diagnosed.[1-3] Most dogs with mammary tumors are old; the average age of affected dogs is 10 to 11 years of age, and the range is 2 to 16 years of age.[1-16] In one study of mammary tumors, all dogs younger than 6 years of age had benign tumors.[1] There is no consensus about which breeds have the highest incidence; however, poodles, terriers, cocker spaniels, and German shepherds are commonly noted as being overrepresented.[2,3] Chihuahuas and boxers reportedly have less risk of developing mammary tumors than other breeds.

Much research has examined risk factors that may be associated with the development of canine mammary neoplasia. Many risk factors associated with mammary tumors in humans do not seem to be significant in dogs. Factors that are not associated with increased risk in female dogs include stage of pregnancy, age at first litter, number of puppies born, and history of abnormal estrous cycles and of pseudopregnancy.[4,5] Sex hormones certainly play a role in development of mammary tumors in the bitch. Exogenous progestogens may instigate tumor development. Approximately 50% of canine mammary tumors are estrogen-receptor positive, and 44% are estrogen- and progesterone-receptor positive.[5-7] Intact females have a seven-fold increased risk of developing mammary cancer compared to neutered females.

The age at which ovariohysterectomy takes place is directly proportional to the risk of developing mammary cancer (Table 5-15).[5] Data clearly indicate the preventive role of spaying prior to the second estrus. Although it has not been proven that spaying at the time of mastectomy improves survival or disease-free interval, no study has evaluated the effect of ovariohysterectomy in dogs with estrogen-receptor–positive mammary tumors. One study[18] did show that ovariecto-

> **KEY POINT:**
>
> *Intact females have a seven-fold increased risk of developing mammary cancer compared to neutered females. Spaying prior to the second estrus reduces the risk of mammary tumor development in dogs.*

MANAGEMENT OF SPECIFIC DISEASES

TABLE 5-15
Relationship between time of ovariohysterectomy and the risk of developing mammary neoplasia[5]

Time of Ovariohysterectomy	Risk of Developing Mammary Tumor
Before first estrus	0.05%
Between first and second estrus	8%
After second estrus	26%

my, even when performed at an advanced age, protects against mammary tumor development. Obesity may be a factor in mammary neoplasia. In one case-controlled study, the risk of mammary gland cancer among spayed dogs was significantly reduced in dogs that had been thin at 9 to 12 months of age. Among intact dogs that were thin at 9 to 12 months, however, risk of mammary cancer was only reduced insignificantly.[17]

Clinical Presentation and History

A diagnosis of mammary neoplasia in dogs may be suspected based on a history that includes factors such as postponed spaying, progestogen therapy, irregular heat cycles, unexplained lactation, and the presence of a lump within the mammary chain. Physical examination can confirm the presence of a mammary mass, which may range in size from a few millimeters to many centimeters. At least 50% of dogs with mammary gland tumors have multiple masses.[1-17] Some studies suggest that the tumors are more common in the caudal mammary glands, whereas other studies report a uniform distribution throughout mammary tissue.

Inflammatory carcinomas represent less than 10% of malignant mammary tumors. Dogs with this type of tumor usually have hot, swollen mammary glands that may be misdiagnosed as mastitis. These animals may have edema of a nearby limb as well as widespread microscopic or measurable metastatic disease. Diagnosis of an inflammatory carcinoma is made by biopsy along with the observation of an inflamed mammary gland. The prognosis is very poor.

Staging and Diagnosis

The two most common sites of metastases are lungs and regional lymph nodes. Therefore, staging should include chest radiographs, complete blood count (CBC), biochemical profile, urinalysis, and an evaluation of regional lymph nodes by palpation, fine-needle aspiration cytology, and (if indicated) biopsy. Chest radiographs have a sensitivity of 65%, a specificity of 97%, and a diagnostic accuracy of 87%.[20] Other common sites of metastases include liver, kidney, adrenal glands, spleen, pancreas, diaphragm, ovaries, heart, bone, and urethra. Although bone metastases may be common in the later stages of the disease, one study using radionuclide bone imaging showed that bone metastases are rare at initial presentation of dogs with mammary cancer.[16] Fine-needle aspiration cytology may help make a definitive diagnosis in some cases; however, because results of cytology can be misleading, an excisional or incisional biopsy is always recommended.

False-positive results from cytology are rare, but as many as one third of cases of mammary neoplasia evaluated cytologically have false-negative results.[8] Excisional or incisional biopsy should always be used to confirm a suspected diagnosis.

Prognostic Factors

Somewhat surprisingly, the prognosis for dogs with mammary cancer is not influenced by either tumor location or number. The following are prognostic factors that predict survival or disease-free interval.

KEY POINT:

Fine-needle aspiration cytology may be helpful in making a definitive diagnosis in some cases; however, results of cytology can be misleading. Excisional or incisional biopsy is always recommended.

MANAGEMENT OF SPECIFIC DISEASES

Breed

One study suggested that German shepherds with mammary cancer had a poorer prognosis than other breeds, such as beagles and dachshunds.[9,10]

Tumor Size

Dogs with mammary tumors less than 3 cm in diameter have a significantly better prognosis than dogs with larger tumors (Figure 5-84).[11]

Degree of Invasion and Ulceration

Dogs with tumors that are fixed to underlying structures or that ulcerate overlying skin have a worse prognosis than those without these clinical features.[12]

Duration of Tumor Presence

One study found that a shorter history of signs prior to surgery was associated with longer survival after surgery.

Histopathology

Several histologic grading schemes are of prognostic significance. Important factors include histologic classification, degree of nuclear differentiation, and the presence of lymphoid accumulation.[1,11–14] In general, the more highly differentiated the tumor, the better the prognosis. Poorly differentiated tumors are much more likely to recur than well-differentiated tumors.[1] The chance of recurrence for poorly differentiated canine mammary tumors is 90%; for moderately differentiated tumors, 68%; and for well-differentiated tumors, 24%. Dogs with precancerous mastopathy have a nine-fold increased risk of developing mammary cancer.[14] Thus, precancerous mastopathy should not be dismissed as benign. Dogs that have mammary cancer but no evidence of lymphoid cellular reactivity at the time of initial mastectomy have a threefold increased risk of developing recurrence within two years compared to those with such reactivity. In one study, 75% of dogs with malignant mammary tumors did not survive more than two years. The type of surgery (simple mastectomy versus en bloc resection) failed to influence survival.[19] Mammary sarcomas have a very poor prognosis compared to carcinomas or mixed malignant mammary tumors.

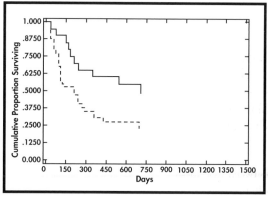

Figure 5-84: *Comparison of the cancer-free interval in dogs with malignant mammary tumors after surgical removal. Stage II tumors that are 3 to 5 cm in diameter (solid line) are compared to stage III tumors that are greater than 5 cm in diameter (dashed line). These data show that size is an important prognostic factor for those dogs that have tumors surgically excised. (From Withrow SJ, MacEwen EG (eds): Tumors of the mammary gland. Clinical Veterinary Oncology. Philadelphia, JB Lippincott, 1989, p 299; with permission.)*

KEY POINT:

Removing regional lymph nodes at the time of surgery may be of prognostic value. Metastases to regional lymph nodes suggest a poor prognosis, but there is no evidence that removal of affected lymph nodes increases survival or disease-free interval.

Lymph Node Involvement

Metastases to regional lymph nodes has been associated with an increase risk for tumor recurrence.[1]

Hormone-Receptor Activity

Dogs with tumors that are estrogen- and/or progesterone-receptor positive have a better prognosis than dogs with tumors that do not have receptors. Receptor-positive tumors are likely to be benign.[6,7]

MANAGEMENT OF SPECIFIC DISEASES

Treatment

Surgery is the treatment of choice for localized mammary tumors.[1,9–15] The extent of surgery influences neither survival nor disease-free interval. Results of several studies suggest that lumpectomy or regional mastectomy of affected glands with resection of available nodes for staging may be the best choice. The tumor and a surrounding "cuff" of normal tissue should be removed. As a general rule, there should be enough normal tissue around the tumor to remove any small unseen "fingers" of tumor tissue that can extend from the primary lesion. The following are procedures that may be considered.

Lumpectomy

This surgical procedure is performed by incising the skin and bluntly dissecting the mammary tissue that surrounds the tumor. It generally is indicated for tumors that are smaller than 5 mm.

Mammectomy

The removal of one gland is indicated for tumors larger than 1 cm. Because glands four and five are often confluent, they are usually removed together. The body wall and skin are removed if they are involved or if the tumor approaches these structures.

Regional or Total Mastectomy

Several glands can be removed if multiple glands contain tumors. For localized tumors, mastectomy does not prolong the disease-free interval or survival compared to lumpectomy or mammectomy.

Lymph Node Removal

Because dogs with lymph node tumors have a poorer prognosis than those without such involvement, it may be appropriate to remove an adjoining lymph node at surgery for prognostic information.

Ovariohysterectomy

As noted earlier, most studies show that concurrent ovariohys-terectomy fails to alter survival and disease-free interval.[1,12,13,15] One study, however, documented that ovariohysterectomy with tumor removal produced a mean survival of 18.5 months compared to 6.1 months for mastectomy alone.[19]

Tamoxifen (0.42 mg/kg BID PO), an antiestrogen drug, is reported as effective for treating dogs with mammary adenocarcinoma.[21] Although not proven in large clinical trials, the combination of doxorubicin (30 mg/m^2 IV on day 1 of a 21-day cycle) and cyclophosphamide (50 mg/m^2 PO on days 3–6 of each 21-day cycle) has been recommended as an effective adjunctive treatment for malignant mammary neoplasia.[19] Two dogs treated with doxorubicin for metastatic mammary neoplasia had a partial remission for 12 and 15 months.[22] Anecdotally, cisplatin may cause regression of some pulmonary metastases. Other drugs that are effective in women with breast cancer that are being evaluated in dogs are mitoxantrone (6 mg/m^2 IV every 21 days) and taxol (165 mg/m^2 IV with appropriate pretreatment with dexamethasone, benadryl, and cimetidine every 21 days). Appropriate clinical studies are essential to document the efficacy of chemotherapy.

MAMMARY TUMORS IN CATS
Incidence, Signalment, and Etiology

Malignancy must be considered in any cat that is presented with a mammary mass. At least 70% to 90% of feline mammary tumors are malignant.[23–25] Mammary tumors are the third most common tumor in cats, after hematopoietic neoplasms and skin tumors.[3,25,26] The incidence of mammary tumors in cats is less than half of that of dogs.[2,3,23–28] Although there is no proven breed predilection for mammary tumors, some investigators have suggested that domestic shorthairs and Siamese have higher incidence rates than other cats.[3,29,30] Siamese may have twice the risk of any other breed of developing mammary tumors.[3]

> **KEY POINT:**
>
> *At least 25% of affected cats have ulcerated masses and at least 80% of all mammary masses are adenocarcinomas.*

MANAGEMENT OF SPECIFIC DISEASES

Mammary neoplasia has been reported in cats from 9 months to 23 years of age; the mean age of occurrence 10 to 12 years.[3,24,27,28,30–32] One study suggests that the disease occurs at an earlier age in Siamese and that the incidence in this breed reaches a plateau at about 9 years of age.[24] The majority of affected cats are intact females, but the disease occasionally affects spayed females and, rarely, male cats.[3,29,30]

More than 80% of feline mammary tumors are histologically classified as adenocarcinomas.[2,28,30] The frequency of diagnosis of the specific types of adenocarcinomas differs slightly among pathologists, but most agree that tubular, papillary, and solid carcinomas are the most common.[30] The majority of adenocarcinomas have a combination of tissue types in each tumor. Sarcomas, mucinous carcinomas, duct papillomas, adenosquamous carcinomas, and adenomas are rare.[3]

The exact cause of mammary tumors in cats is unknown and is an area of considerable research. Hormonal influences may be involved in the pathogenesis of mammary tumors in women, cats, and dogs. One study suggests that intact dogs and cats have a seven-fold greater risk of developing mammary cancer than spayed dogs and cats.[28] Not all investigators agree with this degree of risk, but all agree that intact cats are more likely to develop mammary tumors than spayed cats.[3,28] Studies have been performed to determine the etiologic roles of progesterone, testosterone, and estrogen in feline mammary tumors. Low levels of progesterone receptors have been found in the cytoplasm of some feline mammary tumors.[31,32] Several reports have documented a strong association between the prior use of progesterone-like drugs and the development of benign or

KEY POINTS:

Metastatic lung and thoracic cavity involvement may be extensive without respiratory signs or may cause respiratory insufficiency due to a pleural carcinomatosis with an effusion that often contains malignant cells.

Cats with fibroepithelial hyperplasia are usually young, intact females with very large mammary gland swellings that may cause pain and discoloration of the overlying skin as well as an abnormal gait.

malignant mammary masses in the cats.[3,33] Dihydrotestosterone receptors have not been found in mammary tumors in cats.[31] Only 10% of the feline tumors assayed were positive for estrogen receptors; a much higher percentage of positive tests is seen in dogs and humans. Cystic ovaries and a variety of uterine diseases are found in many mammary tumor patients.[23]

Clinical Presentation and History

Cats with mammary tumors are often presented to the veterinarian five months after tumors were initially noted.[30] Thus, the tumors are usually in an advanced state of development. A feline mammary tumor appears as a locally invasive mass that is firm and nodular. Metastasis has frequently occurred.[3] The neoplasm may adhere to the overlying skin and also can adhere to the underlying abdominal wall. At least 25% of affected patients have ulcerated masses.

The infiltration of lymphatics may be clinically apparent as subcutaneous linear, beaded chains.[29] Swelling due to tumor thrombi or decreased vascular return can cause discomfort, edema, and a change in the temperature in the pelvic limbs. The involved nipples are red and swollen and may exudate a tan or yellow fluid. The tumor can involve any or all mammary glands and is noted equally in the left and right sides.[23,29] A slightly higher incidence has been noted in the cranial two glands by some investigators.[23,29] More than 50% of the affected cats have more than one gland involved.[23,29] These tumors can be associated with chronic mastitis, uterine disease, and other unrelated tumors as well as with anemia, osteoporosis, ascites, and leukocytosis.

MANAGEMENT OF SPECIFIC DISEASES

Staging and Diagnosis

Before diagnostic procedures or therapeutic steps are begun, a biochemical profile, urinalysis, and a CBC should be done to identify any presurgical abnormalities. In several studies, more than 80% of the cats with a mammary malignancy had metastases to the lymph nodes, lungs, pleura, liver, diaphragm, adrenal glands, and/or kidneys at the time of euthanasia.[3,23,24] Thoracic radiographs in both the right and left lateral and ventrodorsal planes should be taken to search for pulmonary, lymph node, and pleural metastases. Pulmonary metastases from mammary tumors appear radiographically as interstitial densities. They range in size from those that are faintly seen, to those that are several centimeters in diameter, to miliary pleural lesions that can produce significant effusion. Sternal lymphadenopathy occasionally occurs. Aging changes in the lungs and pleura as well as inactive inflammatory lesions may mimic metastatic disease. Treatment should not be withheld because of equivocal radiographic findings. Whenever regional lymph nodes can be evaluated, they should be assessed by fine-needle aspiration cytology or biopsy.

Because of the high frequency of malignancy, an aggressive approach should be taken to confirm the diagnosis. A preliminary biopsy is not recommended unless it will change either the owner's willingness to treat the animal or the surgical procedure. Tissue for histopathology is taken at the time of mastectomy and should include the regional lymph nodes. Cytology should be performed on any pleural fluid present to search for malignant cells.

Although uncommon, a variety of nonmalignant lesions must be considered in a differential diagnosis of mammary neoplasia. The most common benign growths are classified as cysts, papillary cystic hyperplasia, lobular hyperplasia, and mastitis.[33–35] Fibroepithelial hyperplasia is a common benign lesion involving one or more glands and is frequently seen one to two weeks after estrus.[33] The gland may be so large that the patient may walk with an abnormal gait. The skin overlying the mass may be discolored, edematous, and painful (Figure 5-85). Cats with

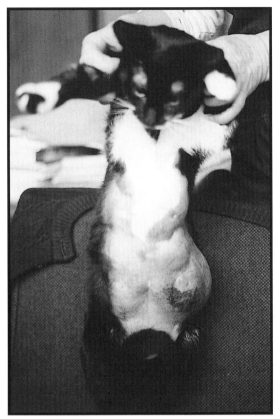

Figure 5-85: *Fibroepithelial hyperplasia is seen in young cycling intact female cats. The greatly enlarged mammary glands bruise easily and may cause an abnormal gait in some cats. Although spaying can resolve clinical signs, cats often return to normal without therapy.*

fibroepithelial hyperplasia are often young, intact females. The signs are similar to those seen with most malignant tumors. Because the benign masses closely resemble malignant neoplasms, they are often treated as malignancies.

Prognostic Factors

Because stromal invasion is almost always present and metastases are frequently present at the time of surgery, the prognosis is guarded to poor. Sixty-six percent of cats with tumors that were surgically excised have a recurrence at the surgical site.[30] The

MANAGEMENT OF SPECIFIC DISEASES

time from tumor detection to the death of the cat is rarely longer than 12 months.[3,23,24] The most significant prognostic factors influencing tumor recurrence and survival for cats with malignant mammary neoplasia are tumor size, the extent of surgery needed to remove the tumors, and histologic grading of the tumors.[34,36]

MacEwen et al[36] has shown that tumor size is the most important of these prognostic factors (Figure 5-86). After surgery, the median for survival of cats with tumors larger than 3 cm in diameter is six months. Cats with tumors 2 to 3 cm in diameter have a median for survival after surgery of two years. Cats with tumors smaller than 2 cm in diameter have a median for survival after surgery of approximately three years.[38] Compared with regional "lumpectomy," radical surgery reduces local tumor recurrence but does not increase the overall survival time. Cats with well-differentiated tumors with few mitotic figures per high-power field live longer than cats with moderately or poorly differentiated tumors.[23,37] The 1-year survival rate was high in cats with a tumor that did not show lymphatic infiltration. There is a good correlation between the grade of malignancy, rate of growth and invasive capacity, and prognosis. Patients with pulmonary metastatic disease rarely survive more than two months.

Treatment

Feline mammary neoplasms have been treated in a variety of ways; however, surgery is the most widely used treatment. There have been no reports documenting the efficacy of radiation therapy or commercially available biological response modifiers for the treatment of this disease. The biological response modifier, liposome-encapsulated muramyltripeptide-phosphatidylethanolamine (L-MTP-PE), may be effective when used in combination with surgery or chemotherapy.

> ### KEY POINT:
>
> *The most significant prognostic factors influencing tumor recurrence and survival for cats with malignant mammary neoplasia are tumor size, the extent of surgery needed to remove the tumor, and histologic grading of the tumor.*

The success of surgery is hindered by the invasiveness and tendency for early metastasis of the disease. Radical mastectomy (i.e., removal of all glands on the affected side) is the surgical method of choice because it significantly reduces the chance of local tumor recurrence[23,25,27,36] (Figures 5-87 and 5-88). This procedure is used regardless of the size of the tumor.

Several surgical principles are observed when performing a mastectomy on feline mammary tumor patients. During or prior to surgery, a bacterial culture and antibiotic sensitivity testing are advisable, because approximately one fourth of mammary carcinomas are ulcerated. An en bloc resection is often employed in such a way that the tumor and draining nodes and vessels are removed by wide surgical excision and a partial or complete resection of the underlying tissue is done.[23,37] If bilateral mastectomy is indicated, the affected glands and their associated lymph nodes are

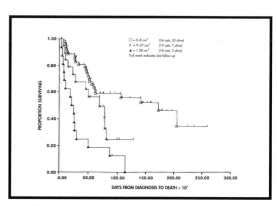

Figure 5-86: *Survival time in relation to tumor size in cats with malignant mammary adenocarcinoma. These data demonstrate that the larger the tumor, the shorter the survival. (From MacEwen EG, Hayes AA, Harvey HJ, et al: Prognostic factors for feline mammary tumors.* JAVMA *185:201–204, 1984; with permission.)*

MANAGEMENT OF SPECIFIC DISEASES

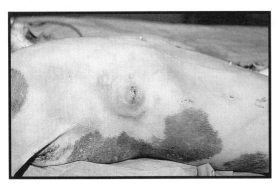

Figure 5-87: *Cat in dorsal recumbency prepared for surgery to remove a single ulcerated mammary tumor. Prior to surgery, it is important to stage the patient to make sure that there is no overt evidence of metastatic disease. Staging is done with a CBC, biochemical profile, urinalysis, chest radiographs, and an assessment of regional lymph nodes.*

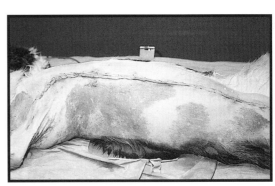

Figure 5-88: *The cat in figure 5-87 after surgery. Note that the entire mammary chain was removed along with an axillary lymph node. If there was evidence of tumor in the contralateral chain, a second mastectomy would be performed in 10 to 14 days.*

removed, and a second surgery is performed 10 to 14 days later. The interim allows the skin to stretch for a complete primary closure at the second surgery. Early vessel ligation is essential; one study noted that patients examined in two thirds of the cases had tumor invasion of lymphatics and veins. Gentle handling of all damaged tissue is essential. After removal of the tumor, copious flushing of the surgery area helps eliminate exfoliated neoplastic cells. Although spaying does not decrease the incidence of recurrence, some believe that it is warranted because of the possibility of coexisting ovarian and uterine disease.[3,30] If the mammary mass is caused by a benign condition, such as fibroepithelial hyperplasia, spaying often results in regression of the hyperplastic tissue. Regression may take as long as five months. This condition may resolve spontaneously within a few weeks of diagnosis, sometimes without an oophorectomy.

Radiation Therapy

Radiation therapy is not used routinely to treat feline mammary tumors. Radiation does not seem to dramatically increase the survival rate of feline mammary tumor patients, but it may reduce local recurrence rates.

Chemotherapy

Chemotherapy, alone or in combination with surgery, is not as successful for feline mammary tumors as it is for other feline tumors, such as lymphoma. Cyclophosphamide has been used alone and in combination with other chemotherapeutic agents and has not consistently helped feline mammary tumor patients.[39] The combination therapy of doxorubicin and cyclophosphamide induces short-term partial and complete responses in 50% of cats with metastatic or nonresectable local disease.[40,41] This chemotherapeutic protocol is toxic in some cats and does not prolong survival. The role of mitoxantrone and taxol is still being elucidated; however, both have some efficacy in cats with malignant neoplasia. Further studies are necessary to quantify the benefit of adjunctive therapy for mammary neoplasia in cats.

> **KEY POINT:**
>
> *Mastectomy is the surgical method of choice for cats with mammary adenocarcinoma because it significantly reduces the chance of local tumor recurrence.*

REFERENCES

1. Kurzman ID, Gilbertson SR: Prognostic factors in canine mammary tumors. *Semin Vet Med Surg (Small Anim)* 1:25–32, 1986.
2. Dorn CR, Taylor DON, Frye FL, et al: Survey of animal neoplasms in Alameda and Contra Costa Counties, California. II. Cancer and morbidity in dogs and cats from Alameda County. *J Natl Cancer Inst* 40:307–318, 1968.
3. Preister WA, Mantel N: Occurrence of tumors in domestic animals. Data from 12 United States and Canadian colleges in veterinary medicine. *J Natl Cancer Inst* 47:1333–1344, 1971.
4. Allen SW, Mahaffey EA: Canine mammary neoplasia: Prognostic indications and response to surgical therapy. *JAAHA* 25:540–546, 1989.
5. Schneider R, Dorn CR, Taylor DON: Factors influencing canine mammary cancer development and postsurgical survival. *J Natl Cancer Inst* 43:1249–1261, 1969.
6. Sartin EA, Barnes S, Kwapien RP, et al: Estrogen and progesterone receptor status of mammary carcinomas and correlation with clinical outcome in dogs. *Am J Vet Res* 53:2196–2200, 1992.
7. MacEwen EG, Patnaik AK, Harvey HJ, et al: Estrogen receptors in canine mammary tumors. *Cancer Res* 42:2255–2259, 1982.
8. Allen SK: Cytologic differentiation of benign from malignant canine mammary tumors. *Vet Pathol* 23:649–655, 1986.
9. Withrow SJ: Surgical management of canine mammary tumors. *Vet Clin North Am Small Anim Pract* 5:95–96, 1975.
10. Harvey HJ. Gilbertson SR: Canine mammary gland tumors. *Vet Clin North Am Small Anim Pract* 7:205–209, 1977.
11. Fidler IJ, Brodey RS: A necropsy study of canine malignant mammary neoplasms. *JAVMA* 151:710–715, 1967.
12. Misdorp W, Hart AAM: Canine mammary cancer. I. Prognosis. *J Small Anim Pract* 20:385–394, 1979.
13. Fowler EH, Wilson GP, Koestner A: Biologic behavior of canine mammary neoplasms based on histogenic classification. *Vet Pathol* 11:212–229, 1974.
14. Gilbertson SR, Kurzman ID, Zachrau RE, et al: Canine mammary epithelial neoplasms: Biologic implications of morphologic characteristics assessed in 232 dogs. *Vet Pathol* 20:127–142, 1983.
15. Misdorp W, Hart AAM: Canine mammary cancer. II. Therapy and causes of death. *J Small Anim Pract* 20:395–402, 1979.
16. Ogilvie GK, Allhans RA, Twardock EG, et al: Use of radionuclide imaging to identify malignant mammary tumor bone metastases in the dogs. *JAVMA* 195:220–226, 1989.
17. Sonnenschein EG, Glickman LT, Goldschmidt MH, et al: Body conformation, diet, and risk of breast cancer in pet dogs: A case control study. *Am J Epidemiol* 133:694–703, 1991.
18. Misdorp W: Canine mammary tumors: Protective effect of late ovariectomy and stimulating effect of progestin. *Vet Q* 10:26–33, 1988.
19. Johnston SD: Reproductive systems, in Slatter D (ed): *Textbook of Small Animal Surgery*, ed 2. Philadelphia, WB Saunders, 1993, pp 2177–2200.
20. Tiemessen I: Thoracic metastases of canine mammary gland tumors in the dog: A radiographic study. *Vet Radiol* 30:349–354, 1989.
21. Kitchell BE, Mammary carcinoma in dogs: An update on biology and therapy. *Proc 12th ACVIM Forum*: 884–886, 1994.
22. Hahn KA, Richardson RC, Knapp DW: Canine malignant neoplasia: Biological behavior, diagnosis, and treatment alternatives. *JAAHA* 28:251–256, 1992.
23. Baker GJ: Treatment of malignant neoplasia: Surgical management. *J Small Anim Pract* 133:373–379, 1972.
24. Dorn CR, Taylor DON, Frye FS, et al: Survey of animal neoplasms in Alameda and Contra Costa Counties, California. I. Methodology and description of cases. *J Natl Cancer Inst* 40:295–305, 1968.
25. Hayes HM Jr, Milne KL, Mandell CP: Epidemiological features of feline mammary carcinomas. *Vet Rec* 108:476–479, 1981.
26. Schmidt RE, Langham RF: A survey of feline neoplasms. *JAVMA* 151:1325–1328, 1967.
27. Patnaik AK, Liu SK, Hurvitz AL, et al: Non-hematopoietic neoplasms in cats. *J Natl Cancer Inst* 54:855–860, 1975.
28. Hayden DW, Neilsen SW: Feline mammary tumors. *J Small Anim Pract* 12:687–697, 1971.
29. Hayes A: Feline mammary gland tumors. *Vet Clin North Am Small Anim Pract* 7:205–212, 1977.
30. Moulton JE: *Tumors in Domestic Animals*, ed 2. Berkeley, CA, University of California Press, 1978, pp 367–369.
31. Elling H, Ungemach FR: Progesterone receptors in feline mammary cancer cytosol. *J Cancer Res Clin Oncol* 100(3):325–327, 1981.
32. Johnston SD, Hayden DW, Kiang DT, et al: Progesterone receptors in feline mammary adenocarcinomas. *Am J Vet Res* 45:379–382, 1984.
33. Hayden DW, Johstons JD, Kiang DT, et al: Feline mammary hypertrophy/fibroadenoma complex: Clinical and hormonal aspects. *Am J Vet Res* 42:1699–1703, 1981.

34. Canellos GP: Carcinoma of the breast, in Wyngaarden JB, Smith IB (eds): *Textbook of Medicine*, ed 7. Philadelphia, WB Saunders, 1982, pp 1282–1286.

35. Nimmo JS, Plummer JM: Ultrastructural studies of fibroadenomatous hyperplasia of mammary glands of two cats. *J Comp Pathol* 91:41–50, 1981.

36. MacEwen EG, Hayes AA, Harvey HJ, et al: Prognostic factors for feline mammary tumors. *JAVMA* 185:201–204, 1984.

37. Silver IA: Symposium on mammary neoplasia in the dog and cat. I. The anatomy of the mammary gland of the dog and cat. *J Small Anim Pract* 7:689, 1966.

38. MacEwen EG, Hayes AA, Mooney S, et al: Evaluation of effect of levamisole on feline mammary cancer. *J Biol Response Mod* 5:541–546, 1984.

39. Hayes AA, Mooney S: Feline mammary tumors. *Vet Clin North Am Small Anim Pract* 15:513–520, 1985.

40. Jeglum KA, DeGuzman E, Young K: Chemotherapy of advanced mammary adenocarcinoma in 14 cats. *JAVMA* 187:157–160, 1985.

41. Mauldin GN, Matus RE, Patnaik AK: Efficacy and toxicity of doxorubicin and cyclophosphamide used in the treatment of selected malignant tumors in 23 cats. *J Vet Intern Med* 2:60–65, 1988.

CLINICAL BRIEFING: TUMORS OF THE BODY CAVITIES

Mesothelioma in Dogs

Common Clinical Presentation	Effusion of body cavities causing abdominal discomfort, tachypnea, and respiratory distress; in decreasing order of incidence, affects pleural, peritoneal, or pericardial cavities
Common Histologic Type	Epithelial-type mesothelioma
Epidemiology and Biological Behavior	Old dogs; exposure to asbestos and pesticide powders may be associated with development of mesothelioma in dogs
Prognostic Factors	None identified
Treatment **Chemotherapy**	Intracavitary cisplatin may provide palliation; responses to intravenous doxorubicin and mitoxantrone have been noted

Thymoma in Dogs

Common Clinical Presentation	Cough; less commonly, dyspnea and lethargy; may have aspiration pneumonia secondary to myasthenia gravis and megaesophagus
Common Histologic Type	Epithelial malignant component associated with mature lymphocytes and mast cells
Epidemiology and Biological Behavior	Old dogs; females possibly predisposed; usually large, invasive, slow-growing tumors with low metastatic rate *Paraneoplastic Syndromes:* Myasthenia gravis is most common; polymyositis, hypercalcemia, and second malignancies may occur
Prognostic Factors	Dogs with megaesophagus have very poor prognosis
Treatment **Surgery**	May be curative for small or encapsulated tumors; dogs with megaesophagus need to be monitored for aspiration pneumonia; most thymomas are unresectable

MANAGEMENT OF SPECIFIC DISEASES

Radiation Therapy	Little information available; may be useful in reducing tumor prior to surgery
Chemotherapy	Little information available; prednisone may be an active agent

Thymoma in Cats

Common Clinical Presentation	Dyspnea due to pleural effusion or large mass
Common Histologic Type	Malignant epithelial component with mature lymphocytes and mast cells
Epidemiology and Biological Behavior	Old cats; no association with FeLV; tumors are usually encapsulated; paraneoplastic syndromes include myasthenia gravis, but this is less common than in dogs
Prognostic Factors	None identified
Treatment	
Surgery	Treatment of choice for cats; may be curative
Radiation Therapy	Not reported
Chemotherapy	Not reported

Other Tumors Reviewed

Mesothelioma in cats	

Normal mesothelial cells line the pleural, pericardial, and peritoneal cavities and the surface of the testes as a single layer. When mesothelial cells become altered by malignancy or inflammation, they take on cytologically similar "reactive" characteristics, making it difficult to distinguish between neoplastic and activated mesothelial cells.

Neoplastic involvement of the visceral or parietal pleura is almost invariably associated with effusion. Pleural and peritoneal fluids are normally present in minute amounts that are controlled by hydrostatic and colloid osmotic pressures. The small amount of protein normally leaked from capillaries is reabsorbed by lymphatic drainage. Neoplastic involvement of the coelomic surfaces disrupts capillary integrity, which allows increased protein exudation. Tumor cells may obstruct lymphatic drainage and cause accumulation of fluid. The process may be accelerated by inflammatory reaction to the tumor cells.

Primary tumors, such as mesothelioma, are rare in dogs and cats. Malignant effusion is often a result of other tumors, such as metastatic primary lung tumors, mammary or prostatic carcinomas, or tumors from other sites. These tumors rarely consist

MANAGEMENT OF SPECIFIC DISEASES

of masses of sufficient size to be visualized by radiography, ultrasonography, or computed tomography (CT) scans, although effusion may be identified.

MESOTHELIOMA IN DOGS
Incidence, Signalment, and Etiology

Mesotheliomas are rare in all species. In humans, the development of mesothelioma after exposure to asbestos by inhalation is well documented, although it may take decades to arise. Some dogs with mesothelioma have higher levels of chrysotile asbestos fibers in their lungs than control dogs.[1,2] Affected dogs seem to have greater environmental exposure to asbestos-related situations than control dogs.[1] Exposure to pesticides is a co-factor that apparently increases the risk of mesothelioma formation,[1] and dogs in an urban environment seem to be at higher risk.[1]

Mesothelioma occurs in old dogs; the average age is 8 years,[1-8] although affected dogs range from 4 to 15 years of age.[2,3,9] The tumor is more common in males than in females.[1-10] There does not seem to be any strong breed predilection, but one study found that Bouvier des Flandres, Irish setters, and German shepherds were at increased risk.[1]

Clinical Presentation and History

Clinical signs largely depend on the site of involvement with mesothelioma. Involvement of such single body cavities as the pleural cavity, the pericardial sac, and the peritoneal cavity are most common. More than one cavity (i.e., both pleural and peritoneal cavities[1,2] or the pericardial sac and pleural[2] or peritoneal cavities[7]) may be involved. Mesothelioma of the tunica vaginalis has been documented.[8] Most reported cases involve the thoracic cavity. This is reflected by the common clinical findings of tachypnea, respiratory distress, decreased exercise tolerance, and cough.[2,3,5] Clinical signs have usually been obvious to the owner for one month.[2] Interestingly, one dog with mesothelioma remained asymptomatic for pleural masses and effusion for 33 months.[9]

On physical examination and auscultation, dogs with thoracic malignant effusion due to mesothe-

lioma often have muffled heart sounds and decreased lung sounds with weak peripheral pulses. Dogs with abdominal mesothelioma are usually presented for abdominal distension and nonspecific signs of lethargy and anorexia. Peritoneal effusion is easily recognized on physical examination.

Staging and Diagnosis

In any dog with malignant effusion, blood work, urinalysis, radiographs, and ultrasonography provide valuable staging information. On radiography, pleural effusion may be extensive. In cases of pericardial involvement, the cardiac silhouette is enlarged and globoid and the trachea is elevated dorsally. Other radiographic findings, depending on the site of the tumor, include pulmonary edema, mild hepatomegaly, and peritoneal effusion. When present, effusion usually obliterates visualization of lymph nodes and other structures in these cavities.

Ultrasonography is useful in determining the involvement of intrathoracic or intra-abdominal viscera, although mesotheliomas rarely penetrate beneath the surface of these organs. It may be difficult to identify any specific cause for the effusion, because mesotheliomas may not form discrete mass lesions, but rather may produce a diffuse thickening of the coelomic surfaces that is not imaged by ultrasonography or computed tomography.

Cytologic evaluation of fluid aspirated from the affected body cavity should be undertaken; however, in any benign or malignant transudative process, mesothelial cells undergo extensive hypertrophy and may exfoliate into the fluid. These cells may be binucleate or even multinucleate; therefore, strict criteria of malignancy may be difficult to impose. In one study, exfoliative cytology was suggestive in only one of six dogs with mesothelioma.[6] Therefore, definitive diagnosis is made by biopsy. Although thoracoscopy- or laparoscopy-guided biopsies are rarely used in veterinary practice, these techniques can provide a definitive histopathologic diagnosis with little morbidity to the patient. Exploratory surgery is an alternative diagnostic method, but it is rarely therapeutic. The exception is pericardial mesothelioma, in which

MANAGEMENT OF SPECIFIC DISEASES

pericardectomy provides palliative relief. Surgery may also allow removal of grossly visible mass lesions, thereby "cytoreducing" the tumor prior to adjunctive therapy.[10]

"Epithelial type" mesothelioma is most common in dogs.[4] It may be confused cytologically or histologically with carcinomatosis. Mesotheliomas do not contain the neutral mucosubstances seen in adenocarcinoma cells and do not stain with mucicarmine or periodic acid–Schiff reaction (PAS) stains.

Visceral metastasis from mesothelioma is rare in dogs, although evidence of lymphatic invasion by tumor cells[2] or involvement of mediastinal and sternal lymph nodes has been described.[6] Widespread metastasis has been reported.[6,7,9]

Treatment

Aggressive surgery is rarely feasible or warranted in dogs with mesothelioma because of extensive serosal involvement (Figure 5-89). Palliation of clinical signs caused by effusion can be achieved by repeated thoracocentesis or pericardiocentesis, which can be tolerated by the patient for several months.[4,5] In most animals treated in this way, it eventually becomes necessary to perform centesis every few days.[3] Obliteration of the pleural space by sclerosis has a palliative benefit in humans, but the role of sclerotherapy in dogs is less clearly defined. Tetracycline or talc has been used with some success in human patients, but in dogs, responses vary, which may be more attributable to technique than to the substance used. In dogs, tetracycline pleurodesis was no better than a placebo for managing experimentally produced pleural effusion.[11] The optimal dose and method have not been established, and this therapy is not recommended for dogs.[12]

Chemotherapy with mitoxantrone (5 mg/m² every 3 weeks) resulted in complete remission for 42 days in one dog with mesothelioma,[13] and doxorubicin (30 mg/m² IV) caused complete remission in one dog for an unstated period.[14] There was no response to vincristine, cyclophosphamide, and prednisone in another dog.[10] Intracavitary cisplatin chemotherapy (50 mg/m² every 3 weeks) was used to treat three

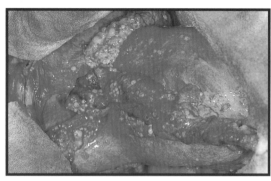

Figure 5-89: *Diagnosis of mesothelioma is rarely made by cytology; however, pleuroscopy or exploratory thoracotomy allows tissue biopsy. A thoracotomy is unlikely to be of therapeutic benefit because of the diffuse nature of this tumor. (Courtesy J. Berg)*

dogs with pleural mesothelioma. Complete control of fluid accumulation was seen in all three dogs for 129 days, 289 days, and 306 days. One dog survived 410 days, and another dog survived more than 306 days; the third dog was lost to follow-up.[10] Intracavitary cisplatin seems to reduce fluid accumulation rapidly if it is going to be effective. If the dog does not respond after one or two treatments, it is unlikely to respond to subsequent treatments. Intracavitary cisplatin is the treatment of choice for mesothelioma in dogs, and concurrent systemic doxorubicin may improve the response rate.

MESOTHELIOMA IN CATS
Incidence, Signalment, and Etiology

Mesothelioma is less common in cats than in dogs, and few details are available regarding the reported cases. Three of four cats with mesothelioma were female. Ages ranged from 1.5 years to 15 years, and three cats were Siamese.[15–18]

Clinical Presentation and History

Mesothelioma in cats has been reported in pleural cavity,[3] pericardium,[16] and peritoneal cavity.[17,18] The most obvious clinical signs are from fluid accumulation. Abdominal swelling, cough, and nonspecific signs of lethargy and anorexia have been reported.[16–18]

MANAGEMENT OF SPECIFIC DISEASES

Two cats with peritoneal mesothelioma had a palpable anterior abdominal mass.[17,18]

Staging and Diagnosis

As with dogs, staging procedures for a cat with malignant effusion should include radiographs and ultrasonography as well as blood work. Also, as for dogs, it is difficult to make a definitive diagnosis of mesothelioma without a biopsy. Metastasis is not described, although one cat with peritoneal mesothelioma seemed to have a lung lesion that arose by direct extension through the diaphragm.[17]

Treatment

Treatment has not been described, and cisplatin is not safe for use in cats. Pericardiectomy was unsuccessful in one cat treated by surgery.[16]

THYMOMA IN DOGS
Incidence, Signalment, and Etiology

Thymomas originate from the thymic epithelium but often contain a significant proportion of mature lymphocytes. Thymomas invariably occur in the cranial mediastinum,[19] although their exact location may vary. These tumors occurs mainly in old dogs with a median age of about 10 years,[19–21] although dogs as young as 2.5 years of age may be affected.[19] No obvious breed predilection has been reported. Forty of 61 reported cases (65%) occurred in female dogs.[19–22]

Clinical Presentation and History

Predictably, most of the clinical signs relating to thymoma in dogs involve the respiratory tract; coughing is the most common sign.[19] Dogs with thymoma may also have dyspnea, listlessness, and decreased exercise tolerance. Decreased appetite and weight loss are nonspecific signs associated with thymoma. Some dogs may show dysphagia or regurgitation, presumably from mechanical obstruction by a large compressive mass or from megaesophagus secondary to myasthenia gravis, which is a paraneoplastic syndrome associated with thymoma.[19,20] Dogs with large compressive tumors may have precaval syndrome and edema of their forelimbs, although this is uncommon and occurred in only 7 (11%) of 61 reported cases.[19–22] Polydipsia and polyuria may occasionally occur secondary to paraneoplastic hypercalcemia.[19] The most common abnormalities detected on physical examination are decreases in heart sounds and in ventral lung sounds on auscultation.[19] Small dogs may have an incompressible cranial thorax on palpation.[22]

Staging and Diagnosis

The high proportion of paraneoplastic diseases in dogs with thymoma makes it necessary to perform specialized diagnostic testing, such as electromyography, in addition to routine staging procedures. Thoracic radiographs are very useful in determining whether a dog has an anterior mediastinal mass. Often, the heart is displaced caudodorsally and the trachea is compressed dorsally. In rare cases, however, the thymoma may be in the craniodorsal anterior mediastinum (Figures 5-90 and 5-91).[19] A small thymoma is occasionally discovered on routine radiographs.[20] Pleural effusion and megaesophagus may be noted, and changes consistent with pneumonia may be present, possibly following regurgitation and aspiration.[20] Pleural effusion may prevent detection of a thymoma on radiographs.[19]

Ultrasonography is the most useful tool for obtaining fine-needle aspirates and needle biopsies while avoiding vessels that may be surrounded or displaced by the thymoma. Both ultrasonography and computed tomography (CT) may be

> **KEY POINTS:**
>
> *Pleural effusion may prevent radiographic detection of a thymoma.*
>
> ———
>
> *Thymomas contain a relatively large number of mature lymphocytes, which may make diagnosis based on cytologic specimens difficult.*

MANAGEMENT OF SPECIFIC DISEASES

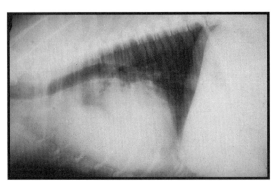

Figure 5-90

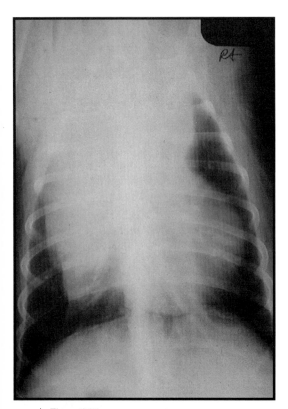

Figure 5-91

Figures 5-90 and 5-91: *Thymoma in dogs is usually visible radiographically as a large, poorly defined anterior mediastinal mass that should be differentiated histologically from lymphoma by an abundance of mature lymphocytes and an obvious malignant epithelial component. (Courtesy of J. Berg)*

useful in determining whether a tumor is encapsulated or invasive; however, for very large tumors, it may be impossible to distinguish between compression and invasion around vital thoracic structures. Thymomas are often described ultrasonographically as being cystic, whereas anterior mediastinal lymphomas are usually poorly echogenic. Distant metastases have not been described in dogs with thymoma.

Fine-needle aspirates may be difficult to evaluate cytologically because of the variable proportion of mature lymphocytes that can be present. As the other most frequent anterior mediastinal tumor in dogs is lymphoma, this presents a diagnostic dilemma. Mast cells are frequently identified in thymomas,[19] and the coincidence of these cells together with numerous mature lymphocytes should increase suspicion for thymoma.

Definitive diagnosis requires a biopsy specimen that demonstrates the malignant epithelial portion of thymoma, which may not be evident on aspiration cytology. Thymomas may be subclassified on the basis of their histologic appearance, dependent on the proportion and differentiation of the epithelial component; however, this is probably of little prognostic significance.[19]

Thymoma is associated with a high proportion of paraneoplastic syndromes. The best described syndrome is myasthenia gravis. The diagnosis of myasthenia gravis was confirmed in 14 of 38 dogs in two recent reviews of dogs with thymoma.[19,20] All but one of these 14 dogs[19] had evidence of megaesophagus. Clinical signs associated with myasthenia, such as exertional muscle weakness and regurgitation, were present for five days to three weeks. One dog, however, had shown signs for more than three years.[20] Diagnosis of myasthenia may be confirmed by demonstrating improvement after administration of edrophonium chloride ("Tensilon test") at a dose of 0.11 to 0.22 mg/kg IV; response should be dramatic but transient. Electromyography may demonstrate multifocal fibrillation or other abnormalities but is not widely available. The most specific test is for the presence of serum acetylcholine-receptor antibody (AchRAb), which is elevated in the majority of dogs with thymoma and myasthenia gravis.[19,20,22] Normal serum concentrations of AchRAb are less than 0.03 nM. Myasthenia gravis may also develop after surgical removal of the thymoma.[19] The reason for this phenomenon is not clear; however, it is possible that immunologic abnormalities persist even after tumor removal.

Polymyositis has been described in dogs in association with thymoma[19,20] and resulted in third-degree atrial-ventricular block in three dogs due to myocardial involvement.[19] Hypercalcemia has been described as a paraneoplastic syndrome in dogs with thymoma[19,21] and may resolve after successful treatment.[19] Anterior mediastinal lymphoma is commonly associated with hypercalcemia, so increased serum calcium cannot be considered as specific for either tumor. Second malignancies have been reported to be common in dogs with thymoma and occurred in 15 of 61 dogs.[19–22] These tumors include lymphoma, osteosarcoma, and various adenocarcinomas.[19,20]

Prognostic Factors

In one study, individual factors associated with prognosis were age, histologic cell type, and the presence or absence of megaesophagus. Old dogs fared better than did young dogs, and dogs with lymphocyte-rich thymomas lived longer. On multivariate analysis, however, only the absence of megaesophagus was associated with longer survival. Eleven dogs with thymoma and megaesophagus had a median survival of 6 days, compared with 14.5 months for seven dogs without megaesophagus.[19]

Treatment

Surgery is potentially curative, but thymoma in dogs is frequently a large and invasive tumor. Even when the tumor is encapsulated, there may be exten-

KEY POINTS:

Dogs with confirmed thymoma should be tested for serum AchRAb. Complete staging may help to rule out the presence of other primary malignancies.

Dogs with thymoma and megaesophagus have a very poor prognosis due to the usual development of aspiration pneumonia.

sive intrathoracic adhesions. The treatment of choice for small thymomas is surgical excision. If surgical margins cannot be assured for larger tumors, incisional biopsy may be preferred to an attempted excision. Other treatment modalities should be considered, particularly if the dog has megaesophagus; careful attention should be given to reduce the risk for aspiration pneumonia.

In one study, 13 dogs were treated with surgery alone, and survival times ranged from 1 day to 45 months, with a median survival of 7 days. Three dogs lived more than one year.[19] In another study, three dogs without paraneoplastic signs were treated with surgery alone. Two dogs died within 2 days of surgery, and one had local recurrence at 4 months.[20] Two of seven other dogs treated with surgery died perioperatively, and four dogs lived for 6 months, 1 year, 4 years, and 5 years, respectively.[21]

Radiation therapy is important in the treatment of thymoma in humans. Its use has been described only in one dog treated with 54 Gy of orthovoltage radiation in nine weekly fractions.[22] This dog had a 60% reduction in tumor mass and normalization of elevated AchRAb levels for six months before signs of myasthenia recurred. The dog was also treated with prednisone (2.2 mg/kg QOD PO), however.[22] Radiation may reduce tumor size to a point at which surgical excision is feasible, but risks of radiation toxicity to lungs and myocardium are dose-limiting.

The most active chemotherapeutic agents for treatment of thymoma in human patients are prednisone and cisplatin. In dogs, chemotherapy has been used alone, usually when thymoma is mistakenly diagnosed as lymphoma. Canine thymoma did not respond to chemotherapy with cyclophosphamide, vincristine, and prednisone (COP).[20,21] In contrast, one dog that received these three drugs after surgery

MANAGEMENT OF SPECIFIC DISEASES

was in complete remission 29 months later,[19] and another dog that received COP for 2 weeks and then prednisone alone maintained stable tumor measurements for 14 months.[19] A dog treated with cisplatin and doxorubicin for osteosarcoma had no change in size of an incidental thymoma.[19] Anecdotally, dogs with thymoma may have reduction in tumor volume after prednisone therapy (40 mg/m² SID PO) (A.S. Moore, G.K. Ogilvie, personal observations, 1994).

The best treatment for canine thymoma has yet to be determined. Surgery should probably be reserved for dogs without megaesophagus that have well-encapsulated tumors. Radiation therapy and chemotherapy may be useful in reducing the size of the tumor so that surgery may be performed, although little information exists as to the success of this approach. Dogs with myasthenia gravis should be treated with prednisone to reduce AchRAb levels, which may ameliorate clinical signs. Dogs with megaesophagus should be monitored closely for aspiration pneumonia, and samples should be obtained by transtracheal aspiration for bacterial culture prior to beginning antibiotic therapy. The prognosis for dogs with thymoma and megaesophagus is very poor.

THYMOMA IN CATS
Incidence, Signalment, and Etiology

Thymoma is a rare disease in cats. It primarily affects old cats that average 9 to 10 years of age. Affected cats, however, can be as young as 3 years of age.[23,24] Most affected cats are domestic shorthairs, although four of 23 reported cats were Siamese.[23,24] There is no gender predilection. FeLV does not seem to play a role in this disease.[23,24]

Clinical Presentation and History

As with dogs, clinical signs of thymoma in cats primarily are related to the respiratory tract; dyspnea due to pleural effusion or to a large compressive mass is the most common sign.[23,24] Other respiratory signs include cough and dysphonia.[23] Nonspecific signs include lethargy and inappetence. Clinical signs usually occur acutely; median time to presentation is four weeks.[23]

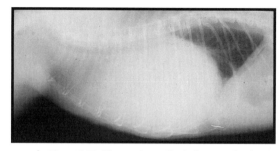

Figure 5-92: *The anterior mediastinal mass in this thoracic radiograph of a cat was determined to be a thymoma. Thymoma in cats may be difficult to distinguish from mediastinal lymphoma on radiography, and biopsy is usually required, although fine-needle aspiration cytology may be suggestive of thymoma.*

On physical examination, bilaterally muffled heart sounds and absent ventral lung sounds are common, and some cats may have an incompressible cranial thorax from a large thymoma.[23]

Staging and Diagnosis

Thoracic radiographs reveal a cranial mediastinal mass that displaces the heart caudally and the trachea dorsally (Figure 5-92). Pleural effusion is common.[23,24] In one cat, effusion was chylous.[24] Ultrasonographic guidance is useful for fine-needle aspiration or needle core biopsy, particularly if pleural effusion is present. Cytology is limited as a diagnostic aid because of numerous lymphocytes and rare malignant epithelial cells. Mast cells are present in up to 50% of aspirates from thymomas in cats. Cytology from an anterior mediastinal mass in an old cat that has a preponderance of small lymphocytes rather than lymphoblasts indicates that the tumor may be thymoma rather than lymphoma. Needle core biopsy was successful in providing a definitive diagnosis of thymoma in 6 of 12 cats (50%), as this method more readily demonstrates the malignant epithelial component. Paraneoplastic syndromes are not as common in cats with thymoma as they are in dogs. In one study, 2 of 12 cats (17%) developed myasthenia gravis after surgical excision of a thymoma. These cats showed clinical signs of weakness, gait abnormalities, neck ventroflexion, and regurgitation, and

MANAGEMENT OF SPECIFIC DISEASES

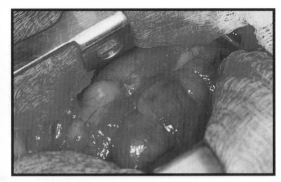

Figure 5-93

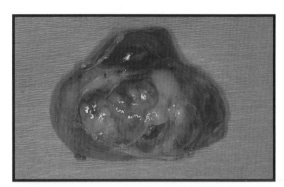

Figure 5-94

Figures 5-93 and 5-94: *At surgery, this thymoma in a cat appeared large and invasive; however, it was well encapsulated, and complete resection was achieved. Unlike dogs, cats with thymoma are often cured by surgery.*

the diagnosis was confirmed in one cat with AchRAb concentrations of 6.5 nM presurgically and 10.5 nM postsurgically (normal = <0.03 nM).[23] In another study, 3 of 11 cats had clinical signs of weakness from polymyositis.[24] Metastasis is rare in cats but occurred to the lungs and kidney of one cat.[25]

Treatment

Surgery is the treatment of choice for feline thymoma (Figures 5-93 and 5-94). The surgical approach is by median sternotomy or intercostal thoracotomy and is described in detail elsewhere.[23] The tumor was well encapsulated in 5 of 12 cats treated with surgery alone, and adhesions to the pericardium, pleura, and cranial vena cava occurred in seven cats.[23] In three of these cats, excision was incomplete. Despite adhesions, nine tumors were histologically encapsulated. Two cats died in the postoperative period (one from bleeding and one from fungal pleuritis), and three cats required transfusions during surgery. Four of the surviving 10 cats died of unrelated diseases without evidence of thymoma, and the other six cats survived for between 3 and 36 months after surgery for a median survival of 16 months.[23] Unlike dogs, cats with thymoma should be offered a good prognosis, particularly if the tumor appears encapsulated.

Two cats that developed myasthenia gravis after surgery responded rapidly to treatment with prednisone (2.2 mg/kg SID PO) and pyridostigmine bro-

mide (0.5 mg/kg BID PO) and were normal 9 and 62 months later, respectively.[23]

REFERENCES

1. Glickman LT, Domanski LM, MacGuire TG, et al: Mesothelioma in pet dogs associated with exposure of their owners to asbestos. *Environ Res* 32:305–313, 1983.
2. Harbison ML, Godleski JJ: Malignant mesothelioma in urban dogs. *Vet Pathol* 20:531–540, 1983.
3. Breeze RG, Lauder IM: Pleural mesothelioma in a dog. *Vet Rec* 96:243–246, 1975.
4. Trigo FJ, Morrison WB, Breeze RG: An ultrastructural study of canine mesothelioma. *J Comp Pathol* 91: 531–537, 1981.
5. Ikede BO, Zubaidy A, Gill CW: Pericardial mesothelioma with cardiac tamponade in a dog. *Vet Pathol* 17:496–501, 1980.
6. Thrall DE, Goldschmidt MH: Mesothelioma in the dog: Six case reports. *J Am Vet Radiol Soc* 19:107–115, 1978.
7. Smith DA, Hill FWG: Metastatic malignant mesothelioma in a dog. *J Comp Pathol* 100:97–101, 1989.
8. Cihak RW, Roen DR, Klaassen J: Malignant mesothelioma of the tunica vaginalis in a dog. *J Comp Pathol* 96:459–462, 1986.
9. Morrison WB, Trigo FJ: Clinical characterization of pleural mesothelioma in seven dogs. *Compend Contin Educ Pract Vet* 6:342–348, 1984.
10. Moore AS, Kirk C, Cardona A: Intracavitary cisplatin chemotherapy experience with six dogs. *J Vet Intern Med* 5:227–231, 1991.
11. Gallagher LA, Birchard SJ, Weisbrode SE: Effects of tetracycline hydrochloride on pleurae in dogs with

MANAGEMENT OF SPECIFIC DISEASES

induced pleural effusion. *Am J Vet Res* 51:1682–1687, 1990.

12. Birchard SJ, Gallagher L: Use of pleurodesis in treating selected pleural diseases. *Compend Contin Educ Pract Vet* 10:826–832, 1988.

13. Ogilvie GK, Obradovich JE, Elmslie RE, et al: Efficacy of mitoxantrone against various neoplasms in dogs. *JAVMA* 198:1618–1621, 1991.

14. Ogilvie GK, Reynolds HA, Richardson RC, et al: Phase II evaluation of doxorubicin for treatment of various canine neoplasms. *JAVMA* 195:1580–1583, 1989.

15. Andrews EJ: Pleural mesothelioma in a cat. *J Comp Pathol* 83:259–263, 1973.

16. Tilley LP, Owens JM, Wilkins RJ, Patnaik AK: Pericardial mesothelioma with effusion in a cat. *JAAHA* 11:60–65, 1975.

17. Raflo CP, Nuernberger SP: Abdominal mesothelioma in a cat. *Vet Pathol* 15:781–783, 1978.

18. Carpenter JL, Andrews LK, Holzworth J: Tumors and tumor-like lesions, in Holzworth J (ed): *Diseases of the Cat. Medicine and Surgery.* Philadelphia, WB Saunders, 1987, pp 406–596.

19. Atwater SW, Powers BE, Park RD, et al: Canine thymoma: 23 cases (1980–1991). *JAVMA* 205:1007–1013, 1994.

20. Aronsohn MG, Schunk KL, Carpenter JL, King NW: Clinical and pathologic features of thymoma in 15 dogs. *JAVMA* 184:1355–1362, 1984.

21. Bellah JR, Stiff ME, Russell RG: Thymoma in the dog: Two case reports and review of 20 additional cases. *JAVMA* 183:306–311, 1983.

22. Hih ME, Shaw DP, Hogan PM, et al: Radiation treatment for thymoma in a dog. *JAVMA* 190:1187–1190, 1987.

23. Gores BR, Berg J, Carpenter JL, Aronsohn MG: Surgical treatment of thymoma in cats: 12 cases (1987–1992). *JAVMA* 204:1782–1785, 1994.

24. Carpenter JL, Holzworth J: Thymoma in 11 cats. *JAVMA* 181:248–251, 1982.

25. Middleton DJ, Ratcliffe RC, Xu FN: Thymoma with distant metastases in a cat. *Vet Pathol* 22:512–514, 1985.

CLINICAL BRIEFING: BONE TUMORS

Osteosarcoma of the Appendicular Skeleton in Dogs

Common Clinical Presentation	Lameness and pain at metaphyseal sites, particularly distal radius, proximal humerus, proximal tibia, and distal femur; lytic and productive bone lesion on radiographs
Common Histologic Type	Osteoblastic osteosarcoma
Epidemiology and Biological Behavior	Large to giant-breed dogs; no sex predilection; usually middle-aged to old dogs; metastasis occurs early but may not be clinically evident
Prognostic Factors	Survival is poor; prognosis is not correlated with gender, tumor site, or whether a presurgical biopsy is performed

Treatment
   Surgery
 	
   Chemotherapy and Surgery
 	
   Biological Therapy
 	
   Radiation Therapy
	
	 With amputation alone, median survival is 162 days; 11% of dogs alive at 1 year; limb sparing provides good limb function for distal radial tumors
	 Cisplatin: Median survival of 300 to 400 days; 40% to 60% of dogs alive at 1 year
	 Doxorubicin: Median survival of 350 days; 50% of dogs alive at 1 year
	 Combinations: Similar results
	 L-MTP-PE: Median survival of 220 days; may be used in combination with chemotherapy
	 Palliative for painful bony lesions

Osteosarcoma of the Axial Skeleton in Dogs (including Multilobular Osteochondrosarcoma)

Common Clinical Presentation	Tumors of the appendicular skeleton are four times more common than axial tumors
Epidemiology and Biological Behavior	Old dogs (except rib tumors, which often affect young dogs); no breed predilection; more females may be affected; highly metastatic, but local recurrence is more of a problem; mandibular osteosarcoma may have lower metastatic rate

MANAGEMENT OF SPECIFIC DISEASES

Prognostic Factors	None identified

Treatment
  Surgery
 	
  Chemotherapy and Surgery
  Radiation Therapy
	
	Difficult due to location of tumors; mandible and rib tumors can be resected
	Cisplatin is recommended for osteosarcoma of all sites
	May be useful adjunct to surgery to reduce local recurrence

Nonosteosarcoma Bone Tumors in Dogs

Common Clinical Presentation	More often affect axial skeleton rather than appendicular skeleton; care required in interpreting incisional biopsy specimens
Common Histologic Types	Chondrosarcoma, fibrosarcoma, and hemangiosarcoma
Epidemiology and Biological Behavior	Old dogs, except oral fibrosarcoma, in which younger dogs predominate; metastases occur at a lower rate than osteosarcoma and may occur late in the course of the disease

Treatment
  Surgery
 	
  Radiation Therapy
  Chemotherapy
	
	Palliative; may be curative in some dogs, although metastases may arise even months to years after surgery
	May improve tumor control
	Not known to be effective

Synovial Cell Sarcoma in Dogs

Common Clinical Presentation	Lameness and palpable mass
Common Histologic Type	Fibroblastic cell type
Epidemiology and Biological Behavior	Middle-aged dogs; medium to large breeds; predominantly male dogs; predilection for the right side
Prognostic Factors	Histologic grade
Treatment Surgery	 *Amputation:* Better than 75% chance of 3-year survival

MANAGEMENT OF SPECIFIC DISEASES

Chemotherapy	Inadequately studied; a combination of doxorubicin and cyclophosphamide may be helpful
Primary Bone Tumors in Cats	
Common Clinical Presentation	Lameness for appendicular tumors (60% of tumors); palpable mass for axial tumors, which most commonly affect the head; primarily lytic lesions
Common Histologic Type	Osteosarcoma
Epidemiology and Biological Behavior	Old cats; no obvious gender predilection; metastatic rate is low

Treatment
  Surgery
 	
  Radiation Therapy
  Chemotherapy
	
	Potential for cure if surgery eliminates all tumor (e.g., amputation)
	Seems to improve local control of osteosarcoma
	Not reported

OSTEOSARCOMA OF THE APPENDICULAR SKELETON IN DOGS
Incidence, Signalment, and Etiology

Osteosarcoma of the limbs is more common in dogs than in any other species and accounts for more than 80% of malignant bone tumors in dogs. These tumors are believed to arise from the medullary cavity, usually at a metaphysis, and expand outward, destroying cortex and disrupting periosteum.

Large- to giant-breed dogs with a body weight of more than 20 kg are most often affected. Giant-breed dogs (>35 kg) are 60 times more likely and large-breed dogs (20 to 35 kg) are eight times more likely to develop osteosarcoma than dogs that weigh less than 10 kg.[1] Rapid early growth and increase in stress on weight-bearing limbs may explain this increased risk. Tumors are more likely to arise in the forelimbs than in the hindlimbs.[2,3] Dogs with osteosarcoma are middle-aged to old animals with a median age of 8 years (range = 8 months to 13 years).[2] The tumor can affect dogs of any age, however, and occurs in giant-breed dogs at a young age. There is no sex predilection.[2–4]

Osteosarcoma has been associated with sites of healed fractures or internal-fixation devices, implying that chronic irritation may play a role in tumor development. This hypothesis is further supported by the occurrence of osteosarcoma in sites that are irradiated for treatment of other tumors. These tumors occur in less than 5% of dogs between 1.5 and 5 years after irradiation. High single-dose radiation (i.e., coarse fractionation) in one study increased the risk of tumor formation.[5]

Clinical Presentation and History

Osteosarcoma most commonly affects the appendicular skeleton, particularly in the metaphyseal region. The most common sites are the distal radius

MANAGEMENT OF SPECIFIC DISEASES

and the proximal humerus ("away from the elbow") (Figure 5-95). Less common sites are the proximal tibia and distal femur ("toward the knee").[2,3] Lameness is often intermittent early in the course of the disease and may be exacerbated by or associated with a traumatic event. Lameness then becomes chronic, and the limb can no longer bear weight. The early fluctuating course is believed to be due, in part, to subperiosteal bleeding and microfractures of the weakened cortex. Initially, there may be no clinically apparent lesion on palpation and radiographs of the limb may show only subtle radiographic changes. As the disease progresses, swelling and lameness may rapidly worsen and the lesion may become painful to the touch. If the tumor is untreated, progressive erosion of the cortex may cause pathologic fracture of the affected limb. The duration of clinical signs may be very short and often ranges from one to three months.

Staging and Diagnosis

Dogs with a suspected primary bone tumor should have high-detail radiographs of the lesion. In addition, routine blood work and urinalysis as well as thoracic radiographs should be performed. Primary bone tumors may have a lytic, productive, or mixed appearance on high-detail radiographs. The signs most suggestive of neoplasia include cortical bone lysis in a lesion that does not cross a joint space. Tumor extension and mineralization form periosteal spicules in the surrounding soft tissues, imparting a "sunburst" appearance on radiographs (Figures 5-96 and 5-97). The margins or extent of neoplastic disease in osteosarcoma may be difficult to define on radiographs. Radiographs tend to underestimate the true extent of the lesion, as bony lysis is not apparent until more than 50% of mineral has been removed. On the other hand, bone scintigraphy overestimates tumor margins in delineating tumor and surrounding reactive bone (Figures 5-97 and 5-98).[6] Tumor margins are important if limb salvage, rather

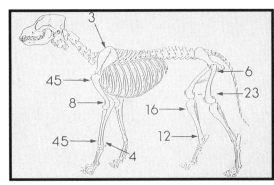

Figure 5-95: *A schematic diagram showing the distribution of appendicular osteosarcoma in 162 dogs. (Courtesy J. Berg)*

than amputation, is contemplated.

Although pulmonary metastases are rarely detectable at the time of diagnosis, thoracic radiographs still should be taken. Right and left lateral views and a dorsoventral view should be obtained. Dogs with clinically detectable pulmonary metastases have a poor prognosis, with or without treatment. Regional lymphadenopathy from tumor metastasis is observed in less than 5% of dogs at the time of presentation, which approximates the incidence of pulmonary metastases.

Synchronous primary osteosarcoma or bony metastases of osteosarcoma have been described but are rarely seen at presentation. In a group of 66 dogs with appendicular osteosarcoma that underwent technetium scintigraphy, none manifested other bony lesions.[7]

Definitive diagnosis is confirmed by histopathology. For old animals with a large lytic metaphyseal bone lesion, osteosarcoma is the most common diagnosis. Differentials include other neoplastic conditions as well as fungal and bacterial infections. In each case, removal of the limb is an acceptable procedure. Therefore, biopsy at the time of amputation is advised. If there is significant doubt as to the cause of the lesion, a preoperative biopsy should

> **KEY POINT:**
>
> *A radiographic bone lesion that includes bone lysis but does not cross a joint space is very suggestive of neoplasia.*

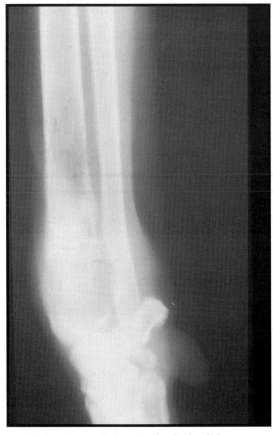

Figure 5-96: Radiograph of a distal radial osteosarcoma showing lysis and medullary extension. Note that the lesion does not cross the joint space. (Courtesy J. Berg)

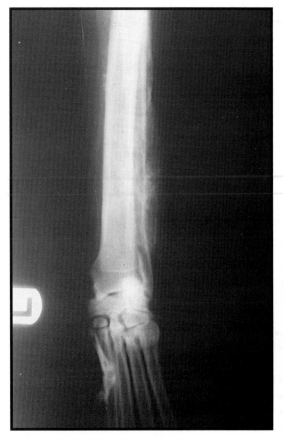

Figure 5-97: Radiograph of a dog with an osteosarcoma of the ulna. It is difficult to define tumor margins accurately, and the radiograph limits are likely to underestimate true tumor margins. (Courtesy J. Berg)

be obtained. Unlike soft tissue tumors, in bone tumors, diagnostic biopsy samples are best obtained from the center of the lesion. Multiple biopsy specimens increase the chance of diagnosis. A Jamshidi bone marrow biopsy needle is an excellent instrument for this purpose (see the chapter on Bone Marrow Aspiration and Biopsy in the Biopsy section). Osteosarcoma frequently includes areas of cartilage and fibrous tissue as well as osteoid and is often surrounded by new bone. For these reasons, a histopathologic diagnosis of chondrosarcoma, fibrosarcoma, or reactive bone should be considered suspect and further samples obtained at amputation or definitive surgery should be submitted for histopathologic examination.

KEY POINT:

Unlike soft tissue tumors, in bone tumors, biopsy samples are most likely to be diagnostic if obtained from the center of the lesion.

Prognostic Factors

Early studies indicated a relatively favorable prognosis for dogs with the fibrosarcomatous variant of osteosarcoma[3]; however, this has not been

MANAGEMENT OF SPECIFIC DISEASES

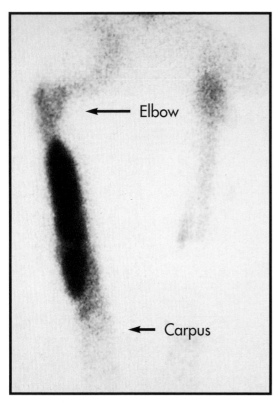

Figure 5-98: *Bone scintigraphy of the same tumor in Figure 5-97 will tend to overestimate the tumor margins, due to imaging of all reactive bone. This is a better guide than radiography if a limb-salvage procedure is anticipated. (Courtesy J. Berg)*

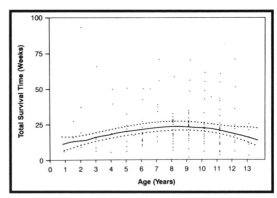

Figure 5-99: *Plot of survival time versus age for 162 dogs with osteosarcoma treated by amputation alone. Dashed lines indicate 95% confidence band. (From Spodnick GJ, Berg J, Rand WM, et al: Prognosis for dogs with appendicular osteosarcoma treated by amputation alone: 162 cases (1978–1988). JAVMA 200:995–999, 1992; with permission.)*

recently substantiated. In a recent study, age at time of diagnosis was important for determining survival in dogs treated with amputation alone.[2] Dogs between the ages of 7 and 10 years had the longest survival times; both old and young dogs fared less well (Figure 5-99).

Prognostic factors that did *not* influence survival are gender, site of the tumor (i.e., distal or proximal; forelimbs or hindlimbs), and whether a presurgical biopsy was performed.[2]

In studies of adjuvant therapy for appendicular osteosarcoma, the percentage of tumor necrosis following doxorubicin chemotherapy correlated with survival.[8] The percentage of necrosis following pre-

operative cisplatin or radiation correlated with local tumor control after limb-sparing surgery but not with survival.[9]

Treatment
Amputation

Amputation usually eliminates the primary tumor, which provides pain relief with little to no reduction in mobility and quality of life for the dog. The procedure is also usually accepted by owners.[10] For lesions in the forelimbs, complete forequarter amputation, including the scapula, provides cosmetically and functionally good results. For distal hindlimb tumors, amputation at the proximal third of the femur is performed. For distal femoral tumors, a hip disarticulation is performed and proximal femoral lesions are treated by hemipelvectomy. Surgical treatment of osteosarcoma by amputation is palliative but rarely increases survival. In one study, the median survival of 65 dogs treated with amputation was 126 days; only 10.7% of dogs were alive one year after surgery.[11] A more recent study of 162 dogs treated with amputation corroborated these data (Figure 5-100).[2] Surgery of any type is only palliative, and dogs with appendicular osteosarcoma should be given chemotherapy.

MANAGEMENT OF SPECIFIC DISEASES

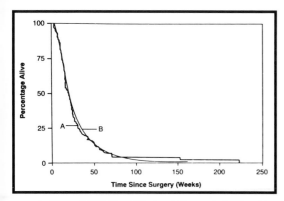

Figure 5-100: *Plot of Kaplan–Meier survival (**A**) and log-normal best fit (**B**) for 162 dogs with osteosarcoma treated by amputation alone. (From Spodnick GJ, Berg J, Rand WM, et al: Prognosis for dogs with appendicular osteosarcoma treated by amputation alone: 162 cases (1978–1988). JAVMA 200:995–999, 1992; with permission.)*

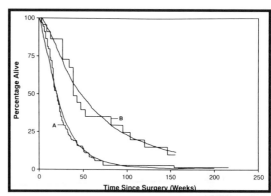

Figure 5-101: *Plot of Kaplan–Meier survival for dogs with osteosarcoma treated by amputation alone (**A** = 162 dogs) or with adjuvant cisplatin chemotherapy (**B** = 22 dogs). (From Berg J, Weinstein J, Schelling SH, Rand WM: Treatment of dogs with osteosarcoma by administration of cisplatin after amputation or limb-sparing surgery: 22 cases (1987–1990). JAVMA 200:2005–2008, 1992; with permission.)*

Limb-sparing surgery is important in human patients, for whom cosmetic appearance and function are impaired by amputation. This procedure may be ideal for dogs that are poor candidates for amputation (e.g., very large dogs or dogs with other orthopedic or neurologic problems) or for dogs whose owners refuse amputation. During limb-sparing surgery, a cortical bone graft is used to replace the widely excised tumor, and arthrodesis of the nearby joint is usually performed. The best results are obtained with distal radial lesions or lesions of the ulna. It is possible to perform limb salvage for proximal humeral or scapular lesions, but function may be more impaired. Good functional results have been reported for partial or complete scapulectomy in dogs with osteosarcoma.[12]

Limb salvage is not an option for large lesions that involve more than 50% of the bone, tumors that invade adjacent soft tissue, and tumors of the hindlimb. Complications of limb salvage include allograft rejection and implant failure. Complications occurred in 86 (55%) of 145 dogs treated with limb salvage.[13] Implant failure was seen in 12 (8%) of these 145 dogs and infection in 71 (49%) dogs. Infection required allograft removal or limb amputation in 16 dogs (11%).[13] Local recurrence of osteosarcoma is a frequent problem with

limb-salvage procedures and affects up to 40% of dogs. Even at institutions that perform limb salvage frequently and use adjunctive chemotherapy, recurrence rates of 17% to 27% are seen.[13]

Before limb salvage is performed, intra-arterial cisplatin, with or without radiation therapy, often increases tumor necrosis and reduces the risk of local recurrence.[9,14] In addition, local implantation of polymer impregnated with cisplatin (open polylactic acid–cisplatin or OPLA–Pt) releases cisplatin slowly into the tumor bed, reducing local recurrence rates from 27% for dogs that do not receive OPLA–Pt to 17% for dogs undergoing limb salvage with OPLA–Pt. The survival and disease-free interval for dogs treated with OPLA–Pt is similar to that of dogs receiving systemic cisplatin, presumably because locally implanted cisplatin is dispersed systemically. Local recurrence is not a problem when amputation is performed.

Chemotherapy

Survival of dogs with osteosarcoma can be significantly prolonged by adjuvant chemotherapy. Cisplatin markedly improves survival rates to a median survival of between 180 and 400 days and 1-year sur-

MANAGEMENT OF SPECIFIC DISEASES

TABLE 5-16
Survival times and rates for dogs with osteosarcoma of the appendicular skeleton treated with surgery and cisplatin chemotherapy

Number of Dogs	Cisplatin (mg/m²)	Treatment Interval (Days)	Number of Courses	Survival of 1 Year (%)	Survival of 2 years (%)	Median Survival (Days)	Reference
17	70 (postoperatively)	21	2	38	18	226	16
19	70 (pre- and perioperatively)	21	2	43	16	177	16
5	40–50 (postoperatively)	28	2–6	Not reported	Not reported	301	15
15	60 (postoperatively)	14 and 35	2	30	7	290	17
16	50 (postoperatively)	28	6+	62	19	413	18
22	60 (postoperatively)	21	1–6	45	21	325	19
162	Surgery only	—	—	11.5	2	134	2

vival rates to between 30% and 62%; 2-year survival rates are between 7% and 21%.[5-19] (Table 5-16).

There are trends toward longer survival times with increasing the number of doses of cisplatin,[13,18] but statistical evaluation is lacking. More than two doses of cisplatin may improve survival (Figure 5-101).[13,19] Preliminary evidence suggests that OPLA–Pt may also influence survival, possibly by providing prolonged, albeit low, plasma levels of cisplatin.[13]

Doxorubicin (30 mg/m²) failed to prolong survival in 14 dogs treated by amputation and receiving postoperative chemotherapy every three weeks.[20] The median survival after surgery was 104 days; 14% of the

> **KEY POINT:**
>
> *Both cisplatin and doxorubicin are active agents in the adjuvant treatment of canine osteosarcoma.*

dogs were alive one year after surgery. More recently, 35 dogs with appendicular osteosarcoma were treated with five biweekly doses of doxorubicin (30 mg/m²).[21] Two or three doses were given prior to surgery, and the subsequent doses were given the day after surgery and two weeks later. Median survival was 366 days; 50% of the dogs were alive at 1 year, and 10% were alive at 2 years, thereby approaching a similar efficacy to that of cisplatin. The higher dose intensity of this protocol, in addition to the timing of chemotherapy, may possibly explain the differences in survival rates between these two studies.[20,21]

A protocol alternating cisplatin (60 mg/m²) with doxorubicin (30

MANAGEMENT OF SPECIFIC DISEASES

mg/m^2) every 21 days for two cycles was delivered after amputation to 19 dogs with appendicular osteosarcoma. The median survival was 300 days (range = 65 to 1320 days), with 37% of dogs alive at 1 year and 26% alive at 2 years. Despite the lower dose intensity of the two drugs compared with single-agent protocols, survival rates were comparable to cisplatin chemotherapy alone.[22]

Methotrexate was given intravenously to five dogs with osteosarcoma at doses ranging from 3 to 6 g/m^2. Leucovorin rescue was used. Methotrexate treatment was preceded by vincristine at 1 mg/m^2. Myelosuppression was the dose-limiting toxicity, and no clinical response was seen.[23] Seventeen dogs with osteosarcoma were treated by local resection and implantation of acrylic cement-containing methotrexate at total doses ranging from 1.6 mg/kg to 16 mg/kg. Gastrointestinal toxicities were seen in four dogs receiving more than 4 mg/kg of methotrexate, and one of these dogs died. Four dogs showed delayed wound healing and sepsis. Ten of 17 dogs were alive without metastases at 8 months; however, no follow-up examination was reported. With the toxicity and uncertain efficacy of methotrexate and the availability of proven alternatives, we cannot recommend treatment with methotrexate at this time.

Carboplatin (300 mg/m^2 IV) was given adjunctively after surgery to 48 dogs.[24] Median survival was 321 days; 35.4% of the dogs were alive one year after surgery. In this study, small dogs (<40 kg) appeared to have longer survival times. Carboplatin seems to be as effective as cisplatin in treating canine appendicular osteosarcoma. Table 5-17 summarizes various protocols applied to osteosarcoma of the appendicular skeleton in dogs.

Biological Response Modifiers

Liposome-encapsulated muramyltripeptide-phosphatidyethanolamine (L-MTP-PE) is a nonspecific activator of monocytes and macrophages that induces tumoricidal activity in these cells. Dogs treated with L-MTP-PE showed prolonged median survival (220 days) over dogs receiving liposomes alone. In a further study, 11 dogs that had received four doses of cisplatin (70 mg/m^2 every 28 days) after amputation were treated with L-MTP-PE. These dogs had a median survival of 438 days.[26]

Metastatic Disease

Once osteosarcoma metastases are clinically or radiographically evident, good response to chemotherapy is rare. In one study, two of three dogs with metastatic osteosarcoma responded partially to cisplatin chemotherapy.[27] In another report, 45 dogs with osteosarcoma metastases were treated with cisplatin (70 mg/m^2 IV), doxorubicin (30 mg/m^2), mitoxantrone (5 mg/m^2 IV), or sequential combinations of these drugs every 3 weeks. Only one dog experienced a partial remission for 21 days with doxorubicin.[28] Cisplatin had been given prior to the development of metastases in 29 of the 45 dogs.

Pulmonary metastatectomy seems to prolong survival in specific circumstances only if the animal develops clinically evident metastases more than 300 days after the initial diagnosis and if fewer than three nodules are radiographically apparent. Median survival time after metastatectomy was found to be 176 days.[29]

Palliative Radiation Therapy

If owners refuse definitive treatment for their pet with osteosarcoma or if an animal is not considered an eligible candidate for amputation or limb sparing, consideration may be given to palliation of tumor pain with radiation therapy.

Fifteen dogs with osteosarcoma of various sites were treated with ^{60}Co teletherapy using three, 10 Gy fractions on a schedule of days 0, 7, and 21.[29] Twelve of these dogs showed improved limb function with increased weight bearing and activity between 7 and 22 days of starting radiation therapy. The median duration of this response was 130 days (range = 17–288 days). Two of the responding dogs developed pathologic fractures, possibly from increased weight bearing following pain relief.

Samarium-153-EDTMP emits β particles and accumulates in areas of increased bony activity, thereby providing high-dose localized radiation therapy.

MANAGEMENT OF SPECIFIC DISEASES

TABLE 5-17
Responses of dogs with osteosarcoma of the appendicular skeleton to chemotherapy

Treatment	Doses (mg/m²)	Comments	Median Survival After Surgery (Days)	Survival Time	Number of Dogs	Reference
Cisplatin	50–70	See Table 5-16	180–400	1 year: 30%–62% 2 years: 7%–21%	94	See Table 5-16
Doxorubicin	30	5 biweekly, 2 before, and the remainder after surgery	366	1 year: 50% 2 years: 10%	35	21
Cisplatin and Doxorubicin	60 30	Alternate 21 days, 2 cycles each	300	1 year: 37% 2 years: 26%	19	22
Carboplatin	300	Every 21 days	321	1 year: 35.4%	48	24
L-MTP-PE	2	Twice weekly for 8 weeks	222	1 year: 28% 2 years: 14%	14	25
L-MTP-PE and Cisplatin	As above 70	As above Every 28 days	438	—	11	26

This compound was given to 28 dogs with osteosarcoma of the appendicular (n = 20) or axial (n = 8) skeleton.[30] Many dogs showed functional improvement; however, the average survival for the 20 dogs with appendicular osteosarcoma was 240 days. This treatment may palliate in a manner similar to external beam radiation.

OSTEOSARCOMA OF THE AXIAL SKELETON IN DOGS
Incidence, Signalment, and Etiology

In a large series of 116 dogs with osteosarcoma of the axial skeleton,[31] the distribution of lesions was mandible, 31 (27%); maxilla, 26 (22%); spine, 17 (15%); cranium, 14 (12%); ribs, 12 (10%); nasal bones, 10 (9%); and pelvis, 6 (5%). In this study, medium to large dogs were the most commonly affected but there was no specific breed predilection. Old dogs were affected (mean age = 9 years) with the exception of rib tumors, which occurred in younger dogs (median age = 5.4 years). The ratio of males to females varied with the site of the osteosarcoma. Overall, these tumors are more common in female dogs than in males; the trend is most pronounced for maxillary and pelvic osteosarcoma, which occur primarily in female dogs.[31] The 116 dogs in this study represented 25% of all dogs with osteosarcoma diagnosed in the specified time period.

MANAGEMENT OF SPECIFIC DISEASES

Clinical Presentation and History

The average duration of signs was 10 weeks in 54 of 116 dogs with axial osteosarcoma, but the range was from days to 2 years. Signs varied depending on the site affected.

Staging and Diagnosis

At the time of presentation, few dogs have evidence of pulmonary metastasis.[31] In one study, the highest rate of pulmonary metastasis occurred with osteosarcoma of the calvarium (2 of 5, or 40%); no metastases were detected with tumors of the maxilla (11 dogs), nasal cavity (4 dogs), and pelvis (2 dogs). Pulmonary metastases were seen with tumors of the rib (2 of 7), spine (1 of 6), and mandible (1 of 19). In another study, only one of eight dogs with nasal osteosarcoma developed metastases.[32] Regional lymphadenopathy, which may have signaled metastasis but was not histologically confirmed, was present in 6 of 85 dogs, all of which had tumors of the head.

Treatment

In most dogs with axial osteosarcoma, tumors recur after surgery and before metastases are clinically evident. This contrasts with appendicular osteosarcoma, where surgical margins are easily obtained but the metastatic rate is very high.[2]

Overall median survival for 38 dogs that underwent attempted surgical removal of an axial osteosarcoma was 22 weeks. Twenty-five percent of the dogs were alive at 1 year, and nearly 20% were alive at 2 years.[31] Untreated dogs died within 1 month.

Maxillary Osteosarcoma

Aggressive resection is warranted for osteosarcoma of the maxilla because recurrence, not metastasis, is usually the cause of death. Local recurrences are common if a limited surgery is performed,[31] and even with partial maxillectomy, recurrence rates are still high.[31,33] The skill of the surgeon and preoperative planning are important to the suc-

cess of surgery, and recurrence rates as low as 25%, with up to 45% of dogs alive one year after surgery, have been reported.[34] Distant metastases may be a late occurrence, with rates of 35% to 50%; however, rates may be higher in dogs that do not have local tumor recurrence and therefore live longer.[33,34] Cisplatin chemotherapy alone or in combination with radiation therapy did not reduce recurrence rates in one study of 10 dogs,[31] and radiation therapy used alone was unsuccessful in preventing rapid tumor regrowth in two dogs.[35]

Nasal Osteosarcoma

Surgical excision was attempted in three dogs, and the tumor recurred within six weeks in two dogs.[31] One dog that received 48 Gy of orthovoltage radiation with low-dose cisplatin (10 mg/m² IV) instead of surgery remained tumor-free for 12 months and died of unrelated causes.[31]

Spinal Osteosarcoma

Five dogs with spinal osteosarcoma had tumor resection by either laminectomy and curettage of three extradural tumors, debulking of a ventral lumbosacral tumor, or removal of a coccygeal vertebra by tail amputation.[31] The dog with tail amputation survived for 2.5 years and died of unrelated causes. None of the other dogs survived more than three days.

Pelvic Osteosarcoma

Hemipelvectomy is the treatment of choice for pelvic osteosarcoma; however, the metastatic rate may be high. Three of eight dogs treated with hemipelvectomy and postoperative cisplatin (70 mg/m² IV) developed pulmonary metastases.[36] Survival in four remaining dogs ranged from 21 days to 200 days with no evidence of recurrence.

Mandibular Osteosarcoma
Incidence, Signalment, and Etiology

One study found no obvious breed

KEY POINT:

Osteosarcoma of the axial skeleton in dogs should, with few exceptions, be considered to act as aggressively metastatically as appendicular osteosarcoma.

MANAGEMENT OF SPECIFIC DISEASES

predilection among 45 dogs[37] with mandibular osteosarcoma, which included seven small dogs (<15 kg). There were 28 female and 17 male dogs, which accords with dogs with axial skeletal osteosarcoma of other sites.[31]

Staging and Diagnosis

Of 45 dogs studied, 13 developed metastases,[37] of which 10 had pulmonary metastases. Other metastatic sites were ribs, skull, subcutaneous tissue, muscle, and lymph node. In another study, only one of 19 dogs had metastatic disease at the time of diagnosis.[31] Mandibular osteosarcoma may not be as aggressive as osteosarcoma of the appendicular skeleton.

Treatment

Mandibulectomy alone may provide good control of this tumor, and recurrence rates after aggressive resection are low[31,37] compared with less aggressive local excision. Seventy percent of 23 dogs treated by mandibulectomy were still alive 1 year after surgery.[37]

For mandibular osteosarcoma, the success of therapy adjunctive to mandibulectomy is equivocal. Additional therapy using chemotherapy with cisplatin and doxorubicin (10 dogs), radiation therapy (3 dogs), or a combination (4 dogs) does not seem to improve survival significantly over mandibulectomy alone.[31,37]

Radiation therapy alone provided long-term control (1229 days) in one dog but failed to control the tumor in another. One dog with mandibular osteosarcoma was treated with samarium-153-EDTMP, a β-particle–emitting compound that accumulates in regions of bony activity.[30] The lesion remained static for more than 3 years after treatment.

Osteosarcoma of the Rib
Incidence, Signalment, and Etiology

Although primary rib tumors are much less common than appendicular osteosarcomas, they behave just as aggressively. Osteosarcoma of the rib was seen primarily in dogs that weighed at least 20 kg.[38] The median age of affected dogs was 7 years. There was no gender predilection.

Clinical Presentation and History

Tumors of the rib are often large at the time of presentation. The median tumor volume is 500 cm³; not surprisingly, this is the most common reason for seeking veterinary advice.[38] In one study, pleural effusion was seen in 4 of 10 dogs with osteosarcoma of the rib.[37]

Staging and Diagnosis

Three of 10 dogs with osteosarcoma of the rib had evidence of lung metastasis at the time of presentation, and two other dogs had metastasis discovered at necropsy.[39] Thus, if osteosarcoma of the rib is suspected, thoracic radiographs, along with preoperative blood work and a surgical biopsy, should be routine.

Treatment

In dogs, osteosarcoma of the ribs develops aggressively, but adjuvant cisplatin chemotherapy seems to prolong survival. When 20 dogs were treated with en bloc surgical resection of affected ribs and received no further therapy, median survival was 90 days, which was similar to previous reports.[38,40] Of another four dogs that had en bloc resection of tumor, the tumor recurred in two dogs and one died in the perioperative period.[31] In another trial, nine dogs received adjuvant chemotherapy after surgery.[40] The chemotherapy consisted of cisplatin (70 mg/m² IV) or an alternating schedule of cisplatin (60 mg/m² IV) and doxorubicin (30 mg/m² IV) every 3 weeks, as described previously for osteosarcoma of the appendicular skeleton. Median survival for this group of dogs was 240 days.

Multilobular Osteochondrosarcoma
Incidence, Signalment, and Etiology

Multilobular osteochondrosarcoma (MLO) is considered the most common tumor of the canine skull and has been described using several names, including chondroma rodens, multilobular osteoma/osteosarcoma/chondroma, and multilobular tumor of bone.

Multilobular osteochondrosarcoma is a tumor of middle-aged to old dogs (7.5[41] to 9.0[42] years of age on

MANAGEMENT OF SPECIFIC DISEASES

average). There is no breed or gender predilection. The tumor is usually found in medium to large dogs as opposed to small or giant breeds. The most common sites are the parietal crest, temporo-occipital region, and zygomatic arch, from which tumors may extend into the sinuses, orbit, or cranial vault.

Clinical Presentation and History

Because of tumor expansion, dogs may be presented for a palpable mass noticed by the owner. Dogs may also be presented for dysphagia and pain in opening the mouth, exophthalmia, or neurologic signs. Radiographically, the lesion is sharply delineated with a lobulated appearance. This tumor usually grows slowly and the progression of signs may be slow.

Staging and Diagnosis

Metastasis at the time of presentation is unusual and was reported in only 1 of 16 dogs in one study[41] and in 1 dog in a different study.[43] Metastasis occurred a median of 14 months after surgical excision in 7 of 12 dogs, however. Interestingly, the median time from detection of metastasis to death was 11 months (range = 5 to 33 months), which concurs with other reports of long survival of dogs even once they have metastatic disease.[44,45] Radiographs of the thorax and tumor site are recommended prior to treatment, and thoracic radiographs should be used to monitor patients after surgery. A computed tomography (CT) scan may assist the surgeon in planning surgery (Figure 5-102).[41]

Treatment

Surgery is the treatment of choice for MLO, although complete excision is rarely accomplished. In one study, wide resection was accomplished in nine dogs with MLO, and there was no recurrence in four dogs that had histologically complete resection (Figure 5-103).[41]

Treatment of MLO with radiation therapy as an adjunct to surgical excision seems justified on the basis of limited data. Although cisplatin seems to give the best chance of preventing metastasis, there are

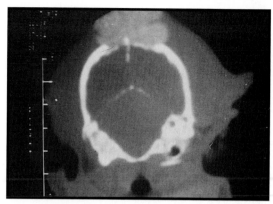

Figure 5-102: Computed tomography (CT) of multilobular osteochondrosarcoma involving the skull of a cocker spaniel (see Figure 5-103). (Courtesy J. Berg)

only preliminary data at this time. More anaplastic MLO tumors are likely to metastasize and thus may warrant adjunctive therapy. One dog that received adjuvant radiation therapy at the time of surgery for MLO had its tumor controlled for 26 months, and one had control until metastasis at 27 months.[41] Orthovoltage radiation therapy (45 Gy) resulted in more than 9 months of control of a tumor that had been resected three times in 8 months.[46] Only one dog received cisplatin (10 mg/m² every week) in addition to radiation therapy and surgery for a recurrent MLO four months after initial surgery. The tumor in this dog progressed, and pulmonary metastases were evident at necropsy.[41] Survival after development of metastasis may be long even with no treatment.

EXTRASKELETAL OSTEOSARCOMA IN DOGS
Incidence, Signalment, and Etiology

Extraskeletal osteosarcomas are extremely rare in dogs. They most often have been reported in the spleen[47,48] but also occur in the adrenal gland, eye, testicle, vagina, kidney, intestine, mesentery, and liver.[48] Dogs with extraskeletal osteosarcoma are old (mean = 11 years of age; range = 9 to 15 years of age[48]). There may be a higher incidence in female dogs.[48] There is no breed predilection.

MANAGEMENT OF SPECIFIC DISEASES

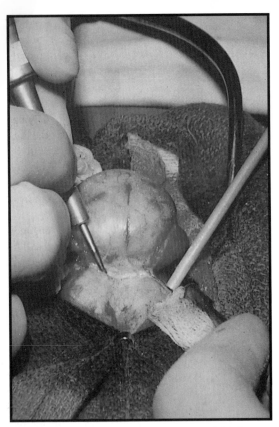

Figure 5-103: *Surgical excision of the multilobular osteochondrosarcoma seen in Figure 5-102. Wide surgical margins may provide long-term control; however, for tumors with an anaplastic histology or if tumor margins cannot be assured, adjuvant radiation therapy should be considered. (Courtesy J. Berg)*

Clinical Presentation and History

Clinical signs vary with the site of involvement. In dogs with splenic tumors, anorexia, lethargy, and abdominal distention are most common.[47]

Staging and Diagnosis

Metastatic disease is common, and most splenic osteosarcoma metastasizes to the liver and omentum. Metastases have been reported for extraskeletal osteosarcoma of the eye, testicle, vagina, intestine, and liver, principally to regional lymph nodes; other extraskeletal osteosarcomas spread by local extension only.

Treatment

Splenectomy does not give a good outcome for splenic osteosarcoma even if evidence of metastatic disease at the time of surgery is lacking.[47] Survival in three dogs with extraskeletal osteosarcomas of other sites ranged from 15 to 124 days.[48] Adjuvant chemotherapy has not been reported for this disease.

NONOSTEOSARCOMA BONE TUMORS IN DOGS
Incidence, Signalment, and Etiology

Primary bone tumors that are not osteosarcomas are rare in dogs. The tumors most commonly described are chondrosarcomas, fibrosarcomas, and hemangiosarcomas. Less common tumors include giant cell tumors, liposarcomas, and synovial cell sarcomas. Synovial cell tumors are not strictly bone tumors and are described separately later in this chapter.

In a series of 26 nonosteosarcoma appendicular bone tumors, the most frequently recognized was fibrosarcoma (9 dogs). Hemangiosarcoma (5 dogs) and chondrosarcoma (2 dogs) were less frequently noted.[49] Chondrosarcoma probably predominates in the axial skeleton.[50] Affected dogs are mostly large breeds. There is no gender predilection, and old dogs are most often affected.[49]

Giant cell tumors are infrequently reported, and there are no data regarding incidence or treatment. This tumor may metastasize.

Clinical Presentation and History

Nonosteosarcoma tumors of the bone differ little from osteosarcomas in either clinical presentation or radiographic appearance. The finding of a bone tumor in the axial skeleton increases the index of suspicion for one of these tumor types.

Staging and Diagnosis

Histopathology from incisional or needle biopsies of bone lesions must be viewed with some skepticism, as osteosarcomas frequently have localized areas that do not contain osteoid and are composed of purely fibrous or cartilaginous tissue. For this reason, a definitive diagnosis should be delayed until a larger

MANAGEMENT OF SPECIFIC DISEASES

biopsy specimen is obtained (e.g., at amputation). In one retrospective study, 6 of 11 dogs with fibrosarcoma were found on further histologic sectioning to have osteosarcoma.[51] This point is particularly important if adjuvant therapy is being considered.

Treatment

Surgery remains the treatment of choice for nonosteosarcoma bone tumors in dogs. Adjunctive chemotherapy has been reported for very few dogs.

Fibrosarcoma
Incidence, Signalment, and Etiology

Fibrosarcomas of bone are rare. They usually involve the axial skeleton.[49,51] These tumors primarily affect mature male dogs.

Staging and Diagnosis

Complete staging for any dog with a bone tumor should include blood work, urinalysis, fine detail radiographs of the lesion, thoracic radiographs, and careful evaluation of regional lymph nodes. In a series of five dogs with mandibular fibrosarcoma, metastasis to the regional lymph node was confirmed in one dog and suspected in two dogs 13, 7, and 10 months after mandibulectomy.[52] In another series of 14 dogs with fibrosarcoma of the maxilla (n = 7) or mandible (n = 7), metastasis occurred in only 14%.[34] Two dogs with fibrosarcoma of the rib developed systemic metastases 120 and 450 days after surgical resection.[38] Metastases were seen in cardiac muscle and pericardium, skin, and patella in three of five dogs with appendicular fibrosarcomas treated by amputation.[51] Metastasis in fibrosarcomas of the axial skeleton may be less prevalent than for appendicular sites and may sometimes occur late in the course of the disease.

Treatment

For appendicular fibrosarcoma in five dogs, survival after amputation ranged from 4 to 40 months; three dogs developed metastatic disease.[51] Three of the dogs also received adjuvant cisplatin (70 mg/m[2] IV or IA every 3 weeks). Two of these dogs developed

metastasis, and one had no evidence of disease 17 months later. One dog that did not receive chemotherapy had no evidence of disease 40 months after surgery.

Median survival for 34 dogs treated for fibrosarcoma by mandibulectomy or maxillectomy was 12 months.[34,52] Local recurrence was seen in 11 dogs. The outlook for a dog with fibrosarcoma of the bone is better than for dogs with osteosarcoma, but the prognosis is still guarded, and local recurrence may be more of a problem with maxillectomy than with mandibulectomy (see also the chapter on Tumors of the Oral Cavity).

Local control rates may be improved by using radiation teletherapy as an adjuvant to surgery. This approach has improved survival times for dogs with soft tissue sarcomas[53,54] and may play a similar role for fibrosarcoma of bone if surgical margins cannot be assured.

Chondrosarcoma
Incidence, Signalment, and Etiology

Chondrosarcomas were found in 41 of 394 bone tumors or tumor-like lesions in dogs. Old dogs were mostly affected in two studies (mean = 8 to 9 years of age; range = 1 to 15 years of age).[55,56] In another group of 35 dogs with chondrosarcomas, the average age was 6 years.[50] Chondrosarcomas most commonly involve the axial skeleton and ribs, nasal turbinates, and pelvis.[50,55,56] This tumor is most common in large-breed dogs.

Chondrosarcomas of the appendicular skeleton are uncommon, accounting for 16 of 97 cases in one study, and seem to involve the hindlimb more frequently (14 of 16).[56]

Staging and Diagnosis

Staging should be performed as described for all bone tumors. Chondrosarcoma is believed to have a low metastatic rate compared to osteosarcoma, although chondrosarcoma of the appendicular skeleton has been associated with widespread systemic metastases.[56] In two studies, 7 of 38 dogs with chondrosarcoma had systemic metastases.[50,55] In another

MANAGEMENT OF SPECIFIC DISEASES

study of 97 dogs with this tumor, 20.5% of the dogs died or were euthanatized with lung metastases.[56] In a large study of 55 dogs with chondrosarcoma, metastasis was noted from all sites except the nasal passages; the highest rates were for tumors of the long bones and rib.[57] Only 1 of 12 dogs with a nasal chondrosarcoma developed metastases in another study.[32]

In a series of 15 dogs with chondrosarcoma of ribs, eight developed pulmonary metastasis.[38] These metastases, however, occurred often long after surgical excision of the primary tumor. Metastasis may occur late (median survival after surgery was more than 3 years in one study[38]); thus, early studies may have reflected less aggressive therapy and death due to recurrence or progression of local disease. Thoracic radiographs to monitor for pulmonary metastasis are warranted, particularly for appendicular and rib chondrosarcomas.

Treatment

Dogs with appendicular chondrosarcoma treated by amputation alone had a median survival of 540 days. All five dogs in one study died of metastatic disease.[56] Three dogs with digital chondrosarcoma treated by amputation survived 135 to 1350 days.[56] Therefore, amputation alone is a good option for treatment of dogs with appendicular chondrosarcoma compared to those with osteosarcoma; however, this surgery cannot be considered curative. In contrast, for a further seven dogs with chondrosarcomas of the appendicular skeleton, the metastatic rate approached 60% and median survival was 160 days.[57]

Surgical resection of rib chondrosarcomas resulted in long-term control and survival in one study in which the median survival for 15 dogs was 1080 days, even though eight dogs developed systemic

metastases.[38] The longest survivor was free of disease 7 years after surgery. In this study, survival for dogs with chondrosarcoma was found to be significantly longer than for dogs with osteosarcoma of the rib. No adjunctive chemotherapy was administered to these dogs.[38] Similarly, in two other studies, although some dogs did not survive the perioperative period (presumably due to the aggressive surgery required for en bloc resection), the remaining dogs had a median survival of 5 years and most dogs lived more than one year. Some of these dogs (2 of 11) had local recurrence, and 2 of 11 developed metastatic disease.[50,56] Wide surgical margins are important in prolonging survival of dogs with rib chondrosarcomas.

In two earlier studies of dogs with rib chondrosarcomas that underwent definitive surgery (14 dogs[58] and 7 dogs[59]), median survival was 300 and 105 days, respectively. This may be because of a higher local recurrence rate and because the occurrence of very large tumors that made resection more difficult.[58] Two dogs with chondrosarcoma of the pelvis were treated with hemipelvectomy, and both survived more than 50 months without developing metastases.[36]

Radiation may be a useful adjunct to treatment of chondrosarcomas. In one series of 55 dogs with chondrosarcoma, the longest median survival (500 days) was in dogs with nasal chondrosarcoma that received radiation therapy.[57] In another study, two of four dogs that received orthovoltage radiation as an adjunct to surgery for nasal chondrosarcoma lived more than two years.[56]

Hemangiosarcoma

Hemangiosarcoma as a primary bone tumor is rare. It may be seen as a result of systemic metastases from a visceral site. It most often affects young adult,

MANAGEMENT OF SPECIFIC DISEASES

large-breed dogs. Hemangiosarcomas are destructive lesions, and bony changes on radiographs are primarily lytic. As in other locations in the body, the metastatic rate of this tumor is high. Of three dogs with hemangiosarcoma of the rib, two had metastatic disease within 5 months of surgery.[38] One dog with appendicular hemangiosarcoma was treated with doxorubicin (30 mg/m² IV) and cyclophosphamide (50 to 75 mg/m² PO) after amputation and died 154 days later from metastatic disease.[60]

SYNOVIAL CELL SARCOMA IN DOGS
Incidence, Signalment, and Etiology

Synovial cell sarcoma is rare in dogs. It arises from the synovioblastic mesenchyme deep in the connective tissue that is adjacent to joints. In a review of 45 reported cases, this tumor was found to occur primarily in male dogs (M:F ratio = 1.5:1.0) at a median age of 7 years (range = 1 to 14 years of age).[61] There was no obvious breed predisposition. A more recent study of 35 dogs found similar demographics.[62] The tumor occurred in middle-aged (median age = 9 years; range = 2 to 15 years) male dogs (M:F ratio = 1.3:1.0). Both series found the disease to be most common in large-breed dogs (median weight = 22 kg).

Synovial cell sarcoma occurred in the stifle in 37 of 80 dogs; the next most commonly affected sites were the hock and elbow (12 dogs each). In addition, tumors were diagnosed in the shoulder, carpus, metatarsus, digit, radius, hip, and femur.[61,62] Interestingly, one study found a 3:1 predilection for the right side among 35 dogs with synovial sarcoma.[62]

Staging and Diagnosis

Of 31 dogs with synovial sarcoma, only two had pulmonary metastases detected at the time of diagnosis.[62] However, five dogs evidenced tumor spread to the regional lymph node, and one tumor metastasized to the kidney. Overall, nearly one quarter of dogs presented with synovial sar-coma had metastatic disease. In another retrospective review,[61] 12 of 37 dogs had metastases detected at presentation and eight other dogs developed metastases between 6 weeks and 18 months after diagnosis. In these 20 dogs, regional lymph nodes and lungs were affected with equal frequency and other sites considerably less frequently. Four dogs developed renal metastases.

Histologically, synovial sarcoma is biphasic,[63] meaning that the tumor has varying degrees of an epithelioid (synovioblastic) component and a fibroblastic component.

Prognostic Factors

In a study of 36 synovial sarcomas in dogs, some histologic criteria were found to have prognostic significance.[63] Dogs with tumors that had a high mitotic rate, a high degree of nuclear pleomorphism, and considerable necrosis had poor survival and their tumors were more likely to recur. A grading system based on these criteria showed that dogs with grade III tumors had a median survival of 210 days compared with 1080 days for dogs with grade I or II tumors. Dogs that had tumors with a high epithelial component, as measured by cytokeratin immunohistochemistry, had considerably less time until the tumor recurred or metastasized (105 days versus 420+ days). Cytokeratin staining may be performed at certain veterinary pathology laboratories.

Treatment

Tumors undergoing marginal resection recur rapidly (median = 4.5 months); however, amputation improves local tumor control. In one study of 21 dogs that were treated by amputation, two had a local stump recurrence, and four developed metastases in a median of 5 months (range = 2 to 13 months). Of the remainder, more than half were free of tumor 3 years after surgery. Results of radiation therapy for this disease have not been reported.

> **KEY POINT:**
>
> *Dogs with synovial sarcoma that histologically have a high mitotic rate, marked nuclear pleomorphism, and necrosis have poor survival.*

MANAGEMENT OF SPECIFIC DISEASES

Chemotherapy using doxorubicin (30 mg/m² IV) has been reported to provide long-term response in dogs with synovial sarcoma.[64,65] In contrast, a group of four dogs that received doxorubicin (1 dog), doxorubicin and cyclophosphamide (1 dog), COP (cyclophosphamide/vincristine/prednisone) (1 dog), or piroxicam (1 dog) showed no measurable tumor responses.

SYNOVIAL CELL TUMORS IN CATS

Too few synovial tumors have been reported in cats to enable comment on their behavior or treatment. All reported cases have been locally invasive and tend to recur after local excision, but wide excision results in long-term control. Synovial tumors have been reported in cats ranging from 6 to 16 years of age.[68] These tumors did not metastasize, even over long periods. One cat developed metastasis to the local lymph node and then systemically within months of amputation (A.S. Moore, personal observation, 1994).

PRIMARY BONE TUMORS IN CATS
Osteosarcoma
Incidence, Signalment, and Etiology

Osteosarcoma is the most common primary bone tumor in cats and occurs in old cats (median age = 11 years)[66] with a predilection for male cats in the United Kingdom[66] and for female cats in the United States.[67,68] In 4 series of cases totalling 106 cats with osteosarcoma, 30 occurred in the skull, 56 occurred in the appendicular skeleton (38 in the hindlimb and 18 in the forelimb), and the remaining 20 involved either vertebrae (8 cats), scapula (2 cats), rib (5 cats), or pelvis (5 cats).[66–69]

Parosteal (juxtacortical) osteosarcomas seem to originate from the surface of the bone without cortical or medullary involvement[70] and are most common on the head.[67] An extraosseous (soft tissue) osteosarcoma arose in the mammary tissue of one cat.[71]

Clinical Presentation and History

Cats with osteosarcoma are usually presented for swelling, although two cats with appendicular tumors presented with pathologic fractures in one

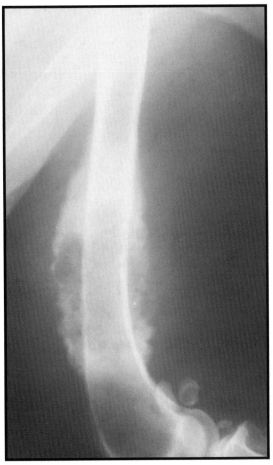

Figure 5-104: *Radiograph of an appendicular osteosarcoma in a cat. Appendicular osteosarcomas in cats are usually metaphyseal and primarily lytic radiographically. The prognosis after amputation is excellent in cats, in contrast to the situation in dogs.*

study.[66] Cats with appendicular tumors are usually presented for lameness and development of a large, painless mass. Growth may be slow and signs are often present for months prior to diagnosis. Radiographically, most tumors of the appendicular skeleton are metaphyseal and primarily lytic (Figure 5-104). Two cats with parosteal osteosarcoma of the limbs were also presented for chronic lameness in another study.[70]

MANAGEMENT OF SPECIFIC DISEASES

Staging and Diagnosis

Metastasis is uncommon in cats with osteosarcoma. In one series, only 1 of 19 affected cats had metastases to the lung[66] and none of 3 other cats with appendicular osteosarcoma had metastases detected.[70] In another series of 15 cats with appendicular osteosarcoma, only one cat developed metastases.[69] Two cats with parosteal osteosarcoma did not develop metastases, despite the tumor being present for 12 months in one of the cats; however, a cat with a soft tissue osteosarcoma developed pulmonary metastasis in less than two months.[71] Metastasis from tumors of the axial skeleton have not been described. Thoracic radiographs should be performed in all cats with primary bone lesions; however, it is unusual for these cats to develop metastases even long after surgery.

Treatment

Four of the five cats with osteosarcoma in one study were successfully treated by amputation. One cat died from metastatic disease 5 months after surgery, but the other cats were alive without metastases up to 26 months after surgery.[67] In 12 other cats with appendicular osteosarcoma treated by amputation, pulmonary metastasis occurred in only one cat; more than half of the cats were alive 64 months after surgery. Of the 5 cats that died, median survival was 50 months.[69] In the same study, 4 cats with osteosarcomas of the axial skeleton did not fare well, as complete surgical excision of the tumor could not be obtained.

The low rate of metastasis implies that radiation therapy may play an important role in the control of incompletely excised osteosarcoma, although published reports are few. Although three cats with osteosarcoma of the skull had recurrence within three months of surgery, one cat that received radiation therapy had local recurrence 16 months after surgery, indicating a possible pallia-

tive role for radiation.[69] Radiation therapy (42 Gy in 7 weekly fractions of orthovoltage teletherapy) controlled an osteosarcoma involving the nasal cavity of a cat for two years.[70]

Adjunctive chemotherapy is rarely warranted for the treatment of feline osteosarcoma because of the low rate of metastasis. Doxorubicin (30 mg/m^2) was given to three cats following amputation for appendicular osteosarcoma.[20] Two of these cats developed pulmonary metastases 133 and 274 days after treatment. Survival times for these 3 cats were 143, 180, and 414 days, which differ little from survival times for amputation alone. A cat with pelvic osteosarcoma received vincristine (0.5 mg/m^2 IV), cyclophosphamide (50 mg/m^2), and methotrexate (2.5 mg/m^2) every 2 weeks and had an 80% reduction in tumor size for 13 months.[69] Cisplatin cannot be safely administered systematically to cats.[72]

Other Bone Tumors

Other primary bone tumors in cats include fibrosarcomas, giant cell tumors, and osteochondromas. Occasionally, tumors will invade bone by extension (i.e., fibrosarcoma, hemangiosarcoma, and synovial cell sarcoma) or as part of systemic disease (i.e., lymphoma and multiple myeloma). Hemangiosarcoma of bone has been noted to spread systemically.[66,70] Two cats with a fibrosarcoma of the appendicular skeleton were still alive with no evidence of metastasis 12 and 18 months after amputation.[73,74]

Squamous cell sarcoma commonly invades the mandible or maxilla in cats and creates a radiographic proliferation lesion that can only be differentiated from osteosarcoma by biopsy.[31]

> ## KEY POINTS:
>
> *Metastasis is uncommon in cats with osteosarcoma, and adjuvant chemotherapy is not usually indicated.*
>
> ---
>
> *Proliferative bony tumors in the mandible or maxilla of cats are more likely to be squamous cell carcinoma than osteosarcoma.*

REFERENCES

1. Tjalma RA: Canine bone sarcoma: Estimation of relative risk as a function of body size. *J Natl Cancer Inst* 36:1137–1150, 1966.
2. Spodnick GJ, Berg J, Rand WM, et al:

Prognosis for dogs with appendicular osteosarcoma treated by amputation alone: 162 cases (1978–1988). *JAVMA* 200:995–999, 1992.

3. Misdorp W, Hart AAM: Some prognostic and epidemiologic factors in canine osteosarcoma. *J Natl Cancer Inst* 62:537–545, 1979.

4. Brodey RS, Riser WH: Canine osteosarcoma: A clinicopathologic study of 194 cases. *Clin Orthop Rel Res* 62:54–64, 1969.

5. Gillette-McChesney S, Gillette EL, Powers BE, Withrow SJ: Radiation- induced osteosarcoma in dogs after external beam or intraoperative radiation therapy. *Cancer Res*:54–57, 1990.

6. Lamb CR, Berg J, Bengston AE: Preoperative measurement of canine primary bone tumors, using radiography and bone scintigraphy. *JAVMA* 196:1474–1478, 1990.

7. Berg J, Lamb CR, O'Callaghan MW: Bone scintigraphy in the initial evaluation of dogs with primary bone tumors. *JAVMA* 196:917–920, 1990.

8. Weinstein MJ, Berg J, Kusazaki K, et al: In vitro assay of nuclear uptake of doxorubicin hydrochloride in osteosarcoma cells of dogs. *Am J Vet Res* 52:1951–1955, 1991.

9. Powers BE, Withrow SJ, Thrall DE, et al: Percent tumor necrosis as a predictor of treatment response in canine osteosarcoma. *Cancer* 67:126–134, 1991.

10. Carberry CA, Harvey HJ: Owner satisfaction with limb amputation in dogs and cats. *JAAHA* 23:227–232, 1987.

11. Brodey RS: Results of surgical treatment in 65 dogs with osteosarcoma. *JAVMA* 168:1032–1035, 1976.

12. Trout NJ, Pavletic MM, Kraus KH: Partial scapulectomy in the treatment of malignant sarcomas in three dogs and two cats. *Vet Surg*, 1994, in press.

13. O'Brien MG, Straw RC, Withrow SJ: Recent advances in the treatment of canine appendicular osteosarcoma. *Compend Contin Educ Pract Vet* 15:939–947, 1993.

14. Withrow SJ, Thrall DE, Straw RS: Intra-arterial cisplatin with or without radiation in limb sparing for canine osteosarcoma. *Cancer* 71:2484–2490, 1993.

15. Shapiro W, Fossum TW, Kitchell BE, et al: Use of cisplatin for treatment of appendicular osteosarcoma in dogs. *JAVMA* 192:507–511, 1988.

16. Straw RC, Withrow SJ, Richter SL, et al: Amputation and cisplatin for treatment of canine osteosarcoma. *J Vet Intern Med* 5:205–210, 1991.

17. Thompson JP, Fugent MJ: Evaluation of survival time after limb amputation, with and without subsequent administration of cisplatin, for treatment of appendicular osteosarcoma in dogs: 30 cases (1979–1990). *JAVMA* 200:531–533, 1992.

18. Kraegel SA, Madewell BR, Simonson E, Gregory CR: Osteogenic sarcoma and cisplatin chemotherapy in dogs: 16 cases (1986–1989). *JAVMA* 199:1057–1059, 1991.

19. Berg J, Weinstein J, Schelling SH, Rand WM: Treatment of dogs with osteosarcoma by administration of cisplatin after amputation or limb-sparing surgery: 22 cases (1987–1990). *JAVMA* 200:2005–2008, 1992.

20. Madewell BR, Leighton RL, Theilen GH: Amputation and doxorubicin for treatment of canine and feline osteogenic sarcoma. *Eur J Cancer* 14:287–293, 1978.

21. Berg J, Weinstein MJ, Springfield DS: Response of osteosarcoma in dogs to surgery and chemotherapy with doxorubicin. *JAVMA*, 1994, in press.

22. Mauldin GN, Matus RE, Withrow SJ, Patnaik AK: Canine osteosarcoma. Treatment by amputation versus amputation plus adjuvant chemotherapy using doxorubicin and cisplatin. *J Vet Intern Med* 2:177–180, 1988.

23. Cotter SM, Parker LM: High-dose methotrexate and leucovorin rescue in dogs with osteogenic sarcoma. *Am J Vet Res* 39:1943–1945, 1978.

24. Bergman PJ, MacEwen EG, Kurzman ID, et al: Amputation and carboplatin for treatment of dogs with osteosarcoma: 48 cases (1991–1993). *JAVMA*, 1994, in press.

25. MacEwen EG, Kurzman TD, Rosenthal RC, et al: Therapy for osteosarcoma in dogs with intravenous injection of liposome encapsulated muramyl tripeptide. *J Natl Cancer Inst* 81:935–938, 1989.

26. MacEwen EG, Helfand SC: Recent advances in the biologic therapy of cancer. *Compend Contin Educ Pract Vet* 15:909–922, 1993.

27. Knapp DW, Richardson RC, Booney PL, Hahn K: Cisplatin therapy in 41 dogs with malignant tumors. *J Vet Intern Med* 2:41–46, 1988.

28. Ogilvie GK, Straw RC, Jameson VJ: Evaluation of single-agent chemotherapy for treatment of clinically evident osteosarcoma metastasis in dogs: 45 cases (1987–1991). *JAVMA* 202:304–306, 1993.

29. O'Brien MG, Straw RC, Withrow SJ, et al: Resection of pulmonary metastases in canine osteosarcoma: Thirty-one cases (1983–1992). *Vet Surg* 22:105–109, 1993.

30. Lattimer JC, Corwin LA, Stapleton J, et al: Clinical and clinicopathologic response of canine bone tumor patients to treatment with samarium-153-EDTMP. *J Nuclear Med* 31:1316–1325, 1990.

31. Heymann SJ, Diefender DL, Goldschmidt MH, Newton CD: Canine axial skeletal osteosarcoma. A retrospective study of 116 cases (1986 to 1989). *Vet Surg* 21:304–310, 1992.

32. Patnaik AK, Lieberman PH, Erlandson RA, Liu SK:

MANAGEMENT OF SPECIFIC DISEASES

Canine sinonasal skeletal neoplasms: Chondrosarcomas and osteosarcomas. *Vet Pathol* 21:475–482, 1984.

33. Wallace J, Matthiesen DT, Patnaik AK: Hemimaxillectomy for the treatment of oral tumors in 69 dogs. *Vet Surg* 21:337–341, 1992.

34. White RAS: Mandibulectomy and maxillectomy in the dog: Long-term survival in 100 cases. *J Small Anim Pract* 32:69–74, 1991.

35. Withrow SJ, Doige CE: En bloc resection of a juxtacortical and three intraosseous osteosarcoma of the zygomatic arch in dogs. *JAAHA* 16:867–872, 1980.

36. Straw RC, Withrow SJ, Powers BE: Partial or total hemipelvectomy in the management of sarcomas in nine dogs and two cats. *Vet Surg* 21:183–188, 1992.

37. Straw RC, Powers BE, Henderson RA, et al: Canine mandibular osteosarcoma. Forty-five cases (1980–1991). *Proc 11th Ann Conf Vet Cancer Soc*:79–80, 1991.

38. Pirkey-Ehrhart N, Straw RC, Withrow SJ, et al: Primary rib tumors in 54 dogs. *JAAHA*, 1994, in press.

39. Feeney DA, Johnston GR, Grindem CB, et al: Malignant neoplasia of canine ribs: Clinical, radiographic, and pathologic findings. *JAVMA* 180:927–933, 1982.

40. Matthiesen DT, Clark GN, Orsher RJ, et al: En bloc resection of primary rib tumors in 40 dogs. *Vet Surg* 21:201–204, 1992.

41. Straw RC, LeCouteur RA, Powers BE, Withrow SJ: Multibular osteochondrosarcoma of the canine skull: 16 cases (1978–1988). *JAVMA* 195:1764–1769, 1989.

42. Pool RR: Tumors of bone and cartilage, in Moulton JE (ed): *Tumors in Domestic Animals*, ed 3. Berkeley, CA, University of California Press, 1990, pp 157–230.

43. Johnston TC: Osteosarcoma of the canine skull (a case report). *Vet Med Small Anim Clin* 71:629–631, 1976.

44. McLain DL, Hill JR, Pulley LT: Multilobular osteoma and chondroma (chondroma rodens) with pulmonary metastasis in a dog. *JAAHA* 19:359–362, 1983.

45. Losco PE, Diters RW, Walsh KM: Canine multilobar osteosarcoma of the skull with metastasis. *J Comp Pathol* 94:621–624, 1984.

46. Pletcher JM, Koch SA, Stedham MA: Orbital chondroma rodens in a dog. *JAVMA* 175:187–190, 1979.

47. Weinstein MJ, Carpenter JL, Schunk-Mehlaff, CJ: Nonangiogenic and nonlymphomatous sarcomas of the canine spleen: 57 cases (1975–1987). *JAVMA* 195:784–788, 1989.

48. Patnaik AK: Canine extraskeletal osteosarcoma and chondrosarcoma: A clinicopathologic study of 14 cases. *Vet Pathol* 27:46–55, 1990.

49. Gibbs C, Denny HR, Lucke VM: The radiological features of nonosteogenic malignant tumors of bone in the appendicular skeleton of the dog. *J Small Anim Pract* 26:537–553, 1985.

50. Brodey RS, Misdorp W, Riser WH, Heul van der RO:

Canine skeletal chondrosarcoma: A clinicopathological study of 35 cases. *JAVMA* 165:68–78, 1974.

51. Wesselhoeft-Ablin L, Berg J, Schelling SH: Fibrosarcoma of the canine appendicular skeleton. *JAAHA* 27:303–309, 1991.

52. Salisbury SK, Lantz GC: Long-term results of partial mandibulectomy for treatment of oral tumors in 30 dogs. *JAAHA* 24:285–294, 1988.

53. McChesney SL, Withrow SJ, Gillette EL, et al: Radiotherapy of soft tissue sarcomas in dogs. *JAVMA* 194:60–63, 1989.

54. Mauldin GN, Meleo KA, Burk RL: Radiation therapy for the treatment of incompletely resected soft tissue sarcomas in dogs: 21 cases. *Proc Vet Cancer Soc 13th Ann Conf*:111, 1993.

55. Liu SK, Dorfman HD, Huruitz AI, Patnaik AK: Primary and secondary bone tumors in the dog. *J Small Anim Pract* 18:313–326, 1977.

56. Popovitch CA, Weinstein MJ, Goldschmidt MH, Shofer FS: Chondrosarcoma: A retrospective study of 97 dogs (1987–1990). *JAAHA* 30:81–85, 1994.

57. Obradovich JE, Straw RC, Powers BE, Withrow SJ: Canine chondrosarcoma: A clinicopathologic review of 55 cases (1983–1990). *Proc 10th Ann Conf Vet Cancer Soc*:29–30, 1990.

58. Matthiesen DT, Clark GN, Orsher RJ, et al: En bloc resection of primary rib tumors in 40 dogs. *Vet Surg* 21:201–204, 1992.

59. Montgomery RD, Henderson RA, Powers RD: Retrospective study of 26 primary tumors of the osseous wall in dogs. *JAAHA* 29:68–72, 1993.

60. Hammer AS, Couto CG, Filppi J, et al: Efficacy and toxicity of VAC chemotherapy (vincristine, doxorubicin and cyclophosphamide) in dogs with hemangiosarcoma. *J Vet Intern Med* 5:160–166, 1991.

61. McGlennon NJ, Houlton JEF, Gorman NT. Synovial sarcoma in the dog: A review. *J Small Anim Pract* 29:139–152, 1988.

62. Vail DM, Powers B, Morrison WB, et al: Clinical aspects of synovial cell sarcoma (SCS) in the canine: A retrospective study of 35 cases. *Proc 10th Ann Vet Cancer Soc Conf*:31–32, 1990.

63. Vail DM, Powers BE, Getsy D, et al: Prognostic importance of histological grade and cytochemical staining patterns for canine synovial cell sarcoma: Preliminary results of a VCOG study. *Vet Cancer Soc Newsletter* 17(1):1–4, 1993.

64. Tilmant LL, Gorman NT, Ackerman N, et al: Chemotherapy of synovial cell sarcoma in a dog. *JAVMA* 188:530–532, 1986.

65. Ogilvie GK, Reynolds HA, Richardson RC, et al: Phase II evaluation of doxorubicin for treatment of various canine neoplasms. *JAVMA* 195:1580–1583, 1989.

MANAGEMENT OF SPECIFIC DISEASES

66. Quigley PJ, Leedale AH: Tumors involving bone in the domestic cat: A review of fifty-eight cases. *Vet Pathol* 20:670–686, 1983.

67. Liu SK, Dorfman HD, Patnaik AK. Primary and secondary bone tumors in the cat. *J Small Anim Pract* 15:141–156, 1974.

68. Carpenter JL, Andrews LK, Holzworth J: Tumors and tumor-like lesions, in Holzworth J (ed): *Diseases of the Cat. Medicine and Surgery.* Philadelphia, WB Saunders, 1987, pp 406–596.

69. Bitetto WV, Patnaik AK, Schrader SC, Mooney SC: Osteosarcoma in cats: 22 cases (1974–1984). *JAVMA* 190:91–93, 1987.

70. Turrel JM, Pool RR: Primary bone tumors in the cat: A retrospective study of 15 cats and literature review. *Vet Radiol* 23:152–166, 1982.

71. Easton CB: Extraskeletal osteosarcoma in a cat. *JAAHA* 30:59–61, 1994.

72. Knapp DW, Richardson RC, DeNicola DB, et al: Cisplatin toxicity in cats. *J Vet Intern Med* 1:29–35, 1987.

73. Levitt L, Doige CE: Primary intraosseous fibrosarcoma in a cat. *JAVMA* 194:1601–1603, 1989.

74. Tischler SA: Ulnar fibrosarcoma in a cat. *Mod Vet Pract* 67:39, 1986.

CLINICAL BRIEFING: TUMORS OF THE SKIN AND SURROUNDING STRUCTURES

Cutaneous Squamous Cell Carcinoma In Dogs

Common Clinical Presentation	Ulcerated cutaneous lesions, most often on limbs (digits); lesions may be induced by sunlight on trunk
Common Histologic Type	Most cutaneous squamous cell carcinomas are well differentiated and rarely metastasize
Epidemiology and Biological Behavior	Large, black-breed dogs prone to subungual tumor, which may metastasize; light-skinned dogs prone to actinically induced tumors
Prognostic Factors	Nasal–planum tumors more aggressive; subungual and skin tumors may metastasize; lymphatic invasion for subungual lesion *does not* influence prognosis for survival
Treatment	*Early Lesions:* Surgical excision, retinoids, topical 5-fluorouracil or carmustine (BCNU) ointments, and cryotherapy if lesions are <1 cm *Invasive Lesions:* Surgery, with or without radiation therapy and intralesional chemotherapy *Metastatic Lesions:* Cisplatin or mitoxantrone chemotherapy

Cutaneous Squamous Cell Carcinoma in Cats

Common Clinical Presentation	Ulcerated cutaneous lesions, most often on head and neck
Common Histologic Type	Most are well-differentiated; metastasis to regional lymph nodes is rare
Epidemiology and Biological Behavior	Cats lacking skin pigment are prone to actinically induced tumors; tumors are locally invasive with a low metastatic rate
Prognostic Factors	None identified
Treatment	*Early Lesions:* Brachytherapy, radiation therapy, local current-field hyperthermia, and cryotherapy if lesions are <1 cm

MANAGEMENT OF SPECIFIC DISEASES

Treatment	*Invasive Lesions:* External beam radiation therapy, surgery, photodynamic therapy, and intralesional chemotherapy

Soft Tissue Sarcoma in Dogs and Cats

Common Presentation	Subcutaneous firm and irregular mass appears (**but is not**) encapsulated
Common Histologic Types	Fibroma, fibrosarcoma, hemangiopericytoma, neurofibroma, neurofibrosarcoma, schwannoma, rhabdomyoma, rhabdomyosarcoma, leiomyoma, leiomyosarcoma, and malignant fibrous histiocytoma
Epidemiology and Biological Behavior	Young cats; may be related to FeSV and FeLV infection; possible correlation with vaccination site in cats; locally invasive with a low metastatic rate
Prognostic Factors	**Wide** surgical excision at first surgery; metastasis is uncommon

Treatment
  Surgery
  Radiation Therapy
 	
  Chemotherapy
	
	Wide surgical excision
	Adjuvant external beam radiation therapy of ≥50 Gy gives control of 70%–90% at 1 year
	Chemotherapy with doxorubicin-based protocols is being evaluated

Cutaneous Melanoma in Dogs

Common Clinical Presentation	Darkly pigmented epidermal lesion, usually raised but not ulcerated
Common Histologic Type	Most are well differentiated (benign); subungual tumors are more aggressive
Epidemiology and Biological Behavior	Adult to aged dogs
Prognostic Factors	Subungual melanoma, 50% metastasize; other cutaneous sites, metastasis is rare

MANAGEMENT OF SPECIFIC DISEASES

Treatment	
Surgery	Surgical excision curative for most cutaneous lesions
Chemotherapy	Cisplatin or carboplatin chemotherapy for metastatic lesions (or possibly as an adjunct to surgery in subungual melanoma)

Mast Cell Tumors in Dogs (see also chapter on Mast Cell Tumors)

Mast Cell Tumors in Cats (see also chapter on Mast Cell Tumors)

Other Tumors Reviewed

Papilloma, basal cell tumors, hair matrix tumors, sebaceous and sweat gland tumors, vascular skin tumors, histiocytoma, plasmacytoma, transmissible venereal tumors, cutaneous lymphoma, mycosis fungoides, and histiocytic diseases

The skin is the major barrier between animals and their environment and thus is exposed to a high level of environmental carcinogens. This exposure is reflected in the high number and variety of primary skin tumors that occur in the skin, subcutis, and adnexa of dogs and cats. The skin is one of the most common sites of tumors in animals. Most skin tumors in dogs are benign. For cats, however, the opposite is true. Tumors that occur on the skin are likely to be discovered by the animal's owner, who is likely to seek veterinary advice. Management of skin tumors (identifying them and deciding whether to remove them and whether further treatment is necessary once a tumor has been removed) is an important part of small animal practice.

Skin tumors occur mostly in cats older than 10 years of age. In one study, the most common skin tumor types in cats, in decreasing frequency, were basal cell tumors, squamous cell carcinomas, and fibrosarcomas.[1] The most common skin tumors in dogs are mast cell tumors (MCTs) (10% to 20%) and histiocytomas (3% to 15%). Some authors have

grouped tumors of the basal cells, sebaceous adenomas, and sebaceous epitheliomas.[2] This classification accounts for between 20% and 30% of all skin tumors.

Some canine breeds are predisposed to develop particular skin tumors (e.g., boxers and MCTs; cocker spaniels and sebaceous tumors). Certain skin characteristics seem to promote other types of tumors (dogs with poorly pigmented, lightly haired ventral abdominal skin are predisposed to developing squamous cell carcinoma and cutaneous hemangiosarcomas).

Skin tumors are often superficial and their margins are often obvious. Infiltrative masses, such as MCTs and soft tissue sarcomas, often have diffuse neoplastic margins that are not easily identified. For skin tumors that attach to underlying tissue or interfere with function, ultrasonography and computed tomography (CT scan) may be useful adjuncts for staging and delineating tumor borders prior to surgical excision. In one series of 26 dogs with cutaneous tumors, these two modalities identified 18 dogs that

MANAGEMENT OF SPECIFIC DISEASES

had more advanced disease than was expected on clinical examination and the surgical plan was subsequently altered.[3] In any case, a pre-operative biopsy is recommended if its results might change either the owner's willingness to treat (benign versus malignant) or the type of treatment that would be offered (e.g., sebaceous adenoma versus a grade III anaplastic mast cell tumor).

EPITHELIAL TUMORS
Papilloma (Warts) in Dogs
Incidence, Signalment, and Etiology

This is a papovavirus-induced benign tumor of stratified squamous epithelium. Many tumors identified clinically as warts are, in fact, such other tumors as sebaceous adenomas. Papillomas are more common in males. Middle-aged and old dogs are most often affected.

Clinical Presentation and History

Papillomas generally are smaller than 1 cm in diameter. These lesions are usually small, solitary, superficial, pedunculated nodules that are hard and have a rough, corrugated surface. They are found mainly on the head, eyelids, feet, and genitalia. Numerous small, fungiform projections arise from a broad, flat base. When subjected to trauma, they may bleed and become secondarily infected.

Treatment

Therapy includes benign neglect, surgical removal, or cryotherapy. If cryotherapy is employed, a 2% lidocaine block is applied subcutaneously and the surface of the tumor is excised for histopathology. The base of the papilloma is then frozen twice with a spray or focal-contact applicator. After surgical excision or cryotherapy, a good prognosis can be given.

Papilloma (Warts) in Cats

There are no known reports in the veterinary literature of viral papillomatosis of cats. Cutaneous papillomas are rare, affect old cats, and are usually solitary.

SQUAMOUS CELL CARCINOMA IN DOGS
Incidence, Signalment, and Etiology

These tumors are firm, nodular masses that may be proliferative and/or erosive and may extend deep into the dermis. Sites exposed to solar radiation are most at risk, especially in dogs with areas of low skin pigmentation. Broad-based erosive squamous cell carcinomas that are presumably actinically (sunlight-) induced have been observed on the bellies of lightly pigmented dogs that like to sunbathe.[4] These tumors are in areas of chronic inflammation that progress to actinic keratoses and eventually malignant tumors. Large, black-breed dogs are predisposed to subungual squamous cell carcinomas (SCCs).

Clinical Presentation and History

Squamous cell carcinomas in dogs most frequently involve the limbs. The trunk, head, and neck are affected at a slightly lower rate. Tumors are often ulcerated and bleed easily, forming crusts and deep erosions; however, they may be proliferative.

Staging and Diagnosis

The majority of SCCs arising in the skin are well differentiated and have a good prognosis after adequate surgical removal. Metastasis is rare. If the lesion is poorly differentiated histologically, however, the regional lymph nodes should be palpated and fine-needle aspiration performed. Highly anaplastic tumors may metastasize to regional lymph nodes and subsequently to the lungs. Therefore, these tumors warrant a guarded prognosis.

Treatment (Figure 5-105)

For solitary SCC, surgical excision is the treatment of choice. Some tumors, particularly actinically induced SCC, may be multiple. For these tumors and for tumors that have metastasized other treatments modalities should be considered.

Retinoids are synthetic derivatives of vitamin A that may reverse preneoplastic or metaplastic changes in human dermatologic conditions. Etretinate (a synthetic retinoid) at a dose of 1 mg/kg orally twice dai-

MANAGEMENT OF SPECIFIC DISEASES

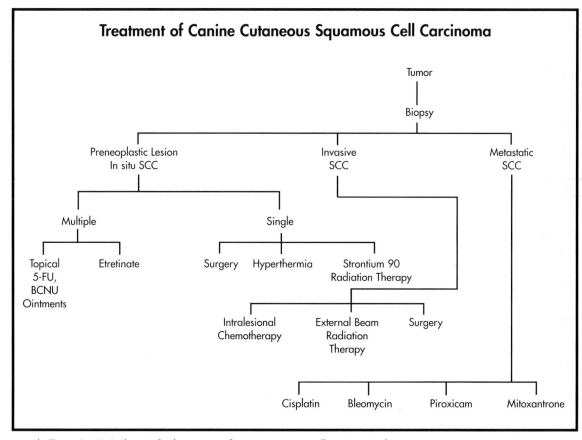

Treatment of Canine Cutaneous Squamous Cell Carcinoma

| Figure 5-105: *A schematic for the treatment of cutaneous squamous cell carcinoma in dogs.*

ly caused complete resolution of some preneoplastic SCC lesions in dogs.[5] This therapy may be beneficial for dogs with multifocal preneoplastic lesions.

Superficial and noninvasive (in situ) lesions may be treated with topical 5-fluorouracil or carmustine (BCNU) ointments. These ointments create an intense inflammatory reaction as part of their antineoplastic effect. Gloves should be worn when applying these ointments.

Cryotherapy may control small (<1 cm) noninvasive lesions; however, treatment may have to be repeated.

Squamous cell carcinoma is con-

sidered radiation-sensitive. For tumors that cannot be excised and have not metastasized, external beam teletherapy should be considered.

Cisplatin has caused objective tumor response in subungual SCCs that have metastasized to lymph nodes and lung. In one dog, an escalating dose produced a partial response at 40 mg/m² and complete response at 60 mg/m².[6] In another dog, partial response occurred at a dose of 60 mg/m², but the patient relapsed after the fourth therapy. Three of five dogs treated with cisplatin for SCC of the head and neck

> ## KEY POINT:
>
> *Because of neurotoxicity, 5-fluorouracil ointment should not be applied to cats.*

had partial responses of 14, 70, and 105 days.[7] It is likely that similar responses may be achieved for metastatic SCC of other sites, and cisplatin is probably the drug of choice for dogs with this tumor. This agent, however, cannot be administered systemically to cats.[8] Bleomycin chemotherapy caused a partial tumor response in one dog with actinically induced SCC.[9] The efficacy of this drug in dogs, however, has not been further investigated. Mitoxantrone at a dose of 4.5 to 5 mg/m² intravenously every 3 weeks caused short-term (42 to 147 days) responses in four of nine dogs with SCC,[10] and may be considered for treatment of metastatic disease.

Intralesional chemotherapy using bovine collagen matrix combined with 5-fluorouracil or cisplatin resulted in 81% of dogs with SCC having a greater than 50% reduction in tumor; 55% had complete tumor resolution.[11] Piroxicam, a nonsteroidal anti-inflammatory drug, was administered orally at 0.3 mg/kg every 24 hours to 10 dogs with nonresectable SCC.[12] Five dogs had a 50% or greater reduction in tumor size for an unstated duration.

Subungual Squamous Cell Carcinoma

Locally destructive SCC of the digit (subungual) is an aggressive tumor. It is usually single but may occur simultaneously in multiple digits. Tumors arising from the digit may destroy the nail and, eventually, the phalanx (Figure 5-106). Large, black dogs, such as giant schnauzers and standard poodles are predisposed to this particular tumor. Nail-bed SCCs have been seen in related giant schnauzers.[13]

Treatment

This tumor is best treated by high digital amputation. Although they commonly invade the lymphatics of the toe, these tumors often have an indolent course. Seventy-five percent of dogs are alive one year after surgery, and 40% survive two years.[14] As mentioned earlier, cisplatin chemotherapy resulted in long-term objective tumor responses in pulmonary

> **KEY POINT:**
>
> *Despite appearing aggressive histologically, subungual squamous cell carcinomas in dogs rarely metastasize.*

metastases from canine subungual SCC.[6]

Nasal Planum Squamous Cell Carcinoma

In dogs, SCC of the nasal planum is an extremely aggressive and erosive disease, in contrast to SCC of the nasal planum in cats.

Treatment

The tumor does not often respond to radiation therapy or to chemotherapy. Wide excision ("nosectomy") may be curative in some cases where the tumor is localized. Owners should be warned of alterations in the appearance of their dog.

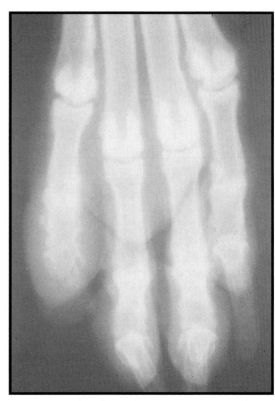

Figure 5-106: *Radiograph showing extensive lysis of the digit in a dog with subungual squamous cell carcinoma. (Courtesy J. Berg)*

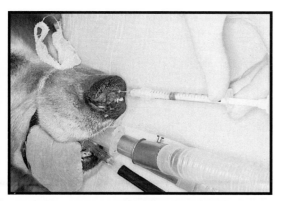

Figure 5-107: Intralesional cisplatin chemotherapy using bovine collagen matrix vehicle is being injected into and around the squamous cell carcinoma on the nose of this dog. This therapy may be palliative for some squamous cell carcinomas and has caused complete remission in some animals.

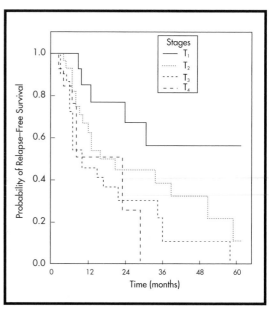

Figure 5-108: The relationship between clinical stage and progression-free survival probability in 90 cats with squamous cell carcinoma of the nasal planum treated with radiation therapy (From Theon AP, Madewell BR, Shearn V, Moulton JE: Irradiation of squamous cell carcinomas of the nasal planum in 90 cats. 13th Ann Conf Vet Cancer Soc; courtesy of Alain P. Theon)

Three dogs with nasal planum SCC were treated with interstitial hyperthermia and intralesional cisplatin in bovine collagen matrix (Figure 5-107). One dog had a complete response for more than 36 weeks; another dog that had a partial response developed distant metastases nine weeks after treatment.[15]

Oral Squamous Cell Carcinoma

Oral SCCs in dogs are aggressive lesions that rarely metastasize. Although they are not skin tumors, they are mentioned here for comparative purposes. The more rostral an oral SCC is located, the better the prognosis; surgery and/or radiation often result in long-term control. Caudal oral tumors, especially of the tonsil, are highly aggressive metastatic tumors that do not respond to surgery, radiation therapy, chemotherapy, or combinations of these modalities.[16] Further details can be found in the chapter on Tumors of the Oral Cavity.

CUTANEOUS SQUAMOUS CELL CARCINOMA IN CATS
Incidence, Signalment, and Etiology

Squamous cell carcinomas occur mostly in adult cats. They are most common around the head and neck, particularly the ears, nose, and eyelids of cats lacking cutaneous pigment. In these locations, the tumor is induced by sunlight in the same manner as described for dogs. Siamese are less likely to develop cutaneous SCC than other felidae.[1] In a series of 90 cats with nasal planum SCC, 66 cats (73%) had some white skin or hair color[17] (Figure 5-108).

Clinical Presentation and History

There is a clear clinical progression of the lesions on the face and ears of cats lacking cutaneous pigment. Initially, the area is erythematous and may have a waxy, dark crust that is easily removed. These lesions appear histologically as either actinic keratosis (precancer) or as carcinoma in situ (noninvasive cancer). Ulceration progresses if the lesion is untreated and there is subsequent invasion and destruction of surrounding structures by the tumor.

TABLE 5-18
WHO staging scheme for cutaneous tumors

Tumor Size	Criteria
T_1	Tumor <2 cm, superficial or exophytic
T_2	Tumor 2–5 cm or minimal invasion
T_3	Tumor >5 cm or invasion of subcutis
T_4	Tumor invading muscle, bone, or cartilage

Staging and Diagnosis

Actinically induced cutaneous SCC in cats rarely metastasizes. In a series of 90 cats with nasal planum SCC, six were found to have metastasis to mandibular lymph nodes and one to lungs,[17] but this usually occurred late in the course of disease. Regional lymph nodes should be palpated, and fine-needle aspiration or biopsy should be performed if tumors are enlarged. Thoracic radiographs usually are not indicated for this tumor in cats. In a study of 90 cats, 17% were found to be in stage T_1, 31% in T_2, 37% in T_3, and 15% in T_4 (Table 5-18).

Prognostic Factors

Tumor proliferative fraction, as measured by immunohistochemical detection of proliferating cell nuclear antigen (PCNA) was prognostic for control of nasal planum SCC in cats treated by radiotherapy,[17] as was tumor stage. Cats with small tumors (T_1) had not reached a median survival (i.e., fewer than half of the cats had tumor recurrence), but the average survival was 53 months. Larger tumors (T_3) were controlled for a median of 9 months[17] (Figure 5-109).

Treatment
Early Lesions

The synthetic retinoid 13 *cis*-retinoic acid did not reverse preneo-

plastic changes for SCC in cats,[18] but newer retinoids, such as etretinate have not yet been evaluated in this species. As etretinate is efficacious in dogs, these newer retinoids may also be valuable in the treatment of feline preneoplastic SCC.

In cats, actinically induced SCC is very sensitive to radiation therapy. Precancerous plaques and early lesions less than 2 mm in depth may be treated with brachytherapy radiation (e.g., ^{90}Sr) at a single, high dose. In a group of 25 cats treated with ^{90}Sr, nearly 90% were free of tumor at 1 year; the average tumor-free period was 34 months.[19]

Local current-field radiation hyperthermia (50°C for 30 seconds) is very effective in causing tumor regression in superficial SCC of cats.[20] Of 19 cats with SCC, 13 (68%) had complete regression. Tumors that did not extend 2 mm or deeper in tissue responded best. Duration of response was observed for only two to six months.

Advanced Lesions

Resection of the pinna for aural SCC is effective in the majority of cats if adequate resection is achieved. The entire pinna should be removed. These tumors may recur locally, as may SCC of the eyelids and nasal planum (Figure 5-110).

For more advanced lesions, external beam teletherapy produces long remission times. It should be remembered, however, that the cat is still susceptible to acquiring new tumors from exposure to sunlight, and its behavior should be appropriately modified. If possible, cats should be protected from sunlight exposure during the middle part of the day. Ninety cats with SCC of the nasal planum were treated with orthovoltage radiation therapy to a dose of 40 Gy in 4-Gy fractions.[17] The median control of tumors for these cats was 14 months. Advanced tumor stage (i.e., large tumors) affected outcome adversely (see Prognostic Factors). Fifteen cats with recurrent tumors were re-irradiated successfully.

Cryotherapy has been recom-

> **KEY POINT:**
>
> *Small, cutaneous squamous cell carcinomas in cats have an excellent prognosis following treatment with radiation therapy.*

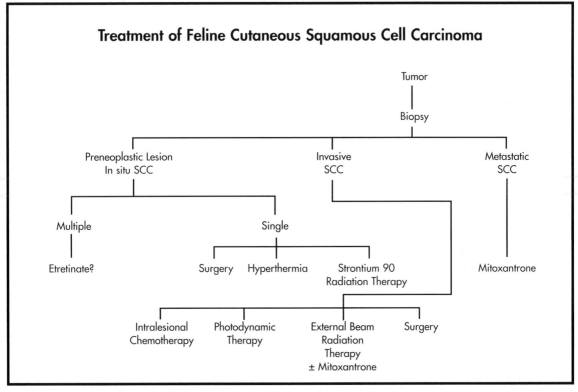

Treatment of Feline Cutaneous Squamous Cell Carcinoma

| *Figure 5-109:* *A schematic for the treatment of cutaneous squamous cell carcinoma in cats.*

mended as a treatment for SCC of the face in cats. In one study, however, this modality was considerably less effective than either surgery or radiation therapy in achieving local tumor control.[21] Eleven of 15 cats had local tumor recurrence within a median of 6 months after cryotherapy. Cryotherapy should not be used as the primary treatment modality on lesions larger than 1 cm or if it will delay more effective forms of treatment.

Photodynamic therapy is effective in controlling this tumor in cats. In one study, 7 of 11 feline SCCs of the pinna or nasal planum completely resolved using a chloroaluminum sulfonated-phthalocyanine photosensitizer, and five of these responses lasted 44 weeks or longer.[22] In another trial using aluminum phthalocyanine tetrasulfonate, long-term (3 to 18 months) responses were seen in 12 of 17 patients.[23]

Toxicities, including one fatality, were more prevalent in this study, however.

Cisplatin cannot be delivered systemically to cats; paradoxically, cisplatin was used successfully in a unique collagen-matrix intralesional implant system to treat 118 feline SCCs.[11] In this study, 83% of cats had a greater than 50% reduction in tumor volume, and 64% had complete resolution after six treatments. The lack of systemic toxicity seen in these cats was ascribed to the depot nature of the treatments and subsequent slow release of cisplatin. Sterilized sesame oil seems to function as a similar vehicle to collagen matrix and may be used at a dose of 2 ml of sesame oil to 10 mg cisplatin dissolved in 1 ml of saline.[24]

Mitoxantrone chemotherapy rarely brings objective response in feline oral SCC but can be considered as an option for metastatic skin lesions.[25] When

MANAGEMENT OF SPECIFIC DISEASES

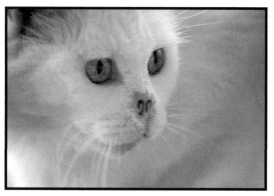

Figure 5-110: Surgical removal of the nasal planum may provide long-term control of squamous cell carcinoma when radiation therapy is not available.

combined with external beam radiation therapy, mitoxantrone has been shown to control oral SCC for a median of 170 days, which is substantially longer than when either modality is used alone.[26] Three cats with dermal SCC showed partial responses of short duration to bleomycin chemotherapy.[9] Carboplatin chemotherapy is currently under investigation for treatment of SCC in cats.

Oral Squamous Cell Carcinoma

In contrast to dogs, oral SCC in cats is a highly aggressive disease that responds poorly to surgical treatment or radiation therapy regardless of its location in the mouth. The longest control and survival rates have been obtained using a combination of radiation therapy and mitoxantrone chemotherapy[26] (see the chapter on Tumors of the Oral Cavity).

BASAL CELL TUMORS (BASAL CELL CARCINOMA, BASAL CELL EPITHELIOMA)
Incidence, Signalment, and Etiology

Basal cell tumors are more com-

mon in cats than in dogs. They are usually benign tumors originating from basal cells of the epidermis, hair follicles, sweat glands, or sebaceous glands. They have a predilection for the head and neck. Middle-aged to old cats are prone to developing these tumors. There is no breed or sex predilection. In cats, basal cell tumors are both the most common skin tumor and the most common melanotic tumor. Dogs with basal cell tumors are middle-aged to old, and the tumor is especially prevalent in cocker spaniels.

Clinical Presentation and History

These tumors usually appear as well-demarcated, small, firm nodules that sharply elevate the overlying epidermis. On cut surface, they are usually white and may appear lobulated; however, cystic spaces and a darkly pigmented appearance are not uncommon.

Staging and Diagnosis

Basal tumors are considered benign. Occasionally, a truly malignant basal cell tumor may be diagnosed, but metastasis of basal cell tumors is rare. Therefore, chest radiographs may be indicated for old animals but are probably optional. Resection is generally all that is needed for staging and diagnosis.

KEY POINT:

Use of 5-fluorouracil ointment is contraindicated in cats because of acute, fatal neurotoxicity. In addition, cisplatin causes acute fatal pulmonary edema in cats given therapeutic doses, and this drug is not recommended for intravenous use.

Treatment

Local recurrence is rare after adequate surgical removal. For incompletely excised or metastatic lesions, the use of radiation therapy and chemotherapy may be appropriate but has not been reported in the veterinary literature. The therapeutic approach outlined for SCC is probably appropriate for basal cell tumors as well.

TUMORS THAT FORM SPACES OR "CYSTS"

This group of tumors form cystic structures that may be filled with glandular secretions, keratin, or other epidermal/dermal structures.

MANAGEMENT OF SPECIFIC DISEASES

Most are benign, and their differentiation is mainly of pathologic, rather than clinical, interest. For most of these tumors, rupture, whether iatrogenic or trauma by the patient, may cause a dramatic inflammatory reaction and require excision.

Intracutaneous Cornifying Epithelioma (Keratoacanthoma)
Incidence, Signalment, and Etiology

This benign neoplasm of epidermal origin is most common in young, male dogs. Two distinct patterns of this tumor are found:

1. The solitary type, which occurs with a higher incidence in purebred dogs, is located mostly on the back, neck, thorax, and shoulders.
2. The generalized form, seen in Norwegian elkhounds, shows numerous growths in various stages of development within the skin.
   A pore leading into the mass may be observed.

Clinical Presentation and History

This tumor appears as a dermal or subcutaneous nodule from 0.5- to 5-cm in diameter that may elevate the overlying epidermis and give it a tannish-brown appearance. Rupture produces a severe pyogranulomatous dermatitis in reaction to the keratin contents of the cysts.

Treatment

Surgical resection of solitary tumors is curative; for multiple tumors, surgery is often impractical. Anecdotally, retinoids, such as etretinate (1 mg/kg BID PO), have been useful in treating multicentric keratoacanthomas.

Trichoepithelioma (Hair Matrixoma)
Incidence, Signalment, and Etiology

Trichoepitheliomas are derived from primitive hair-matrix cells that differentiate into either mature or incompletely developed hair follicles. Most trichoepitheliomas occur in dogs (rarely in cats) older than five years of age, with no breed or sex predilection.

Clinical Presentation and History

These tumors often resemble basal cell tumors, but they may be cystic and contain keratin. The tumor is most frequently found on the back, although other areas of the body have been reported. The overlying epidermis is atrophic, hairless, and, often, ulcerated as a result of trauma. These tumors are slow growing, minimally invasive, and usually well encapsulated.

Treatment

Recurrence after adequate surgical excision is rare.

Pilomatricomas (Pilomatrixomas and Necrotizing and Calcifying Epitheliomas)
Incidence, Signalment, and Etiology

Pilomatricomas are tumors which originate from the small, dark-staining cells of the pilar (hair) matrix. Kerry blue terriers and poodles have a higher prevalence than other breeds. Old dogs are most commonly affected.

Clinical Presentation and History

These are firm, well-defined nodules composed of either multiple cysts filled with tan, pasty material or of cysts containing a gritty, granular mineralized material. Most cases are confined to the skin of the rump and shoulder area.

Staging and Diagnosis

These tumors are slow growing and well encapsulated. Rarely, malignant pilomatricomas metastasize to local lymph nodes and internal organs.

Treatment

Surgical excision should be curative if adequate margins are resected. There are no reports of therapy for metastatic tumors.

Epidermoid Cysts (Epidermal Cyst, Epidermal Inclusion Cyst)
Incidence, Signalment, and Etiology

Epidermal cysts are believed to arise in response to degenerative changes in hair follicles, cystic changes in ducts or cells of sebaceous glands, or traumatic displacement of epidermal fragments. The lesions usually are acquired; they are rarely congenital. They may be single or multiple, and are most common on the head, neck, and sacral region. They are very common in dogs and may occur in any breed (especially boxers, Kerry blue terriers, cocker spaniels, springer spaniels, fox terriers, and German shepherds). Middle-aged to old animals usually are affected.

Clinical Presentation and History

These cysts appear as a single, soft, fluctuant nodule that is freely movable in the dermis and beneath the elevated overlying skin. The cut surface of the cyst is thin-walled and contains tan to yellow pasty material.

Treatment

As with other cystic tumors, when an epidermal cyst ruptures and the contents of the cyst are released into the dermis, a severe foreign body reaction occurs. Surgical excision is usually curative.

Sebaceous Gland Tumors
Incidence, Signalment, and Etiology

These tumors represent 6% to 35% of all skin tumors in dogs, but they are rare in cats. Sebaceous gland tumors are often misdiagnosed as sebaceous "cysts." They are similar in appearance to basal cell tumors and trichoepitheliomas. Sebaceous glands are found in many different areas of the body, and the tumors are named accordingly. For example, there are tumors of the meibomian glands or tumors of the perianal (circumanal or hepatoid) glands.

Tumors of sebaceous glands can be subdivided into three major categories according to the level of maturation of the cells involved: adenomatous hyperplasia of sebaceous glands, sebaceous gland adenomas, and sebaceous gland adenocarcinomas. Adenomatous hyperplasia of sebaceous glands is most common. Adenomas are more common than carcinomas, which are rarely encountered in the skin of dogs. Spaniel breeds are at higher risk of developing all

forms of sebaceous gland tumor. All three categories of sebaceous tumors affect old dogs and most often occur on the head.

Adenomatous Hyperplasia
Clinical Findings and History

Adenomatous hyperplasia often presents as multiple lesions and appears as small (<1 cm), superficial, rubbery nodules covered by a thin, shiny, hairless epithelium. They may be multilobulated and are grossly indistinguishable from adenomas. Old dogs, especially males and spayed females (which indicates a possible connection to androgen), are predisposed. The most common site is the meibomian glands of the eyelid.

Treatment

Treatment consists of local resection, followed by cryotherapy if excision is incomplete. Dogs are likely to develop new areas of hyperplasia.

Sebaceous Adenomas
Clinical Findings and History

Adenomas are seen in dogs of either sex and of any breed (especially cocker spaniels, springer spaniels, Boston terriers, and wirehaired terriers). They tend to occur in old dogs and at any site, especially the head. There are often multiple tumors, coexisting with other skin tumors. Adenomas are usually small (2 to 10 mm in diameter), raised, multilobulated, domed or pedunculated, well circumscribed, and greasy. Tumors may ooze "toothpaste" material when squeezed. If perianal gland adenomas occur in females, hyperadrenocorticism should be suspected; the excess production is trophic for these adenoma cells.

Treatment

Treatment consists of local resection, followed by cryotherapy if excision is incomplete. Perianal gland adenomas are androgen responsive and usually regress after castration. External beam radiation at low doses will shrink perianal adenomas; however, this modality is probably best used when the tumor is unresponsive to hormonal manipulations or if rapid tumor reduction is required.

Sebaceous Adenocarcinomas
Clinical Findings and History

Sebaceous gland carcinomas can be distinguished from benign adenomas by their rapid rate of growth and early ulceration through the skin. Malignant tumors are large, usually solitary, poorly circumscribed, ulcerated, and invasive. Sebaceous adenomas are usually slow growing and only rarely recur after surgical removal, whereas sebaceous adenocarcinomas may metastasize to local lymph nodes and to the lungs.

Treatment

If surgical removal is inadequate, local recurrence may be a problem. In castrated male and in female dogs, most perianal adenocarcinomas metastasize early to the sublumbar lymph nodes. Radiation therapy may cause adenomas to regress, but it has a little role, other than palliation, for adenocarcinomas because of their high metastatic rate. There are anecdotal reports that cisplatin causes regression of metastatic lymph node lesions in dogs.

Sweat Gland Tumors
Incidence, Signalment, and Etiology

Sweat gland tumors are less common than sebaceous gland tumors in dogs and are equally rare in cats.[27] The sweat glands of the skin in dogs and cats are mainly apocrine glands; eccrine glands are found only on the footpads. Therefore, most tumors of sweat gland origin are of apocrine type. Apocrine glands are found in many different parts of the body, and their tumors are named accordingly. In the ear, for example, they are called ceruminous gland tumors. In a survey of ear canal tumors, ceruminous adenocarcinoma was the most common malignancy in both dogs and cats.[28] Distant metastasis is rare in dogs. It cats, it is not much more common, but the tumors tend to be quite invasive in this species. Other apocrine tumors include mammary gland tumors, anal sac tumors, and tumors of the glands at the anal mucocutaneous junction. Mammary gland tumors are described in the chapter on Mammary Neoplasia, and anal sac tumors are dealt with in the chapter on Gastrointestinal Tumors.

Sweat gland adenomas most often affect dogs older than eight years of age. They may be most common in males. Golden retrievers and spaniel breeds reportedly have an increased incidence of these tumors.[27] Sweat gland adenomas develop most frequently on the head and neck. Carcinomas arise on the ventral abdomen, neck, and legs in the axilla and inguinal area.

Clinical Presentation and History

Adenomas are small, elevated, well demarcated nodules. They often have an ulcerated surface as a result of trauma. The tumors generally are firm but may have cystic areas.

Malignant tumors of sweat gland origin are often indistinguishable from adenomas. Some sweat gland tumors, however, present as firm, poorly circumscribed masses diffusely infiltrating the skin, producing an ulcerated, moist, and, sometimes, hemorrhagic skin surface that is frequently misdiagnosed as acute dermatitis. In both dogs and cats, adenocarcinomas of the sweat glands are more common than adenomas[27] (Figure 5-111).

Staging and Diagnosis

Sweat gland carcinomas may metastasize. Metastasis occurs primarily via the lymphatics to regional lymph nodes, but hematogenous spread to the lungs has been noted. In two studies, approximately 20% of carcinomas metastasized in both dogs and cats.[27,29] Therefore, after a minimum data base (consisting of CBC, biochemistry panel, and urinalysis) is established, thoracic radiographs should be obtained. Because of the difficulty in clinically distinguishing between adenomas and

> **KEY POINT:**
>
> *Ceruminous gland adenocarcinomas may be bilateral.*

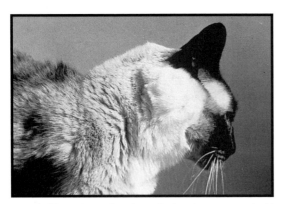

Figure 5-111: *Ceruminous gland carcinomas, as seen in this cat, are derived from modified sweat glands in the ear. Aggressive surgery, with or without adjuvant radiation therapy, is required to control this tumor. (Courtesy A. Evans)*

adenocarcinomas, the veterinarian should consider either presurgical biopsy or a wide surgical excision as an initial therapeutic approach. Ceruminous gland adenocarcinoma may be bilateral.[29]

Treatment

Surgical removal of sweat gland adenomas is usually curative, but carcinomas may recur locally after surgical removal. Aggressive surgery is required for successful treatment of ceruminous gland adenocarcinoma in cats. Sixteen cats treated by ear canal ablation and bulla osteotomy had a 42-month median remission and a 25% recurrence rate, whereas six cats treated with lateral ear resection had a 10-month median remission and four cats had recurrence.[30] For localized tumors (i.e., no lymphatic or vessel invasion and no metastasis), radiation therapy may be palliative, although the few animals treated preclude definitive recommendations. Ceruminous gland adenocarcinomas frequently are incompletely excised because they encroach upon the middle ear.[21,31] In this situation, radiation therapy may improve local control, and in dogs without metastases, radiation may significantly improve survival. Megavoltage radiation therapy (48 Gy in 12 fractions) was used to treat five dogs and six cats with ceruminous gland carcinoma. Six animals had been treated surgically with incomplete

margins; therefore, radiation was adjuvant. Four animals (2 dogs and 2 cats) had recurrence. Metastasis to lymph nodes, lung, and intra-abdominal organs each occurred in one animal. Tumor-free survival was estimated as 39 months for all animals, which is comparable to aggressive surgery alone.[29]

Chemotherapy for metastatic tumors is anecdotal only, although cisplatin may be a useful agent in dogs. Three of five dogs with circumanal gland malignancies treated with doxorubicin had objective responses (2 CR, 1 PR), although the duration of these responses was not documented.[32] One cat with an apocrine gland carcinoma had a short-term (21 days) response to mitoxantrone chemotherapy.[25]

MESENCHYMAL TUMORS
Lipoma
Incidence, Signalment, and Etiology

Lipomas are benign tumors of adipose cells and are most common in adult to old dogs. There is no breed predisposition. Females are affected twice as frequently as males. The tumor may occur anywhere, although the chest, abdomen, legs, and axillae are the most frequent sites.

Clinical Presentation and History

Lipomas are usually solitary, of variable size and shape, slow growing, well circumscribed, subcutaneous, and very common. They usually feel soft, but lipomas that develop between muscle planes may feel quite firm. These tumors are very slow growing and enlarge by expansion rather than by invasion (Figure 5-112).

Infiltrative lipomas can cause pain and pressure atrophy of muscles, and they can interfere with movement. In one study of 11 dogs with infiltrative lipoma, five were Labrador retrievers, and most of the others were large-breed dogs.[33] In most cases, the tumor was present for one year or more before presentation to a veterinarian.

Treatment

Excision of a lipoma is warranted if it interferes with function and mobility, if it is rapidly growing, or if it is bothersome to the owner. In most cases, surgery is curative. Infiltrative lipoma should be treated with aggressive, initial surgery; even then, recurrence is likely. Radiation therapy may be indicated postoperatively for infiltrative lipomas if residual disease is suspected.

Soft Tissue Sarcomas of the Skin and Surrounding Structures

Nomenclature for this group of tumors largely depends on microscopic appearance. As this may change depending on site of biopsy or stage of growth, the same tumor may be given different names at different stages. This is initially frustrating to clinicians; however, there is very little difference in biological behavior between these tumors. Thus, whether a tumor is labelled fibroma, fibrosarcoma, hemangiopericytoma, neurofibroma, neurofibrosarcoma, schwannoma, rhabdomyoma, rhabdomyosarcoma, leiomyoma, leiomyosarcoma, or malignant fibrous histiocytoma may not matter as much as the site of tumor and the thoroughness of excision. Some of these tumors may initially be characterized as benign, but the term "benign tumor" may be a misnomer; it is more clinically correct to consider these as histologic "gradations" of a single tumor type. Local recurrence is a common problem for any soft tissue sarcoma that has not been excised with **wide margins**! Soft tissue sarcomas often spread locally but rarely metastasize.

In this section, the incidence, signalment, and etiology for each tumor type is discussed separately. Treatment of all soft tissue sarcomas is identical and is discussed at the end of the section.

Fibroma/Fibrosarcoma in Dogs
Incidence, Signalment, and Etiology

Fibrosarcomas are relatively com-

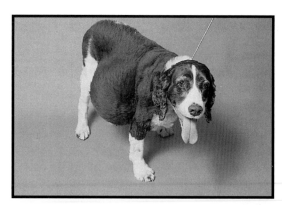

Figure 5-112: *Cutaneous lipoma is a biologically benign tumor, but it may reach a large size and interfere with ambulation. Tumors such as this lipoma in a 13-year-old dog should be removed before they cause problems.*

mon in dogs. They usually occur in adult or aged animals. There are no breed or sex predilections. They may occur anywhere but are most common on the trunk, mammary glands, limbs, and face. Fibrosarcomas are usually solitary, variably sized, poorly circumscribed, irregular and nodular, nonencapsulated, firm to fleshy, with soft, friable/ ulcerated areas. They may be located subcutaneously or dermoepidermally. On cut surface, there may be a pattern of interweaving bands of white tissue with foci of hemorrhage and necrosis.

Fibroma/Fibrosarcoma in Cats
Incidence, Signalment, and Etiology

Fibrosarcomas account for 12% to 25% of feline skin tumors. Multiple fibrosarcomas occur in cats concurrently infected with feline sarcoma virus (FeSV) and feline leukemia virus (FeLV). FeSV alone will not cause neoplasia and is not transmitted horizontally; to replicate, it

> ## KEY POINTS:
>
> *Excision of a lipoma is warranted if it interferes with function and mobility, if it is rapidly growing, or if it is bothersome to the owner.*
>
> ---
>
> *Soft tissue mesenchymal tumors are rarely biologically benign, and wide surgical margins should be taken regardless of histologic appearance.*

requires FeLV as a "helper" virus. Fibrosarcomas in cats older than 5 years of age are usually solitary and rarely caused by FeSV. In cats younger than 5 years of age that are FeLV positive, FeSV-induced sarcoma must be considered, especially if multiple sites are affected.

Vaccine-Related Fibrosarcoma in Cats

The limbs are the most common site of occurrence for feline fibrosarcoma,[1] but recent reports of fibrosarcoma arising on the trunk at sites of previous vaccination have prompted suspicion that this tumor may be induced by vaccine adjuvants and its resultant inflammation. Until further information is available, it is prudent to administer vaccines in areas that may be amenable to wide surgical excision in case of tumor formation (e.g., limbs or tail), rather than the more commonly used area between the scapulae (see also the chapter on Vaccine-Associated Sarcomas in Cats).

Nerve Sheath Tumors

These tumors are also known as neurofibroma/neurofibrosarcoma, schwannoma, neurolemmoma, or perineural fibroblastoma.

Incidence, Signalment, and Etiology

These tumors arise from nerve sheaths and usually involve spinal or cranial nerve roots in the dog but behave clinically like any soft tissue sarcoma (relatively low probability of metastasis and aggressive local invasion of surrounding tissue). Primary cutaneous nerve sheath tumors are rare, but they occasionally arise in the subcutaneous tissues of dogs and cats and can be either benign or malignant. They occur in adult to aged animals. There are no sex or breed predilections. These tumors may occur anywhere but are most common on the trunk and limbs. Nerve sheath tumors may be solitary (most) or multiple (tortuous and nodular enlargement of nerve or "chains of nodes," which is termed *neurofibromatosis*). They often grow large rapidly and tend to be firm, poorly demarcated, adherent to overlying skin, and ulcerative.

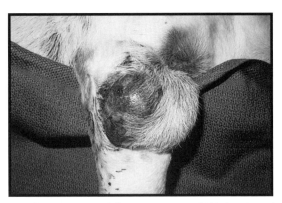

Figure 5-113: *Soft tissue sarcomas are highly invasive and often recur after surgery. The metastatic rate for soft tissue sarcomas is low, and wide surgical margins may provide a cure. The hemangiopericytoma on the elbow of this 8-year-old dog is best treated by amputation. (Courtesy G.H. Theilen)*

Myxoma/Myxosarcoma
Incidence, Signalment, and Etiology

These tumors consist of mucin-producing altered fibroblasts and, as such, act clinically like all soft tissue sarcomas. They are rare. They usually occur in adult or aged animals. There are no breed, sex, or site predilections.

Myxosarcomas usually are infiltrative growths with no definite shape (e.g., soft, slimy, and nonencapsulated). They are often grayish-white, with clear, viscid, honey-like areas visible on the cut surface. The tumors are difficult to remove totally but rarely metastasize.

Hemangiopericytoma (Spindle Cell Sarcoma, Dermatofibrosarcoma)
Incidence, Signalment, and Etiology

These tumors are more common in dogs than in cats and tend to occur in adult to old animals. There is no sex predilection. Any breed may be affected, although boxers, German shepherds, and cocker spaniels seem predisposed. These tumors frequently occur on the limbs as masses that are solitary, subcutaneous, smooth to lobulated, firm, slow growing, and poorly circumscribed (Figure 5-113). As for other soft tissue sarcomas, the metastatic rate is low (15% to 20%).

MANAGEMENT OF SPECIFIC DISEASES

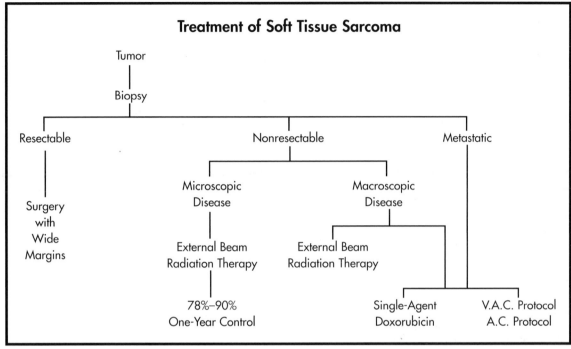

Figure 5-114: *A schematic for the treatment of soft tissue sarcomas in dogs and cats.*

Liposarcomas
Incidence, Signalment, and Etiology

Liposarcomas are rare. They are usually solitary; vary in shape, size, and consistency; and are poorly demarcated, subcutaneous, and invasive. They are, however, rarely metastatic. In a study of 20 cases of liposarcoma, only one patient developed metastasis to regional lymph nodes and the lung.[34]

Leiomyoma/Leiomyosarcoma
Incidence, Signalment, and Etiology

These tumors are extremely rare in the cutaneous tissues; benign or malignant tumors arise from arrector pili muscles.

Malignant Fibrous Histiocytoma and Giant Cell Sarcoma
Incidence, Signalment, and Etiology

These soft tissue sarcomas are more common in cats than in dogs. Their symptoms resemble that of other soft tissue sarcomas.

Treatment of Soft Tissue Sarcomas
(Figure 5-114)

Therapy for all soft tissue sarcomas should consist of early surgical excision. The best time to cure these tumors is with the *first* definitive surgery. Because wide surgical margins in all directions are essential for cure, a preoperative biopsy can be of great value in planning this surgery. These tumors are frequently incompletely excised. Excision should be wide and deep, as sarcomas are surrounded by a pseudocapsule of tumor cells undergoing pressure necrosis. Despite the pressure, these cells are perfectly viable and are capable of forming local recurrent tumors. Soft tissue sarcomas send microscopic, finger-like projections into tissue surrounding the pseudocapsule, increasing the likelihood of incomplete excision. In contrast to many other cutaneous malignancies, these tumors rarely metastasize. If metastasis occurs, it is usually late in the course of disease. Therefore, local therapies, such as surgery and radiation are potentially curative if used appropriately and early. The surgeon attempting to resect a soft tissue sarcoma should try to resect margins that include one fascial plane below the clinically detectable tumor or margins of 2 to 3 cm. Margins should always be examined histopathologically, and tagging surgically "close" margins will allow the pathologist to identify and examine the areas where the surgeon is concerned about incomplete excision (Figure 5-115).

Radiation therapy is a useful adjunct to incomplete surgery for all of these mesenchymal tumors. The tumor is relatively resistant to low doses of radiation, however. Remission durations for dogs with soft tissue sarcomas treated with radiation therapy depend on the dose of radiation delivered. For one group of dogs, a total dose of 45 Gy controlled tumor growth in 48% of dogs for one year; 67% of dogs treated with 50 Gy experienced similar control.[35] By two years, only 50% of the dogs treated with 50 Gy still experienced tumor control. More recent data suggest

> **KEY POINT:**
>
> *The response of soft tissue sarcomas to radiation therapy is dependent on the total dose delivered. Higher doses give longer control.*

that at a dose of 52 Gy, 78% of dogs treated had local control of disease one year after surgery and radiation. With higher doses of radiation and with accelerated fractionation (i.e., more frequent treatments), response rates for soft tissue sarcoma improve. In a study using a megavoltage (^{60}Co) radiation total dose of 63 Gy to the surgical site of incompletely excised soft tissue sarcomas, only 4 of 21 tumors recurred in the radiation field. The 4-year survival rate was 86%.[36] Radiation doses of greater than 60 Gy apparently controlled soft tissue sarcoma in dogs effectively. Of 22 dogs with hemangiopericytoma that received orthovoltage radiation after surgical debulking, 41% were free of tumor at 2 years (range = 1.5 to 55 months).[37] Dogs with tumors of the frontlimb had significantly shorter survival times than those with hemangiopericytoma of the hindlimbs. Radiation therapy is probably the adjunctive therapy of choice for incompletely excised soft tissue sarcomas.

For the rare cases in which this tumor metastasizes, reports concerning chemotherapeutic agents are too sparse to enable valid generalization. In human patients with soft tissue sarcoma, doxorubicin is the adjunctive treatment of choice. Doxorubicin treatment caused three complete responses and two partial responses in 29 dogs with soft tissue sarcomas.[32] Doxorubicin and cyclophosphamide used in combination has produced good results in synovial sarcoma in one dog.[38] It is possible that similar responses could follow from its combination in cats and dogs with cutaneous soft tissue sarcomas. Mitoxantrone was used to treat 16 dogs with soft tissue sarcomas. Two dogs achieved complete responses, and two dogs had partial responses; however, these responses were for a median of 21 days (range = 16 to 63 days).[10] A cat with an oral fibrosarcoma had complete regression of the tumor for 30 weeks after treatment with vincristine alone.[39] Of six cats with soft tissue sarcomas treated with mitoxantrone chemotherapy, only one achieved a complete remission, which lasted 90 days.[25]

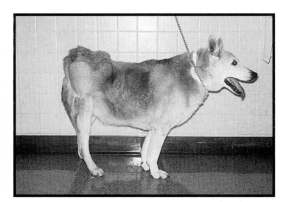

Figure 5-115: After multiple, incomplete surgical excisions, soft tissue sarcomas may recur throughout the previous surgical sites, creating a huge, unresectable tumor, as in this aged crossbreed dog. (Courtesy J. Berg)

MANAGEMENT OF SPECIFIC DISEASES

Intralesional chemotherapy using a bovine collagen matrix depot of cisplatin followed by methotrexate resulted in significant tumor reduction in 18 of 21 cats with fibrosarcoma. In five of these cats, the tumor resolved completely.[11] Similarly administered intralesional cisplatin treatment in combination with radiation therapy seemed to enhance antitumor response to radiation alone.[40]

Cutaneous Hemangioma in Dogs
Incidence, Signalment, and Etiology

Hemangiomas are benign tumors of endothelial cells that occur in old dogs without breed or gender predilection. Cutaneous hemangiomas are about three times more common than their malignant counterparts.[41] The increased incidence of dermal hemangioma and hemangiosarcoma on the ventral abdomen of dogs with glabrous (nonpigmented, lightly haired) skin suggests an association between these tumors and solar radiation in a manner similar to that described for SCC.[4,40,41]

Clinical Presentation and History

Hemangiomas are variably sized, usually solitary, well circumscribed, nonencapsulated, dermo-epidermal to subcutaneous, soft and spongy, and shaded red to black. Hemangiomas arise most commonly in the loose skin of the trunk or neck; they also occur on the face and eyelids.

Treatment

Surgical excision of cutaneous hemangioma should be curative.

Cutaneous Hemangiosarcoma in Dogs
Incidence, Signalment, and Etiology

See also the chapter on Hemangiosarcoma. These tumors occur in old dogs and are more common in females than in males. Breeds with lightly pigmented, poorly haired skin are most often affected.[41,43] In

---

KEY POINT:

Hemangioma and hemangiosarcoma on the ventral abdomen of dogs with glabrous skin are often sunlight induced and are rarely metastatic.

---

addition, cutaneous hemangiosarcomas may be associated with or metastatic from primary tumors of the right atrium or spleen.

Clinical Presentation and History

Hemangiosarcomas grow rapidly and frequently ulcerate through the skin at an early stage. They are usually larger and situated in dermis rather than subcutis. Hemangiosarcomas are soft or spongy, poorly circumscribed, infiltrating, friable masses.

Staging and Diagnosis

It is difficult to determine the primary site of origin of hemangiosarcoma. It often occurs at multiple sites, including the spleen, liver, heart, skin, and bone. If the cutaneous site is primary, the prognosis is probably improved[41,43]; however, local recurrence and metastasis from hypodermal hemangiosarcomas may be more common than in soft tissue sarcomas. Any dog with cutaneous lesions should be thoroughly staged for existing systemic tumors.

Prognostic Factors

The presence of solar elastosis in the skin adjacent to hemangiosarcomas was related to long survival in one study, implying that solar-induced cutaneous hemangiosarcoma may be less aggressive than other hemangiosarcomas.[41]

Treatment

Surgery alone may be sufficient to resolve cutaneous hemangiosarcoma. Of 84 dogs with cutaneous hemangiosarcoma treated by surgical excision, 25 died of tumor-related causes. Of these, only 11 tumors recurred at the site of surgery.[41] This is a considerably lower recurrence and mortality rate than is seen with hemangiosarcoma of systemic origin. Metastasis was uncommon in another group of dogs with cutaneous hemangiosarcoma.[43]

Dogs treated with combination chemotherapy in

addition to surgery have long survival times.[44] As stated earlier, however, dogs with cutaneous hemangiosarcoma have a good prognosis with surgery alone. Further studies are needed to delineate the role of adjunctive chemotherapy in this disease.

Hemangioma/Hemangiosarcoma in Cats
Incidence, Signalment, and Etiology

Cutaneous hemangiomas and hemangiosarcomas are rare in cats and mainly affect old animals. This tumor is similar to SCC in that it is actinic, or sunlight induced.[45–47]

Clinical Presentation and History

Feline hemangiomas appear as solitary tumors in the dermis and subcutis without any site predilection. In contrast, feline hemangiosarcomas may have a predilection for the head (i.e., ear tips and nasal planum) and may also have a predilection for non-pigmented skin.[45] They are usually solitary.

Treatment

Surgical excision of cutaneous hemangioma usually has a good prognosis, although local recurrence after surgical excision of cutaneous hemangiosarcoma is frequent. Metastasis is rare; therefore, it is appropriate to treat this tumor in the same manner as a soft tissue sarcoma in cats. Aggressive initial surgery is the best therapeutic approach.

Lymphangioma and Lymphangiosarcoma
Incidence, Signalment, and Etiology

Lymphangiomas and lymphangiosarcomas are tumors composed of lymph vessels forming capillary, cavernous, or cystic spaces. In a large study, lymphangioma was described in 57 dogs and 13 cats. There was no gender predilection for either species. The median age of affected dogs was 7 years. For cats, the median age was 7 to 10 years. Golden retrievers

accounted for seven cases. Four Siamese and one Persian were included in the feline cases. Lymphangioma most often occurred in the lymphatic vessels, but 19 canine cases and four feline cases arose in the skin.[48] In another study of cats, this tumor was most common in the skin or subcutis of the abdominal wall or distal limbs.[49] This tumor may be associated with, and a sequela to, chronic lymphatic obstruction (i.e., following radical surgical procedures, such as a radical mastectomy for mammary tumors).

Treatment

No treatment has been described for this rare tumor in dogs and cats. Nonetheless, a therapeutic approach similar to that described for hemangiosarcoma is recommended.

Cutaneous Melanoma in Dogs
Incidence, Signalment, and Etiology

Melanomas occur in adult to aged dogs. There is no sex predilection. Although any breed may be affected, Scottish terriers, Airedales, Boston bullterriers, and cocker spaniels seem predisposed. In dogs, melanomas are usually solitary, and the oral mucosa and the skin are the most common sites. The most frequent sites for cutaneous melanoma in dogs are the face (especially the eyelids), the trunk, and the extremities. The behavior of canine melanomas differs strikingly depending on their location. Oral melanomas are invariably malignant, whereas most cutaneous melanomas are benign. Melanoma of the digits is a notable exception and may be highly malignant.

KEY POINT:

Most cutaneous melanomas are benign, while oral and digital tumors are often highly malignant.

Clinical Presentation and History

Melanomas range from inconspicuous black macules to large, rapidly growing masses that may be either amelanotic or dark brown to gray or black in color. The appearance of a melanoma varies depending on its stage of development. Initially, they can appear as flat, black macules.

They may progress into elevated and firm nodules and can be either smooth or rough.

Dermal melanomas usually range from 0.5 to 2.0 cm in diameter; are darkly pigmented; dome-shaped; and have a smooth, hairless surface. On cut surface, the tumors usually are well defined but are seldom encapsulated. Malignant melanomas are normally large, and the overlying skin is frequently ulcerated and secondarily infected. Their color may vary from black to brown to light gray.

Staging and Diagnosis

Although most cutaneous melanomas are benign, malignant melanomas can metastasize via lymph channels and blood. Regional lymph nodes are commonly the first sites affected, and the lung is the most common site of visceral involvement. Therefore, chest radiographs, blood work, and cytologic evaluation of regional and enlarged lymph nodes are prudent, particularly for melanomas of the digits.

Treatment

Therapy includes wide surgical excision of any melanotic tumor.[50] Tumors arising on the lip and other mucocutaneous junctions always have a poor prognosis. There is no accepted adjunctive therapy for melanomas, although platinum compounds (i.e., cisplatin and carboplatin) may provide palliation in some dogs (see the chapter on Tumors of the Oral Cavity).

Melanocytic tumors of the distal limbs in 28 dogs were reviewed.[50] Two of 14 tumors recurred locally, and 10 of 14 metastasized to lymph nodes or lung. Lung metastasis occurred from 1 to 33 months after surgery; the mean time to metastasis was 13 months. Involvement of the nail bed in any dog suggests malignant melanoma, but histopathologic examination is the only reliable method of diagnosis. The role of adjuvant therapy in this disease is uncertain, but carboplatin and cisplatin are probably the most active agents. Although immunotherapy may improve survival for dogs with oral melanoma,[51] clinical trials have not been performed in dogs with cutaneous tumors.

Cutaneous Melanoma in Cats
Incidence, Signalment, and Etiology

Cutaneous melanoma is extremely rare in cats and accounted for only five of 29 feline melanomas in one study. Oral melanomas occurred with equal frequency. Nineteen of 29 melanomas occurred in the eye. Two of the five cats with cutaneous melanoma were Siamese.[52]

Clinical Findings and History

Cutaneous melanoma has been reported in the digit, head, and lumbar skin.[52] Ocular melanomas are mainly intraocular (rather than palpebral) and frequently metastasize to the mandibular lymph nodes[52] (see the chapter on Ocular and Retrobulbar Tumors).

Treatment

Surgery is the treatment of choice for feline cutaneous melanoma. Metastasis occurred in one of five cats, but three of five were alive and apparently disease-free more than one year after surgery.

ROUND (DISCRETE) CELL TUMORS

This group of tumors may equally be called discrete cell tumors, and cytologically they appear as clumps or individual cells that have no obvious attachment to other cells. Round cell tumors include mast cell tumors (MCTs), histiocytoma, lymphoma, plasmacytoma, and transmissible venereal tumor (TVT).

Mast Cell Tumors in Dogs
(see also Chapter on Mast Cell Tumors)
Incidence, Signalment, and Etiology

Mast cell tumors are most common in old dogs, with no sex predilection.[52] Hereditary factors present in boxers and Boston terriers may predispose them to developing MCTs.[54]

Clinical Presentation and History

Most cutaneous MCTs present as intracutaneous nodules which vary markedly in their appearance. Some show ulceration of the overlying epidermis; others present as single or multiple elevated, erythematous nodules with alopecia of the overlying skin.

Mast cell tumors without skin involvement are uncommon in dogs in contrast to cats, in which the disease frequently is only visceral. Approximately 11% of affected dogs have multiple cutaneous tumors.[54]

Staging and Diagnosis

Staging procedures for MCTs prior to definitive treatment include lymph node aspiration (if the node is enlarged), buffy coat smears, bone marrow aspiration, and abdominal radiographs and ultrasonography.[54] Other round cell tumors lack the blue-to-purple cytoplasmic granules seen on presurgical fine-needle aspiration of MCTs. Eosinophils are often seen in aspirates of MCTs as a result of eosinophil chemotaxis.

Histopathologic grading of the tumor correlates with both recurrence and survival. Although well-differentiated tumors recur, undifferentiated (anaplastic) tumors have a higher recurrence rate.[55] Dogs with neoplasms of the extremities have longer tumor-free times and longer survival than dogs with tumors on the trunk.

Treatment

Control of canine MCTs involves the use of surgery, chemotherapy, or radiation therapy used either individually or in combination. Surgical excision is indicated if the tumor is solitary and there is no evidence of lymph node involvement or systemic spread. Excision should be wide *and deep* to a minimum margin of 3 cm around the perceived borders of the tumor and one fascial plane below.[57] If the tumor cannot be completely excised or is moderately or poorly differentiated, further therapy is indicated. Animals should be evaluated for radiation therapy, when available. Dogs treated with radiation therapy after surgical debulking have significantly longer tumor control and survival than other dogs.[56,58,59]

In cases of MCTs in which metastasis or systemic spread has occurred, localized forms of therapy, such as

> **KEY POINT:**
>
> *Histologic differentiation of mast cells in canine cutaneous tumors correlates with the recurrence rate after surgery as well as survival.*

surgery or radiation therapy are not appropriate except as purely palliative procedures for discomfort or mechanical obstruction. For these dogs, the most frequently recommended drugs are corticosteroids. Oral prednisone (2 mg/kg/day for 2 weeks, then 1 mg/kg/day for 2 weeks, then 1 mg/kg every other day for 6 months) is given as long as tumor progression is not observed.[60] Anecdotally, other chemotherapeutic agents, such as L-asparaginase, chlorambucil, and vincristine, have been used to treat MCTs; however, no objective responses have been repeatedly observed or published. To prevent gastric ulceration in patients with widespread or bulky disease, antagonists of H_2-antihistamines should be prescribed for 24 to 48 hours prior to and during chemotherapy.

Mast Cell Tumors in Cats
(see also chapter on Mast Cell Tumors)
Incidence, Signalment, and Etiology

Mast cell tumors were the only cutaneous tumor diagnosed in cats younger than one year of age in one study.[1] In the same study, Siamese were three times more likely to develop cutaneous MCTs than other breeds. Tumors in Siamese are usually subcutaneous and composed of "histiocytic" cells. These tumors may regress without therapy.[61]

Clinical Presentation and History

Cutaneous mast cell tumors in cats are usually histologically well differentiated and have a benign clinical course[2]; however, in some studies, cutaneous tumors are associated with malignant disease evidenced by visceral involvement.[62,63]

Staging and Diagnosis

In cats with cutaneous MCTs, the tumor may be metastic from visceral disease; therefore, cats should be evaluated for systemic MCTs. A CBC, buffy coat evaluation, and bone marrow aspiration as well as abdominal ultrasound and thoracic radiographs should be performed in cats with mast cell tumors. Sites for lymphoreticular MCTs in cats are the spleen, mediastinum (with resultant pleural effusion), and lymph nodes.

Treatment

The treatment of choice for cutaneous MCTs in cats is surgery; for solitary tumors, a good prognosis usually can be given. Some cats develop multiple well-differentiated tumors, and these cats may be treated with multiple palliative surgeries or corticosteroids (1 mg/kg prednisone daily). For invasive or incompletely excised MCTs, radiation therapy apparently is a successful adjunct to surgery; however, data regarding tumor control and patient survival are not as well established as for dogs.

Mitoxantrone caused a partial response in a feline MCT, but the drug has not been evaluated further for the treatment of this disease.[25]

Histiocytoma

Incidence, Signalment, and Etiology

Cutaneous histiocytoma is a neoplasm that is unique to the canine skin. It has no similarities to the cutaneous histiocytoma found in humans, nor is it encountered in any other species. It may be misdiagnosed by "human" pathologists as histiocytic lymphoma. This tumor should *not* be confused with malignant fibrous histiocytoma, which is a soft tissue sarcoma, or with systemic histiocytosis. Histiocytomas are far more common in young than in old dogs. Fifty percent of cases occur in dogs younger than two years of age. Purebred dogs have a higher incidence than mixed-breed dogs, and boxers and dachshunds are predisposed.

The cause of the tumor is unknown. Intracytoplasmic reticular aggregates, suggestive of viral causation, have been found on electron microscopic examination of tumor cells. No causative agent has been isolated, however, and attempts to transmit the tumor have been unsuccessful.

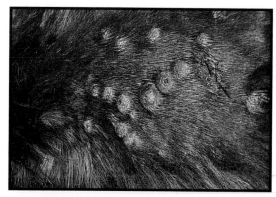

Figure 5-116: Multiple cutaneous histiocytomas, as seen in this 8-month-old Scottish terrier, usually regress spontaneously.

Clinical Presentation and History

The tumors are most common on the head (especially the pinna of the ears), hindlegs, feet, and trunk. The neck, forelegs, and tail are sometimes involved. Histiocytomas are rapidly developing, circular, dome-shaped lesions in the skin.[2] The surface of the skin is shiny and alopecic or ulcerated. Although erythematous in appearance, these tumors cause no discomfort to the animal. Tumors range in size from 0.5 to 4.0 cm in diameter; the majority are 1 to 2 cm.

Treatment

Although rapid growth and high mitotic index are highly suggestive of a malignant tumor, these are benign tumors that usually regress spontaneously with lymphoid infiltration. Rarely, new tumors arise at the site of excision or at other sites on the body.

Multiple histiocytomas have rarely been reported. These tumors also resolve without therapy over 8 to 12 weeks, although their disappearance may not be synchronous[64] (Figure 5-116).

Cutaneous Plasmacytoma
Incidence, Signalment, and Etiology

Canine cutaneous plasmacytomas show no breed or sex predilection

> ### KEY POINT:
>
> *Canine cutaneous histiocytoma usually regresses spontaneously after lymphoid infiltration.*

MANAGEMENT OF SPECIFIC DISEASES

(large breeds are affected slightly more often). Tumors are usually solitary in middle-aged to old dogs (mean age = 9.7 years). Cocker spaniels may be overrepresented. A more complete discussion is found in the chapter on Plasma Cell Tumors.

Clinical Presentation and History

There is a tumor predilection for skin of digits, lips, and ears.[67,68] Tumors appear as single, soft to firm, raised, circumscribed nodules. These are benign neoplasms and are usually not associated with the syndrome of multiple myeloma.[66] Dogs sometimes have distant recurrences after surgical excision. This may be due to unrelated or asynchronous primary tumors rather than to metastasis.[69]

Treatment

These tumors are locally infiltrative and recur if excision is incomplete. Occasional vessel invasion has been reported, but there is no systemic spread. Excision has been curative in nearly all reported dogs, although tumors of the oral cavity may be more difficult to excise. Individual reports of tumor response after chemotherapy with doxorubicin[71] and (anecdotally) responses to prednisone and melphalan imply that these drugs may be useful for the treatment of nonresectable or widespread disease.

Transmissible Venereal Tumors
Incidence, Signalment, and Etiology

Transmissible venereal tumors (TVTs) can occur in dogs of any age (especially during sexually active years), sex, or breed. This tumor is common in dogs in the southwestern and southeastern United States and is enzootic in Puerto Rico and in the Bahamas, where it is the most common tumor of dogs (see also the chapter on Tumors of the Reproductive System).

Tumor cells are transmitted by coitus or other contact and grow until immune mechanisms cause regression of the tumor or until the growth or its metastases kill the host. Dogs are immune to recurrence after recovery.

Clinical Presentation and History

Transmissible venereal tumors are solitary or multiple and are almost always located on the external genitalia. There have been a number of reports of venereal tumors in extragenital sites of skin. Most metastatic lesions, particularly in the skin, occur from trauma and mechanical implantation of tumor cells from the genital areas.

Treatment

Therapy may include surgical excision, radiation, and/or chemotherapy with vincristine. Vincristine (0.5 mg/m^2 IV every week) is considered *curative* in nearly all cases. Tumor responses can be expected within 2 to 6 weeks. Vinblastine also may be an active agent for the treatment of TVTs. Cyclophosphamide treatment does not improve the response to vincristine.[71–73]

Cutaneous Lymphoma
Incidence, Signalment, and Etiology

This disease may primarily involve the skin or it may be part of the generalized manifestations of lymphoma. Cutaneous lymphoma is more common in old dogs. There is no significant breed or site predilection (see also Chapter on Lymphoma).

Clinical Presentation and History

Cutaneous lymphoma can present as solitary or multiple dermal masses of recent onset or as a chronic unresolved or progressive case of dermatitis in which a positive diagnosis is rendered on histopathologic examination of skin biopsy specimens. Pruritus is common. Chronic unresolved dermatitis eventually may produce multiple skin nodules or show the formation of generalized plaques, pustules, or ulcerative skin disease. The dermal nodules vary in size from several millimeters to several centimeters in diameter. The covering skin may show partial or complete alopecia. Some of the nodules are covered by a thick, dry crust, which reveals a pink healing epidermis upon removal. Other areas show epidermal ulceration with a peripheral rim of erythema. Most dogs with mycosis fungoides, a specific form of cuta-

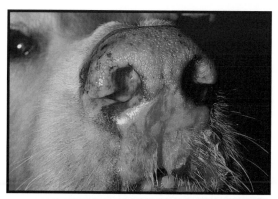

Figure 5-117: Mycosis fungoides is a specific T cell variant of lymphoma that occurs within the epidermis. Ulceration and pruritus are common with this disease, and the lesion seen on the nasal planum of this 13-year-old golden retriever is typical.

neous lymphoma in which the malignancy involves T cells, have only plaque-like or nodular lesions and a chronic history of progressive skin disease (see next section on Mycosis Fungoides).

Treatment

Biological behavior is extremely variable with this type of tumor. Some dogs with a solitary mass that was surgically excised show no evidence of recurrence, progression to other skin sites, or internal metastasis. Other dogs with solitary nodules that were surgically removed develop additional skin nodules and show progression of the disease. Solitary lesions may be treated with radiation therapy and usually respond rapidly and completely. Chemotherapy is recommended as an adjunct to surgery and/or radiation therapy, because lymphoma is always considered to be a systemic disease. Combination chemotherapy protocols are most likely to result in clinical response. Response to lymphoma chemotherapy protocols varies, but remissions are usually shorter than those that occur with multicentric lymphoma.

Mycosis Fungoides (Cutaneous T Cell-like Lymphoma)
Incidence, Signalment, and Etiology

Mycosis fungoides (MF) is a primary cutaneous lymphoma in humans as well as dogs and, rarely, cats. The neoplastic cell has been immunologically determined to be a helper T cell. The tumor tends to occur in the epidermis, superficial dermis, and periadnexally (epidermotrophic). There are characteristic "micro-abscesses" of tumor cells within the skin (Pautrier micro-abscesses). A similar disease has been described in both dogs and cats. The T cell origin of the tumor has been documented in both cats and dogs. In dogs, MF tends to occur in old animals (mean age = 11 years), and no sex predilection is seen. There is a possible overrepresentation of poodles and cocker spaniels. In a reported series of 22 cases of cutaneous lymphoma, two dogs (9%) demonstrated MF lesions. The disease is rare in cats.

Clinical Presentation and History

Mycosis fungoides has a protracted clinical course with three apparent clinical stages:

1. *Premycotic Stage (Erythroderma Stage):* Skin lesions are characterized by eczema, erythema (erythroderma), pigmentation or depigmentation, telangiectasis, atrophy, alopecia, and variable pruritus. Skin lesions usually start over the trunk or neck and may progress to involve more of the body. Lesions sometimes show a primarily mucocutaneous-junction distribution.
2. *Mycotic Stage (Plaque Stage):* Skin lesions are characterized by erythematous, raised, thickened, firm plaques. Lesions may be ulcerated and exudative. These lesions may develop where previous skin lesions existed or in new areas (Figure 5-117).
3. *Tumor Stage:* Skin lesions are characterized by distinct, proliferative, protruding nodules, and the skin may be ulcerated. Malignant spread to lymph nodes or other organs may occur.

Sezary syndrome is a leukemic variant of MF characterized by circulating, malignant, helper T cells with similar morphology and antigenic markers as malignant cells in skin lesions. This syndrome can occur during any stage of MF and does not alter the usual progression of the disease or long-term progno-

MANAGEMENT OF SPECIFIC DISEASES

sis. Mycosis fungoides complicated with Sezary syndrome is characterized by splenomegaly, lymphadenopathy, and cyclic episodes of generalized erythroderma. The number of peripheral Sezary cells increases immediately prior to episodes of erythroderma and declines rapidly during the episodes. This suggests migration of these cells from blood to skin and sequestration of Sezary cells in the skin. Most animals with MF are euthanatized prior to the development of overt tumors due to difficulty of controlling skin lesions.

A solitary variant of MF occurs in the oral mucosa of dogs. This may progress to systemic MF, but it often has an indolent course over many years.

Staging and Diagnosis

Definitive diagnosis is made by biopsy. Multiple and serial biopsy specimens should be taken until the diagnosis is confirmed; a single lesion may not contain all the histologic characteristics necessary to confirm the diagnosis. Earlier lesions in the premycotic and mycotic stages are better samples for histology. Because of the possibility of disease elsewhere, a CBC, biochemical profile, urinalysis, radiographs, and bone marrow aspirate are appropriate.

Lymph node enlargement may occur at any stage of MF, but it usually represents a reactive response to chronic dermatitis rather than malignant spread of the tumor (dermatopathic lymphadenopathy). Enlargement is nevertheless an indication for lymph node biopsy. Secondary pyodermas are common with MF and may complicate diagnosis and treatment.

Treatment

Many different treatments have been used for MF. None has proven entirely satisfactory, but some success has been achieved with each. If the lesions are limited to the skin, a variety of therapies seem efficacious.

Topical nitrogen mustards, such as mechlorethamine or carmustine (BCNU), have been the most widely used treatment in both animals and

humans. These compounds are potent carcinogens, however, which is of more concern to humans contacting the chemicals than for the animals treated. These ointments should not be used in cats.

A treatment widely used in humans for MF is such vitamin A analogues as 13-*cis*-retinoic acid and other synthetic compounds, such as isotretinoin (Accutane® [Roche], 1 to 3 mg/kg SID PO). The mechanism of action of these compounds is by inducing terminal differentiation of tumor cells, and improvement has been reported in dogs using the dose given above.[72]

Electron beam therapy has been used extensively in humans for MF with good results. This technology is limited in availability for veterinary medicine, although radiation therapy may play a role in palliation of the disease. For the solitary variant of mycosis fungoides found in the oral cavity, external beam radiation therapy may provide long-term remission and occasional cures for lesions that cannot be excised.

A technique called PUVA (Psoralen UVA) has been reported as a treatment for MF in humans. A compound called 8-methoxypsoralen is given orally and is converted to psoralen in the body. Psoralen is activated by UV-A light and binds to the DNA of cells in the epidermis and superficial dermis where UV light has penetrated. Therefore, an antineoplastic effect is localized to the areas exposed to and penetrated by UV light. The use of this method has not yet been reported in veterinary medicine.

Intravenous and local injections of fibronectin were used in one cat with MF, and the size of the lesion was significantly reduced. Fibronectin is believed to act as an opsonin in areas of disrupted tissue, chemotactically attracting macrophages.

One dog was treated with intradermal injections of placental lysate and prednisone orally, and clinical remission of severe skin lesions was achieved for 25 months. No skin lesions were seen at necropsy. In this

> ## KEY POINT:
>
> *Cutaneous lymphoma and mycosis fungoides are frequently nonresponsive to systemic combination chemotherapy.*

dog, skin lesions relapsed if either medication was removed from the protocol. The treatments just prescribed have proven useful only in controlling the skin lesions of MF. They have no efficacy in controlling systemic disease. The use of systemic chemotherapy protocols as described in the chapter on Lymphoma have been suggested for cases in which the disease has disseminated; however, these tumors have proven to be poorly responsive to most commonly used chemotherapeutic agents. Anecdotally, L-asparaginase may be more effective than other commonly used drugs (A.S. Moore, personal observations, 1994).

HISTIOCYTIC DISEASES

These diseases recently have been reported in dogs and, rarely, in cats. Histiocytic diseases should be distinguished from canine cutaneous histiocytoma, which is benign, and from malignant fibrous histiocytoma, which is a soft tissue sarcoma.

Systemic Histiocytosis
Incidence, Signalment, and Etiology

This is an uncommon disease that occurs most frequently in Bernese mountain dogs in what may be an inherited manner.[76] It principally affects middle-aged male dogs. No etiologic agent has been identified, but systemic histiocytosis is considered to be a nonneoplastic disease.

Clinical Presentation and History

Dogs with systemic histiocytosis are usually depressed, anorexic, and have multiple cutaneous masses up to 4 cm in diameter that are ulcerated, crusted, or alopecic. Cutaneous lesions are most common on the face. Systemic spread has been noted to regional and distant lymph nodes and abdominal organs, which are infiltrated with macrophages/histiocytes. The clinical course is prolonged and is often punctuated by periods of clinical remission.

Treatment

Dogs with systemic histiocytosis have multiple episodes of clinical disease punctuated by periods when they are asymptomatic. Definitive treatment has not been reported; however, anecdotally, responses have occurred to thymic extract, prompting suspicion that the disorder may be at least partly immunoregulatory in nature.[75]

Malignant Histiocytosis
Incidence, Signalment, and Etiology

This is an uncommon disease that has been reported most frequently in Bernese mountain dogs, in which it is suspected to have an inherited basis.[75] The disease also has been noted in rottweilers, Doberman pinschers, Labrador retrievers, flat-coated retrievers, and golden retrievers as well as in cats.[76] The disease occurs with equal frequency in both sexes and is most common in old dogs.

Clinical Findings and History

The tumor frequently involves the lung as solitary or multiple nodular opacities on thoracic radiographs. It occasionally may occur as diffuse pulmonary infiltrates, with or without hilar lymph node involvement.[76] Although respiratory signs predominate, neurologic signs are common and include posterior paresis, paralysis, or seizures. Bone marrow is frequently involved, with resultant cytopenias and their sequelae. In addition, the spleen, liver, and, occasionally, other abdominal organs may be involved.[75]

Staging and Diagnosis

Complete clinical staging includes thoracic and abdominal radiographs as well as routine blood work, urinalysis, and a bone marrow aspirate. Abdominal ultrasonography may enable needle (Tru-Cut®) biopsies to obtain a definitive diagnosis. Care should be taken when biopsying dogs with bone marrow infiltrative and consequent cytopenias, as thrombo-

> **KEY POINT:**
>
> *Systemic histiocytosis is characterized by cutaneous mass lesions, while malignant histiocytosis frequently involves the lungs, bone marrow, and central nervous system.*

cytopenia may be marked and the patient may be prone to bleeding. Dogs with liver involvement may have low serum albumin and peripheral edema, which can complicate treatment.

Treatment

There are anecdotal reports of clinical remission after treatment with cyclophosphamide, vincristine, and prednisone or doxorubicin-based chemotherapy protocols used for the treatment of lymphoma (see Lymphoma chapter), but these remissions are of relatively short duration. Supportive treatment in the form of blood transfusions, plasma transfusions, or the use of dextrans and hetastarch for hypoproteinemic dogs may be as important as chemotherapy in prolonging survival of severely affected dogs.

REFERENCES

1. Miller MA, Nelson SL, Turk JR, et al: Cutaneous neoplasia in 340 cats. Vet Pathol 28:389–395, 1991.
2. Pulley LT, Stannard AA: Tumors of the skin and soft tissues, in Moulton JE (ed): Tumors in Domestic Animals, ed 3. Berkeley, CA, University of California Press, 1990, pp 23–87.
3. Hahn KA, Lantz GC, Salisbury K, et al: Comparison of survey radiography with ultrasonography and x-ray computed tomography for clinical staging of subcutaneous neoplasms in dogs. JAVMA 196:1795–1798, 1990.
4. Nikula KJ, Benjamin SA, Angleton GM, et al: Ultraviolet radiation, solar dermatosis, and cutaneous neoplasia in beagle dogs. Radiat Res 129:11–18, 1992.
5. Marks SL, Song MD, Stanard AA, Power HT: Clinical evaluation of etretinate for the treatment of canine solar-induced SCC and preneoplastic lesions. J Am Acad Dermatol 27:11–16, 1992.
6. Himsel CA, Richardson RC, Craig JA: Cisplatin chemotherapy for metastatic squamous cell carcinoma in two dogs. JAVMA 189:1575–1578, 1986.
7. Shapiro W, Kitchell BE, Fossum TW, et al: Cisplatin for treatment of transitional cell and squamous cell carcinomas in dogs. JAVMA 193:1530–1533, 1988.
8. Knapp DW, Richardson RC, DeNicola DB, al et: Cisplatin toxicity in cats. J Vet Intern Med 1:29–35, 1987.
9. Buhles WC, Theilen GH: Preliminary evaluation of bleomycin in feline and canine squamous cell carcinoma. Am J Vet Res 34:289–291, 1973.
10. Ogilvie GK, Obradovich JE, Elmslie RE, et al: Efficacy of mitoxantrone against various neoplasms in dogs.

11. Orenberg EK, Luck EE, Brown DM, Kitchell BE: Implant delivery system: Intralesional delivery of chemotherapeutic agents for treatment of spontaneous skin tumors in veterinary patients. Clin Dermatol 9:561–568, 1992.
12. Jones SE, Knapp DW, Hogenesch H, DeNicola DB: Pilot study of piroxicam therapy of non-resectable squamous cell carcinoma in dogs. Proc Vet Cancer Soc 13th Annual Conf:53–54, 1993.
13. Paradis M, Scott DW, Breton L: Squamous cell carcinoma of the nail bed in three related giant schnauzers. Vet Rec 125:322–324, 1989.
14. O'Brien MG, Berg J, Engler SJ: Treatment by digital amputation of subungual squamous cell carcinoma in dogs: 21 cases (1987–1988). JAVMA 201:759–761, 1992.
15. Theon AP, Madewell BR, Moore AS, et al: Localized thermo-cisplatin therapy: A pilot study in spontaneous canine and feline tumors. Int J Hyperthermn 7:881–892, 1991.
16. Brooks MB, Matus RE, Leifer CE, et al: Chemotherapy versus chemotherapy plus radiotherapy in the treatment of tonsillar squamous cell carcinoma in the dog. J Vet Intern Med 2:206–211, 1988.
17. Theon AP, Madewell BR, Shearn V, Moulton JE: Irradiation of squamous cell carcinomas of the nasal planum in 90 cats. Proc 13th Ann Conf Vet Cancer Soc:147–148, 1993.
18. Evans EG, Madewell BR, Stannard AA: A trial of 13-cis-retinoic acid for treatment of squamous cell carcinoma and preneoplastic lesions of the head in cats. Am J Vet Res 46:2553–2557, 1985.
19. VanVechten MK, Theon AP: Strontium-90 plesiotherapy for treatment of early squamous cell carcinomas of the nasal planum in 25 cats. Proc 13th Annual Conf Veterinary Cancer Soc:107–108, 1993.
20. Grier RL, Brewer WG, Jr, Theilen GH: Hyperthermia treatment of superficial tumors in cats and dogs. JAVMA 177:227–233, 1980.
21. Atwater SW, Powers BE, Straw RC, Withrow SJ: Squamous cell carcinoma of the pinna and nasal planum. Fifty-four cats (1980–1991). Proc Vet Cancer Soc 11th Ann Conf:35–36, 1991.
22. Roberts WG, Klein MK, Loomis M, et al: Photodynamic therapy of spontaneous cancers in felines, canines, and snakes with chloro-aluminum sulfonated phthalocyamine. J Natl Cancer Inst 83:18–23, 1993.
23. Peaston AE, Leach MW, Higgins RJ: Photodynamic therapy for nasal and aural squamous cell carcinoma in the cat. JAVMA 202:1261–1265, 1993.
24. Theon AP, Pascoe JR, Carlson GP, Krag DN: Intratumoral chemotherapy with cisplatin in oily emulsion in

horses. *JAVMA* 202:261–266, 1993.

25. Ogilvie GK, Moore AS, Obradovich JE, Elmslie RE, et al: Toxicoses and efficacy associated with the administration of mitoxantrone to cats with malignant tumors. *JAVMA* 202:1839–1844, 1993.

26. LaRue SM, Vail DM, Ogilvie GK, et al: Shrinking-field radiation therapy in combination with mitoxantrone chemotherapy for the treatment of oral squamous cell carcinoma in the cat. *Proc 11th Ann Conf Vet Cancer Soc*:99, 1991.

27. Kalaher KM, Anderson WI, Scott DW: Neoplasms of the apocrine sweat glands in 44 dogs and 10 cats. *Vet Rec* 127:400–403, 1990.

28. London CA, Dubielzig RR, Ogilvie GK, et al: Ear canal tumors of dogs and cats: Preliminary results of a VCOG retrospective study. *Proc Vet Cancer Soc 13th Ann Conf*:59–60, 1993.

29. Theon AP, Barthez PY, Madewell BR, Griffey S: Radiation therapy of ceruminous gland carcinomas in dogs and cats. *JAVMA*, 1994, in press.

30. Marino DJ, MacDonald JM, Matthiesen DT, Patnaik AK: Results of surgery in cats with ceruminous gland adenocarcinoma. *JAAHA* 30:54–58, 1994.

31. Little CJL, Pearson GR, Hurvitz AI: Neoplasia involving the middle ear cavity of dogs. *Vet Rec* 124:54–57, 1989.

32. Ogilvie GK, Reynolds HA, Richardson RC, et al: Phase II evaluation of doxorubicin for treatment of various canine neoplasms. *JAVMA* 195:1580–1583, 1989.

33. Bergman PJ, Withrow SJ, Straw RC, Powers BE: Canine infiltrative lipoma: 11 cases (1981–1990). *Proc Vet Cancer Soc 11th Ann Conf*:39, 1991.

34. Strafuss AC, Bozarth AJ: Liposarcoma in dogs. *JAAHA* 9:183–187, 1973.

35. McChesney SL, Withrow SJ, Gillette EL, et al: Radiotherapy of soft tissue sarcomas in dogs. *JAVMA* 194:60–63, 1989.

36. Mauldin GN, Meleo KA, Burk RL: Radiation therapy for the treatment of incompletely resected soft tissue sarcomas in dogs: 21 cases. *Proc Vet Cancer Soc 13th Ann Conf*:111, 1993.

37. Evans SM: Canine hemangiopericytoma: A retrospective analysis of response to surgery and orthovoltage radiation. *Vet Radiol* 28:13–16, 1987.

38. Tilmant LL, Gorman NT, Ackerman N, et al: Chemotherapy of synovial cell sarcoma in a dog. *JAVMA* 188:530–532, 1986.

39. Hahn KA: Vincristine sulfate as single-agent chemotherapy in a dog and a cat with malignant neoplasms. *JAVMA* 197:796–798, 1990.

40. Theon AP, Madewell BR, Ryu J, Castro J: Concurrent irradiation and intratumoral chemotherapy with cis-

platin: A pilot study in dogs with spontaneous tumors. *Int J Radiat Oncol Biol Phys* 29:1027–1034, 1994.

41. Hargis AM, Ihrke PJ, Spangler WL, Stannard AA: A retrospective clinicopathologic study of 212 dogs with cutaneous hemangiomas and hemangiosarcomas. *Vet Pathol* 29:316–328, 1992.

42. Er J, Sutton RH: A survery of skin neoplasms in dogs from the Brisbane region. *Aust Vet J* 66:225–227, 1989.

43. Ward H, Fox LE, Calderwood-Mays MB, et al: Cutaneous hemangiosarcoma in 25 dogs: A retrospective study. *J Vet Intern Med* 8:345–348, 1994.

44. Sorenmo KU, Jeglum KA, Helfand SC: Chemotherapy of canine hemangiosarcoma with doxorubicin and cyclophosphamide. *J Vet Intern Med* 7:370–376, 1993.

45. Miller MA, Ramos JA, Kreager JM: Cutaneous vascular neoplasia in 15 cats: Clinical, morphologic and immunohistochemical studies. *Vet Pathol* 29:329–336, 1992.

46. Scavelli TD, Patnaik AK, Mehlaff CJ, Hayes AA: Hemangiosarcoma in the cat: Retrospective evaluation of 31 surgical cases. *JAVMA* 187:817–819, 1985.

47. Carpenter JL, Andrews LK, Holzworth J: Tumors and tumor-like lesions, Holzworth J (ed): *Diseases of the Cat. Medicine and Surgery*. Philadelphia, WB Saunders, 1987, pp 406–596.

48. Lawler DF, Evans RH: Multiple hepatic cavernous lymphangioma in an aged male cat. *J Comp Pathol* 109:83–87, 1993.

49. Stobie D, Carpenter JL: Lymphoangiosarcoma of the mediastinum, mesentery and omentum in a cat with chylothorax. *JAAHA* 29:78–80, 1993.

50. Aronson EG, Carpenter JL: Distal extremity melanocytic nevi and malignant melanomas in dogs. *JAAHA* 26:605–612, 1990.

51. MacEwen EG, Patnaik AK, Harvey HJ, et al: Canine oral melanoma: Comparison of surgery versus surgery plus *Corynebacterium parvum*. *Cancer Invest* 4:397–402, 1986.

52. Patnaik AK, Mooney S: Feline melanoma: A comparative study of ocular, oral and dermal neoplasms. *Vet Pathol* 25:105–112, 1988.

53. Patnaik AK, Ehler WJ, MacEwen EG: Canine cutaneous mast cell tumor: Morphologic grading and survival time in 83 dogs. *Vet Pathol* 21:469–474, 1984.

54. Macy DW: Canine and feline mast cell tumors: Biologic behavior, diagnosis and therapy. *Semin Vet Med Surg (Small Anim)* 1:72–83, 1986.

55. O'Keefe DA, Couto CG, Burke-Schwartz C, Jacobs RM: Systemic mastocytosis in 16 dogs. *J Vet Intern Med* 1:75–80, 1987.

56. Hottendorf GH, Nielson SW: Pathologic study of 300 extirpated canine mastocytomas. *Zentralbl Veterin-

armed [A] 14:272–281, 1967.

57. Bostock DE: The prognosis following surgical removal of mastocytomas in dogs. *J Small Anim Pract* 14:27–41, 1973.

58. Turrel JM, Kitchell BE, Miller LM, Theon A: Prognostic factors for radiation treatment of mast cell tumor in 85 dogs. *JAVMA* 193:936–940, 1988.

59. Al-Sarraf R, Mauldin GN, Meleo KA, Patnaik A: A prospective study of radiation therapy for the treatment of incompletely resected grade 2 mast cell tumors in 32 dogs. *Proc 13th Ann Conf Vet Cancer Soc:*64, 1993.

60. Frimberger AE, Moore AS, LaRue SM, et al: Radiotherapy of incompletely resected intermediately differentiated mast cell tumors in the dog: 37 cases (1989–1993). *JAVMA*, 1994, in press.

61. McCaw DL, Miller MA, Ogilvie GK, et al: Response of canine mast cell tumors to treatment with oral prednisone. *Proc 11th Ann Conf Vet Cancer Soc:*28, 1991.

62. Wilcock BP, Yager JA, Zink MC: The morphology and behavior of feline cutaneous mastocytomas. *Vet Pathol* 23:320–324, 1986.

63. Scott DW: Feline dermatology 1900–1978: A monograph. *JAAHA* 16:331–459, 1980.

64. Garner FM, Lingeman CH: Mast cell neoplasms of the domestic cat. *Pathol Vet* 7:517–530, 1970.

65. Liska WD, MacEwen EG, Zaki FA, Gavery M: Feline systemic mastocytosis: A review and results of splenectomy in seven cases. *JAAHA* 15:589–597, 1979.

66. Bender WM, Muller GH: Multiple, resolving, cutaneous histiocytoma in a dog. *JAVMA* 194:535–537, 1989.

67. Rakich PM, Latimer KS, Weiss R, Steffens WL: Mucocutaneous plasmacytomas in dogs: 75 cases (1980–1987). *JAVMA* 194:803–810, 1989.

68. Baer KE, Patnaik AK, Gilbertson SR, Hurvitz AI: Cutaneous plasmacytomas in dogs: A morphologic and immunohistochemical study. *Vet Pathol* 26:216–221, 1989.

69. Clark GN, Berg J, Engler SJ, Bronson RT: Extramedullary plasmacytomas in dogs: Results of surgical excision in 131 cases. *JAAHA* 28:105–111, 1992.

70. Brunnert SR, Dee LA, Herron AJ, Altman NH: Gastric extramedullary plasmocytoma in a dog. *JAVMA* 200:1501–1502, 1992.

71. Boscos C: Canine transmissible venereal tumor: Clinical observations and treatment. *Anim Famil* 3:10–15, 1988.

72. Amber EI, Henderson RA, Adeyanju JB, Gyany EO: Single-drug chemotherapy of canine transmissible venereal tumor with cyclophosphamide, methotrexate, or vincristine. *J Vet Intern Med* 4:144–147, 1990.

73. Amber EI: Low dose cyclophosphamide therapy of canine venereal tumor. A preliminary study. *Proc 9th Ann Conf Vet Cancer Soc:*1989.

74. Moore PF: Systemic histiocytosis of Bernese mountain dogs. *Vet Pathol* 21:554–563, 1987.

75. Moore PF, Rosin A: Malignant histiocytosis of Bernese mountain dogs. *Vet Pathol* 23:1–10, 1986.

76. Schmidt ML, Rutteman G, Wolvekamp P: Canine malignant histiocytosis (MH): Clinical and radiographic findings. *Tijdschr Diergeneesk* 117(Suppl 1):43–44, 1992.

CLINICAL BRIEFING: MAST CELL TUMORS

Mast Cell Tumors in Dogs

Common Clinical Presentation	Raised or ulcerated intracutaneous mass; may be hairless or haired; may be single or multiple. Mast cell tumors can look and feel like anything!
Common Histologic Type	Moderately differentiated (grade II)
Epidemiology and Biological Behavior	Boxers, Boston terriers, and golden retrievers predisposed, but can occur in any breed, at any age; metastasis similar to other hematopoietic tumors: to regional lymph nodes as well as to liver, spleen, and bone marrow
Prognostic Factors	Tumors on limbs have better prognosis than trunk (especially perineum); slow growth and long duration of presence may be favorable; most important prognostic factor is histologic grade *Histologic Grade:* Recurrence rate 6 months after surgery Well-differentiated: 25% Moderately differentiated: 44% Poorly differentiated: 76%
Treatment	*Well-Differentiated to Moderately Differentiated Tumors:* **Wide** surgical excision; adjunctive radiation therapy (88% achieve 5-year control for moderately differentiated tumors); chemotherapy only with disseminated disease, although efficacy is unknown *Poorly Differentiated Tumors:* Surgery, with or without radiation therapy, is palliative; H_2 blockers, prednisone, and vincristine chemotherapy may be helpful

Mast Cell Tumors in Cats

Common Clinical Presentation	*Cutaneous:* Single or multiple raised hairless masses *Lymphoreticular:* Splenomegaly and chronic vomiting *Intestinal:* Chronic vomiting and/or diarrhea

MANAGEMENT OF SPECIFIC DISEASES

Common Histologic Types	Cutaneous tumors are usually well differentiated; lymphoreticular and intestinal tumors are malignant
Epidemiology and Biological Behavior	Histiocytic cutaneous mast cell tumors in Siamese may regress spontaneously; lymphoreticular and intestinal tumors are always malignant; cutaneous tumors are often benign, even for multiple tumors; may occur in young animals
Prognostic Factors	None identified
Treatment	*Cutaneous:* Surgery; radiation therapy, with or without corticosteroids, for invasive lesions *Lymphoreticular:* Splenectomy gives 12-month median survival *Intestinal:* Wide resection, with or without corticosteroids, but survival is poor

Normal mast cells are derived from hematopoietic and connective tissue cells. They are present throughout the body in perivascular locations, particularly skin and subcutaneous tissue, lung parenchyma, and digestive tract and liver, where they play an integral role in allergic reactions and inflammatory processes. Mast cells are only occasionally seen in bone marrow and almost never in the systemic circulation. Following binding of IgE to the cell surface, mast cells elicit an immediate hypersensitivity response by releasing vasoactive amines, such as histamine and heparin both locally and into the circulation, causing vasodilation, blood stasis, and edema. Histamine chemotactically attracts eosinophils, which neutralize histamine.

MAST CELL TUMORS IN DOGS
Incidence, Signalment, and Etiology

In dogs, mast cell tumors (MCTs) are most commonly found in the cutaneous tissue, particularly in the skin of the trunk and hindquarters and sometimes in the skin of the extremities.[1] Mast cell tumors are least common in cutaneous sites around the head and neck. In most dogs, tumors are solitary, but in about 10%, the tumors are multiple. Tumors usually occur in old dogs (mean age = 9 years) with no sex predilection. Mast cell tumors, however, may also be seen in dogs as young as 6 months of age. Boxers, Boston terriers, bullmastiffs, and English setters are at high risk for developing MCTs.[1,2] Mast cell tumors in boxers and, possibly, in golden retrievers are usually of a lower (well-differentiated) histologic grade than MCTs in other breeds. In dogs, MCTs have been experimentally transmitted using cell-free extracts, which suggests a viral origin. Ultrastructural examination of numerous MCTs of different species has failed to reveal viral particles, however.

Clinical Presentation and History

It is uncommon to diagnose MCTs without skin involvement in dogs. Mast cell tumors vary greatly in appearance, and no estimate of their malignancy or prediction of their behavior can be made on clinical appearance alone. Some MCTs may be present for months to years before rapidly disseminating; others act aggressively from the beginning.

Most cutaneous MCTs present as intracutaneous nodules that vary from 1 to 10 cm in diameter, but

MANAGEMENT OF SPECIFIC DISEASES

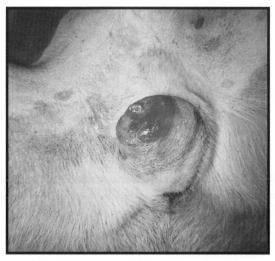

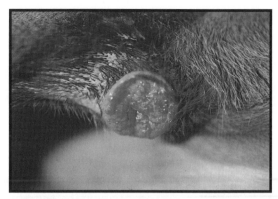

| *Figure 5-119*

Figure 5-118: Mast cell tumors in the inguinal area are usually aggressive and have a high rate of systemic spread. Shown is a scrotal tumor in a male Boston terrier. (Courtesy G.H. Theilen)

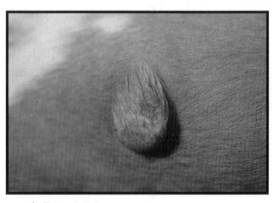

Figure 5-120

Figures 5-119 and 5-120: Mast cell tumors with vastly different appearances found on the same weimaraner. External appearance does not indicate a diagnosis. (Courtesy A. Evans)

they may become larger. Some cause ulceration of the overlying epidermis; others present as single or multiple elevated, erythematous nodules with alopecia of the overlying skin. Mast cell tumors may be edematous on palpation or present as firm, intracutaneous nodules. The tumor usually arises in the dermis and frequently extends into the underlying subcutaneous tissue and musculature. Extension occurs most frequently with rapidly growing tumors (Figures 5-118 to 5-120).

Occasionally, mechanical manipulation during examination of this tumor causes degranulation of mast cells, producing erythema and wheal formations. This phenomenon has been observed in both dogs and cats (the "Darier's sign") and is considered of diagnostic significance. Owners may report that the tumor enlarges rapidly and then diminishes in size over a period of about 24 hours. Such a history should increase the clinician's suspicion of mast cell tumor.

> **KEY POINT:**
>
> *Mast cell tumors may "grow" and "shrink" rapidly due to inflammation caused by mast cell degranulation.*

Staging and Diagnosis

The clinical appearance of MCTs in dogs may vary widely but is relatively easy to diagnose using aspiration cytology. Presurgical aspiration of these tumors provides a cytology specimen characterized by *round cells* that may have well-stained and large cytoplasmic granules (well-differentiated) or that may be more anaplastic with small, poorly staining cytoplasmic granules (see Biopsy section). Other

MANAGEMENT OF SPECIFIC DISEASES

TABLE 5-19
Survival of dogs with mast cell tumors following surgical excision

Grade of Mast Cell Tumor	Study 1[7]		Study 2[6]	
	Number of Dogs	Number (%) Alive at 1500 days	Number of Dogs	Number (%) Alive at 210 days
Well-differentiated	30	28 (93)	39	30 (77)
Moderately differentiated	36	16 (44)	30	14 (45)
Poorly differentiated	17	1 (6)	45	6 (13)
All tumors	83	45 (54)	114	50 (44)

examples of round cell tumors are lymphoma, cutaneous plasmacytoma, histiocytoma, transmissible venereal tumor (TVT), and melanoma. Cells from these tumors lack the blue-to-purple cytoplasmic granules of MCTs. Eosinophils are often seen in aspirates of MCTs because of eosinophil chemotaxis to histamine release.

Diagnosis of MCT often can be made by fine-needle aspiration cytology; but excisional biopsy is required for accurate histologic grading of the tumor. Histopathologic grading of the tumor correlates with both recurrence and survival. Follow-up examinations of 300 animals from which MCTs were excised disclosed recurrence in 25% of well-differentiated tumors.[3] This percentage increased to 44% for moderately differentiated tumors and to 76% for undifferentiated (anaplastic) tumors (Table 5-19). Dogs with neoplasms of the extremities have longer tumor-free times and longer survival than dogs with tumors on the trunk.

All dogs with MCTs should be staged to determine the extent of their disease. This is especially important for dogs being considered for radiation therapy. A standard staging scheme includes the following:

1. *Complete Blood Count (CBC)*
   A CBC is valuable in assessing animals with MCTs because animals with systemic mastocytosis occasionally have peripheral eosinophilia and basophilia in addition to circulating mast cells. Mastocythemia is more common in cats than in dogs. The CBC may also reveal anemia or a regenerative or degenerative left shift that could suggest gastrointestinal bleeding or perforation, respectively. Either may arise from chronic histamine release from the tumor.

2. *Buffy Coat Smears*
   The presence of mast cells in peripheral blood provides evidence that systemic spread has occurred. Care must be exercised in interpreting buffy coat smears, because mastocythemia has been reported in a variety of canine acute inflammatory diseases, including parvovirus infections.

3. *Bone Marrow Aspirates*
   The presence of more than 10 mast cells/1000 nucleated cells indicates systemic spread of the neoplasm. Because mast cells may be accompanied by eosinophils, the presence of eosinophilia in the marrow should alert the clinician to search carefully for mast cells.[4]
   In a study involving 16 dogs with systemic mastocytosis, bone marrow aspiration was deemed superior to either buffy coat or blood-smear examination.[5]

KEY POINT:

Pulmonary metastasis from canine cutaneous mast cell tumors is extremely rare; therefore, thoracic radiographs are rarely useful for staging.

MANAGEMENT OF SPECIFIC DISEASES

4. Lymph Node Aspirates

The clinician should perform fine-needle aspiration of the regional lymph node if the node is enlarged. The presence of mast cells (and eosinophils) is an indication that the MCT is no longer confined to the primary site.

5. Radiographs and Ultrasonography

Splenomegaly or hepatomegaly may indicate spread of MCTs systemically. Enlarged regional nodes (especially sublumbar nodes for perineal tumors) may be identified. Fine-needle aspiration may confirm the suspicion of metastasis. Pulmonary metastasis of MCTs is rare.

6. Miscellaneous Tests

There were signs of systemic illness in 8 of 16 (50%) dogs with systemic disease. Of the eight dogs with systemic signs, five were necropsied, and three of these dogs had gastric ulceration.[5] Histamine release by MCTs and subsequent histamine binding at H_2-receptor sites has been shown to stimulate hydrochloric acid secretion by gastric parietal cells. Occult blood tests may be useful in evaluating patients with mast cell disease. The stools of dogs with MCTs should be examined for evidence of gastrointestinal bleeding produced by ulceration that results from histamine release. In many cases, feces may contain small amounts of blood that are insufficient to produce melena. Evidence of gastrointestinal bleeding in a patient with a MCT should prompt the clinician to treat with medications that block the effects of mast cell hyperhistaminemia (i.e., H_2 blockers, such as cimetidine).

Prognostic Factors

The most important prognostic factors for canine MCTs are the histologic grade of the tumor and the completeness of excision (i.e., whether the surgical margins are "dirty"). In addition, tumor location is often considered to be an important prognostic indicator. Dogs with tumors on the extremities survive longer than those with tumors on the trunk. Tumors in the inguinal and perineal regions have a poor prognosis regardless of histologic grade, but they are usually undifferentiated on histopathology. Also, dogs with tumors that grow at a rate greater than 1 cm per week have only a 25% chance of surviving for 30 weeks.[6]

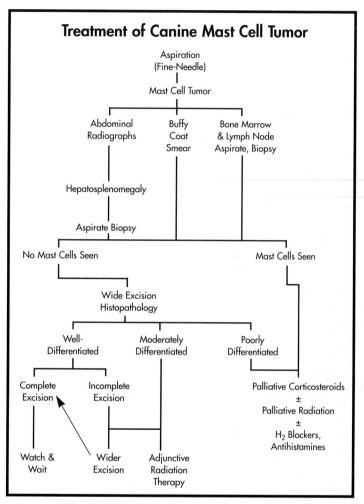

Figure 5-121: *A schematic flow chart for the treatment of mast cell tumors in dogs.*

MANAGEMENT OF SPECIFIC DISEASES

Treatment

Control of canine MCTs involves the use of surgery, chemotherapy, or radiation therapy, either individually or in combination (Figure 5-121).

Surgery

Surgical excision is indicated if the tumor is solitary and evidence of lymph node involvement or systemic spread is lacking. Excision should be wide *and deep* to a minimum margin of 3 cm around the perceived borders of the tumor and one fascial plane below. Even with this aggressive surgical approach, approximately one third of MCTs recur after surgery.[6]

The percentage of dogs alive following surgical excision of MCTs was studied in two case series. The results are in Table 5-19.

As previously stated, surgical excision should be aggressive. All excised tissue should be examined histologically for completeness of tumor excision. Extension of the tumor beyond the surgical borders should prompt either wider excision or radiation therapy of the tumor bed and surrounding tissue. If the tumor is well differentiated and excision is complete, no further treatment is necessary. If the tumor is well differentiated and incompletely excised, then a wider excision should be performed. A second excision should include the previous excision site **plus** margins of 3 cm around this tissue. If the tumor cannot be completely excised or if it is moderately or poorly differentiated, further therapy is indicated. The animal should be evaluated for radiation therapy, if available.

Radiation Therapy

Mast cell tumors are quite sensitive to the effects of radiation therapy, even at moderate doses. In one study, 44% of 23 dogs had satisfactory responses to radiation therapy with tumor control of greater than 12 months and an average longevity of 24 months.[8] Another study using external beam radiation to treat 95 MCTs on 85 dogs, found mean and median tumor-free times of 63 and 17 months, respectively;

> ## KEY POINT:
>
> *The most important prognostic factor for canine mast cell tumors is histologic grade of the tumor.*

79% of dogs were tumor-free at 1 year, and 77% were tumor-free at 2 years.[9] In this study, survival was shorter in dogs that had higher tumor grade and both recurrence and survival were affected by tumor location. Dogs with neoplasms on the limbs had longer tumor-free times and survived longer than dogs with tumors on the trunk. Dogs with moderately differentiated tumors survived longer than dogs with undifferentiated tumors.

The long control and survival times in this study[9] are at least in part owing to inclusion of dogs that had no measurable evidence of disease after surgical removal of MCTs but which had *incomplete* excision on histologic examination of excised tissues. This group of dogs has significantly longer tumor control and survival than other dogs; thus, postsurgical radiation therapy for incompletely excised tumors seems beneficial. Mast cell tumors of the extremities often present the greatest challenge for complete surgical excision. For well- or moderately differentiated tumors in these locations, combined modalities of less aggressive surgical "debulking" followed by radiation therapy may be a more acceptable treatment— both functionally and cosmetically. In a recent study, 32 dogs with intermediate-grade (grade II) MCTs that were incompletely excised received adjunctive ^{60}Co radiation therapy to a cumulative dose of 54 Gy.[10] Tumor-free survival rates were 96% at 1 year and 88% at 2 through 5 years. Similar results were achieved using orthovoltage or linear accelerator radiation to doses of 48 Gy.[11] Adjunctive radiation therefore seems to be the treatment of choice for incompletely excised intermediate-grade MCTs.

Radiation "reactions" occur at a higher incidence and with greater severity in dogs with MCTs, possibly because of mast cell degranulation and release of proteolytic enzymes and vasoactive amines. Reactions can be of great significance in the distal extremities where the skin is thin, and great care to prevent self-injury should be taken with dogs undergoing this therapy.[9] Radiation therapy may alleviate symptoms

MANAGEMENT OF SPECIFIC DISEASES

of extensive or systemic disease. When the tumor is poorly differentiated or metastasis is already confirmed, the use of high-dose intermittent radiation treatments may improve the quality of life by stopping bleeding or reducing the size of a bulky or irritating tumor. In these cases, a fully fractionated course would be costly and reduce the amount of time spent by owners with the dog. A coarsely fractionated series of three 10-Gy treatments on a schedule of day 0, 7, and 21, however, provides relief from symptoms, although it will not increase life span. Systemic therapy, as outlined later, can be considered.

Other Local Therapies

Injection of de-ionized water into the site of incomplete surgical resection seems to reduce local recurrence of MCTs. For moderately differentiated MCTs examined in one study, 7 of 27 tumors injected recurred locally.[12] Injections were painful, and dogs required heavy sedation or anesthesia. The injection of de-ionized water is discouraged because it may delay or preclude more appropriate therapy.

Anecdotally, intralesional injections of triamcinolone at a dose rate of 1 mg/cm diameter of tumor every 2 weeks gives good palliative local tumor control.

Systemic Therapy

When MCTs have metastasized or spread systemically, localized therapies, such as surgery or radiation, are appropriate only as palliation for discomfort or mechanical obstruction. For these dogs, the most frequently recommended drugs are corticosteroids. Corticosteroids are primarily palliative, but some long-term responses do occur. Oral prednisone (2 mg/kg/day for 2 weeks, then 1 mg/kg/day for 2 weeks, then 1 mg/kg every other day for 6 months) is given as long as the tumor does not progress.

The exact mechanism by which glucocorticoids exert their cytotoxic effects on MCTs in unknown, although the process may parallel the effects of glucocorticoids on lymphocytes. Glucocorticoid receptor sites were found in the cytoplasm of canine mast cells; these sites may be involved with the susceptibility of MCTs to glucocorticoids. Although receptors for progesterone and estrogen have been described in the tumor cells of dogs with canine MCTs, the role of sex steroids in the treatment of canine MCTs has yet to be investigated. The type of glucocorticoid administered is immaterial, but intralesional application of corticosteroids may be more effective than systemic therapy. Fewer cushingoid side effects have been seen with such short-acting glucocorticoids as prednisone. Remission times are usually 10 to 20 weeks. Anecdotally, dogs that are tumor-free after six months have a lower incidence of recurrence; therefore, therapy is usually discontinued at this time. The only controlled study using prednisone found that 5 of 21 dogs (24%) showed an objective response (1 complete and 4 partial).[13] Of the five dogs that responded, two had solitary tumors, two had multiple tumors, and one had regional lymph node metastasis. L-asparaginase has been recommended as an active agent in treating MCTs. In one study, three of six dogs with cutaneous MCTs showed an objective response (whether complete or partial was not specified) for the short interval of one to two months.[14] One of two other dogs treated with L-asparaginase showed an objective response to therapy for six months.[15]

Anecdotally, other chemotherapeutic agents, such as chlorambucil and vincristine, have been used to treat MCTs. Prospective studies are underway to evaluate vincristine, and preliminary data suggest that it may be an active agent.

Palliation of Systemic Disease

Ancillary drug therapy is important with canine MCTs. Animals with mastocytosis or bulky mast cell disease should receive H_2 antagonists, as rapid degranulation of neoplastic mast cells may follow surgery or chemotherapy. Cimetidine reduces gastric acid production by competitive inhibition of the action of histamine on H_2 receptors of the gastric parietal cells. Ranitidine, a newer H_2 antagonist that may require less frequent administration, may be used for a similar effect. The objective of the therapy is to prevent gastrointestinal ulceration associated

MANAGEMENT OF SPECIFIC DISEASES

with elevated levels of histamine and to treat ulcers already present. Some new evidence indicates that cimetidine may also alter the immune response to tumors. Dogs with evidence of gastrointestinal ulceration and bleeding may benefit from sucralfate therapy at a dose of 0.5 to 1.0 g TID PO. Sucralfate reacts with stomach acid to form a highly condensed, viscous, adherent, paste-like substance that binds to the surface of both gastric and duodenal ulcers. The barrier formed protects the ulcer from potential ulcerogenic properties of pepsin, acid, and bile, allowing the ulcer to heal. Such H_1 antagonists as benadryl should be considered for use along with cimetidine before and after surgical removal of canine MCTs to help prevent the negative effects of local histamine release on fibroplasia and wound healing.

MAST CELL TUMORS IN CATS

Mast cell tumors in cats are almost as common in the visceral organs than the skin, in contrast to the situation in dogs. In one survey of feline neoplasms, MCTs were the second most common skin tumor, the most common hematopoietic tumor of the spleen, and the third most common intestinal tumor after lymphoma and adenocarcinoma.[16]

Cutaneous Mast Cell Tumors
Incidence, Signalment, and Etiology

Skin tumors generally occur in old cats (mean age = 9 years). There is no gender predilection. In one study, MCTs were the only cutaneous tumor diagnosed in cats younger than one year of age.[17] In the same study, Siamese were three times more likely than other breeds to develop cutaneous MCTs, which may indicate a breed predilection. Tumors in Siamese are usually subcutaneous and are composed of "histiocytic" cells.[18] These tumors may regress without therapy.

Clinical Presentation and History

The most common reason for pre-

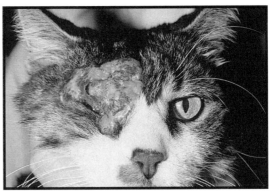

Figure 5-122: *Plaque-like mast cell tumor on the head of an 11-year-old cat.*

sentation of cats with cutaneous MCTs is as single, firm, and circumscribed dermal nodule; the next most common reason for presentation is of multiple similar masses.[19] Some tumors are plaque-like (Figure 5-122). These tumors are usually histologically well differentiated and have a benign clinical course.[20]

In contrast to dogs, most cats develop cutaneous MCTs in the skin of the head and neck, particularly the periorbital skin and pinnae. Most cutaneous MCTs in cats are benign, but tumors of the skin may have metastasized from malignant visceral disease.

Staging and Diagnosis

Mast cell tumors in cats are usually composed of well-differentiated cells that can be diagnosed by aspiration cytology. Eosinophils are rarely found in well-differentiated tumors, but they may be present in poorly differentiated or diffuse tumors.[16] Any cat with a cutaneous MCT, particularly if there are multiple lesions, should be evaluated for systemic involvement. Abdominal palpation, abdominal ultrasonography to evaluate the spleen and liver, a complete blood count, and (possibly) a bone marrow aspiration (as outlined for staging of dogs with

KEY POINT:

Cimetidine reduces gastric acid production and ulceration that results from degranulation of bulky or disseminated mast cell tumors.

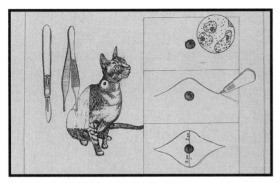

Figure 5-123: *After fine-needle aspiration of a cutaneous mast cell tumor, a wide and deep excision is made. Cats usually have well-differentiated tumors, and surgical excision may be curative. (From Elmslie RE, Ogilvie GK: Variables in behavior and management of mast cell tumors, in August JR (ed):* Consultations in Feline Internal Medicine, *ed 2. Philadelphia, WB Saunders, 1994, p 571; with permission.)*

cutaneous MCTs on pages 505–507) should be performed.

Treatment

The treatment of choice for feline cutaneous MCTs is surgery. For solitary tumors, a good prognosis usually can be given (Figure 5-123). Some cats develop multiple, well-differentiated tumors. These cats may be treated with multiple palliative surgeries or corticosteroids (1 mg/kg prednisone daily). For invasive or incompletely excised MCTs, radiation therapy is a successful adjunct to surgery but data regarding tumor control and patient survival are not as well established as they are for dogs.

In one study, mitoxantrone caused a partial response in a feline MCT, but the drug has not been further evaluated for the treatment of this disease.[21]

Lymphoreticular Mast Cell Tumors
Incidence, Signalment, and Etiology

The most commonly affected tissues in the viscera are in the "lymphoreticular" system; the spleen,

mediastinum, and lymph nodes are affected in decreasing incidence. This disease affects old cats (mean age = 10 years). There is no breed or gender predilection. There is no association between feline MCTs and FeLV.

Clinical Presentation and History

Lymphoreticular MCTs are often seen in cats. *Marked* splenomegaly is the most common finding. Diffuse cutaneous disease may occur with this form of MCT, and mastocythemia with bone marrow involvement is often noted. The presenting signs of vomiting and anorexia are presumably caused by tumor degranulation and release of histamine into the circulation. As with dogs, gastric and duodenal ulceration may result from hyperhistaminemia and vomiting may become chronic.

On clinical examination, the splenic enlargement caused by the tumor may be extraordinary. Borders of the organ may be smooth and rounded or they may be nodular. Peritoneal effusion may be present as a clear or a bloody exudate; mast cells and/or eosinophils are usually present.

Cats with cranial mediastinal MCTs present with signs similar to those of cats with mediastinal lymphoma. The most common presenting sign is dyspnea resulting from either a large mediastinal mass or pleural effusion.

Staging and Diagnosis

Definitive diagnosis is readily accomplished by cytologic examination of percutaneous fine-needle aspirates from involved organs (i.e., spleen, anterior mediastinum, or lymph nodes). Ultrasonography may be helpful in directing an aspirate or biopsy but is often unnecessary, particularly when the spleen is very enlarged and may be immobilized by hand. Smears from peritoneal or pleural effusions may contain mast cells, eosinophils, or both. Eosinophils in pleural effusion may occur with lymphoma, so their presence alone is not a criterion for diag-

> ### KEY POINT:
> *Most cutaneous mast cell tumors in cats are benign, although they can be multiple.*

MANAGEMENT OF SPECIFIC DISEASES

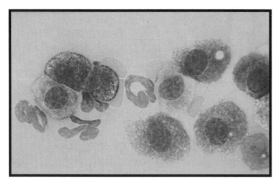

Figure 5-124: *A buffy coat smear concentrates the circulating white cells and allows rapid evaluation for mast cells; 60% of this 10-year-old cat's circulating white cells were mast cells. (Courtesy S.M. Cotter)*

nosis, and biopsy is required to confirm the diagnosis. Mast cells may be present in aspirates from a thymoma, but other cytologic features should help to distinguish these tumors. Cats with MCTs of the viscera often have a high number of circulating mast cells as well as anemia and other cytopenias due to bone marrow infiltration and erythrophagocytosis by malignant cells[22] (Figure 5-124). Therefore, a complete blood count, bone marrow aspirate, and other staging procedures described for dogs should be performed on affected cats (see pages 505–507).

Treatment

Splenectomy is the treatment of choice for feline MCTs of the spleen; cats often survive for long periods even in the absence of other therapy. Median survival of cats after splenectomy is between 11[23] and 12 months; some survive more than three years from the time of splenectomy. Response to splenectomy seems greater than would be explained by simple tumor-mass reduction, as hematologic and other organ involvements apparently resolve.

KEY POINTS:

Splenectomy alone for visceral mast cell tumors in cats results in long survival times.

Cats with a splenic mast cell tumor can be treated prior to splenectomy with cimetidine and diphenhydramine to reduce the risks associated with mast cell degranulation during surgery.

It is possible that splenic suppressor cell activity may be reduced after splenectomy, allowing for some control of the tumor by the immune system. For this reason, the use of postoperative corticosteroids in these cats is controversial.[16,23]

Most cats with MCTs of the viscera vomit continually from duodenal and gastric ulceration following chronic hyperhistaminemia. Intraoperative deaths have been reported after manipulation of the spleen during splenectomy, probably from release of vasoactive amines. For this reason, cats with MCTs should be treated prior to splenectomy with cimetidine (25 mg/kg QID PO) and diphenhydramine hydrochloride (2 mg/kg TID PO or IV) to reduce the risks of deleterious effects after mast cell degranulation.

Combination chemotherapy using such agents as vincristine, cyclophosphamide, and methotrexate has not been shown to improve survival time in cats with lymphoreticular MCTs, and the use of chemotherapy has only an anecdotal role in the palliation of this disease.[16]

There are no reports of treatment for mediastinal MCTs in cats, although external beam radiation therapy may be palliative.

Intestinal Mast Cell Tumors
Incidence, Signalment, and Etiology

Mast cell tumors occur in the intestinal tract at about the same frequency as they do in the lymphoreticular system and are seen in old cats (mean age = 13 years). There is no gender predilection. One survey found no purebred cats among 46 cats with intestinal MCTs.[16]

Clinical Presentation and History

As would be expected, cats with intestinal MCTs have a history of intermittent vomiting, diarrhea, and anorexia. Most cats have a palpable

MANAGEMENT OF SPECIFIC DISEASES

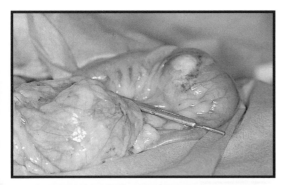

Figure 5-125: Exploratory surgery reveals an intestinal mast cell tumor, which was resected with 5 to 10 cm of "normal" bowel on either side of the lesion. These tumors are highly malignant. (Courtesy J. Berg)

abdominal mass that can be localized by ultrasonography or contrast radiography to the intestinal wall. Tumors are usually solitary but may be multiple. Unlike cats with "lymphoreticular" MCTs, cats with intestinal MCTs have no circulating mast cells.

Staging and Diagnosis

These tumors are usually poorly differentiated on histopathology, and aspiration cytology may give no conclusive information. Intestinal MCTs should be considered malignant. Ultrasonography is helpful in identifying cats that have tumor metastases to regional lymph nodes, spleen, or liver. In one series, 18 (65%) of 28 cats had involvement of one or more of these sites as well as lung or bone marrow metastases in some cats.[16]

Treatment

To treat intestinal MCTs, it is necessary to resect 5 to 10 cm of bowel with the tumor and to check the regional lymph nodes, liver, and spleen carefully for metastasis (Figure 5-125). There is often systemic involvement. Corticosteroid therapy may be palliative in these animals,[24] but the prognosis for survival beyond four months is poor.

REFERENCES

1. Macy DW: Canine and feline mast cell tumors: Biologic behavior, diagnosis and therapy. *Semin Vet Med Surgery (Small Anim)* 1:72–83, 1986.
2. Goldschmidt MH, Shofer FS: Mast cell tumors, in Goldschmidt MH, Shofer FS (eds): *Skin Tumors of the Dog and Cat.* Oxford, UK, Pergamon, 1992, pp 231–251.
3. Hottendorf GH, Nielson SW: Pathologic study of 300 extirpated canine mastocytomas. *Zentralbl Veterinärmed [A]* 14:272–281, 1967.
4. Bookbinder PF, Butt MT, Harvey HJ: Determination of the number of mast cells in lymph node, bone marrow and buffy coat cytologic specimens from dogs. *JAVMA* 200:1648–1650, 1992.
5. O'Keefe DA, Couto CG, Burke-Schwartz C, Jacobs RM: Systemic mastocytosis in 16 dogs. *J Vet Intern Med* 1:75–80, 1987.
6. Bostock DE: The prognosis following surgical removal of mastocytomas in dogs. *J Small Anim Pract* 14:27–41, 1973.
7. Patnaik AK, Ehler WJ, MacEwen EG: Canine cutaneous mast cell tumor: Morphologic grading and survival time in 83 dogs. *Vet Pathol* 21:469–474, 1984.
8. Slusher R, Roengik WJ, Wilson GP: Effect of x-irradiation on mastocytoma in dogs. *JAVMA* 151:1049–1054, 1967.
9. Turrel JM, Kitchell BE, Miller LM, Theon A: Prognostic factors for radiation treatment of mast cell tumor in 85 dogs. *JAVMA* 193:936–940, 1988.
10. Al-Sarraf R, Mauldin GN, Meleo KA, Patnaik A: A prospective study of radiation therapy for the treatment of incompletely resected grade 2 mast cell tumors in 32 dogs. *Proc 13th Ann Conf Vet Cancer Soc*:64, 1993.
11. Frimberger AE, Moore AS, La Rue SM, et al: Radiotherapy of incompletely resected intermediately differentiated mast cell tumor in the dog. 37 cases (1989–1993). *JAVMA*, 1994, in press.
12. Grier RL, DiGuardo G, Schaffer CB, et al: Mast cell tumor destruction by deionized water. *Am J Vet Res* 51:1116–1119, 1990.
13. McCaw DL, Miller MA, Ogilvie GK, et al: Response of canine mast cell tumors to treatment with oral prednisone. *Proc 11th Ann Conf Vet Cancer Soc*:28, 1991.
14. Hardy WD, Old LJ: L-asparaginase in the treatment of neoplastic disease of the dog, cat and cow. *Cancer Res* 33:131–139, 1970.
15. Legrand JJ, Carlier B, Parodi A-L: Apport de la cytologie au dignostic, au pronostic et au suivi therapeutique du mastocytoma chez le chien. *Bull Acad Vet France* 60:269–278, 1987.
16. Carpenter JL, Andrews LK, Holzworth J: Tumors and tumor-like lesions, in Holzworth J (ed): *Diseases of the Cat. Medicine and Surgery.* Philadelphia, WB Saun-

ders, 1987, pp 406–596.

17. Miller MA, Nelson SL, Turk JR, et al: Cutaneous neoplasia in 340 cats. *Vet Pathol* 28:389–395, 1991.

18. Wilcock BP, Yager JA, Zink MC: The morphology and behavior of feline cutaneous mastocytomas. *Vet Pathol* 23:320–324, 1986.

19. Scott DW: Feline dermatology 1900–1978: A monograph. *JAAHA* 16:331–459, 1980.

20. Pulley LT, Stannard AA: Tumors of the skin and soft tissues, in Moulton JE (ed): *Tumors in Domestic Animals*, ed 3. Berkeley, CA, University of California Press, 1990, pp 23–87.

21. Ogilvie GK, Moore AS, Obradovich JE, et al: Toxicoses and efficacy associated with the administration of mitoxantrone to cats with malignant tumors. *JAVMA* 202:1839–1844, 1993.

22. Madewell BR, Gunn CR, Gribble DH: Mast cell phagocytosis of red blood cells in a cat. *Vet Pathol* 20: 638–640, 1983.

23. Liska WD, MacEwen EG, Zaki FA, Gavery M: Feline systemic mastocytosis: A review and results of splenectomy in seven cases. *JAAHA* 15:589–597, 1979.

CLINICAL BRIEFING: VACCINE-ASSOCIATED SARCOMAS IN CATS

Common Clinical Presentation	Mass near site of previous vaccination
Common Histologic Types	Fibrosarcoma or other soft tissue sarcoma; other histologic types have been reported
Epidemiology and Biological Behavior	Tumor develops months to years after vaccination; multiple vaccinations at the same site at one time increase risk of tumor development; locally aggressive; frequent recurrence after surgery; rare distant metastases
Prognostic Factors	None identified

Treatment
    Surgery
 	
    Radiation Therapy
    Chemotherapy
	
	Treatment of choice; wide and deep surgical margins are essential for all vaccine-induced sarcomas
	May be effective before or after surgical removal
	Unproven, but doxorubicin may be effective, with or without surgery and radiation therapy

VACCINE-ASSOCIATED SARCOMAS IN CATS

Recently, awareness of vaccine-associated sarcomas in cats has been increasing.[1-6] This highly aggressive malignancy has been associated with a wide variety of vaccines. These sarcomas are difficult to treat because of their invasive nature. Vaccine-associated sarcomas primarily occur in areas of the cat most commonly vaccinated: the cervical interscapular and femoral regions.

Incidence, Signalment, and Etiology

In a recent epidemiologic study,[2] sarcomas were temporally associated with previous injection of various vaccines into specific body locations. Feline leukemia virus (FeLV) vaccination, rabies vaccination, and development of fibrosarcomas at the injection site within one year after vaccination were statistically associated. This study demonstrated a 5.5%

increased risk of developing sarcomas in response to FeLV vaccination and a two-fold increase in risk of development of sarcomas after rabies vaccination. The actual incidence of the tumor was estimated to be approximately one sarcoma per 10,000 administered FeLV and rabies vaccines. No association between sex, breed, and concurrent viral infections in the development of these sarcomas was found. Another study showed that although many vaccines were administered to cats that developed tumors in the site of vaccination, only the FeLV vaccine was statistically associated with an increased risk of developing sarcomas.[5] Cats with vaccine-associated sarcomas were young, and their tumors were more aggressive and had more frequent recurrences than cats with non-vaccine–associated sarcomas.

The aluminum adjuvant in many of these vaccines may be associated with development of vaccine-associated sarcomas.[2,4,5] Kass et al[2] demonstrated, howev-

MANAGEMENT OF SPECIFIC DISEASES

er, that certain aluminum-free vaccines may also be associated with development of these soft tissue sarcomas. Increase in risk of developing soft tissue sarcoma after one vaccination was 50%, after two vaccinations simultaneously administered at the same location was 127%, and after three or four vaccines simultaneously administered at the same location was approximately 175%.[2] Therefore, there seems to be a multifactorial association between vaccines and growth of sarcomas.[1,5] The development of sarcomas in response to vaccines, especially those that contain aluminum as an adjuvant, may suggest an association between foreign bodies and the growth of these neoplasms. This is not a new observation. Indeed, other metals, such as arsenic, chromium, and nickel have been shown under an array of conditions to induce sarcoma formation.[1,7,8]

Histologically, vaccine-associated sarcomas are enveloped in dense, fibrous connective tissue and infiltrated with inflammatory lymphocytes and macrophages. Macrophages often contain bluish-gray foreign material that electron-probe x-ray microanalysis identifies as aluminum and oxygen.[2,4] Other tumors develop in apparent association with other foreign bodies. For example, ocular sarcomas have been associated with foreign material in the eye.[7] Osteosarcomas also have been associated with metallic implants.[8] Despite this compelling information, no specific etiology has been determined for the development of these sarcomas, only causal association. Additional research must answer the question of etiopathogenesis.

Clinical Presentation and History

Cats with vaccine-associated sarcomas present with a mass in areas of vaccination. Some owners may note

---

KEY POINTS:

Vaccine-associated sarcomas in cats are highly invasive and are associated with rabies and FeLV vaccines. The risk of developing a tumor increases with the number of vaccinations administered in a location at one time.

All diagnostic steps should be carried out in such a way as to avoid disseminating the tumor beyond the local site.

---

that this mass has persisted since vaccination. The lesions generally are not painful but may be fixed to underlying structures. The clinician should remember that soft tissue sarcomas extend microscopically, far beyond the palpable mass.

Staging and Diagnosis

Vaccine-associated soft tissue sarcomas are frequently located in areas of previous vaccination, such as between the shoulder blades and in the hindleg. A diagnosis is made by fine-needle aspiration cytology or, preferably, incisional biopsy. The clinician should keep in mind that these soft tissue sarcomas are encased in a pseudocapsule that is actually compressed tumor tissue. In addition, tendrils of tumor extend far beyond the site of palpable tumor.

If vaccine-associated sarcoma is suspected, the affected area should be radiographed for evidence of bone lysis or of extension of the tumor along other tissue planes. Other staging steps

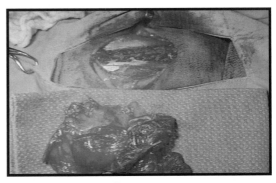

Figure 5-126: *A 1-cm diameter subcutaneous vaccine associated sarcoma was removed with very wide surgical margins. In this surgery, 2- to 3-cm margins were obtained laterally. In addition, all epaxial muscles and the dorsal spinous processes were removed en bloc so that the tumor and a large "cuff" of normal tissue was removed around the tumor.*

MANAGEMENT OF SPECIFIC DISEASES

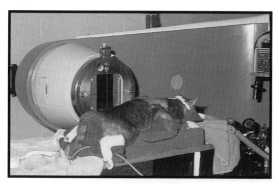

Figure 5-127: *Preoperative or postoperative radiation therapy may be effective for the treatment of vaccine-associated sarcomas. This cat was irradiated with very wide margins two months after the tumor was surgically removed (see Figure 5-126).*

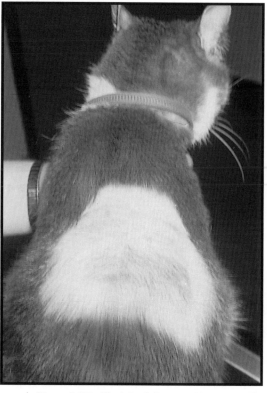

Figure 5-128: *The hair of the cat in Figure 5-127 has turned white in response to the radiation therapy.*

include CBC, biochemical profile, urinalysis, FeLV status and, if appropriate, thyroid evaluation (T_4). These tests ensure that general health is adequate. Metastatic disease is not common but thoracic radiographs should be obtained in each case.

Prognostic Factors

To date, no prognostic factors are known to influence outcome. As noted previously, the more vaccines that are injected in a local site at one time, the greater the risk of developing soft tissue sarcoma in the vaccinated area.

Treatment

Treatment must be aggressive regardless of tumor size. These soft tissue sarcomas grow rapidly and extend far beyond the palpable mass. The most effective treatment is not known, but surgery should be employed whenever possible. In each case, extremely wide and deep surgical margins (>3 cm), including all the soft tissue structures and any bony structures in the region of the postvaccinal sarcoma, should be obtained (Figure 5-126). Essentially, the tumor and a large "cuff" of nor-

> **KEY POINT:**
>
> *A well-planned surgery designed to take wide margins is essential for tumor control. Radiation therapy and chemotherapy should be considered as adjunctive treatments for this aggressive soft tissue sarcoma.*

mal tissue surrounding the mass should be removed en bloc. All lateral and deep margins should be marked and submitted for histopathology to determine presence of residual neoplastic disease. In some veterinary oncology centers, presurgical radiation therapy is routine to minimize the amount of viable tumor around the palpable tumor (Figures 5-127 and 5-128). If surgical excision is found to be incomplete, postoperative adjunctive radiation therapy to an area that includes wide margins around the tumor site should be considered. In addition, doxorubicin may be effective for controlling local disease for a time. In some centers, surgery, radiation therapy, and chemotherapy are used in conjunction to control this type of tumor.

Until more effective treatments are known, the following recommendations may help prevent development of postvaccinal sarcomas: (1) avoid administering multiple vaccines in the same site, (2) administer vaccines in extremities or at the base of the tail to allow future amputation as an effective treatment, and (3) remove postvaccinal granulomas that persist several months after vaccination. Research on different adjuvants to reduce the development of vaccine-induced sarcomas should be continued.

REFERENCES

1. Hendrick MJ, Kass PH, McGill D, Tivard IR: Postvaccinal sarcomas in cats. *J Natl Cancer Inst* 86:335–341, 1994.
2. Kass PH, Barnes WG, Spangler WL, et al: Epidemiologic evidence for a causal relation between vaccination and fibrosarcoma tumorigenesis in cats. *JAVMA* 203: 396–405, 1993.
3. Esplin DG, McGill LD, Meninger AG, et al: Postvaccinal sarcomas in cats. *JAVMA* 202:1245–1247, 1993.
4. Hendrick MJ, Brooks JJ: Postvaccinal sarcomas in the cat: Histology and immunohistochemistry. *Vet Pathol* 31:126–129, 1994.
5. Macy DM: Vaccine-associated sarcomas. *Proc 12th Ann Vet Med Forum ACVIM*:854–856, 1994.
6. Hendrick MJ, Shofer FS, Goldschmidt MH, et al: Comparison of feline fibrosarcomas at vaccination sites: Signalment, causative factors, biological behavior, and prognosis: 239 cases (January 1991–June 1992). *JAVMA*, 1994, in press.
7. Sinibaldi K, Rosen H, Liu S, et al: Tumors associated with metallic implants in animals. *Clin Orthop Rel Res* 118:257–266, 1976.
8. Ryu RKN, Bovill EG, Skinner HB, et al: Soft tissue sarcoma associated with aluminum oxide ceramic total hip arthroplasty: A case report. *Clin Orthop Rel Res* 216:270–275, 1987.

INDEX

f = figure
t = table

2,4D	2,4 dichlorophenoxyacetic acid	antibody 231
5-FU	5-fluorouracil	cm — centimeter(s)
5-HT-3	5-hydroxytryptamine	CML — chronic myeloid leukemia
6-MP	6-mercaptopurine	CNS — central nervous system
AchRAb	acetylcholine-receptor antibody	Co — cobalt
ACT	activated clotting (coagulation) time	CO_2 — carbon dioxide
ACTH	adrenocorticotropic hormone (corticotropin)	COAP — cyclophosphamide (Cytoxan®), vincristine (Oncovin®), ara-c (cytosine arabinoside), prednisone
ADH	antidiuretic hormone	
AG	alopecia, gastrointestinal toxicity	COP — cyclophosphamide (Cytoxan®), vincristine (Oncovin®), prednisone
AIGR	amended insulin:glucose ratio	
ALL	acute lymphoblastic leukemia	
ALP	alkaline phosphatase	COPA — cyclophosphamide (Cytoxan®), vincristine (Oncovin®), prednisone, doxorubicin
ALT	alanine aminotransferase	
AML	acute myeloid leukemia	
AMM	anterior mediastinal mass	CPR — cardiopulmonary resuscitation
ANLL	acute nonlymphoid leukemia	CR — complete response (remission)
APTT	activated partial thromboplastin time	Cs — cesium
ara-C	cytosine arabinoside	CSF — cerebrospinal fluid
AST	aspartate aminotransferase	CT — computed (computerized) tomography
AT	adrenal tumor	
AT-III	antithrombin III	CTZ — chemoreceptor trigger zone
ATLS	acute tumor lysis syndrome	DEA — dog erythrocyte antigen
ATP	adenosine triphosphate	DHM3 — bi(3,5-dimethyl-5-hydromethyl-2-oxomorpholin-3-yl)
AV	atrioventricular	
BAG	bone marrow suppression, alopecia, gastrointestinal toxicity	DIC — disseminated intravascular coagulopathy (coagulation)
BCG	bacillus Calmette-Guerin	dl — deciliter(s)
BCNU	carmustine	DMSO — dimethylsulfoxide
BER	basal energy requirement	DNA — deoxyribonucleic acid
BID	twice a day	DPG — diphosphoglycerate
BRM	biological response modifier	DTIC — dacarbazine
BSA	body surface area	ECG — electrocardiogram
BUN	blood urea nitrogen	EDTA — ethylenediamine tetraacetic acid
°C	celsius	e.g. — for example
CBC	complete blood count	et al — and others
CCNU	lomustine	etc. — et cetera
cDNA	copy DNA	FDP — fibrin degradation product
CLL	chronic lymphocytic leukemia	FeLV — feline leukemia virus
CL/MAb 231	canine lymphoma monoclonal	FeSV — feline sarcoma virus

FIV	feline immunodeficiency virus	LDDS	low-dose dexamethasone-suppression
FOCMA	feline oncornavirus-associated cell membrane antigen	L-MTP-PE	liposome-encapsulated muramyltripeptide-phosphatidyethanolamine
Fr	French	LRS	lactated Ringer's solution
g	gram(s)	M	distant metastasis (TNM classification)
ga	gauge		
G-CSF	granulocyte colony-stimulating factor	m^2	square meters
GH	growth hormone	m^3	cubic meters
GI	gastrointestinal	mCi	millicurie
GM-CSF	granulocyte-macrophage colony-stimulating factor	MCT	mast cell tumor
		MCV	mean corpuscular volume
Gy	gray	MDR	multiple drug resistance
H	hydrogen	MDS	myelodysplasia
HDDS	high-dose dexamethasone-suppression	M:E	myeloid:erythroid ratio
		mEq	milliequivalent
HDL-CH	high-density lipoprotein cholesterol	MeV	million electron volts
Hg	mercury	MF	mycosis fungoides
HIV-1	human immunodeficiency virus-1	mg	milligram(s)
hr	hour	μg	microgram(s)
I	iodine	μl	microliter(s)
i.e.	that is	μm	micrometer(s)
IER	illness energy requirement	μU	micro unit(s)
IgA	immunoglobulin gamma A	min	minute(s)
IgE	immunoglobulin gamma E	ml	milliliter(s)
IgG	immunoglobulin gamma G	MLO	multilobular osteochondrosarcoma
IgM	immunoglobulin gamma M	mm	millimeter(s)
IL-1	interleukin-1	MOPP	mechlorethamine, vincristine (Oncovin®), procarbazine, prednisone
IL-2	interleukin-2		
IL-3	interleukin-3		
IM	intramuscularly	MRC	Medical Research Council
IP	intraperitoneally	MRI	magnetic resonance imaging
IU	international unit(s)	n	number
IV	intravenously	N	lymph node metastasis (TNM classification)
K	potassium		
Kcal	kilocalorie	Na	sodium
KCl	potassium chloride	NaCl	sodium chloride
kg	kilogram(s)	$NaPO_4$	sodium phosphate
L	liter(s)	Nd:YAG	neodymium: yttrium-aluminum-garnet
lb	pound		

ng	nanogram(s)	SD	stable disease
nM	nanomole(s)	SIADH	syndrome of inappropriate secretion of antidiuretic hormone
no.	number		
NSAID	nonsteroidal anti-inflammatory drug	SID	once a day
OAF	osteoclast-activating factor	SQ	subcutaneously
o,p'-DDD	mitotane	Sr	strontium
OPLA–Pt	open polylactic acid–cisplatin	T	tumor size (TNM classification)
OSHA	Occupational Safety and Health Administration	T_3	triiodothyronine
		T_4	thyroxine
OSPT	one-step prothrombin time	TCC	transitional cell carcinoma
OSPTT	one-step partial thromboplastin time	TID	three times a day
P	phosphorus	TNF	tumor necrosis factor
PAS	periodic acid–Schiff reaction	TSH	thyroid-stimulating hormone (thyrotropin)
PCNA	proliferating cell nuclear antigen		
PCV	packed cell volume	TVT	transmissible venereal tumor
PD	progressive disease	U	unit(s)
PDH	pituitary-dependent hyperadrenocorticism	VCM	vincristine, cyclophosphamide, methotrexate
PEG	polyethylene glycol	WBC	white blood cell
pH	negative logarithm of hydrogen ion activity	WHO	World Health Organization
		wt	weight
PO	orally		
PR	partial response (remission)	α	alpha
PRN	according to circumstances	β	beta
PT	prothrombin time	γ	gamma
PTHrP	parathyroid hormone-related peptide	μ	micro
PTU	propylthiouracil	$\circ$	degrees
PUVA	psoralen ultraviolet-A	/	per
PVC	polyvinylchloride	%	percent
	every	=	equals
	four times a day	>	greater than
	every other day	$\geq$	greater than or equal to
	red blood cell	<	less than
	recombinant canine granulocyte colony-stimulating factor	$\leq$	less than or equal to
		+	plus; positive
	recombinant human granulocyte colony-stimulating factor	−	minus; negative
		$\pm$	plus or minus
	ribonucleic acid	$\times$	times; by
	squamous cell carcinoma	$\div$	divided by